ALZHEIMER'S DISEASE:
A CENTURY OF SCIENTIFIC AND CLINICAL RESEARCH

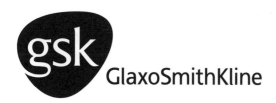

Compliments of GlaxoSmithKline

GlaxoSmithKline is dedicated to research and development of safe and effective treatments to meet unmet medical need in Alzheimer's disease.

Alzheimer's Disease: A Century of Scientific and Clinical Research

Edited by

George Perry
Case Western Reserve University, USA

Jesús Avila
Universidad Autónoma de Madrid, Spain

June Kinoshita
Alzheimer Research Forum, USA

and

Mark A. Smith
Case Western Reserve University, USA

IOS Press

Amsterdam • Berlin • Oxford • Tokyo • Washington, DC

© 2006, IOS Press and the authors

All rights reserved. No part of this book may be reproduced, stored in a retrieval system, or transmitted, in any form or by any means, without prior written permission from the publisher.

ISBN 1-58603-619-X
Library of Congress Control Number: 2006927920

This is the book edition of the *Journal of Alzheimer's Disease*, Volume 9, No. 3 Supplement (2006), ISSN 1387-2877

Publisher
IOS Press
Nieuwe Hemweg 6B
1013 BG Amsterdam
The Netherlands
fax: +31 20 687 0019
e-mail: order@iospress.nl

Distributor in the UK and Ireland
Gazelle Books
Falcon House
Queen Square
Lancaster LA1 1RN
United Kingdom
fax: +44 1524 63232

Distributor in the USA and Canada
IOS Press, Inc.
4502 Rachael Manor Drive
Fairfax, VA 22032
USA
fax: +1 703 323 3668
e-mail: iosbooks@iospress.com

LEGAL NOTICE
The publisher is not responsible for the use which might be made of the following information.

PRINTED IN THE NETHERLANDS

Contents

List of contributors

Preface, Alzheimer's disease: A century of scientific and clinical research 1
    George Perry, Jesús Avila, June Kinoshita and Mark A. Smith

Historical Perspective

Progress in the history of Alzheimer's disease: The importance of context 5
    Jesse F. Ballenger

100 Years of Alzheimer's disease (1906-2006) 15
    José Manuel Martínez Lage

Neuropathology

The essential lesion of Alzheimer disease: A surprise in retrospect 29
    Melvyn Ball

Vulnerability of cortical neurons to Alzheimer's and Parkinson's diseases 35
    Heiko Braak, Udo Rüb, Christian Schultz and Kelly Del Tredici

Neurodegeneration and hereditary dementias: 40 Years of learning 45
    Bernardino Ghetti

Topographic study of Alzheimer's neurofibrillary changes: A personal perspective 53
    Asao Hirano and Maki Iida

Clinicopathological analysis of dementia disorders in the elderly – An update 61
    Kurt Jellinger

The history of the paired helical filaments 71
    Michael Kidd

Synaptic Changes

Vulnerability to Alzheimer's pathology in neocortex: The roles of plasticity and columnar organization 79
    Margaret Esiri and S.A. Chance

Synaptic remodeling during aging and in Alzheimer's disease 91
    Eliezer Masliah, Leslie Crews and Lawrence Hansen

Alzheimer's disease-related alterations in synaptic density: Neocortex and hippocampus 101
    Stephen Scheff and Douglas A. Price

My own experience in early research on Alzheimer disease 117
    Robert D. Terry

Amyloid

Molecular basis of memory loss in the Tg2576 mouse model of Alzheimer disease 123
    Karen Ashe

Soluble amyloid-β in the brain: The scarlet pimpernel 127
Massimo Tabaton and Pierluigi Gambetti

Mice as models: Transgenic approaches and Alzheimer's disease 133
Dora Games, Manuel Buttini, Dione Kobayashi, Dale Schenk and Peter Seubert

Alzheimer's disease: The amyloid cascade hypothesis: An update and reappraisal 151
John Hardy

Pathways to the discovery of the Aβ amyloid of Alzheimer's disease 155
Colin Masters and Konrad Beyreuther

Amyloid β-peptide is produced by cultured cells during normal metabolism: A reprise 163
Dennis Selkoe

Tau

Tau protein, the main component of paired helical filaments 171
Jesús Avila

Immunological demonstration of tau protein in neurofibrillary tangles of Alzheimer's disease 177
Jean-Pierre Brion

The natural and molecular history of Alzheimer's disease 187
André Delacourte

Tau protein, the paired helical filament and Alzheimer's disease 195
Michel Goedert, Aaron Klug and R. Anthony Crowther

Neurofibrillary tangles/paired helical filaments (1981-83) 209
Yasuo Ihara

Discoveries of tau, abnormally hyperphosphorylated tau and others of neurofibrillary degeneration: A personal historical perspective 219
Khalid Iqbal and Inge Grundke-Iqbal

Tau phosphorylation and proteolysys: Insights and perspectives 243
Gail Johnson

Traveling the tau pathway: A personal account 251
Kenneth Kosik

Progress from Alzheimer's tangles to pathological tau points towards more effective therapies now 257
Virginia M.-Y. Lee and John Q. Trojanowski

Disease Mechanisms

A long trek down the pathways of cell death in Alzheimer's disease 265
Peter Davies

Inflammation, anti-inflammatory agents and Alzheimer disease: The last 12 years 271
Patrick L. McGeer, Joseph Rogers and Edith G. McGeer

Lysosomal system pathways: Genes to neurodegeneration in Alzheimer's disease 277
Ralph A. Nixon and Anne M Cataldo

Aluminium and Alzheimer's disease, a personal perspective after 25 years 291
Daniel Perl and Sharon Moalem

Solving the insoluble 301
George Perry

Oxidative stress and iron imbalance in Alzheimer disease: How rust became the fuss! 305
Mark A. Smith

GSK-3 is essential in the pathologenesis of Alzheimer's disease 309
Akihiko Takashima

Frameshift proteins in Alzheimer's disease and in other conformational disorders:
Time for the ubiquitin-proteasome system 319
F.W. van Leeuwen, E.M. Hol and D.F. Fischer

Genetics

Studies on the first described Alzheimer's disease amyloid β mutant, the Dutch variant 329
Efrat Levy, Frances Prell and Blas Frangione

Segregation of a missense mutation in the amyloid β-protein precursor gene with familial
Alzheimer's disease 341
Alison Goate

The discovery and mapping to chromosome 21 of the Alzheimer amyloid gene. My story. 349
Dmitry Goldgaber

On the discovery of the genetic association of Apolipoprotein E genotypes and common late-onset
Alzheimer disease 361
Allen Roses

Early Alzheimer's disease genetics 367
Gerard Schellenberg

Mutations in the tau gene (MAPT) in FTDP-17: The family with Multiple System Tauopathy with
presenile Dementia (MSTD) 373
*Maria Grazia Spillantini, Jill R. Murrell, Michel Goedert, Martin Farlow, Aaron Klug
and Bernardino Ghetti*

Genetic complexity of Alzheimer's disease: Successes and challenges 381
Ekaterina Rogaeva, Toshitaka Kawarai and Peter St George-Hyslop

Genetics and pathology of alpha-secretase site AβPP mutations in understanding of
Alzheimer's disease 389
C. van Broeckhoven and Samir Kumar-Singh

Diagnosis and Treatment

Preclinical characterization of amyloid imaging probes with multiphoton microscopy 401
Jesse Skoch, Bradley T. Hyman and Brian J. Bacskai

Diagnosis of Alzheimer's disease: Two-decades of progress 409
Zaven Khachaturian

Consensus guidelines for the clinical and pathologic diagnosis of dementia with Lewy bodies (DLB): Report of the consortium on DLB international workshop 417
Ian McKeith

Immunotherapy for Alzheimer's disease 425
David Morgan

Alzheimer's disease immunotherapy: From *in vitro* amyloid immunomodulation to *in vivo* vaccination 433
Beka Solomon

Tacrine, and Alzheimer's treatments 439
William Summers

Quality of Life: The bridge from the cholinergic basal forebrain to cognitive science and bioethics 447
Peter Whitehouse

Keyword index 455

Contributor's Index

Ashe, K.H., University of Minnesota, USA and Minneapolis Veterans Affairs, Medical Center, USA	123
Avila, J., Universidad Autónoma de Madrid, Spain	1, 171
Bacskai, B.J., Massachusetts General Hospital, USA	401
Ball, M.J., Oregon Health & Science University, USA	29
Ballenger, J.F., Pennsylvania State University, USA	5
Beyreuther, K., The University of Heidelberg, Germany	155
Braak, H., J.W. Goethe University, Germany	35
Brion, J.-P., Université Libre de Bruxelles, Belgium	177
Buttini, M., Elan Pharmaceuticals, USA	133
Cataldo A.M., McLean Hospital, USA	277
Chance, S.A., University of Oxford, UK	79
Crews, L., University of California, San Diego, USA	91
Crowther, R.A., MRC Laboratory of Molecular Biology, UK	195
Davies, P., Albert Einstein College of Medicine, USA	265
Del Tredici, K., J.W. Goethe University, Germany	35
Delacourte, A., Unit Inserm 422, France	187
Esiri, M.M., University of Oxford, UK and Oxford Radcliffe NHS Trust, UK	79
Farlow, M., Indiana University of Medicine, USA	373
Fischer, D.F., Vrije Universiteit and VU Medical Center, The Netherlands	319
Frangione, B., New York University School of Medicine, USA	329
Gambetti, P., Case Western Reserve University, USA	127
Games, T., Elan Pharmaceuticals, USA	133
Ghetti, B., Indiana University School of Medicine, USA	45, 373
Goate, A., Washington University School of Medicine, USA	341
Goedert, M., MRC Laboratory of Molecular Biology, UK	195, 373
Goldgaber, D., State University of New York at Stony Brook, USA	349
Grundke-Iqbal, I., New York State Institute for Basic Research in Developmental Disabilities, USA	219
Hansen, L., University of California, San Diego, USA	91
Hardy, J., National Institute on Aging, USA	151
Hirano, A., Montefiore Medical Center, USA	53
Hol, E.M., Netherlands Institute for Brain Research, The Netherlands	319
Hyman, T., Massachusetts General Hospital, USA	401
Ihara, Y., University of Tokyo, Japan	209
Iida, M., Montefiore Medical Center, USA	53
Iqbal, K., New York State Institute for Basic Research in Developmental Disabilities, USA	219

Jellinger, K.A., Institute of Clinical Neurobiology, Austria	61
Johnson, G.V.W., University of Alabama at Birmingham, USA	243
Kawarai, T., University of Toronto, Canada	381
Khachaturian, Z.S., Khachaturian, Radebaugh & Associates (KRA), Inc., Potomac, USA	409
Kidd, M., University of London, UK	71
Kinoshita, J., Alzheimer Research Forum, USA	1
Klug, A., MRC Laboratory of Molecular Biology, UK	195, 373
Kobayashi, D., Elan Pharmaceuticals, USA	133
Kosik, K.S., University of California, Santa Barbara, USA	251
Kumar-Singh, S., University of Antwerp, Belgium	389
Lage, J.M.M., University of Navarre Medical School, Spain	15
Lee, V.M.-Y., The University of Pennsylvania School of Medicine, USA	257
Levy, E., New York University School of Medicine, USA	329
Masliah, E., University of California, San Diego, USA	91
Masters, C.L., The University of Melbourne, Australia	155
McGeer, E.G., University of British Columbia, Canada	271
McGeer, P.L., University of British Columbia, Canada	271
McKeith, I.G., Newcastle General Hospital, UK	417
Moalem, S., Mount Sinai School of Medicine, USA	291
Morgan, D., University of South Florida, USA	425
Murrell, J.R., Indiana, University School of Medicine, USA	373
Nixon, R.A., Nathan S. Kline Institute, New York University, USA	277
Perl, D.P., Mount Sinai School of Medicine, USA	291
Perry, G., Case Western Reserve University, USA	1, 301
Prelli, F., New York University School of Medicine, USA	329
Price, D.A., University of Kentucky College of Medicine, USA	101
Rogaeva, E., University of Toronto, Canada	381
Rogers, J., Sun Health Research Institute, USA	271
Roses, A.D., GlaxoSmithKline Research and Development, USA	361
Rüb, U., J.W. Goethe University, Germany	35
Scheff, S.W., University of Kentucky College of Medicine, USA	101
Schellenberg, G., University of Washington, USA	367
Schenk, D., Elan Pharmaceuticals, USA	133
Schultz, C., J.W. Goethe University, Germany	35
Selkoe, D.J., Brigham and Women's Hospital and Harvard Medical School, USA	163
Seubert, P., Elan Pharmaceuticals, USA	133
Skoch, J., Massachusetts General Hospital, USA	401
Smith, M.A., Case Western Reserve University, USA	1, 305

Solomon, B., Tel-Aviv University, Israel	433
Spillantini, M.G. University of Cambridge, UK	373
St George-Hyslop, P., University of Toronto, Canada	381
Summers, W.K., ALZcorp, USA	439
Tabaton, M., University of Genova, Italy	127
Takashima, A., Riken, Brain Science Institute, Japan	309
Terry, R.D., University of California, San Diego, USA	117
Trojanowski, J.Q., The University of Pennsylvania School of Medicine, USA	257
Van Broeckhoven, C., University of Antwerp, Belgium	389
Van Leeuwen, F.W., Netherlands Institute for Brain Research, The Netherlands	319
Whitehouse, P.J., Case Western Reserve University, USA	447

Preface

Alzheimer's disease: A century of scientific and clinical research

George Perry, Jesús Avila, June Kinoshita and Mark A. Smith

The centennial of Alois Alzheimer's original description of the disease that would come to bear his name offers a vantage point from which to commemorate the seminal discoveries in the field. To identify the breakthroughs, we used citation analysis, milestone papers identified by current researchers, and our own suggestions. Our process took into account the perspectives of individuals who recall the impact of findings at the time they were made, as well as of scientists today who have the advantage of hindsight in weighing the lasting influence of these findings. Because modern Alzheimer disease research was triggered by the seminal work of Tomlinson, Blessed, and Roth some four decades ago, we are especially fortunate that the vast majority of these milestone authors are still with us.

Each contributor was invited to discuss what made their particular article a milestone in the context of its time. Furthermore, contributors were asked to provide a highly personal perspective, by recounting the tale of how each discovery unfolded and by frankly describing the contradictions among studies and the debates that once took place in whispered tones in remote corners of seminar rooms and conference halls.

These writings bring to the practitioner, student and interested lay person a perspective not only on the past but also on where the Alzheimer disease field is likely to go in the future. Only time will tell whether these milestones have charted the future accurately, but they are unquestionably the foundation upon which the future will be built.

N.B. The photo's displayed on the title page of the papers show the (corresponding) author.

Historical Perspective

Progress in the history of Alzheimer's disease: The importance of context

Jesse F. Ballenger
Pennsylvania State University, University Park, PA, USA

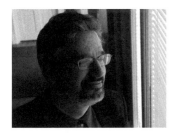

Abstract. The history of Alzheimer's disease (AD) is typically formulated as the history of great doctors and scientists in the past making great discoveries that are in turn taken up by great doctors and scientists in the present – all sharing the aim of unraveling the mysteries of the disease and discovering how it can be prevented or cured. While it can certainly be edifying to study the "great men" and how their contributions laid the foundation for current work, there are problems with this approach to history. First, it oversimplifies the actual historical development of science. Second, using history to legitimate the present can keep us from asking critical questions about the aims and limits of contemporary research. This chapter urges a broader view of the history of AD, one that recognizes that context is as important as the great doctors to the historical development of the concept of AD. Thought of this way, I argue that it is useful to divide of the history of AD into three periods. First there was the period in which Alzheimer and Kraepelin laid the clinical and pathological foundations of the disease concept. Then there is our own period, which began in the late 1970s and has emphasized the biological mechanisms of dementia. In between, there is the period – almost completely ignored in most histories of AD – that conceptualized dementia in psychodynamic terms. It is true that the psychodynamic model of dementia did not directly contribute to the concepts and theories that dominate AD research today. But it did change the context of aging and dementia in important ways, without which AD could not have emerged as a major disease worthy of a massive, publicly supported research initiative.

1. Introduction

Without a doubt, the history of Alzheimer's disease (AD) is a history of progress. As it is usually formulated, progress in medicine means the history of great doctors and scientists in the past making great discoveries that are in turn taken up by great doctors and scientists in the present – all sharing the aim of unraveling the mysteries of disease and discovering how it can be prevented or cured. In this way of looking at the history of science and medicine, the research of previous generations is noticed only to the degree to which it anticipated or contributed to current concepts and research initiatives. In the case of AD, this produces a historical narrative that begins with Alzheimer's first description in 1906 and Kraepelin's naming of the disease in 1910 as the historical foundation, then virtually ignores the next five decades as a veritable dark age – mentioning only a handful of articles that were "ahead of their time" in seeming to anticipate current concepts and concerns (e.g., [37,38]), then skipping ahead to the history of current research projects rooted in the 1970s or later.

It can certainly be edifying to study the "great men" and how their contributions laid the foundation for current work. And it seems appropriate and noble on the occasion of the 100th Anniversary of Alzheimer's first description of the disease to acknowledge that, as the cliché goes, "if we see farther now it is because we stand on the shoulders of giants." But there are problems with this approach to history. First, it oversimplifies the actual historical development of science – and as I will argue below that is certainly true in the case of AD. Second, using history to legitimate the present can keep us from asking critical questions about the aims and limits of contemporary research. If our present course seems foreordained, the logical and inevitable fruit of historical progress, we may be unwilling to consider its pitfalls, and unaware of potential alternatives.

Thus, as a historian, I want to use the attention to history that the 100th Anniversary of AD will garner, to urge a broader view that understands that context is as important as the great doctors to the historical development of the concept of AD. As an alternative to the metaphor of "standing on the shoulders of giants," I would suggest that we view the evolution of scientific and medical ideas about dementia as a garden, and the social and cultural context important factors in the climate and soil that favor the growth of some ideas over others. Changes in that context may of course create opportunities for different sorts of ideas to thrive. Thought of this way, progress in medicine becomes a more complex matter. Progress can be seen when some particularly idea takes deep root and grows over a long period of time, e.g., the original clinical-pathological entity described by Alzheimer, but it can also occur when ideas die and wither away, changing the quality of the soil and atmosphere, and perhaps making conditions ripe for new ideas to emerge.

Thought of this way, I argue that it is useful to divide of the history of AD into three periods. First there was the period in which Alzheimer and Kraepelin laid the clinical and pathological foundations of the disease concept. Then there is our own period, which began in the late 1970s and has emphasized the biological mechanisms of dementia. In between, there is the period – almost completely ignored in most histories of AD – that conceptualized dementia in psychodynamic terms. It is true that the psychodynamic model of dementia did not directly contribute to the concepts and theories that dominate AD research today. But it did change the context of aging and dementia in important ways, without which AD could not have emerged as a major disease worthy of a massive, publicly supported research initiative.

2. Alzheimer, Kraepelin and the foundations of AD

Alois Alzheimer and Emil Kraepelin are usually seen as the founders of the modern concept of AD [52]. There is good reason for this view – Alzheimer did provide a thorough, unified description of the clinical symptoms of AD and what have remained its essential pathological features [34]. But the context in which they worked was much different, and this different context seemed to lead them *away* from conceiving of it as we do – one of the most devastating diseases afflicting the elderly. Although there is great need for a detailed history of Alzheimer and Kraepelin's work on the dementias, thinking about how they conceptualized AD and senile dementia in the context of psychiatry at that time can help us understand what today seems most puzzling about their work in this area – why, despite their insights about the clinical and pathological nature of the dementias, they viewed AD as a rare and relatively insignificant disorder.

As is well known, Alzheimer first described the disease that would eventually be named for him at a meeting of the South West German Psychiatrists in Tübingen in 1906. It was a brief report of the case of a 51-year old woman who developed progressive dementia, accompanied by focal signs, hallucinations and delusions. On post-mortem, her brain was found to contain numerous senile plaques and a newly observed pathological structure – densely twisted bundles of neurofibrils, or neurofibrillary tangles, which were made visible to microscopic observation through a newly developed silver-staining technique. In 1910, Alzheimer's mentor Emil Kraepelin bestowed the eponym in the 8th edition of his influential psychiatric textbook, and, as the story goes, the foundation of AD as a disease entity was established, waiting to be built upon by subsequent research [34].

However, the idea that this episode marked the foundation of the scientific study of one of the most important diseases of the twentieth century would have left Alzheimer and his contemporaries more than a little surprised. Indeed, what seems most remarkable about the episode from today's vantage point is how insignificant it seemed at the time. Alzheimer's initial report drew no reaction or enthusiasm from the audience of psychiatrists who heard him give it, nor did its publication in 1907 draw any significant attention [33]. Kraepelin devoted only a few pages of his massive textbook to it, and his naming of it was somewhat offhand and equivocal:

> The clinical interpretation of this Alzheimer's disease is still confused. While the anatomical findings suggest that we are dealing with a particularly serious form of senile dementia, the fact that this disease sometimes starts already around the age of 40 does not allow this supposition. In such cases we should assume at least a 'senium praecox,' if

not perhaps a more or less age-independent unique disease process [8, pp. 77–78].

Perhaps most surprisingly, given the importance of AD today, after Alzheimer death in 1915, few of the many tributes to him written by his colleagues even made any reference to AD. Alzheimer was remembered by his contemporaries, including Kraepelin, for his clinical and histopathological acumen and intensive work ethic, not for having discovered the "disease of the century" for which his name is a household word today [33].

The insignificance of AD to Alzheimer and his contemporaries is easier to understand when put in historical context. At the turn of the twentieth century, there was a feeling that scientific medicine's ability to define the pathogenesis and etiology of discrete disease entities through bacteriological and pathological research was leaving clinical psychiatry behind [40]. The one exception was the discovery by German psychiatrists in 1857 that general paresis, one of the most common forms of insanity, was connected to syphilitic infection. The example of general paresis raised new hope that clinical-pathological correlations would lead to etiological theories, and ultimately therapeutic interventions, for other forms of mental illness [1,12,46].

Although these grand hopes never materialized, in the first decade of the twentieth century, Kraepelin and his protégés, Alois Alzheimer and Franz Nissl, nearly made AD the second major mental disorder for which a clear pathological basis had been established. The effort failed because of the inability to resolve the issue of whether the clinical symptoms and pathological structures constituted a disease entity or a part of the normal processes of aging. Ironically, Kraepelin, known as the Linnaeus of psychiatry because he established a simple and rational nosological system based on careful observation of the natural history of mental diseases, exacerbated the confusion by creating the entity "AD" to distinguish the relatively rare cases in which dementia developed before the age of 65 (pre-senile dementia) from the common occurrence of dementia in more advanced ages (senile dementia). Kraepelin made this distinction despite the fact that the pathological hallmarks, clinical symptoms, and natural history of both pre-senile and senile dementia were virtually identical. Age of onset appeared to be the only criteria on which the distinction was made. In grappling with Kraepelin's classification of the dementias, subsequent researchers had to puzzle not only about the relationship of AD to senile dementia, but about whether both of them were related to aging in the same way or at all [6].

Alzheimer himself appeared to be ambivalent about whether AD should in fact be considered a disease distinct from senile dementia. In a longer 1911 paper on such cases he wrote that:

> As similar cases of disease obviously occur in the late old age, it is therefore not exclusively a presenile disease, and there are cases of senile dementia which do not differ from these presenile cases with respect to the severity of the disease process. There is then no tenable reason to consider these cases as caused by a specific disease process. They are senile psychoses, atypical forms of senile dementia. Nevertheless, they do assume a certain separate position, so that one has to know of their existence ... in order to avoid misdiagnosis [2, p. 93].

As German Berrios concludes, it seems that all Alzheimer meant to emphasize in describing these cases in both the 1907 and 1911 publications was that senile dementia could occur in a younger person [7].

So why then did Kraepelin create and assert the existence of the new entity? It has been theorized that he did so as part of a struggle against the inroads being made by Freud and psychoanalysis, hoping to create in AD a second example (general paresis being the first) of a mental illness with a clearly defined pathological substrate [50]; that he did so in order to garner prestige for his department, which was in a rivalry with that of Arnold Pick in Prague [3]; that he did so in order to justify the creation of Alzheimer's expensive pathology lab in Munich [35]; finally, that he did so with full intellectual honesty out of the assumption that differences in age of onset was a sufficient reason to make the distinction, and that in any case, he was reserving final judgment for more decisive evidence [6]. All of these explanations may be true, but until more detailed historical research is done on Kraepelin and Alzheimer, they remain somewhat speculative.

What does seem clear is that for Kraepelin it made no sense to call senile dementia a disease since the pathological processes of old age were understood to be "normal," while dementia occurring at earlier ages, even though associated with the same brain pathology, seemed to suggest a disease. As many historians have pointed out, this assumption that mental and physical deterioration were normal in old age was deeply embedded in medicine and Western culture more broadly, and remains powerful today [19,27]. This assumption remained powerful, and seemed to be the reason that the psychiatric literature maintained the distinction between AD as a rare disorder distinct from senile dementia through the 1970s, despite the fact that researchers were well aware of, and puzzled by, their similarity [24, 25]. But beginning in the 1930s, a different orientation towards dementia in psychiatry and the emergence of social gerontology would challenge these assumptions, setting the context for the emergence of the current understanding of AD in the late 1970s.

3. The psychodynamic model of dementia, the rise of social gerontology, and the fight against senility

In the 1930s, the age-associated dementias posed two kinds of problems for psychiatrists. They continued to pose the sort of vexing nosological puzzles described above, and new questions were raised about the role of the associated brain pathology. A large autopsy series published in 1933 reported that the correlation between the clinical symptoms of dementia and the presence of brain pathology post-mortem was surprisingly loose [4, 15]. In some cases, the senile plaques and neurofibrillary tangles that were found in the brains of patients suffering from dementia were also found in the brains of patients who had shown no sign of dementia in life. In other cases, the brains of patients who died severely demented were found at autopsy to be relatively intact.

But the age-associated dementias posed a second, more practical sort of problem as well, at least for psychiatrists in the United States. In the late-nineteenth century, reforms in public policy made care of the mentally ill the responsibility of state rather than local governments. An unintended result of this was that local welfare officials were given a strong financial incentive to regard the old people who could no longer live independently in the community as insane so that they would be institutionalized in the state mental hospitals at the expense of state governments As a result, both the absolute and proportional number of aged patients admitted to the state hospitals increased dramatically, and the mental hospitals remained the institutional center of psychiatry in the United States during this period [16, 17]. Because psychiatry regarded senile dementia as incurable, its rising prevalence in the state mental hospital patient population undermined the therapeutic environment that the state hospitals were supposed to provide. Because the overall population was aging, the problem was regarded by many as an impending crisis – a demographic avalanche that would bury the state hospital as a viable institution, and the professional legitimacy of psychiatry along with it [4]. This remained a concern for psychiatry through the mid-1950s, when American psychiatrists began to increasingly move toward office-based practice in the community. In 1965, provisions in the Medicare and Medicaid legislation made the federal government responsible for funding nursing-home care of the elderly, resulting in the shift of many thousands of elderly patients out of the mental hospitals and into nursing homes and various community care arrangements [18].

In the mid-1930s, American psychiatrists, led by David Rothschild of the Worcester State Hospital, developed a new theory of dementia that seemed to answer both sets of problems. The new concept of dementia emphasized psychosocial factors over brain pathology in the etiology of dementia – thus bringing the age-associated dementias into mainstream psychiatry. The basis of this re-conceptualization was an inability to establish a definitive correlation between dementia and brain pathology, as reported by Gellerstedt and by Rothschild himself [15,42,43,45]. Rothschild and his followers argued that the lack of correlation between clinical and pathological data could best be accounted for by a differing ability among individuals to compensate for organic lesions. Seen this way, age-associated dementia was more than the simple and inevitable outcome of a brain that was deteriorating due to disease and/or aging. Rather, dementia was a dialectical process between the brain and the psychosocial context in which the aging person was situated. Factors such as pre-morbid personality structure, emotional trauma, disruptions of family support and social isolation were regarded as at least as important in explaining dementia as the biological processes within the brain that produced plaques and tangles [4].

For psychodynamically oriented American psychiatrists, the psychodynamic approach was a more satisfying theory of dementia, and provided a logical basis for making meaningful therapeutic interventions. Thus it is no surprise that there was a surge of interest in age-associated dementias within American psychiatry during this period. In the 10 years from 1926–1935, there had only been nine articles concerning senile dementia and/or AD published in the *American Journal of Psychiatry* and the *Archives of Neurology and Psychiatry*, the two leading professional journals; in the following decade, 36 articles appeared. Much of this literature concerned the use of therapies that had previously been considered inappropriate for aged patients – including psychotherapy, ECT, hormones, vitamins, and other drug treatments. From 1935 to 1959, thirty-five articles reporting on the use of therapies including group psychotherapy, hormone treatments, appeared in these two journals. These reports were generally enthusiastic about the results, but this probably said as much about how badly clinicians wanted meaningful treatments for dementia as about the efficacy of these approaches. In any case, these initial studies were generally not extensive or rigorous, and positive results were usually not replicated when more careful studies began to be conducted in the 1970s [4].

But the psychodynamic model offered more than an end-run around nosological problems and a rationale for the therapeutic efforts of desperate psychiatrists in the state hospitals. It also seemed to provide insight into the entire experience of aging in post-World War II America. In the 1940s and 1950s, virtually all American psychiatrists working on senile dementia, including Rothschild himself, who had developed his model on extensive post-mortem evidence, stopped investigating brain pathology. Nor did they attempt to delineate various disease entities based on pathological lesions, but folded Alzheimer-type dementia, cerebral arteriosclerosis, and functional mental disorders into a broad concept of senile mental deterioration, whose pathological hallmarks were not brain deterioration but modern social relations. The locus of senile mental deterioration was no longer the aging brain, but a society that, through mandatory retirement, social isolation and the disintegration of traditional family ties, stripped the elderly of their role in life. Bereft of any meaningful social role and suffering the effects of intense social stigma, it was not surprisingly that the elderly began to deteriorate mentally. As Rothschild argued, "in our present social set-up, with its loosening of family ties, unsettled living conditions and fast economic pace, there are many hazards for individuals who are growing old," he wrote. "Many of these persons have not had adequate psychological preparation for their inevitable loss of flexibility, restriction of outlets, and loss of friends or relatives; they are individuals who are facing the prospect of retirement from their life-long activities with few mental assets and perhaps meagre material resources." [44, p. 125] Other psychiatrists pushed the turn to the social much further than Rothschild, going so far as to argue that that social pathology should in fact be regarded as the *cause* of brain pathology. Maurice Linden and Douglas Courtney argued that "senility as an isolable state is largely a cultural artifact and that senile organic deterioration may be consequent on attitudinal alterations" [32, p. 912], though the authors acknowledged that this hypothesis was difficult to prove. David C. Wilson was less circumspect, arguing that the link between social pathology and brain deterioration was simply a matter of waiting for "laboratory proof" to support what was adequately demonstrated by clinical experience – that the "pathology of senility is found not only in the tissues of the body but also in the concepts of the individual and in the attitude of society." Wilson cited the usual evidence of pathological social relations in old age: the break-up of the traditional family, mandatory retirement, and social isolation. "Factors that narrow the individual's life also influence the occurrence of senility," he asserted. "Lonesomeness, lack of responsibility, and a feeling of not being wanted all increase the restricted view of life which in turn leads to restricted blood flow" [53, p. 905]. Social pathology could even be discerned, it seemed, within the constricted blood vessels of the aging brain.

Because it brought together cultural anxieties about the isolation, emptiness and stigma of aging in modern society with the frightening symptoms of dementia, the broad concept of senile mental deterioration gained currency far beyond professional psychiatry. It figured especially in popular and professional discourse that sought to make retirement a meaningful and desirable stage of life by making it financially secure and emotionally satisfying. To the emerging field of social gerontology, the high prevalence of senile mental deterioration, as construed by psychiatrists like Rothschild, was an indictment of society's failure to meet the needs of the elderly [5, Chapter 3].

The "adjustment" of the individual to aging was the key concept for social gerontologists in the 1940s and 50s. This adjustment could be negative, resulting in senile mental deterioration, or it could be positive, resulting not only in the preservation of mental health, but the discovery of new and satisfying interests and activities to replace those that had been lost with age [11,14,22,39,47]. Though adjustment to old age was ultimately a personal matter, prominent gerontologists argued that "in modern America the community must carry the responsibility of creating conditions that make it possible for the great majority of older people to lead the independent and emotionally satisfying lives of which they are capable" [21, p. 17]. The community's responsibility went beyond altruism, for if their needs were not met the burgeoning aging population would result in a catastrophic increase in senility. As Jerome Kaplan, an advocate for recreation programs argued, "with the number of people who are over 65 increasing significantly each year, our society is today finding itself faced with the problem of keeping a large share of its population from joining the living dead – those whose minds are allowed to die before their bodies do" [26,

p. 3] The solution was a program to provide older people with meaningful activities to fill the remainder of their lives.

Broadly construed, this was the program of social gerontology for reconstructing old age. And whatever the scientific merits of this model of the social production of "senility" as an account of the pathogenesis of dementia, those who embraced it were generally successful in winning a series of significant policy changes that helped to transform the experience of aging in America. By the 1970s, much of this program had in fact been accomplished. The material circumstances of old age had been markedly improved, though not to an equal extent for all older people; significant legal protections had been won against age discrimination; negative stereotypes in popular and professional discourse were increasingly challenged, and, perhaps most importantly, the elderly themselves organized for effective political advocacy an action on their own behalf [10, 20]. In this context, the problem of age-associated dementia became more visible and tragic. As noted above, after 1965 deinstitutionalization increased the burden that dementia posed to communities and families, while heightened expectations for old age made senile dementia an even more devastating prospect [5].

4. The biomedical deconstruction of senility and the emergence of Alzheimer's disease

The expansive concept of senility that had been the basis of psychodynamic psychiatry and gerontology in the 1940s and 50s no longer seemed appropriate in the new era of aging that was taking place in the 1970s. "Ageism" replaced "adjustment" as the key term in social gerontology for a more aggressive and politicized generation of gerontologists in the 1970s. The term ageism was coined by Robert Butler in 1968 to describe the "process of systematic stereotyping of and discrimination against people because they are old, just as racism and sexism accomplish this with skin color and gender" [9, p. 12]. One of the worst aspects of the stereotypical view of aging, in Butler's view, was the belief that the process of aging entailed inevitable physical and mental decline. Butler and other gerontologist argued that virtually all of the physical and mental deterioration commonly attributed to old age was more properly understood as the product of disease processes distinct from aging. "Senility" in this view was not a medical diagnosis, but a "wastebasket term" applied to any person over sixty with a problem. Worse, it rationalized the neglect of those problems by assuming that they were inevitable and irreversible. "'Senility' is a popularized layman's term used by doctors and the public alike to categorize the behavior of the old," Butler argued. "Some of what is called senile is the result of brain damage. But anxiety and depression are also frequently lumped within the same category of senility, even though they are treatable and often reversible." Because both doctors and the public found it so "convenient to dismiss all these manifestations by lumping them together under an improper and inaccurate diagnostic label, the elderly often did not receive the benefits of decent diagnosis and treatment" [9, pp. 9–10]. Butler did not discount the reality of irreversible brain damage, as had an earlier generation of psychiatrists. Rather, he argued that the refusal to systematically distinguish the various physical and mental disease processes from each other and from the process of aging itself was a manifestation of the ageism that kept society from taking the problems of older people serious. In this context, a group of clinical neurologists and psychiatrists, neuropathologists and biochemists who entered the field in the 1960s and 1970s worked to recast age-associated dementia in old age as a number of disease entities distinct from aging.

The first step in this was to put the connection between pathology and the clinical manifestation of dementia on a firmer foundation. The British research group of Martin Roth, Bernard Tomlinson and Gary Blessed accomplished this by developing procedures for quantifying both the clinical manifestation of dementia and the number of plaques and tangles found in the brain, enabling them to calculate the degree of correlation between them. In a series of heavily-cited articles [41,48,49] the group provided statistically significant correlations between plaques and scores on a number of dementia scales. In their initial article in *Nature*, they proclaimed that "far from plaques being irrelevant for the pathology of old age mental disorder, the density of plaque formation in the brain proves to be highly correlated with quantitative measures of intellectual and personality deterioration" [41, p. 110]. The authors ultimately claimed that fully 90% of the cases in their demented group could be satisfactorily accounted for by pathological changes that distinguished them from the control group. That 10% of the cases of dementia could not be explained pathologically was not surprising to the authors, for perfect correlation "would mean that the pathological associations of all dementias in old age are recognized." Though occasional anomalies no doubt occurred, the authors concluded that there was no evidence to support Rothschild's claim that equally severe pathological destruction could be found in normal old age as found in senile or arteriosclerotic dementia [49, pp. 234–235]. Although the study did not completely resolve all issues regarding the relative importance of pathology [31], from the time in which it was published it was widely regarded as providing authoritative evidence for a strong and probably causal relationship between pathology and dementia [29].

The second step was to clarify the nosological position of AD. One aspect of this was distinguishing between irreversible age-associated progressive dementias produced by conditions like AD, and reversible dementias produced by treatable conditions [36]. More importantly, it involved recasting irreversible progressive dementia in old age as a number of disease entities distinct from aging, the most important of them being AD. In a 1976 editorial in the *Archives of Neurology*, neurologist Robert Katzman argued that distinction between AD and senile dementia should be dropped since at both the clinical and pathological level they were identical. This dramatically increased the number of cases of AD. Extrapolating from a number of small community studies that had been done in the 1950s and 1960s, Katzman estimated that there were as many as 1.2 million cases of AD in the United States in 1976, and 60,000–90,000 deaths a year from it – making it the fourth or fifth leading cause of death in the United States [28]. In 1978, Katzman along with Robert Terry and Katherine Bick enlisted the support of the directors of the National Instituted of Neurological Disorders and Stroke, the National Institute of Mental Health, and the newly established National Institute on Aging (NIA) to convene a major workshop conference on AD to address nosological issues and encouraging talented researchers from a variety of fields to being working on the disease [30]. An essential outcome of Katzman's editorial and the conference was consensus not only that AD and senile dementia was a unified entity – Senile Dementia of the Alzheimer Type – but that this entity was not part of the normal aging process aging. Rather, it was a disease whose mechanisms could be unraveled through basic research leading eventually to effective treatments and ultimately prevention [29].

This re-formulation of AD was politically powerful, allowing researchers, aging advocates, and policymakers committed to AD research to make a convincing case that public resources should be allocated for research into Alzheimer's disease. Perhaps the most prominent advocate for AD research was Robert Butler, who was appointed the first director of the NIA when it was established in 1974. Butler made AD the focal point of the fledgling institute, following a disease-specific lobbying strategy that had worked for other institutes within the National Institutes of Health. Butler's strategy was highly successful; by the end of the 1980s, the NIA budget for Alzheimer's disease research had increased more than 800% [13]. Federal funding for AD research has continued to grow, even in an era characterized by budgetary constraints, reaching $700 million in 2005.

5. Conclusion

The reformulation of AD as a distinct disease entity, separate from the process of normal aging, provided a rich intellectual, social and political environment in which many ideas and approaches to AD have flourished. The flowering of AD research in the modern era is well described in the chapters of this volume. But we would be wise to consider that the context of aging and dementia will continue to change. Globalization, our ongoing experience with an aging population, and the difficulty we have had in finding meaningful medical interventions may create a context that favors different conceptions of AD. The call to situate dementia in the broader context the biological, cultural and social processes of aging [51] and increased attention to the role of intellectual and physical exercise in preventing dementia among the elderly [23] may be indications that such changes are already underway. The one certainty is that the complex process of making "progress" on this condition will continue.

References

[1] E.H. Ackerknecht, *A short history of psychiatry*, New York, Hafner Pub. Co, 1959.

[2] A. Alzheimer and H. Forstl et al., On certain peculiar diseases of old age, *Hist Psychiatry* **2**(5 Pt 1) (1991), 71–101.

[3] L.A. Amaducci, W.A. Rocca et al., Origin of the distinction between Alzheimer's disease and senile dementia: how history can clarify nosology, *Neurology* **36**(11) (1986), 1497–1499.

[4] J.F. Ballenger, Beyond the Characteristic Plaques and Tangles: Mid-Twentieth Century US Psychiatry and the Fight Against Senility, in: *Concepts of Alzheimer Disease: Biological, Clinical and Cultural Perspectives*, P. Whitehouse, K. Maurer and J.F. Ballenger, Baltimore, Johns Hopkins University Press, 1999.

[5] J.F. Ballenger, *Self, Senility and Alzheimer's Disease in Modern America*, Baltimore, Johns Hopkins University Press, 2006.

[6] T.G. Beach, The history of Alzheimer's disease: Three debates, *Journal of the History of Medicine and Allied Sciences* (1987).

[7] G.E. Berrios, Alzheimer's Disease: A Conceptual History, *International Journal of Geriatric Psychiatry* **5** (1990), 355–365.

[8] K.L. Bick, L. Amaducci et al., *The early story of Alzheimer's disease: translation of the historical papers by Alois Alzheimer, Oskar Fischer, Francesco Bonfiglio, Emil Kraepelin, Gaetano Perusini*, Padova, Liviana Press, 1987.

[9] R.N. Butler, *Why survive? Being old in America*, New York, Harper & Row, 1975.

[10] R.B. Calhoun, *In search of the new old; redefining old age in America, 1945–1970*. New York, Elsevier, 1978.

[11] W.T. Donahue, C. Tibbitts et al., *Planning the older years*, Ann Arbor, University of Michigan Press, 1950.

[12] E.J. Engstrom, *Clinical psychiatry in imperial Germany: a history of psychiatric practice*, Ithaca, Cornell University Press, 2003.

[13] P. Fox, From senility to Alzheimer's disease: the rise of the Alzheimer's disease movement, *Milbank Q* **67**(1) (1989), 58–102.

[14] E.A. Friedmann and R.J. Havighurst, The meaning of work and retirement, [Chicago], University of Chicago Press, 1954.

[15] N. Gellerstedt, Zur Kenntnis der Hirnveranderungen bei der normalen Altersinvolution, *Upsala Lakareforenings Forhandlingar* **38** (1933), 193–408.

[16] G.N. Grob, *Mental illness and American society, 1875–1940*, Princeton, N.J., Princeton University Press, 1983.

[17] G.N. Grob, Explaining Old Age History: The Need for Empiricism, in: *Old Age in a Bureaucratic Society*, D.D. Van Tassel and P.N. Stearns, New York, Greenwood Press, 1986.

[18] G.N. Grob, *From asylum to community: mental health policy in modern America*, Princeton, N.J., Princeton University Press, 1991.

[19] C. Haber, *Beyond sixty-five: the dilemma of old age in America's past*, Cambridge, Cambridge University Press, 1983.

[20] C. Haber and B. Gratton, *Old age and the search for security: an American social history*, Bloomington, Indiana University Press, 1994.

[21] R.J. Havighurst, Social and Psychological Needs of the Aging, *Annals of the American Academy of Political and Social Science* **279** (1952), 11–17.

[22] R.J. Havighurst and R.E. Albrecht, *Older people*, New York, Longmans, Green, 1953.

[23] H.C. Hendrie, M.S. Albert et al., NIH Cognitve and Emotional Health Project: Report of the Critical Evaluation Study Committee, *Alzheimer's and Dementia* **2** (2006), 12–32.

[24] M. Holstein, Alzheimer's disease and senile dementia, 1885–1920: An interpretive history of disease negotiation, *Journal of Aging Studies* **11**(1) (1997), 1–13.

[25] M. Holstein, Aging, Culture, and the Framing of Alzheimer Disease, in: *Concepts of Alzheimer Disease: Biological, Clinical and Cultural Perspectives*, P.J. Whitehouse, K. Maurer and J.F. Ballenger, Baltimore, Johns Hopkins University Press, 2000.

[26] J. Kaplan, *A social program for older people*, Minneapolis, University of Minnesota Press, 1953.

[27] S. Katz, *Disciplining old age: the formation of gerontological knowledge*, Charlottesville, University Press of Virginia, 1996.

[28] R. Katzman, Editorial: The prevalence and malignancy of Alzheimer disease. A major killer, *Arch Neurol* **33**(4) (1976), 217–218.

[29] R. Katzman and K.L. Bick, The Rediscovery of Alzheimer Disease During the 1960s and 1970s, in: *Concepts of Alzheimer Disease: Biological, Clinical and Cultural Perspectives*, P. Whitehouse, K. Maurer and J.F. Ballenger, Baltimore, Johns Hopkins University Press, 2000.

[30] R. Katzman, R.D. Terry et al., Alzheimer's disease: senile dementia and related disorders, New York, Raven Press, 1978.

[31] T. Kitwood, Explaining Senile Dementia: The Limits of Neuropathological Research, *Free Associations* **10** (1987), 117–138.

[32] M. Linden and D. Courtney, American Journal of Psychiatry, 109: 906 915, 1953 (1953), The Human Life Cycle and its Interruptions: A Psychologic Hypothesis, *Am J Psychiatry* **109** (1987), 906–915.

[33] K. Maurer and U. Maurer, *Alzheimer: the life of a physician and the career of a disease*, New York, Columbia University Press, 2003.

[34] K. Maurer, S. Volk et al., Augusta D.: The History of Alois Alzheimer's First Case, *Concepts of Alzheimer Disease: Biological, Clinical and Cultural Perspectives*, P.J. Whitehouse, K. Maurer and J.F. Ballenger, Baltimore, Johns Hopkins University Press, 2000.

[35] T. Myfanwy and M. Isaac, Alois Alzheimer: A Memoir, *Trends in Neuroscience* **10** (1987), 306–307.

[36] National Institute on Aging, C. T. F. Senility reconsidered. Treatment possibilities for mental impairment in the elderly. Task force sponsored by the National Institute on Aging, *Jama* **244**(3) (1980), 259–263.

[37] M. Neumann and R. Cohn, Incidence of Alzheimer's Disease in a Large Mental Hospital: Relation to Senile Psychosis and Psychosis with Cerebra; Arteriosclerosis, *Archives of Neurology and Psychiatry* **69** (1953), 615–636.

[38] R.D. Newton, The Identity of Alzheimer's Disease and Senile Dementia and Their Relationship to Senility, *Journal of Mental Science* **94** (1948), 225–249.

[39] O. Pollak and G. Heathers, *Social adjustment in old age; a research planning report*, New York, Social Science Research Council, 1948.

[40] C.E. Rosenberg, The Crisis in Psychiatric Legitimacy: Reflections on Psychiatry, Medicine, and Public Policy, *Exploring Epidemics and Other Essays in the History of Medicine*, New York, Cambridge University Press, 1992.

[41] M. Roth, B.E. Tomlinson et al., Correlation between scores for dementia and counts of senile plaques in cerebral grey matter of elderly subjects, *Nature* **209**(18) (1966), 109–110.

[42] D. Rothschild, Alzheimer's Disease: A Clinicopathologic Study of Five Cases, *American Journal of Psychiatry* **91** (1934), 485–519.

[43] D. Rothschild, Pathologic Changes in Senile Psychoses and Their Psychobiologic Significance, *American Journal of Psychiatry* **93** (1937), 757–787.

[44] D. Rothschild, The Practical Value of Research in the Psychoses of Later Life, 8: 123, 1947, 125, *Diseases of the Nervous System* **8** (1947), 123–128.

[45] D. Rothschild and J. Kasanin, Clinicopathologic Study of Alzheimer's Disease: Relationship to Senile Conditions, *Archives of Neurology and Psychiatry* **36** (1936), 293–321.

[46] E. Shorter, *A history of psychiatry: from the era of the asylum to the age of Prozac*, New York, John Wiley & Sons, 1997.

[47] C. Tibbitts and W.T. Donahue, *Aging in today's society*, Englewood Cliffs, N.J., Prentice-Hall, 1960.

[48] B.E. Tomlinson, G. Blessed et al., Observations on the brains of non-demented old people, *J Neurol Sci* **7**(2) (1968), 331–356.

[49] B.E. Tomlinson, G. Blessed et al., Observations on the brains of demented old people, *J Neurol Sci* **11**(3) (1970), 205–242.

[50] R.M. Torack, Adult dementia: history, biopsy, pathology, *Neurosurgery* **4**(5) (1979), 434–342.
[51] P.J. Whitehouse, The end of Alzheimer disease, *Alzheimer Dis Assoc Disord* **15**(2) (2001), 59–62.
[52] P.J. Whitehouse, K. Maurer et al., *Concepts of Alzheimer disease: biological, clinical, and cultural perspectives*, Baltimore, Johns Hopkins University Press, 2000.
[53] D.C. Wilson, 111: 902, 1955, The Pathology of Senility, *Am J Psychiatry* **111** (1955), 902–906.

100 Years of Alzheimer's disease (1906–2006)

José Manuel Martínez Lage*
Department of Neurology, University of Navarre Medical School, Pamplona, Spain

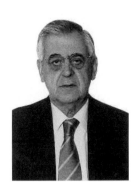

Abstract. As we commemorate the first centennial since Alzheimer's disease (AD) was first diagnosed, this article casts back into the past while also looking to the future. It reflects on the life of Alois Alzheimer (1864–1915) and the scientific work he undertook in describing the disorder suffered by Auguste D. from age 51 to 56 and the neuropathological findings revealed by her brain, reminding us of the origin of the eponym. It highlights how, throughout the 1960's, the true importance of AD as the major cause of late life dementia ultimately came to light and narrates the evolution of the concepts related to AD throughout the years and its recognition as a major public health problem. Finally, the article pays homage to the work done by the Alzheimer's Association and the research undertaken at the Alzheimer's Disease Centres within the framework of the National Institute on Aging (NIA) Program, briefly discussing the long road travelled in the fight against AD in the past 25 years and the scientific odyssey that we trust will result in finding a cure.

1. Introduction

It is a curious irony that the professional and popular discourses surrounding Alzheimer's disease (AD) proceed with little awareness of its past, as Whitehouse et al. mention in the preface to an excellent collection of essays [35]. It is my hope, in writing this article commemorative of the centennial of AD crucial discovery, to contribute to a global understanding and a much needed assessment of this irony. My idea is not simply to preserve the past for its own sake, but to better understand where we are and where we may be going. As quoted by Bick [5], Thomas Carlyle, at the beginning of 19th century, pondered the symbiosis between the search for knowledge and knowledge of history. He went on to invoke reasoning and belief as equally essential as action and passion. The reader will note that action, emotion, and reasoning have their impact on my view of this mythical disease.

2. Alois Alzheimer: The "Psychiatrist with the Microscope"

An overview of Dr. Alois Alzheimer's life and work, all meticulously compiled in a book published originally in German in 1998 and subsequently translated into English [21], is most certainly a worthwhile venture. Born at dawn on 14 July 1864, in Markbreit, a town in the German region of Lower Franconia, he was the son of the second marriage of Eduard Alzheimer to Theresia, his first wife's sister. The Alzheimer family moved to Aschaffenburg to give the children the opportunity to attend a prestigious high school. Alois "was praised for his profound understanding of the natural sciences but he was excused from gymnastics". He completed these studies in 1883. Imbued with the desire to serve others, a traditional trait in a family comprised of teachers and clerics, Alois decided to become

*Address for correspondence: José Manuel Martinez Lage, Vuelta del Castillo 11, 2AB, 31007 Pamplona, Spain. Tel.: +34 948 250 312; Fax: +34 948 29 65 00; E-mail: jmmarlage@unav.es.

a doctor. In the autumn of that same year, he commenced his medical studies at the University of Berlin, at that time the epicentre of medical science. In 1884, he transferred to the University of Würzburg, where he was an active participant in student life. There, in the lab of Kolliker, he learned the histological techniques and use of the microscope that would be key in his future career. He studied at the University of Tubinga in 1886–1887, but later returned to Würzburg to continue perfecting his work with the microscope. He graduated in May 1888, and completed his doctoral thesis at the same university over the following months, studying the wax-producing glands of the ear.

In December 1888, Alzheimer applied for a position as a resident at the The Municipal Asylum for the Insane and Epileptic in Frankfurt am Main and although still very young, was awarded a place by Professor Emil Sioli, Director of the Asylum, on the strength of his outstanding academic achievements. Just a few months after starting work in Frankfurt, Franz Nissl, discoverer of the new nerve staining technique that bears his name, joined the hospital staff. Alzheimer and Nissl took to each other immediately and became close friends and collaborators. Together with Sioli, they formed a triumvirate that transformed the asylum into a sound Psychiatric Clinic where two primary concerns were foremost: firstly, to avoid the use of physical restraint to reduce patient agitation; and secondly, to promote research by doing as many autopsies and neurological studies as possible.

Alois Alzheimer published significant studies on a variety of neuro-psychiatric topics, including vascular dementia and neurosphyillis. His professional prestige continued to grow, and his colleagues nicknamed him "the psychiatrist with the microscope", for the way he focused his work. By day he examined his patients with painstaking care and tenderness, and by night he sat at his microscope to study the samples he had prepared. He was convinced that mental disorders were actually diseases of the brain, a view that was in sharp contrast to the prevailing freudian psychoanalytical theory of the times, which traced psychological problems to traumatic childhood experiences.

His marriage to Cecilie Geisenheimer, the rich widow of a banker, in 1895, gave him enough money to support himself working as an assistant professor without a salary. The couple had three children before she died in 1901.

Alzheimer, "an obsessed doctor and scientist", continued to reap triumph after triumph. In 1902, he left Frankfurt and moved to Heidelberg to do research with Emil Kraepelin, whom he followed to Munich a year later. He was appointed Director of the famous Cerebral Anatomical Laboratory, which trained distinguished physicians from Italy, Poland, Spain, Germany, Russian, and Switzerland. Alzheimer was also a magnet that drew eminent students from overseas. In the words of Perusini, "all of us were seeking to discover the neuropathology of psychosis" [5].

Alzheimer received his qualification as a university professor in 1904. Two years later he discovered the characteristic lesions that cause the disease that have borne his name since 1910. In 1912, he was appointed as Professor in Psychiatry at the University of Breslau, but his health had been seriously weakened by rheumatic fever with endocarditis, which led to his death of renal failure on 15 December 1915, at age 51 [21].

Alzheimer is buried in the central cemetery in Frankfurt. His birthplace was discovered in 1989 by Konrad Maurer, his wife Ulrike and other colleagues from the Department of Psychiatry and Psychotherapy at the Unviersity Joham Wolfgang Goethe in Frankfurt, during a symposium held in Markbreit to commemorate the 125th anniversary of his birth. It was purchased in 1995 by the Eli Lilly company and, thanks to the meticulous work of Ulrike, is now a museum and conference centre [34].

3. Patient Auguste D[eter]: A historical case report and brain donation

On 4 June 1997, the newspaper Frankfurter Runddschau published the following news item: "For two years Drs. Maurer, Volk and Gerbaldo have systematically but unsuccessfully searched the files of the State, the City Historical Institute and the Psychiatric Unit at the University Clinic in Frankfurt for the files on Auguste D[eter], examining all the case histories of patients registered under the initials A.D., in reference to the patient who contributed to the scientific discovery of a new disease". Twelve different files marked with those initials were found, but none of them proved to be related to the patient they were seeking. However, the element of chance came to their assistance. The medical files they searched for were found stored in the basement of the University Clinic, in a section set aside for a completely different year. They had lain there for years, misfiled with the case histories of other patients treated after 1920. Thus, by a stroke of luck, the doctors finally came upon what they had been searching for so assiduously, in their last attempt, on 21 December 1995 [21].

The documents found comprised 32 well-preserved pages in a dark blue folder tied up in string. The cover shows the patient's personal data: Auguste D., wife of a railway worker, born on 16 May 1850, of the Reformed faith. Admitted on 25 November 1901.

Maurer and Maurer comment on the document as if discussing a novel: The assistant physician, Dr. Nitsche, examined Auguste on the day she was admitted and informed Alzheimer that the patient showed unusual clinical symptoms. Alzheimer interviewed her the following day, as recorded on the first page that he personally wrote, transcribing his conversation with the patient.

- What is your name? was his first question.
- *Auguste.*
- And your surname?
- *Auguste.*
- What is your husband's name?
- *Auguste, I think.*
- I am asking for your husband's name . . .
- *Oh, my husband!*
- Are you married?
- *To Auguste.*
- Are you Mrs. D[eter]?
- *Yes, to Auguste.*
- How long have you been here?
- *Three weeks.*

3.1. An extraordinary case history

The file records the onset, symptoms, and course of the disease, the cause of death and the autopsy findings. There are six pages written by Alzheimer. Four of them, dated between 26 and 30 November 1901, describe conversations between the doctor and his patient, and include samples of the patient's writing. Four photographs of Auguste taken by Rudolph, the hospital photographer, were also found. According to Maurer and Maurer [21], the case history, pieced together with the information provided by the husband, was as follows:

"D., Auguste, 51 and one half years-old. Her mother suffered convulsive attacks after menopause, during which she did not lose consciousness; she died of pneumonia at the age of 64. Her father died of throat anthrax at age 45. She has three healthy siblings. There is no family history of alcoholism or mental disorders. Auguste has never been ill prior to this time. She lived quite happily, married in 1873, had a healthy daughter and no miscarriages. She was a polite, hard-working, shy and slightly anxious woman. There is no data that leads us to believe that either she or her husband have a syphilitic infection."

On approximately 18 March 1901, Auguste began to suffer from the delusion that her husband was seeing a neighbor woman. Soon after, she began having trouble remembering things. Two months later, she was making serious mistakes in her cooking and constantly wandering restlessly through the house for no apparent reason. Little-by-little, she became indifferent to everything and lost all sense of the value of money. These symptoms worsened progressively. She believed a train conductor who frequented the house was attempting to harass her. She thought that everyone was talking about her. At times, she was terrified that she was dying and trembled violently. She rang her neighbours' doorbells for no reason. She was unable to find objects that she herself had put away.

The following is another example of a dialogue between Alzheimer and Auguste while she was eating cauliflower and pork [21].

- What are you eating?, Alzheimer asked her.
- *Spinach.*

She chewed, rather than ate the meat. And then she said:
First I eat the potatoes and then the radishes.

He showed her various objects. After a short lapse, she did not remember having seen them. Meanwhile she talked and said repeatedly:

- *Mister Twin, I know Mr. Twin, twins.*
- Write Mrs. D[eter] here, Alzheimer requested.

She wrote: *Mrs*, but not her surname. She could write her full name when it was dictated to her. Instead of *Auguste,* she wrote *Auguse*.

The patient found it difficult to write ordered phrases and sentences, and showed signs of compulsive verbal repetition. When reading, she jumped from line to line and repeated the same sentence up to three times. She did not appear to understand what she was reading.

Her general medical exam was normal. The alterations lay in memory, language, thought and behaviour.

Later, she frequently became agitated and cried out. She seemed to be panicking and repeated incessantly:

- *I don't want them to hurt me; I don't want to hurt myself.*

From that day on, her behaviour became hostile, she cried out frequently and attacked whoever tried to examine her. She was repeatedly given sedatives, which were effective only at times. She was also given therapeutic baths, sometimes with cold water, sometimes with hot, nearly every day. She was distracted in the common room and touched and hit the other patients in the face. It was difficult to imagine exactly what she wanted and she had to be isolated from the rest of the patients. When attempts were made to speak to her, she said:

– *I don't want to, I haven't time.*

The symptoms worsened month by month. Three years after she was admitted, there is a note dated 11 November 1904 indicating that she lay in foetal position on her bed, curled up under the blankets in the midst of her feces. She no longer cried out as she did previously. Another note made on 12 July 1905 remarked that she appeared completely dazed and lay constantly on her bed in her urine and feces with her knees drawn up, totally silent. She was also visibly losing weight. The last 15 lines describe her final days: at the beginning of 1906 she developed bed sores. Her physical deterioration was progressive. Throughout the month of March of this year, she had a fever of up to 40 °C. She was diagnosed with pneumonia and continued to be very agitated, crying out loudly. In early April, her stupor increased and her fever rose to 41 °C. Finally, at quarter past six on 8 April 1906, she died.

Her illness had lasted just over five years.

3.2. Initial autopsy report

This morning, *exitus letalis*. Cause of death: Septicaemia as a result of the bed sores; blood poisoning. Anatomical diagnosis: Slight external-internal hydrocephalus. Cerebral atrophy. Arteriosclerosis of the small cortical vessels? Pneumonia of both lower lobes. Nephritis.

The doctors in Frankfurt called Alzheimer to give him the news of Auguste's death. Alzheimer asked Professor Sioli to send him the autopsy samples in Munich. When he received them, he wrote up the epicrisis of the illness and recorded it in the corresponding volume under number 181, dated 28 April 1906, twenty days after her death [7].

3.3. Presentation of the case. The lesions

Of course, AD existed prior to its description in 1906. But no one had written up the symptomatology as accurately as Alzheimer did on his patient. Moreover, he was the first to describe the microscopic lesions, later known as neurofibrillary tangles, in full detail. From 1901 on, Alzheimer was convinced that Auguste's case was extraordinary, and he quickly began the study of her brain. He used Bielchowsky's silver impregnation staining technique, and had access to both the most powerful microscopes made by Zeiss and the best camera lucida available in day. He contrasted his findings with Perusini and Bonfiglio, who also examined the samples. All three firmly believed that this was a very unusual case history and that the neuropathology involved had not yet been described. The lesions that appeared were similar to those sometimes found in the brains of 70 and 80-year olds who suffered dementia. But the most surprising findings were that in Auguste's case, the lesions were much more marked and the onset of the illness occured when the patient was just 51. Thus, just six months after her death, on d November 1906, Alzheimer presented his clinico-pathological observations at the 37th Assembly of the Southwest German Psychiatrists in Tübingen. Alzheimer had put a great deal of thought and preparation into his presentation entitled "*On a Peculiar, Severe Disease Process of the Cerebral Cortex*" [21].

Once again, Maurer and Maurer tell the story as if they had been present: "The autopsy showed generalised cerebral atrophy without other visible macroscopic lesions. The large cerebral arteries had undergone atherosclerotic changes. Histological samples showed significant changes in the neurofibrils. Inside each neuron, including those that appeared to be normal, one or more fibrils stood out for their thickness and impregnability. Upon further examination, fibrils that run parallel were seen to change in the same way. Then the merge into thick bundles and gradually rise to the surface of the cells. Finally, the nucleus decays, and the cells, and only a crumpled bundle of fibrils indicates the place on which a ganglial cell had lain. Given that these fibrils were stained differently from normal neurofibrils, it was clear that these structures had undergone a chemical change. This may well explain why these pathological neurofibrils survived the neuronal destruction. These alterations appeared in the majority of the neurons in the cerebral cortex. Many of the neurons in the upper layers had completely disappeared". "Spread over the entire cortex, especially numerous in the upper layers, one finds millet seed-size lesions, which are characterized by the deposit of a peculiar substance in the cerebral cortex". "The glia have formed substantial threads, and alongside them, many glial cells show large fatty deposits". "Taken as a whole, I believe I have just presented a clearly defined and hitherto unrecognised disorder". There were no comments from the audience. Alzheimer had to be disappointed. Did his colleagues not understand? [21].

3.4. Publication of the case

Alzheimer published the Auguste's observation in 1907 [1]. He described his findings of neurofibrillary degeneration. Use of the Bielschowsky silver stain clearly showed characteristic changes in the neurofibrils. The nucleus disappeared and only a tangled bundle remained in the cytoplasm where there once had been a neuron. The transformation of the fibrils was accompanied by the storage of a pathological by-product of neuron metabolism. These alterations appeared in one third or one fourth of the neurons in the cerebral cortex. Many of the neurons had disappeared completely.

He then went on to describe the plaques. A profusion of milliary foci in the cortex showed the areas where the abnormal substance was deposited in abundant dispersion throughout the entire cortex, particularly in the upper layers. These were located outside the neurons and were recognisable even without staining, although their presence was even more evident after staining.

Alzheimer ended his observations by remarking, "As a whole, it is clear that this disorder which, over the course of five years, caused profound dementia in a young adult, represents an entirely new clinico-pathological entity" [21].

3.5. Alzheimer's findings confirmed ninety years later

For some time it was speculated that Auguste's disorder could be of a vascular nature, given that the autopsy report indicated atherosclerotic changes; some even maintained that it could possibly have been a leukodystrophy. Thus, the tissue slides taken from Auguste herself were sought out with great interest. Fortunately, they were found at the Institute of Neuropathology of the University of Munich in 1997 [VI] and do not contain any data that indicates the presence of ischemic or other types of lesions. As Alzheimer had shown 91 years earlier, the slides totally corroborated the existence of abundant neurofibrillary tangles and a profusion of amyloid plaques, particularly in the upper layers of the cerebral cortex. Interestingly enough, these slides did not include the hippocampus nor the entorhinal cortex, where the disorder typically begins. Auguste was not a carrier of the genetic risk factor APOE E4 [9].

4. The Eponym

There were various hypotheses regarding the origin of the eponym. The most likely of these is that the eponym was born in the close collaboration between Kraepelin and Alzheimer, as well as in Kraepelin's awareness of the pre-senile cases published by Alzheimer in 1907 and by Perusini in 1909 [22].

When Kraepelin began his revision of Chapter 8 of the eighth edition of his Treatise on Psychiatry published in 1910 entitled "Dementia at the Degenerative Age", he was already familiar with the publications mentioned above and the clinical observations on the four other patients, similar to Auguste, then studied in Munich. A new version of this highly-demanded book was urgently needed, and the rapid growth of the psychiatric sciences now made a second volume necessary. The first of these reached the bookshops in February 1909. The second, devoted to "Clinical Psychiatry" and the most important of the two, appeared in July 1910. In it Kraepelin's gratitude to Alzheimer was expressed in Chapter 7, entitled "Pre-senile and senile dementia". There, in the table of contents is the name Alzheimer's Disease [20]. On page 624 Kraepelin wrote: "Alzheimer described a group of cases that showed severe neuronal alterations" Interestingly enough, when Alzheimer published his article on a second patient, Johann F., in 1911, he made no reference to the fact that the disease had been baptised by Kraepelin with his surname. – Alzheimer's disease (AD). According to Berrios [3], Alzheimer did not claim to have "discovered" the disease that became named after him.

5. Confounding concepts between presenile and senile dementia

After the classical period, in which the clinical and histopathological acumen of Alzheimer and Perusini brought the disease into scientific focus, Kraepelin made the inscrutable decision to distinguish between presenile and senile dementia, confounding research for generations [2]. It was accepted that AD was a type of premature cerebral senility, and it was generally assumed that "senile dementia" was a different disorder. By 1912 only 13 cases had been written up. The patients were an average of 50 years-old, the mean duration of the illness was seven years, six patients were male and seven were female [5]. From 1907 until the 1950's, AD went practically unnoticed.

At that time, autopsy studies in search of new cases of AD were only done on patients under 65 with presenile dementia. In addition to the fact that very few people lived longer at that time (the average life expectancy was almost half what it is today), the purpose of the studies was to confirm whether the findings of the Munich school were actually sound. However, staining techniques gradually improved and microscopes attained greater optical capacity. Thus, over time, more and more cases of AD were discovered, but always in non-senile patients. Nonetheless, by 1931, the debate regarding the relationship linking AD, senility and normal aging was already underway [10], even into the 1950s it was not easy to understand the intellectual disarray about late-life cognitive changes. There was a failure to establish a clear clinopathological relationship between intellectual impairment and either brain weight or abundance of plaques and tangles [16].

5.1. Cognitive decline in the elderly and AD pathology – The first prospective study: Newcastle

The turn in the tide of opinion, which demonstrated the true importance of AD as the major cause of late life dementia, arose throughout the 1960's. Martin Roth, a professor of psychiatry in Newcastle upon Tyne, designed a study that was decisive in revealing that this disease was actually the greatest and most frequent cause of in senile dementia [11]. A neuropsychological test was developed to measure the mental status (memory, concentration, orientation, etc.) of elderly patients without symptoms of dementia admitted to general hospitals for a variety of reasons, and of other elderly patients in psychiatric hospitals with overt signs of dementia. Garry Blessed developed and administered the test to the two patient groups and later had access to the autopsy reports on both groups of subjects. Pathologist Bernard Tomlinson created a scale for the quantitative assessment of the lesions inherent to AD. In their study published in 1968, the British authors firmly established that neuritic plaques and neurofibrillary tangles were the main cause of what was then known as senile dementia [6]. In a study of all the brains, including those with areas of cerebral infarctions and other diagnoses, they found that 50% showed the histological characteristics of AD without vascular lesions; 17% showed only cerebral infarctions and 18% showed a combination of vascular disease and AD. This, then, meant the end of the belief that most cases of senile dementia were caused by arteriosclerosis, or "lack of circulation in the brain". By proving that the majority of patients with senile dementia had AD, this disorder, hitherto seen as very rare, became a central focus of attention. In a way, it can be said that the disease was actually "rediscovered" [16].

6. Recognition of the public health importance of AD

Robert Katzman, inspired both by a personal involvement with AD and by an awareness of the demographics – the greying America – considers that his most important contribution has been to focus our attention (scientists, doctors, and the general public) on the fact that AD is one of the most common diseases that afflicts mankind and so demands our most intense efforts to combat its ravages [4]. He wrote the 1976 editorial in the Archives of Neurology, his most cited paper [19]. Combining the epidemiological data obtained in small studies on the elderly with the data reported by Blessed et al. affirmed that between 48 and 58% of elderly patients with senile dementia actually had AD, and estimated that there were between 800,000 and 1,200,000 patients suffering from this disorder in the United States. This has had an enormous impact on public opinion.

In 1977, the first meeting organised under the auspices of the NIH was the trigger for extensive research into the disorder, the creation of an appropriate social response, and the demand for reliable diagnosis. Katzman took up the standard for a genuine crusade toward the discovery of the causes and treatment of AD, and of a social movement that maintained that "senility" was not merely a consequence of growing old, but rather a disease that should be studied and dealt with like any other.

In view of Katzman's insistence, the NINCDS organised a conference with the support of the NIA and the NIMH. The driving force behind this conference was Katherine Bick, who worked in the offices of the NINCDS and later played a very active role in Association of Alzheimer's Patients' Families set up in 1979. Thus began the great scientific adventure of funding research projects that have since thrown so much light on the intricacies of AD and its possible treatment.

6.1. Alzheimer's Association

The next important step Katzman took was to create health organisations comprised of volunteers interested in the disease. As always in this type of venture, certain key figures tend to emerge. In this case, Lonnie Wollins, who lost his father to AD in the 70's. Wollins, an expert in non-profit foundations, wanted to found an association. When he met with Katzman and asked him, "What can we do about this disease?" Katzman answered "What we really need is an organisation of health volunteers. You, Lonnie, are a lawyer with expertise in this field – why don't you organise an association for Alzheimer's?" Wollins did not actually take the initiative until some years later, when his father's brother died and the autopsy revealed that he had also suffered from AD. Of Lonnie Wollins' father's six brothers, five died from AD with onset from age 60 to 78. Thus, his motivation for starting up the Alzheimer's Disease Society in New York, a body devoted entirely to research, education, services, etc., was patently clear. Katzman pointed out that what was truly needed were wealthy people interested in the project, who could support it with their donations. Multi-millionaire Jerome Stone, whose wife suffered from AD for 17 years, from age 50 until her death in 1983, was the first philanthropist to become fully committed to the Association [17].

In addition to the association in New York, there were seven similar organizations in Washington, Seattle, San Francisco, Columbus, Ohio, Pittsburgh, Boston and Minneapolis. On 29 October 1979, all these organisation joined together under the auspices of the NIH. It was agreed to found the Alzheimer's Disease and Related Disorders Association (ADRDA), which would later be called simply the Alzheimer's Association, now the most important organization worldwide devoted to the care of AD patients and to conquering this disease.

Many celebrities have contributed to general public awareness of the devastation caused by AD. Rita Hayworth, the unforgettable Gilda, was the first. In 1981, the New York papers reported that the film star suffered from alcoholism. It was said that she was constantly drunk, and neighbors at her luxury apartment in Central Park West asked her to move out of the building and leave them in peace. Dr. Katzman was able to explain that Hayworth's behavior disorders were actually due to AD, not to alcohol ingestion [4,17]. Rita's daughter, Princess Yasmin Aga Khan, became an active fund-raiser for AD. When Hayworth died in 1987 at the age of 68, then-President Ronald Reagan, her co-star in various films, remarked: "The courage and sincerity shown by Rita and her family have done us a great public service by calling the world's attention a disease that all of us hope will soon be curable". It was then that Stone encouraged Princess Yasmin to join the Board of Directors of the Association. She accepted the challenge and later was appointed as Alzheimer's Association Chairwoman. Years later, she also presided over the umbrella organization known as Alzheimer's Disease International (ADI).

For over 20 years, the Alzheimer's Association has provided reliable information, set up support and service programmes for families, substantially increased the funding for research and influenced political decisions related to AD.

7. Alzheimer's Disease Centers Program

In the mid-1980s, the Director of NIA, T. Franklin Williams, established the Office of Alzheimer's Disease, and with the support of NIH Director James Wyngaarden began to consolidate the NIA's coordination of AD research [24]. In 1984, the leaders at the NIA decided it was time to develop a national, interdisciplinary research program specifically focused on the causes and course of AD and the differences between AD and normal aging. The concept of a network of centers on AD (ADCs) began to germinate. Zaven Khachaturian, as Associate Director, Neuroscience and Neuropsychology of Aging Program and the first Director of the Office of Alzheimer's Research, is widely regarded as the architect of ADCR program. Such a network created the necessary infrastructure to promote longitudinal clinical-pathological studies; integrate basic and clinical research; standardize clinical assessment tools method, and clinical trials; and establish national data banks to share resources for clinical, neuropathlogical, and genetic studies. For twenty years, nearly all significant advances in the research on AD have had their origins in these ADCs.

8. Ronald Reagan and AD

On Thanksgiving Day 1982, President Ronald Reagan called for a national awareness week about AD. One of the guests at the reception held in the White House on this occasion was George Glenner, the man who in 1984 would discover the amino acids of the amyloid peptide. Years later, Glenner told a journalist from a San Diego newspaper that President Reagan had looked him in the eye and asked him: "What is Alzheimer's disease?" Glenner explained that it was caused by the formation of neuritic plaques and neurofibrillary tangles in the cerebral cortex, causing the death of numerous neurons, the clinical result of which is dementia, behavior disorders and functional incapacity. Reagan smiled and said: "All I know is that my mother was very elderly and living in an old people's home when she died, and at the last she didn't even recognize me" [31]. His official biographer, Edmund Morris, confirms that Nelle Reagan suffered dementia at her death, most probably due to AD.

In 1993, Reagan underwent a full medical examination at the Mayo Clinic in Rochester, Minnesota and was diagnosed as suffering from AD. On 5 November 1994, he published a famous, hand-written letter in which he informed his fellow citizens that he was "just one more of the millions of Americans suffering from Alzheimer's. Upon learning this news, Nancy and I had to decide whether as private citizens we would keep this a private matter or whether we would make this news known in a public way. [...] So now, we feel it is important to share it with you. In opening our hearts, we hope this might promote greater awareness of this condition. Perhaps it will encourage a clearer understanding of the individuals and families who are affected by it". The letter did society a great service. Reagan commenced the journey that led him, in his own words, to the sunset of his life, but not without first, in 1995, establishing the Ronald and Nancy Reagan Research Institute within the Alzheimer's Association. Reagan died in 2004, 10 years after the he was diagnosed with the disease.

9. The modern era of AD research. The scientific odyssey

The modern period of AD research began during the 1960s with technological and conceptual breakthroughs and the pressure of an aging population created explosive interest and progress. A synopsis of the remarkable progress that has been achieved in the time since that 1977 gathering is in the epilogue of the Katzman and Bick book [15].

9.1. Electron microscope studies

Michael Kidd was the first researcher to apply the electron microscope to the study of the neurofibrillary tangles and neuritic plaques using his own technique of the vibratome [13]. In January 1963, he was the first to report in Nature the paired helical filament structure of AD neurofibrillary tangles. A year later, he described the ultrastructure of the plaques in brain. Also in 1963, Robert Terry used this same technique in a study of biopsied and autopsied tissue. He observed that the neurofibrillary tangles were comprised of paired microtubules organized in a double helix and subsequently published these findings. One year later, he established that the nucleus of the neuritic plaques was made of amyloid protein [18]. Decades after the discoveries made by Kidd and Terry, others showed that the neurofibrillary tangles are made of phosphorylated tau protein and that the nucleus of plaques is comprised of amyloid-beta peptide with 40–42 amino acids.

9.2. First animal experiments

Henry Wisniewski developed an experimental encephalopathy in rabbits by administering aluminium and verifying that plaques and tangles subsequently appeared in their brains [12]. This gave fuel to the idea that this light metal perhaps influenced the onset of AD, a theory that was later ruled out. Wisniewski also showed that plaques identical to those existing in humans also appear in the brains of older dogs and monkeys. However, although the monkeys showed tangles, the dogs did not.

AD appears to be exclusive to human beings [8]. This suggests a relationship between the disease and genetic, functional and structural changes that have taken place throughout the evolution of the human brain.

9.3. The cholinergic hypothesis

Research directly addressing the study of AD and the discovery of a suitable treatment commenced in 1976, by David Bowen, Elaine and Robert Perry, and Peter Davies, whose respective discoveries occurred almost simultaneously [14].

L-dopa, the first drug to be successful in controlling the symptoms of Parkinson's disease, appeared in 1968. For years, it was widely known that in this disease, the striatum stops synthesising dopamine due to nigrostriatal degeneration. L-dopa, a precursor of dopamine, counteracted this dopamine deficiency. Thus, a broad range of substitute therapies emerged, similar to what occurred with insulin in the treatment of diabetes. The key, then, was to find what was missing in the brain in AD and to attempt to correct it.

David Drachman devoted his efforts to the in-depth study of memory and to research in the field of AD [14]. In 1974, he began to study the effects of scopolamine, a substance used as an anaesthesia in surgery, which erases memory during surgical procedures in healthy young adults. He was well aware that scopolamine neutralises the action of acetylcholine, which is an essential element in the formation of memories, retrieval of information and learning processes. A subject under the effects of scopolamine will show memory disorders very similar to those common in the elderly, particularly elderly AD patients. Therefore, he hypothesized that an acetylcholine deficiency could be present in AD.

Through the study of autopsy tissue and cerebral biopsies provided by Nick Corcellis, David Bowen discovered that AD involves a lack of cholinacetyltransferase (CAT). From that moment on, it was clear that the therapeutic target for AD research was to attempt to correct this neurotransmitter deficiency. The cholinergic hypothesis was proven definitively some years later, when research demonstrated a loss of 75% of the cholinergic neurons in the cerebral cortex and the substantia innominata, where an abundance of neuritic plaques and neurofibrillary tangles also appears [34].

9.4. The first drugs

The research mentioned was the trigger for a "cholinergic war", a fever that burned in researchers to find a way to correct the cerebral acetylcholine deficiency. First attempts included the use of choline and lecitine, precursors to acetylcholine and found in various food supplements. Wurtman undertook a series of tests but his work unfortunately did not meet with success.

Anaesthetists in the 1970's who used scopolamine also used a drug called tacrine to counteract the effects of the scopolamine after surgery. Hence, research began on tacrine as a possible drug to be used in treatment of AD, given its anti-scopolamine effects. In 1986, Summers published the first results obtained with tacrine in the New England Journal of Medicine [30]. Some of his results seemed to point to the possibility of a miracle cure. This theory seemed so noteworthy that the prestigious journal devoted an editorial to his work. Summers' research was repeated by other scientists but only modest improvements were obtained with tacrine in more rigorous testing, and the patients treated with this drug showed very high transaminases, evidence of the drug's hepatoxicity.

Nonetheless, tacrine, which soon was set aside, was the first of the approved drugs in the first generation of anticholinesterase inhibitors. New, well-tolerated and more efficient second generation anticholinesterase inhibitors, such as donepezil (1996) and rivastigmine (1998) subsequently made their appearance; later in 2000, galantamine was brought out. This drug, in addition to being an anticholinesterase inhibitor, also activates the nicotinic cholinergic receptors. All of these drugs provide temporary relief of symptomology, but do not halt the progress of the disease [26].

The disease also causes a glutamatergic hyperfunction which produces excitotoxicity and neuronal death. The use of memantine, an NMDA receptor antagonist, to treat patients in moderate to severe stages of the disease was approved in 2002 [25].

9.5. Peptide amyloid-β sequence

The nature of amyloid was not to be definitively discovered until 1984. On realizing the difficulty involved in examining the substance in the cerebral cortex, George Glenner opted for studying it in the meninges and its vessels. Together with Wong, he was able to dissolve it and found two different proteins, which he and his colleague named alpha and beta. With the help of a Bekman analyzer, they discovered the sequence of the amino acids comprising the substance. It is a 40–42 amino acid peptide, the now classic amyloid-β. They published their findings on 16 May 1984 in Biochemical and Biophysical Research Communications magazine. A year later, Australian researcher Colin Masters and German scientist Konrad Beyreuther isolated amyloid-β from the cerebral plaques themselves in patients with Down's syndrome, where lesions identical to those found in AD disease appear between the ages of 40 and 50 [31].

These discoveries led to characterizing the amyloid precursor protein (APP), a molecule with 771 amino acids in its longest form, and locating its encoding gene.

9.6. Tau protein

The protein that makes up the paired helical filaments in the neurofibrillary tangles was finally isolated in 1986, a breakthrough Terry had been pursuing for 15 years [18]. With the assistance of Khalid Iqbal and Inge Grundke-Iqbal, both specialists in protein chemistry, he identified the protein associated to the microtubules that comprise the tangles. He called it tau, the last letter in the Hebrew alphabet, because it was the last to be discovered.

9.7. Genetics of the disease

The next step in AD research was to seek out the genes related to the disease and to discover the function of the proteins encoded by these genes. Since 1990, enormous progress has been made in understanding the genetic and non-genetic causes of AD, the mechanisms involved and the possibilities for a cure that lie on the horizon. One of the key figures in this process, Rudy Tanzi, set out his story enthusiastically and in great detail [31].

Familial early onset AD accounts for no more than 2% of all cases and is autosomally dominantly inherited. The family trees in these cases will show family members affected in every known generation. A causative genetic mutation is detected in 50% of these families. It is important to keep this genetically caused form of the disease in mind when confirming that at least three members of the patient's close family in two different generations have been affected. There are some 2,000 families worldwide known to have a proven mutation. The onset of symptoms occurs early, between the ages of 30 and 60, the clinical progress of the disease is rapid, its manifestations are severe and death occurs within a few years. Known mutations are not detected in the other 50% of familial early onset AD, so it is possible that new mutations may be discovered in the future. The same may be said of sporadic early onset AD not caused by currently known mutations.

Late onset AD is the prototypical form of the disease, and accounts for 98% of all cases. The late onset familial form (with at least one close relative also affected) comprises 50% of the cases, although not through autosomic dominant inheritance. The genetic analysis of this form suggests that various genes, rather than determining mutations, cause susceptibility to the disease. The most significant of these is the $E4$ allele on the $APOE$ gene that codes apolipoprotein E (ApoE). ApoE is a plasma protein synthesized in the liver, astrocytes and oligodendrocytes. It is responsible for the intracellular transport of cholesterol and lipids, plays a significant role in neuronal maintenance and has a key function in the development of the process. The lack of the $E4$ allele in approximately 50% of the cases of late onset AD of any type leads researchers to believe that there may be other genetic polymorphisms involved in susceptibility to the disease.

Rudy Tanzi joined the research team led by Jim Gusella, which discovered the gene causing Huntington's disease located on chromosome 4 in 1983 [31]. He was encouraged to study chromosome 21, as he wanted to learn more about Down's syndrome, given that Down's subjects are carriers of an extra copy of this chromosome. Chromosome 21 is the shortest of the 23 pairs of human chromosomes, making its detailed study more feasible. Similar to those appearing in AD, Down's patients also form amyloid plaques and neurofibrillary tangles in their brains after age 40 to 50. Hence, this chromosome could also shed some light on AD. Tanzi soon had the cell lines for various members of a Canadian family with early onset AD studied by Ronald Polinsky and Linda Nee in Bethesda, and thus was able to begin searching for mutations on chromosome 21. He did the same with an Italian family from the province of Calabria, also with familial early onset AD, the members of which had settled throughout Italy, France and the US. At that time, Glenner continued to assure that "the genetic defect responsible for Alzheimer's disease is located on chromosome 21". All bets backed the idea that AD was a cerebral amyloidosis. Later, Massachusetts General Hospital received new cell lines from two additional families with early onset AD, a very extensive one from Germany, and another from Russia. Peter St. George-Hyslop commenced their study.

In 1987, the Massachusetts General team, with Jie Kang as primary author, and other Australian, German and American researchers, published findings showing that the gene that codes AβPP is located on chromosome 21 in position D21S1 and is comprised of 3,200 pairs of bases. Isolation of the amyloid-β gene was a crucial step, but still fell short of proving that this gene was actually the cause of AD. The four families studied by Tanzi showed no mutation whatsoever in this gene. The same conclusion was reached by John Hardy and Christine Van Broeckhoven (who discovered the genetic mutation responsible for hereditary cerebral hemorrhage with amyloidoisis-Dutch type on chromosome 21 in 1990). Nonetheless, the concept of a mutation on chromosome 21 in certain families with early onset AD was widely believed by all the researchers.

At the same time, enormous progress was being made in gaining in-depth knowledge of the molecular basis of the disease. The biology of AβPP, the production of amyloid-β and its deposition in the brain were gradually brought to light.

Finally, John Hardy and molecular geneticist Alison Goate found a family in London with familial early onset AD that showed the much sought-after mutation on chromosome 21. The study on the "London mutation" was published in February 1991. This first AD-causing mutation consisted of a simple change in the position of the amino acids in AβPP: valine occupied the position that should have been occupied by isoleucine. This same mutation appeared in the DNA of another family whose tissue samples had been in Hardy's laboratory for the previous two years, sent by Allen Roses, from Duke University. At that time, Roses (who would later discover the *APOE* gene that causes susceptibility to sporadic or familial late onset AD) did not believe that amyloid-β played a integral role in the disease. Hardy "could not" tell Roses about the discovery of the first mutation found in the London family and the family supplied by Duke. Furthermore, an additional 22 samples of DNA from families with early onset AD that Hardy had in his laboratory did not show the mutation that his team had just discovered. Thus, it was evident that there had to be other mutations in other genes on other chromosomes, and they it was imperative to find them. Peggy Perikak-Vance, who worked in Roses' laboratory at Duke, had found that certain cases of late onset AD were related to a gene located on chromosome 19. Surprisingly enough, in the autumn of 1992, this gene was found to be responsible for coding apoE. This *APOE* gene has three possible alleles, named with the Greek letter epsilon (ε) and numbered 2, 3 and 4. The predisposition, although not the determining genetic cause, for AD is located precisely on allele ε4.

In 1995, a mutation of the gene that codes the protein presenilin 1, located on chromosome 14, was discovered by Robin Sherrington, Peter Hyslop's right-hand man at his laboratory in Toronto. Tanzi also had a hand in this success [31].

A group of German families, known as the "Volga Germans", settled on the fertile banks of the Volga River in the 18th century; later, members of these families emigrated to the US and Italy. Amongst these Volga Germans, there were various families with early onset AD, and their DNA samples held great interest for researchers. Once again, Tanzi's team found the genetic mutation responsible for causing the early onset AD in the Volga Germans, which was isolated on the gene that codes presenilin 2 protein on chromosome 1 [31].

The discoveries of these three genetic mutations, the *AβPP* gene, the *PS1* gene and the *PS2* gene, were enormously valuable in learning how the lesions of AD are created and how to avoid them. Specifically, they enabled the creation of experimental models of AD in mice, which are microinjected with the mutated human gene (hence, their name, transgenic mice). After injection, their brains develop the lesions of AD and they show learning disorders. These transgenic mice also serve to carry out important therapeutic tests.

Rudy Tanzi recently stated that we are still very much in the dark regarding 70% of the genetics of AD [32]. In any event, research continues to seek a way to define the individual profile of genetic polymorphisms in each patient to be able to draw up a predictive, and eventually preventive, risk pattern.

10. Alzheimer 2006: Discernible control of the disease

Nearly all of the etiopathogenesis of AD has now been revealed, thereby opening the door to the hope that curative treatments that control the progression of the disease may be on the horizon. "If science can halt the deposit of amyloid-β in the brain, it can prevent the appearance of Alzheimer's or halt its progression" [27–29].

In July 2005, the First International Conference on Early Diagnosis and Treatment of Alzheimer's Disease was held in Washington D. C convened by the Alzheimer's Association. There appeared clear that new research brings AD early detection closer to reality and that innovative therapies show promises. Drugs treatment and lifestyle-based interventions shared the spotlight at this first ever prevention conference.

The event was filled with an air of optimism with respect to the possibility of predicting the future appearance of the disease in the cognitively healthy elderly. Two diagnostic indicators have emerged in this respect: hypometabolism of the enthorrinal cortex in the FDG-PET scan and a decrease in the Aβ42/Aβ40 plasma quotient. Those who voluntarily submit to these tests and show signs of anomalies in the scan and analytical findings may be advised by their physicians to commence preventive treatment. This early treatment model, beginning in the pre-symptomatic stage, could conceivably be similar to the current practices used to control arterial hypertension or hypercholesterolemia, and is being popularized by Newsweek magazine [33]. The profusion of new techniques for studying DNA, protein biology, molecular genetics, cellular biology, biochemistry, transgenic mice, scans for protein aggregates, etc. have already made it possible to reach phase III in clinical testing of agents that prevent the aggregation of amyloid-β (Alzhemed), reduce the production of fibrillogenic Aβ42 (Flurizan) or remove it from the brain through passive immunization. Furthermore, genes interact with the environment and patients' lifestyle, and thus, it is essential to reduce the external risk factors that have been proven to increase susceptibility to AD. These include: a reduction in cholesterol and homocysteine levels; b) maintenance of blood pressure within the normal range; c) control of diabetes; d) regular exercise; and, e) participation in intellectually stimulating activities [23].

References

[1] A. Alzheimer, Über einen eigenartigc Erkrankung der Hirnrinde, *Allgemeine Zeitschrift für Psyciatrie und Psychisch-Gerichtliche Medizin* **64** (1907), 146–148.

[2] J.F. Ballenger, Beyond the characteristic plaques and tangles. Mid-twentieth century US Psychiatry and the fight against senility, in: *Concepts of Alzheimer's Disease*, Biological, clinical, and cultural perspectives, P.J. Whitehouse, K. Maurer and M.A. Ballenger, eds, Baltimore, Johns Hopkins University Press, 2000, 83-83-103.

[3] G.E. Berrios, Dementia: historical overview, in: *Dementia*, (Second edition), J. O'Brien, D. Ames and A. Burns, eds, London, Arnold, 2000, pp. 3–13.

[4] K. Bick, Interview with Robert Katzman, in: *Alzheimer disease*, The changing view, R. Katzman and K. Bick, eds, San Diego, Academic Press, 2000, pp. 252–271.

[5] K.L. Bick, The early story of Alzheimer disease, in: *Alzheimer Disease*, R.D. Terry, R. Katzman and K.L. Bick, eds, New York, Raven Press, 1994, pp. 1–8.

[6] G. Blessed, B.E. Tomlinson and M. Roth, The association between quantitative measures of dementia and of senile changes in the cerebral matter of elderly subjects, *Br J Psychiat* **114** (1968), 797–811.

[7] H. Braak and E. Braak, Neurofibrillary changes. The hallmark of Alzheimer disease, in: *Concepts of Alzheimer's Disease*, Biological, clinical, and cultural perspectives, P.J. Whitehouse, K. Maurer and M.A. Ballenger, eds, Baltimore, Johns Hopkins, 2000, pp. 53–77.

[8] E. Bufill and R. Blesa, Alzheimer's diseqase and brain evolution: Is Alzheimjer's disease an example of antagonistic pleiotropiy? *Rev Neurol* **42** (2006), 25–33.

[9] M.B. Graeber, S. Kösel, E. Grasbon-Frodl, H. Möller and P. Mehraein, Histopathology and APOE genotype of the first Alzheimer's disease patient Auguste D, *Neurogenetics* **1** (1998), 223–228.

[10] R. Katzman and K. Bick, *Alzheimer Disease*, The changing view. San Diego, Academic Press, 2000, 387.

[11] R. Katzman and K. Bick, Cognitive decline in the elderly and AD pathology – The first prospective study: Newcastle, in: *Alzheimer disease*, The changing view, R. Katzman and K. Bick, eds, San Diego, Academic Press, 2000, pp. 46–66.

[12] R. Katzman and K. Bick, Experimental models. Henry Wisniewski, in: *Alzheimer Disease*, R. Katzman and K. Bick, eds, San Diego, Academic Press, 2000, pp. 11–28.

[13] R. Katzman and K. Bick, Mikel Kidd, in: *Alzheimer Disease*, The changing view, R. Katzman and K. Bick, eds, San Diego, Academic Press, 2000, pp. 28–46.

[14] R. Katzman and K. Bick, The cholinergic story: Hope for the patient and family, in: *Alzheimer Disease*, The changing view, R. Katzman and K. Bick, eds, San Diego, Academic Press 2000, pp. 167–210.

[15] R. Katzman and K. Bick, The next act, in: *Alzheimer Disease*, The changing view, R. Katzman and K. Bick, eds, San Diego, Academic Press, 2000, pp. 353–378.

[16] R. Katzman and K. Bick, The rediscovery of Alzheimer disease during the 1960s and 1970s, in: *Concepts of Alzheimer's Disease*, Biological, clinical, and cultural perspectives, P.J. Whitehouse, K. Maurer and M.A. Ballenger, eds, Baltimore, Johns Hopkins University Press, 2000, pp. 104–114.

[17] R. Katzman and K. Bick, The rise of the Alzheimer's Association, in: *Alzheimer Disease*, The changing view, R. Katzman and K. Bick, eds, San Diego, Academic Press, 2000, pp. 312–351.

[18] R. Katzman and K. Bick, The ultrastructure of AD. Robert Terry, in: *Alzheimer Disease*, The changing view, R. Katzman and K. Bick, eds, San Diego, Academic Press, 2000, pp. 11–28.

[19] R. Katzman, The prevalence and malignancy of Alzheimer's disease, *Arch Neurol* **33** (1976), 299–308.

[20] E. Kraepelin, *Psychiatric: Ein Lehrbuch für Studierende und Ärtze*, Leipizg, Barth, 1910, 1129–1136.

[21] K. Maurer and U. Maurer, *The Life of a Physician and the Career of a Disease*, Translated by N Levi with A Burns. New York, Columbia University Pres, 2003, 270.

[22] K. Maurer, S. Volk and H. Gerbaldo, Auguste D and Alzheimer's disease, *Lancet* **349** (1997), 1546–1549.

[23] National Institute of Aging, Can Alzheimer's disease be prevented? NIH Publications No. 05-5503, May 2005.

[24] National Institute on Aging. Alzheimer's disease Education & Referral Center, Alzheimer's disease Centers Program celebrates 20th anniversary, *Connections* **12**(3–4) (2004–2005), 1–8.

[25] B. Reisberg, R. Doody, A. Stoffler, F. Schmitt, S. Ferris and H.J. Mobius, Memantine Study Group. Memantine in moderate-to-severe Alzheimer's disease, *N Engl J Med* **348**(14) (3 Apr. 2003), 1333–1341.

[26] L.S. Schneider, Inhibidores de la colinesterasa: presente y futuro, in: *En Alzheimer XXI: Ciencia y Sociedad*, J.M. Martínez Lage and Z.S. Kachaturian, eds, Barcelona, Masson, 2001, pp. 245–262.

[27] D.J. Selkoe, Alzheimer disease: mechanistic understanding predits novel therapies, *Ann Intern Med* **140** (2004), 627–638.

[28] D.J. Selkoe, Alzheimer's disaease: genes, proteins, and therapy, *Physiological Reviews* **81** (2001), 742–766.

[29] D.J. Selkoe, Defining molecular targets to prevent Alzheimer Disease, *Arch Neurol* **62** (2005), 192–195.

[30] W.K. Summers, L.V. Majovski, G.M. Marsh, K. Tachiki and A. Kling, Oral tetrahydroaminoacridine in long-term treatment of senile dementia, Alzheimer type, *N Engl J Med* **315**(20) (13 Nov. 1986), 1241–1245.

[31] R.D. Tanzi and A.B. Parson, *Decoding Darkness*, The search for the genetic causes of Alzheimer's disease. Cambridge, Mass., Perseus, 2000, 281.

[32] R.D. Tanzi, Genetics basis of cerebral amyloidosis, *Alzheimer & Dementia* **1**(Supl1) (2005), 1, Abstract AM-01.

[33] A. Underwood, 7 Ways to save a Brain, Newswek Special Issue. The future of medicine, Summer 2005, 32.

[34] P.J. Whitehouse, D.L. Price, R.G. Struble, A.W. Clark, J.T. Coyle and M.R. Delon, Alzheimer's disease and senile dementia: loss of neurons in the basal forebrain, *Science* **215**(4537) (5 Mar 1982), 1237–1239.

[35] P.J. Whitehouse, K. Maurer and M.A. Ballenger, eds, *Concepts of Alzheimer's Disease*, Biological, clinical, and cultural perspectives. Baltimore, Johns Hopkins University Press, 2000, 341.

Neuropathology

The essential lesion of Alzheimer disease: A surprise in retrospect

Melvyn J. Ball
Department of Pathology L-113, Oregon Health & Science University, 3181 SW Sam Jackson Pk. Rd., Portland, OR 97239-3098, USA
Tel.: +1 503 709 3946; Fax: +1 503 452 1229; E-mail: ballm@ohsu.edu or emball@teleport.com

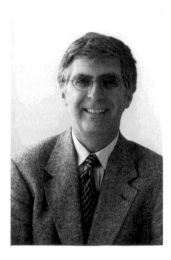

Abstract. In the absence of any naturally occurring animal model of Alzheimer's disease (AD), the British conviction in the 1970's that clinico-pathological investigations of human cases offered the best approach to unraveling the pathogenesis of AD rapidly influenced clinical neuroscientists, neuropathologists and funding agencies in Canada and the USA. But as with my confreres, years of our quantifying AD lesions in autopsy brains have yet to yield definitive conclusions about what is the most important neuronal abnormality. However, during my elusive search, evidence has been slowly gathered that reactivation of latent *Herpes simplex* virus, traveling from trigeminal ganglia into neighbouring mesial temporal cortex, might best explain the limbic predilection for and earliest site of neurofibrillary tangle formation. This maturing hypothesis may serendipitously prove to have been a more essential byproduct of generating the voluminous data than all the publications from our laboratory that reflected endless hours of quantitative morphometry.

Keywords: Alzheimer's disease, morphometry, neurofibrillary tangles, Herpes simplex virus, hippocampus

1. Introduction

While on sabbatical leave in 1972 from the University of Western Ontario, London, Canada, it was my honour to spend a study year abroad at the National Hospital for Nervous Diseases, Queen Square, in the Neuropathology Department of the University of London. There Dr. Anthony Dayan, a Faculty member under Professor William Blackwood,[1] and who was one of the first to apply the new tool of morphometry to what had hitherto been largely descriptive techniques of pathological anatomy, had agreed to tutor me in the nuances of quantitative histopathology.

During that exciting year, I was deeply impressed with the guidelines just issued by the Medical Research Council (MRC) of Great Britain for how best the research community might address the burgeoning challenge of dementia of the elderly, or as the foremost disorder in the "epidemic" of organic dementias became better known, "SDAT" (senile dementia Alzheimer type), or simply "AD" (Alzheimer's disease). The MRC's call for action was greatly influenced by the modern "father of AD neuropathology", Professor Bernard Tomlinson of the University of Newcastle-upon-Tyne, later Sir Bernard, whose pre-retirement reflection upon problematic aspects of AD pathology remains amongst the most thoughtful publications in the entire field [27].

Dr. Tomlinson, who at an international conference in New York had also employed the term *"multi-infarct" dementia* for the second most common cause of chronic

---
[1] ... then busily editing the latest edition of "Greenfield's Neuropathology".

organic neurodegeneration,[2] had already begun to promulgate the understandably appealing notion that one particular lesion seen in the Alzheimer victim's brain would ultimately prove to be the most robust explanation for patients' cognitive deterioration.

Hence his landmark papers with psychiatrist Sir Martin Roth and with Dr. Gary Blessed (who did the actual lesion-counting) on the correlation between number of senile (neuritic) plaques and severity of dementia [7, 28,29] ... although the statistical strength of that putatively linear correlation Tomlinson did acknowledge was somewhat over-stated [26]. Nevertheless, his inherently attractive theory provided considerable momentum for the MRC's published advice that longitudinal clinicopathological studies, tracking many patients until death and brain autopsy, would soon (if not eventually) reveal exactly which of the plethora of striking cellular abnormalities observed more plentifully in AD brains (senile plaques, neurofibrillary tangles, granulovacuoles, rod-like bodies of Hirano, nerve cell dropout) was "the key lesion" of blame.

It thus transpired that I returned to Canada sufficiently buoyed by this concept, and so naively enthusiastic to promote and commence trying the approach, that in short order my very first grant application ever submitted to the National Institutes of Health, USA (a programmatic proposal from the Dementia Study Group which I founded at the University of Western Ontario) met with surprising fiscal success.[3] Dr. Zaven Khachaturian, one of the first NIH administrators to capitalize upon the aging phenomena besetting geriatric members of the United States Congress, so avidly supported our prototype of a comparative investigation of normal subjects and dementing individuals, that very soon thereafter roughly twoscore such academic "Alzheimer research centres" sprouted all across America, funded chiefly by the National Institute on Aging. Who could have forecast in those halcyon days what a tempest of confusion lay in wait for devotees of this modus operandi?

2. Locus minoris resistentiae?

Much to my amazement, my morphometric paper appearing in Acta Neuropathologica of 1977 [1] has proven, if not more durable, at least more quoted than any others I have been privileged to publish. Yet around the same time, innovative observations being made on the basal forebrain by the Johns Hopkins University cadre led Dr. Donald Price and colleagues [32] to insist that the primary trouble in the Alzheimer brain lay in the nucleus basalis of Meynert ... a locus formerly so obscure that in those days four out of five neuroanatomists at the University of Western Ontario[4] were unable to tell any of us its location. (Exactly how the Baltimore group could adequately visualize intraneuronal tangles from cresyl violet-stained Nissl preparations of five demented subjects' brains retrieved from the Yakovlev archives was a similar curiosity.)

The debate about which was the most important neuronal lesion in AD thereupon widened not long afterwards to include predictions about what was the most important *site* of such a lesion in the entire central nervous system (CNS). Hence my Acta Neuropathologica article, arguing for the primacy of neurofibrillary tangle formation and, with tangle-bearing neurones having shown us smaller nucleoli [9], for related hippocampal nerve cell loss, was followed very soon by our still louder contention that histopathological perturbations afflicting the hippocampal formation were far more germane than anything going on in the basal forebrain [4]. Labouring under the boundless audacity of middle age, I proposed in that publication a new term for AD, "a hippocampal dementia". Yet the relative paucity of citations of this later screed possibly reflects the fact that our Lancet paper, while rich in anecdotal histological and biochemical observations, was devoid of abundant hard data. Still, Dr. A. Damasio and co-workers in Iowa came out virtually simultaneously with a similar, though far more eloquently phrased insistence upon the critical role of mesial temporal lobe degeneration, including the entorhinal cortex adjacent to hippocampus proper, in the pathogenesis of AD dementia [16].

As this Alzheimer Centenary issue of the Journal of Alzheimer's Disease calls for reflection on what has happened since the "seminal" paper each of us published, I bemoan the fact that a comprehensive review I was invited to contribute for a rarely referenced European book edited by Ulrich [5] has never been cited with anywhere near the same frequency. For it was in that publication that I proferred the following forecast (paraphrased): "... Once we can explain *why* neurofib-

---

[2] ... popularized by the clinical Ischemic rating scale developed by Dr. Vladimir Hachinski [11].

[3] Some would opine that the American peer review system, unlikely the British, was (at least in those times) not infrequently as much seduced by size of Grant proposal as by quality.

[4] Where Professor Murray Barr had described the juxtanuclear "Barr body" or female sex chromatin [6].

rillary tangles always make their C N S debut specifically here, in the hippocampal formation, we will be within reach of unravelling the etiology of AD". The subsequent "staging" schema advanced by Heiko and Eva Braak [8], which cited neither Damasio's nor our own convictions about tangles in the mesial temporal cortex, surely reiterates all the same just how vital such early entorhinal and adjacent temporal lobe lesions must be ... even though if misused as a post-hoc predictor of clinical severity their pathological staging pattern falls short of the mark [22].

Moreover, a goodly number of more contemporary papers recurrently underscores the fact that limbic pathology both in Mild Cognitive Impairment (MCI) [23] and in early AD remains persistently the favoured patho-anatomic (and neuroimaging) basis for distinguishing normal aging without cognitive decline from preclinical and from earliest dementia of the Alzheimer type [15,21,24,25].

At this juncture, then, rather than stirring yet again the roiling caldron of "Plaque-advocates versus tangle-proponents", or of "Tauists versus B'APPtists" (? Beta-amyloidopathists), I feel it far more useful to rephrase the critical conundrum thusly: What is it about mesial temporal lobe that renders it the *locus minoris resistentiae*, always the very first place we find neurofibrillary tangles?

3. Is herpes simplex virus the culprit?

Thanks to the unflagging tenacity of Professor Ruth Itzhaki and her associates at the University of Manchester, England [14,19], the possibility which I originally fancied in 1982 [2] and which our *in situ* hybridization data reinforced in Dr. Anne Deatly's 1990 autopsy study [10], is nowadays enjoying a renaissance – i.e., that reactivation of *Herpes simplex* virus type 1 (HSV-1), latently residing in the trigeminal ganglia of nearly all adults, may touch off the pathological cascade eventuating in the limbic predilection of and earliest site for neurofibrillary induction, and even in the eventual dementia of AD. To date my explication remains unbending, that the reactivated HSV-1 virus utilizes for its route of entry into the mesial temporal lobe those small Vth cranial nerve sensory fibres from the Gasserian ganglion which track (not down to the site of a recurrent cold sore, but) up towards the basal meninges of the middle cranial fossa; each trigeminal ganglion, mysteriously filled from birth through old age with chronic inflammatory (immunosurveillance) cells [3] lies only

a few mm. away from the entorhinal and hippocampal cortices.

Ruth Itzhaki has been waging a painfully slow, uphill battle for grant support from British agencies, but of late some fiscal acknowledgment apprises us that critics now suspect she could in actuality be on the right track.

Equally refreshing is the very recent modicum of NIH support for my colleague Professor James Hill's virological investigations commencing at Louisiana State University, New Orleans [13], where tissues dutifully harvested from several hundred autopsies during a decade of my directing the Oregon Brain Bank in Portland are to be analyzed with appropriate molecular probes, evaluating this delicious hypothesis still further. Cholesterol-lowering statin drugs, I have posited, may even diminish the risk for AD by limiting lipid raft-dependent viral endocytosis, thus decreasing the trans-neuronal spread of HSV-1 [12].

4. Through the retrospectoscope ...

Thus it seems, nearly thirty years later, that a large pot of money and a huge investment of microscopy have been thrown at the moving target, "Which is the essential lesion causing A D's dementia?" Additionally, no less than three (inter)national Working Groups have grappled with the conundrum of, "Which minimum histopathological criteria ought we to concur are those needed to diagnose A D upon brain examination?" [17, 18,20].

Yet each successive endeavour apparently leaves us more with untidiness than with tightly consensual insight into how to untangle the neuropathological concatenation ... an elusive goal not unlike trying to define the camel, also called "a horse designed by a committee". On rare occasion, thorough neuropathological examination of the brain of an Alzheimer victim may even fail to find *any* light-microscopic lesions at all to account for the typical clinical history [30], although assuredly the measurement of significant neocortical neuronal depletion is a daunting task, especially if not using laborious, unbiased stereological methods [31].

If there is any overarching lesson one might garner from George Perry's tempting each of this issue's contributors to re-examine the "success" of our most quoted disquisition, perchance it is this: that quiet, rare intuition, such as softly strikes one in the pre-arousal wee hours of the morning, may more solidly advance the progress of biomedical research than most of the multi-center, hugely expensive mega-Projects which

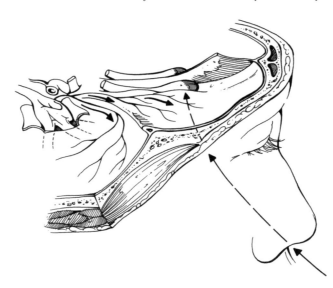

Fig. 1. Small sensory nerve fibres can be seen leaving the Trigeminal Ganglion (at left), proceeding towards the basilar meninges of the middle and anterior cranial fossae (see SOLID arrows). Reproduced with permission from R.T. Johnson, "Viral Infections of the Nervous System", 2nd ed., Fig 6.3, page 142, Lippincott-Raven Press, Philadelphia, 1998.

have been steamrolling across this continent, too frequently discouraging those young investigators who feel they have a really bright, novel and worthy idea to pursue.

Whether *Herpes simplex* virus will ultimately prove a major AD trigger, it is my fervent hope to stay tuned in long enough to learn. And as with all scientific pursuits, maybe the journey itself truly is more important than its final destination.

Acknowledgements

The author thanks all those gracious mentors who guided my way through the thickets of clinical neurology and speculative neuropathology, but especially the late Professor Jerzy ("George") Olszewski, whose gentle nature belied his encyclopedic knowledge.

References

[1] M.J. Ball, Neuronal Loss, Neurofibrillary Tangles and Granulovacuolar Degeneration in the Hippocampus with Ageing and Dementia – a Quantitative Study, *Acta Neuropathologica* **37** (1977), 111–118.

[2] M.J. Ball, Limbic Predilection in Alzheimer's Disease: Is reactivation of Latent Herpes Virus a Cause of Senile Dementia?, *Can. J. Neurol Sci* **9** (1982), 303–306.

[3] M.J. Ball, K. Nuttall and K.G. Warren, Neuronal and Lymphocytic Populations in Human Trigeminal Ganglia: Implications for Ageing and for Latent Virus, *Neuropath. Appl. Neurobiol.* **8** (1982), 177–187.

[4] M.J. Ball, M. Fisman, V. Hachinski, W. Blume, A. Fox, V.A. Kral, A.J. Kirshen, H. Fox and H. Merskey, A New definition of Alzheimer's Disease: a Hippocampal Dementia, *Lancet* **1** (1985), 14–16.

[5] M.J. Ball, Hippocampal Histopathology – a Critical Substrate for Dementia of the Alzheimer Type, Chap. 2 in: *Histology and Histopathology of the Aging Brain*, J. Ulrich, ed., Karger, Basel, 1988, pp. 16–37.

[6] M.L. Barr, L.F. Bertram and H.A. Lindsay, The morphology of the nerve cell nucleus, according to sex, *Anatomical Record* **107** (1950), 283–297.

[7] G. Blessed, B.E. Tomlinson and M. Roth, The Association between Quantitative Measures of Dementia and of Senile Change in the Cerebral Grey Matter of Elderly Subjects, *Br. J. Psychiat.* **114** (1968), 797–811.

[8] H. Braak and E. Braak, Neuropathological stageing of Alzheimer- related changes, *Acta Neuropath* **82** (1991), 239–259.

[9] A.D. Dayan and M.J. Ball, Histometric Observations on the Metabolic Activity of Tangle-Bearing Neurones, *J. Neurol. Sci.* **19** (1973), 433–436.

[10] A. Deatly, A.T. Haase, P.H. Fewster, E. Lewis and M.J. Ball, Human Herpes Virus Infections and Alzheimer's Disease, *Neuropathol. Appl. Neurobiol.* **16** (1990), 213–223.

[11] V.C. Hachinski, L.D. Iliff, E. Zihka et al., Cerebral blood flow in dementia, *Arch Neurol.* **32** (1975), 632–637.

[12] J.M. Hill, I. Steiner, K.E. Matthews, S.G. Trahan, T.P. Foster and M.J. Ball, Statins lower the risk of developing Alzheimer's disease by limiting lipid raft endocytosis and decreasing the neuronal spread of Herpes simplex virus type 1, *Med. Hypoth.* **64** (2005), 53–58.

[13] J.M. Hill, B.M. Gebhardt, A.M. Azcuy, K.E. Matthews, W.J. Lukiw, I. Steiner, H.W. Thompson and M.J. Ball, Can a herpes simplex virus type 1 neuroinvasive score be correlated to other risk factors in Alzheimer's disease? *Med. Hypoth.* **64** (2005), 320–327.

[14] R.F. Itzhaki, W.R. Lin, D.H. Shang, G.K. Wilcock, B. Faragher and G.A. Jamieson, Herpes simplex virus type 1 in brain and risk of Alzheimer's disease, *Lancet* **349** (1997), 241–244.

[15] J.A. Kaye, T. Swihart, D. Howieson, A. Dame, M.M. Moore, T. Karnos, R. Camicioli, M. Ball, B. Oken and G. Sexton, Volume Loss of the Hippocampus and Temporal Lobe in Healthy Elderly Persons Destined to Develop Dementia, *Neurology* **48** (1997), 1297–1304.

[16] B.T. Hyman, G.W. Van Hoesen, A.R. Damasio and C.L. Barnes, Alzheimer's disease: cell specific pathology isolates the hippocampal formation, *Science* **225** (1984), 1168–1170.

[17] B.T. Hyman and J.Q. Trojanowski, Consensus recommendations for the postmortem diagnosis of Alzheimer disease from the National Institute on Aging and the Reagan Institute Working Group on diagnostic criteria for the neuropathological assessment of Alzheimer disease, *J. Neuropath. Exp. Neurol.* **56** (1997), 1095–1097.

[18] Z.S. Khachaturian, Diagnosis of Alzheimer's disease, *Arch. Neurol.* **42** (1985), 1097–1105.

[19] W.R. Lin, M.A. Wozniak, R.J. Cooper, G.K. Wilcock and R.F. Itzhaki, Herpesviruses in brain and Alzheimer's disease, *J. Pathol.* **197** (2002), 395–402.

[20] S.S. Mirra, A. Heyman, D. McKeel et al., The Consortium to Establish a Registry for Alzheimer's Disease (CERAD), II: standardization of the neuropathological assessment of Alzheimer's disease, *Neurology* **41** (1991), 479–486.

[21] L. Musconi, D. Perani, S. Sorbi, K. Herholz, B. Nacmias, V. Holthoff, E. Salmon, J.-C. Baron, M.T.R. De Cristofaro, A. Padovani, B. Borroni, M. Franceschi, L. Bracco and A. Pupi, MCI Conversion to Dementia and the ApoE Genotype – a prediction study with FDG-PET, *Neurology* **63** (2004), 2332–2340.

[22] Zs. Nagy, N.J. Hindley, H. Braak, E. Braak, D.M. Yilmazer-Hanke, C. Schultz, L. Barnetson, E.M.-F. King, K.A. Jobst and A.D. Smith, The Progression of Alzheimer's Disease from Limbic regions to the Neocortex: clinical, radiological and pathological relationships, *Dement. Geriatr. Cogn. Disord.* **10** (1999), 115–120.

[23] R.C. Peterson, R. Doody and A. Kurz, Current concepts in mild cognitive impairment, *Arch Neurol* **58** (2001), 1985–1992.

[24] H. Rusinek, Y. Endo, S. De Santi, D. Frid, W.H. Tsui, S. Segal, A. Convit and M.J. de Leon, Atrophy rate in medial temporal lobe during progression of Alzheimer disease, *Neurology* **63** (2004), 2354–2359.

[25] J. Saxton, O.L. Lopez, G. Ratcliff, C. Dulberg, L.P. Fried, M.C. Carlson, A.B. Newman and L. Kuller, Preclinical Alzheimer disease – Neuropsychological test performance 1.5 to 8 years prior to onset, *Neurology* **63** (2004), 2341–2347.

[26] B.E. Tomlinson, The Pathology of Dementia, in: *Dementia*, C.E. Wells, ed., Davis, Philadelphia, 1977, pp. 113–153.

[27] B.E. Tomlinson, The neuropathology of Alzheimer's disease – Issues in need of resolution, *Neuropath. Appl. Neurobiol.* **15** (1989), 491–512.

[28] B.E. Tomlinson, G. Blessed and M. Roth, Observations on the Brains of Non-demented Old People, *J. Neurol. Sci.* **11** (1968), 331–356.

[29] B.E. Tomlinson, G. Blessed and M. Roth, Observations on the Brains of Demented Old People, *J. Neurol. Sci.* **11** (1970), 205–242.

[30] M. Velickovic, G. Lesser, D. Purohit, R.R. Neufeld, C.Y. Tarshish and L.S. Libow, unpublished data (cited in *J. Amer. Dir. Assoc.* **5** (2004), 407–409).

[31] M.J. West and P.D. Coleman, "How to Count" (editorial), *Neurobiol. Aging* **17** (1996), 503.

[32] P.J. Whitehouse, D.L. Price, R.G. Struble, A.W. Clark, J.T. Coyle and M.R. Delon, Alzheimer's disease and senile dementia: loss of neurons in the basal forebrain, *Science* **215** (1982), 1237–1239.

Vulnerability of cortical neurons to Alzheimer's and Parkinson's diseases

Heiko Braak*, Udo Rüb, Christian Schultz and Kelly Del Tredici
Institute for Clinical Neuroanatomy, J.W. Goethe University, Frankfurt am Main, Germany

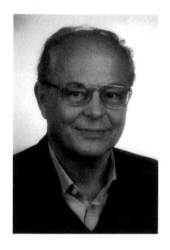

Abstract. Alzheimer's disease (AD) and sporadic Parkinson's disease (PD) are the most frequently occurring degenerative illnesses of the human nervous system. Both involve multiple neuronal systems, but only a few types of nerve cells are prone to develop the disease-associated intraneuronal alterations. In AD affected neurons produce neurofibrillary tangles and neuropil threads, while in PD they develop Lewy bodies and Lewy neurites. In both illnesses select types of projection cells that generate long, unmyelinated or sparsely myelinated axons are particularly susceptible. This kind of selective vulnerability induces a distinctive lesional pattern which evolves slowly over time and remains remarkably consistent across cases. In the present review, lesions developing in the cerebral cortex are described against the backdrop of the internal organisation and interconnectivities linking involved cortical areas and subcortical nuclei. In AD, six and in PD, three stages can be distinguished, reflecting the predictable manner in which the proteinaceous intraneuronal inclusions spread through the cerebral cortex. In AD stages I–II and in PD stage 4, the pathological process makes inroads into the anteromedial temporal mesocortex, entorhinal allocortex, and Ammon's horn; thereafter, in AD stages III–IV and in PD stage 5, it proceeds into the adjoining high order association areas of the basal temporal neocortex. In AD stages V–VI and in PD stage 6, the damage affects additional neocortical association areas including first order association areas and eventually extends into the primary areas of the neocortex. The gradually evolving lesional pattern in AD and PD mirrors the ground plan of the cerebral cortex. The highest densities of lesions occur in the anterior mesocortical transitional zone between allo- and neocortex. From there, the involvement diminishes by degrees and extends into both the hippocampal formation and the neocortex. The severity of the neocortical lesions decreases in inverse proportion to the trajectories of increasing cortical differentiation and hierarchical refinement.

*Corresponding author: Prof. Heiko Braak, MD, Institute for Clinical Neuroanatomy, Theodor Stern Kai 7, D-60590 Frankfurt/Main, Germany. Tel.: +49 69 6301 6900; Fax: +49 69 6301 6425; E-mail: Braak@em.uni-frankfurt.de.

1. Preliminary remarks

Alzheimer's disease (AD) and spontaneously occurring Parkinson's disease (PD) are the most common degenerative disorders of the human nervous system. Both disorders affect multiple neuronal systems and involve pathological aggregation of potentially dangerous proteins in select neuronal types [14]. In AD, susceptible nerve cells develop an abnormal fibrillary material chiefly consisting of altered microtubule-associated tau protein, which appears in the form of somatic neurofibrillary tangles (NFTs) and neuropil threads (NTs) in cellular processes [8,29,45], whereas in PD intraneuronal inclusion bodies predominantly composed of the misfolded α-synuclein protein occur as Lewy bodies (LBs) and Lewy neurites (LNs) [2,21,23,24,46]. In both illnesses, the vulnerability of specific nerve cell groups is reflected in a characteristic topographical distribution pattern of the lesions throughout the cerebral cortex that remains remarkably consistent across cases [4,11,16]. The aim of the present study is to review some phylo- and ontogenetic trajectories that pertain to the problem of selective vulnerability in both AD and PD [15].

2. Neuronal constituents and myelinated axonal plexuses of the cerebral cortex

The cerebral cortex consists of many types of projection cells with a relatively long axon and a variety of short-axoned local circuit neurons [9,37]. Functional maturity of projection cells occurs only after the axon has undergone myelination [18,47,48]. With age, lipofuscin granules accumulate within the nerve cell somata, varying in amount and distribution pattern in different cortical layers and areas [9,10].

The outer and inner lines of Baillarger in neocortical layers IV and Vb are chiefly comprised of a plexus of myelinated axonal collaterals belonging to suprajacent projection neurons. Sublayer IIIb with its affiliated myelinated plexus, the line of Kaes Bechterew, tends to separate from IIIc, foreshadowing an evolutionary shift toward an increase in the number of layers and myelinated lines in the neocortex [33].

3. Three fundamental subdivisions of the cerebral cortex

The various areas of the human cerebral cortex are hierarchically arranged reflecting phylogenetic and ontogenetic trends of differentiation. The two most fundamental subdivisions are the small allocortex and the expansive neocortex (Fig. 1a) [9,50]. The neocortex is principally the interface between the individual organism and the outside world. It constantly receives somatosensory, auditory, and visual data and, at the same time, regulates somatomotor impulses that impact on the environment (Fig. 1a, d). The allocortex includes the olfactory bulb and related areas as well as superordinate centers of the limbic system, such as the entorhinal region, presubicular region, and hippocampal formation. These limbic system centers are important for learning and memory and, among other functions, act as a neuronal bridge that links the external and internal worlds (Fig. 1a, d) [34].

Transitional zones between the neocortex and the allocortex comprise the periallo- and proneocortex, which together form a singularly late-maturing architectonic entity, the mesocortex (Fig. 1a, d). Its temporal portion is remarkably broad among higher primates and especially in humans [9].

The neocortex of the parietal, occipital, and temporal lobes is divided in each instance into a highly refined primary field with particularly dense input from specific thalamo-cortical projections. Each of these fields is flanked by somewhat less highly differentiated first order sensory association areas or premotor fields, and these fields, in turn, are interconnected with large high-order sensory association areas or prefrontal fields (Fig. 1a, d) [34].

A gradual increase in cortical differentiation is observable if one follows an imaginary line from the simply organized temporal mesocortex through prefrontal or high-order sensory association areas and premotor or first order sensory association areas into the highly refined primary fields of the neocortex. This architectonic hierarchy is reflected by an equally hierarchical arrangement of the major interconnecting fiber tracts [34].

Exteroceptive data is relayed from primary sensory fields to the primary motor field and allocortex (Fig. 1d). Visual, auditory, and somatosensory information flows upstream from the primary sensory fields through first order to succeeding high-order association areas and from there via long and sparsely myelinated cortico-cortical projections to the prefrontal cortex. Short, downstream pathways lead away from the prefrontal areas to premotor areas and the primary motor field which acts as a major gateway for motor programs being relayed to brain stem and spinal premotor and motor neurons. The striatal and the cerebellar loops (Fig. 1d, semicircular arrows) function as the main routes for this return pathway and integrate the basal ganglia, many lower brain stem nuclei, and the cerebellum into the regulation of cortical output.

Superordinate limbic system centers participate in this data flow at that juncture where exteroceptive input is transferred from the high-order sensory association

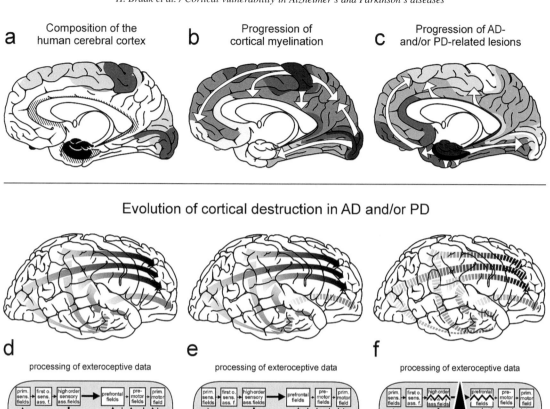

Fig. 1. (a) Composition of the human cerebral cortex. The allocortex (black) consists of the olfactory bulb, entorhinal region, hippocampal formation, and associated areas. The mesocortex (cross-hatching) mediates toward the much larger neocortex. The latter consists of primary sensory or motor fields (dark gray), first order sensory association areas or premotor areas (light gray), and related high-order sensory association areas or prefrontal fields (white). (b) Neocortical myelination begins in the primary sensory and motor fields (dark gray) and progresses (white arrows) via first order sensory association areas and premotor areas (medium gray) to the related high-order sensory association and prefrontal areas (lighter gray tones, indicated by arrows). This results in dense myelination of the primary sensory and motor fields in the human adult. With increasing distance from the primary fields, the average myelin content gradually lessens and is minimal in anterior portions of the mesocortex. (c) An inverse relationship between the myelination process and the destruction of the neocortex exists in AD and/or PD. The first cortical lesions occur in the anterior temporal mesocortex and extend into adjoining high-order association areas, eventually reaching the first order association areas and primary fields of the neocortex (arrows). (d–f) Diagrams showing main subdivisions of the cerebral cortex and components of the limbic loop. Via the afferent trunk of the limbic loop, data are funneled through the anterior temporal mesocortex to both the temporal allocortex and amygdala. The efferent trunk of the limbic loop includes the ventral striatum, ventral pallidum, and mediodorsal thalamus; it directs data to the prefrontal areas. (d) Initial changes in AD stages I–II and/or PD stage 4 mildly hamper the data flow from sensory association areas to superordinate centers of the limbic system. (e) Moderately severe lesions in AD stages III–IV and/or PD stage 5 tend to disconnect the superordinate centers of the limbic system from the neocortex. (f) The destruction in AD stages V–VI and/or PD stage 6 disconnect the neocortical sensory association fields from the prefrontal cortex as well. Abbreviations: endocrine syst. – endocrine system, first o. sens. ass. f. – first order sensory association fields, MD – mediodorsal nuclei of the thalamus, olfact. input – olfactory input, prim. sens. fields – primary sensory fields, ventr. pall. – ventral pallidum, ventr. str. – ventral striatum.

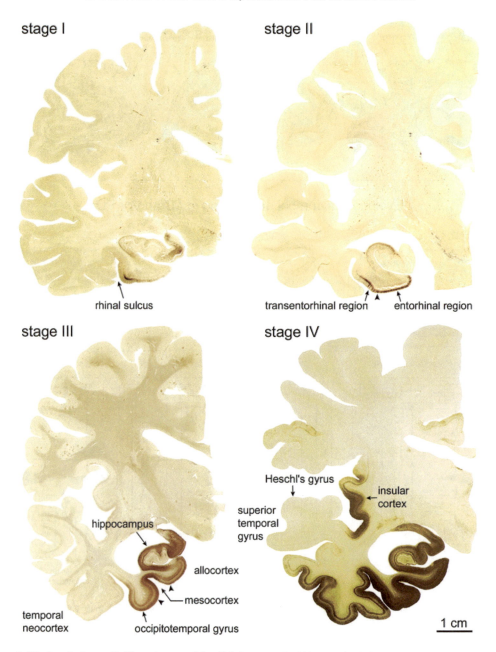

Fig. 2. Stages I–IV of cortical neurofibrillary changes of the Alzheimer type in 100 μm polyethylene glycol-embedded hemisphere sections immunostained for abnormal tau (AT8, Innogenetics). Stage I: involvement is slight and all but confined to the transentorhinal region (part of the temporal mesocortex), usually located on the medial surface of the rhinal or collateral sulcus (arrow). This section originates from a non-demented 80 year-old female. Stage II: Additional immunoreactivity occurs in layer pre-α or layer II of the entorhinal region (arrow). The layer gradually sinks into a deeper position in the transentorhinal region (arrow). The border between entorhinal and transentorhinal regions is clearly recognizable in these early stages (arrowhead). The section was obtained from a non-demented 80 year-old male. Stage III: The lesions make headway into the hippocampal formation (arrow), layers pre-α and, additionally, pri-α of the deep entorhinal layers, the temporal mesocortex (arrow) – largely buried (between the arrowheads) in the banks of the rhinal sulcus, and eventually reach into the adjoining high order sensory association areas of the temporal neocortex. The lesions do not extend beyond the occipitotemporal (arrow) and lingual gyri. The section comes from a 90 year-old female. Stage IV: The third and fourth sectors of the Ammon's horn and a large portion of the insular cortex (arrow) become affected. The involvement of the neocortical high order sensory association cortex of the temporal lobe now extends up to the medial temporal gyrus and stops short of the superior temporal gyrus. The primary fields of the neocortex (see gyrus of Heschl, marked by an arrow) and to a large extent also the premotor and first order sensory association areas of the neocortex remain spared of the pathology. This section was taken from an 82 year-old demented female. Scale bar applies to stage I–IV.

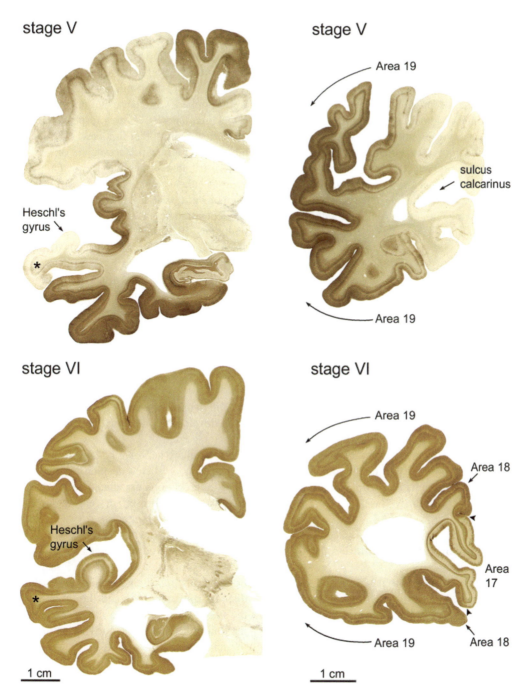

Fig. 3. Stages V–VI of cortical neurofibrillary changes of the Alzheimer type in 100 μm polyethylene glycol-embedded hemisphere sections immunostained for abnormal tau (AT8, Innogenetics). Stage V: In addition to the presence of AD-related lesions in all of the regions mentioned in Fig. 2, pathological changes appear in the superior temporal gyrus (asterisk) and even encroach to a mild degree upon the premotor and first order sensory association areas of the neocortex. In the occipital lobe, the peristriate region (Brodmann area 19) shows varying degrees of affection, and lesions occasionally can even be seen in the parastriate area (Brodmann area 18). These sections were obtained from a 90 year-old female with dementia. Stage VI: Strong immunoreactivity can be detected even in the first order sensory association areas (e.g., the parastriate area, Brodmann area 18, arrows) and the primary areas of the neocortex (e.g., the striate area, Brodmann area 17, between arrowheads) of the occipital neocortex. Compare the superior temporal gyrus (asterisk) and transverse gyrus of Heschl at stage V with the same structures at stage VI. Both stage VI sections originate from a severely demented 70 year-old female Alzheimer patient who died of aspiration pneumonia. Left hand scale bar applies to both hemisphere sections, right hand scale bar to both occipital sections.

areas to the prefrontal cortex. Via the limbic loop, data diverge from the mainstream and proceed through the mesocortex, eventually converging upon the entorhinal region and amygdala, thereby making the neocortex the main source of input to the human limbic system. In addition to this exteroceptive data, the superordinate centers of the limbic system receive input from internal organs (Fig. 1d). As a result, the system is equipped to select from the incoming exteroceptive and interoceptive data the information needed to produce an appropriate response to any given situation. It influences the voluntary motor system via the prefrontal cortex as well as the nuclei that regulate endocrinal and autonomic functions [20,38].

4. Cortical evolutionary trends

The primary fields are the departure points of neocortical evolution and, as such, occupy the most space in the neocortex of lower mammals and early primates. Then follow the less expansive and more simply organized first order sensory association and premotor areas. Least voluminous are the most simply organized high-order sensory association and prefrontal areas. In the course of primate evolution, the association areas expand disproportionately to the primary fields, so that with growing distance from the primary neocortical fields and increasing proximity to the anterior mesocortex, the neocortex exhibits increasingly prominent features of structural immaturity [3,12].

5. Cortical myelination and pigmentation

The phylo- and ontogenetic trends reviewed above can be assessed not only in Nissl sections of the adult human cortex but also in material processed for intraneuronal lipofuscin deposits or myelin.

Myelination is the final step in brain maturation and, in the human cortex – particularly in the lines of Baillarger and Kaes Bechterew – the process is a late-onset one that progresses in a predetermined sequence and persists well into adulthood [39,49].

Initial myelin traces appear in the primary neocortical fields. Thereafter, myelination continues into the premotor and first order sensory association areas and, subsequently, into the prefrontal and high-order sensory association areas (Fig. 1b). The last region to myelinate belongs to the anterior mesocortex. Exceptionally dense myelination of the primary fields is the end-result in the human adult. With increasing distance from the primary fields, however, myelin density falls off gradually (Fig. 1b), so that the anterior mesocortex is very poorly myelinated [39,47].

The brain of the human adult also is particularly well supplied with intraneuronal lipofuscin or neuromelanin deposits. In this respect, it differs notably from the brain of other primates. The lipofuscin granules within cortical projection neurons are usually losely distributed throughout the soma. Local circuit neurons either remain free (or almost free) of such deposits or are packed with granules. Cortical lipofuscin deposition begins in early adulthood and continues with aging [9,10,19,22,25,44]. The degree of lipofuscin accumulation in projection cells of various cortical layers and cortical areas represents the opposite trend of cortical myelination: projection neurons in heavily myelinated areas and densely myelinated layers display far fewer lipofuscin granules than those in the late-myelinating temporal mesocortex that is one of the most richly pigmented regions of the human cortex [9,10].

6. The propensity of select cortical neuronal types to develop AD- and/or PD-related pathology

Of the many neuronal types within the human nervous system, only a few develop the abnormal proteinaceous aggregations associated with AD and PD. By contrast, other directly adjacent nerve cells maintain their morphological integrity.

Neuronal constituents of the cerebral cortex prone to become involved in one or both disease processes have two properties in common. First, all are projection neurons [9,50] and, among these, only cells with disproportionately long and thin axons in relation to the size of the parent soma show a tendency to develop the lesions [36]. Short-axoned projection cells, such as the spiny stellate cells of the fourth neocortical layer or those in the presubicular parvocellular layer, resist the pathology.

Short-axoned local circuit neurons likewise remain untouched by the pathological processes [27,28], with the occasional exception of chandelier cells, which, in AD, display a soluble, abnormal tau material characteristic of the pretangle phase [8] but vanish from the tissue without developing NFTs. To date, PD-related α-synuclein-aggregations have not been seen to occur in cortical local circuit neurons. In sum, AD- and/or PD-related intracellular lesions of the cortex seemingly develop only in projection cells with a long and thin axon.

The vulnerable nerve cell types share a second feature: namely, their long and thin axons remain unmyelinated or have only a thin myelin sheath. By contrast, cortical projection neurons with a heavily myelinated axon resist the formation of AD- and/or PD-related pathologies [16,20]. Pertinent examples are Betz cells in the primary motor cortex and Meynert pyramidal cells in the striate area.

A mature myelin sheath reduces the metabolic demands placed on the parent nerve cell for the transmission of impulses [26]. Thus, rapid-firing projection neurons with unmyelinated or incompletely myelinated axons may be subjected to higher energy turnovers and exposed to greater oxidative stress, a probable contributory factor to the pathogenesis of AD and/or PD [1,7, 30,31,43]. In addition, heavily myelinated projection cells are more stable and more resistant to pathological sprouting [32]. Oligodendrocytes may well be capable of producing as yet unknown protective agents that interact with the axon.

Vulnerable cortical projection neurons develop cross-linked aggregates of the tau protein or of α-synuclein that usually are concentrated in the vicinity of lipofuscin granules. Both the pigment granules and the proteinaceous aggregations are stable and inert. For this reason, no special fixatives are necessary and the material can be assessed at autopsy even after considerable post-mortem delay. Cortical projection neurons are rugged and can survive for decades despite large accumulations of such pathological material. Nevertheless, the functional capabilities of nerve cells filled with NFTs/NTs or LBs/LNs probably decline long before actual cell death [16,36].

7. Progression of AD- and/or PD-associated cortical lesions

Within the cortex, the neurodegenerative process(es) of AD and/or PD first affects a single highly vulnerable area, the periallocortical transentorhinal region, within the anteromedial temporal lobe. Additional areas and ever larger expanses of the cortex become involved (Fig. 1c). A continuum can be said to exist from the first AT8 or α-synuclein-immunopositive changes to the fully-developed cases of AD or PD seen at autopsy in [11,13,16]. For practical purposes, the six stages recommended for the cortical AD-related neurofibrillary pathology can be subsumed under three general subunits (I–II, III–IV, V–VI). Initial diagnosis as to whether abnormal tau inclusions are detectable in the temporal mesocortex (stages I–II), limbic allocortex and amygdala (stages III–IV), or in the neocortex (stages V–VI) simplifies the subsequent task of differentiation. These subunits correspond to the three PD stages where cortical affection also is evident (stages 4–6) [16].

7.1. Mesocortical AD stages I–II and PD stage 4

The neuronal damage that occurs in the early AD stages I–II and in PD stage 4 slightly impairs the transmission of neocortical sensory information – via anteromedial temporal mesocortex – to the superordinate allocortical centers of the limbic system and amygdala (Fig. 1d).

AD Stage I: The transentorhinal region (periallocortex) becomes involved first (Fig. 2). The most vulnerable cells are projection neurons in the superficial entorhinal layer (layer pre-α), which, in the transentorhinal region, gradually slopes downwards on the medial surface of the rhinal sulcus (Fig. 2).

AD Stage II: The lesions in the transentorhinal region are more severe. The pathology now extends into the superficial cellular layer (layer pre-α or layer II) of the entorhinal region (Fig. 2). Additionally, the first and second sectors of the hippocampal formation become involved to a variable degree (Fig. 2).

PD Stage 4: Inclusion bodies appear for the first time in the cerebral cortex, specifically in the anteromedial temporal mesocortex. A network of LNs forms in the superficial layers, while projection neurons in the deep layers develop LBs [16].

7.2. Limbic AD stages III–IV and PD stage 5

The damage typical of the intermediate AD stages III-IV and of PD stage 5 impairs the transmission of neocortical sensory information – via the entorhinal region and hippocampal formation – to the prefrontal neocortex (Fig. 1e).

AD Stage III: The lesions in previously involved stage II sites worsen. The deep entorhinal layer pri-α shows additional affection. From the temporal proneocortex, the disease process gradually encroaches upon the adjoining mature neocortex that covers the occipitotemporal and lingual gyri (Fig. 2).

AD Stage IV: Lesional density increases and the disease process progresses more widely than previously into neocortical high order association areas. In the temporal lobe, it gradually extends up to the superior temporal gyrus (Fig. 2).

PD Stage 5: From the temporal mesocortex, the pathological process extends into related mesocortical insular and anterior cingulate areas, and thereafter into prefrontal and high order sensory association areas of the neocortex. The density of LNs is low in the superfical neocortical layers, and LB-bearing projection cells prevail in their deep layers [16].

7.3. Neocortical AD stages V–VI and PD stage 6

The destruction seen in the late AD stages V–VI and in PD stage 6 cases disconnects not only the allocortex and amygdala from the neocortical fields but also the sensory association areas from the prefrontal neocortex (Fig. 1f).

AD Stage V: From sites involved at stage IV, the neocortical pathology fans out frontally, superolaterally, and occipitally. In the occipital lobe, the patches of NFTs extend into portions of the peristriate region (Brodmann area 19) (Fig. 3).

AD Stage VI: The secondary and primary areas of the neocortex become involved. In the occipital lobe, the pathological process encroaches through the parastriate area (Brodmann area 18) to the striate area (Brodmann area 17) (Fig. 3).

PD Stage 6: The lesions occur in the premotor and first order sensory association areas of the neocortex. A few LBs and LNs even develop in neocortical primary areas, e.g., Heschl's gyrus [16].

8. Progression of the cortical pathology in AD and PD is congruent with the pattern of pigmentation and recapitulates the myelination process in reverse order

The sequential appearance of AD and/or PD-related neocortical lesions is the reverse of the cortical myelination process (compare Fig. 1c with Fig. 1b) – thereby corroborating the earlier observation that regressive changes tend to repeat the maturation process but in reverse order [5,6,12,35,40–42] – and parallels both the sequence and degree of lipofuscin accumulation in cortical projection neurons. Whereas the sparsely pigmented projection cells of the primary neocortical fields (only exception: Betz cells) are heavily myelinated and become involved only in the end stages of both disorders, meso- and neocortical areas that undergo myelination late and whose projection neurons begin lipofuscin accumulation early are especially vulnerable and develop neurofibrillary changes or Lewy body pathology earlier in the disease process and at greater densities [17]. In fact, the lesions commence formation in the vicinity of the lipofuscin granules and the poorly myelinated anteromedial temporal mesocortex is the site of the earliest AD- and/or PD-related lesions in the cerebral cortex. By contrast, cortical nerve cells that remain virtually free of lipofuscin deposits even at an advanced age resist the pathological processes associated with AD and/or PD regardless of the axon's myelin status (e.g., the solitary cells of Cajal). Similarly, heavily myelinated projection neurons do not develop NFTs or LBs even in the presence of considerable lipofuscin deposition [17].

9. Future considerations

It is unclear whether or when the myelination process in human high-order associations areas ends and under the influence of which factors. Were it possible to modify the maturation process so that vulnerable cortical neurons could myelinate more effectively, they might become more resistant to the AD- and PD-related inclusion body pathologies [6]. To have an impact on the prevalence of both disorders, it appears necessary to prevent or at least postpone the beginning of the underlying disease process. Strategies designed to improve cortical myelination and delay the possibly detrimental accumulation of intraneuronal lipofuscin would have to be implemented in early childhood and large numbers of such individuals followed longitudinally.

Acknowledgements

This paper was supported by the Deutsche Forschungsgemeinschaft. We gratefully acknowledge the skillful assistance of Ms. Birgit Meseck-Selchow (tissue preparation and immunohistochemistry) and Ms. I. Szász-Jacobi (graphics).

References

[1] J.E. Ahlskog, Challenging conventional wisdom: the etiologic role of dopamine oxidative stress in Parkinson's disease, *Mov. Disord.* **20** (2005), 271–282.

[2] H. Apaydin, E. Ahlskog, J.E. Parisi, B.F. Boeve and D.W. Dickson, Parkinson disease neuropathology, *Arch. Neurol.* **59** (2002), 102–112.

[3] T. Arendt, M.K. Brückner, H.J. Gertz and L. Marcova, Cortical distribution of neurofibrillary tangles in Alzheimer's disease matches the pattern of neurons that retain their capacity of plastic remodelling in the adult brain, *Neuroscience* **83** (1998), 991–1002.

[4] S.E. Arnold, B.T. Hyman, J. Flory, A.R. Damasio and G.W. van Hoesen, The topographical and neuroanatomical distribution of neurofibrillary tangles and neuritic plaques in the cerebral cortex of patients with Alzheimer's disease, *Cerebral Cortex* **1** (1991), 103–116.

[5] J. Bachevalier and M. Mishkin, Ontogenetic development and decline of memory functions in nonhuman primates, in: *Neurodevelopment, Aging and Cognition,* I. Kostovic, S. Knezevic, H.M. Wisniewski and G.J. Spillich, eds, Birkhäuser, Boston, 1992, pp. 37–59.

[6] G. Bartzokis, J.L. Cummings, D. Sultzer, V. Henderson, K.H. Nuechterlein and J. Mintz, White matter structural integrity in healthy aging adults and patients with Alzheimer's disease, *Arch. Neurol.* **60** (2003), 393–398.

[7] M.F. Beal, Aging, energy, and oxidative stress in neurodegenerative diseases, *Ann. Neurol.* **38** (1995), 357–366.

[8] E. Braak, H. Braak and E.M. Mandelkow, A sequence of cytoskeleton changes related to the formation of neurofibrillary tangles and neuropil threads, *Acta Neuropathol.* **87** (1994), 554–567.

[9] H. Braak, *Architectonics of the Human Telencephalic Cortex,* Springer, Berlin, 1980.

[10] H. Braak, Architectonics as seen by lipofuscin stains, in: *Cerebral Cortex,* (Vol. 1), E.G. Jones and A. Peters, eds, Plenum, New York, 1984, pp. 59–104.

[11] H. Braak and E. Braak, Neuropathological stageing of Alzheimer-related changes, *Acta Neuropathol.* **82** (1991), 239–259.

[12] H. Braak and E. Braak, Development of Alzheimer-related neurofibrillary changes in the neocortex inversely recapitulates cortical myelogenesis, *Acta Neuropathol.* **92** (1996), 197–201.

[13] H. Braak and E. Braak, Temporal sequence of Alzheimer's disease-related pathology, in: *Cerebral Cortex,* (Vol. 14), A. Peters and J.H. Morrison, eds, Plenum, New York, 1999, pp. 475–512.

[14] H. Braak, R.A.I. de Vos, E.N.H. Jansen, H. Bratzke and E. Braak, Neuropathological hallmarks of Alzheimer's and Parkinson's diseases, *Prog. Brain Res.* **117** (1998), 267–285.

[15] H. Braak, K. Del Tredici, C. Schultz and E. Braak, Vulnerability of select neuronal types to Alzheimer's disease, *Ann N.Y. Acad. Sci.* **924** (2000), 53–61.

[16] H. Braak, K. Del Tredici, U. Rüb, R.A.I. de Vos, E.N.H. Jansen Steur and E. Braak[†], Staging of brain pathology related to sporadic Parkinson's disease, *Neurobiol. Aging* **24** (2003), 197–210.

[17] H. Braak, E. Ghebremedhin, U. Rüb, H. Bratzke and K. Del Tredici, Stages in the development of Parkinson's disease-related pathology, *Cell Tissue Res.* **318** (2004), 121–134.

[18] S.T. Brady, A.S. Witt, L.L. Kirkpatrick, S.M. de Waegh, C. Readhead, P.H. Tu and V.M.Y. Lee, Formation of compact myelin is required for maturation of the axonal cytoskeleton, *J. Neurosci.* **19** (1999), 7278–7288.

[19] U.T. Brunk and A. Terman, Lipofuscin: mechanisms of age-related accumulation and influence on cell function, *Free Radical Biol. Med.* **33** (2002), 611–619.

[20] K. Del Tredici and H. Braak, Idiopathic Parkinson's disease: staging an α-synucleinopathy with a predictable pathoanatomy, in: *Molecular Basis of Parkinson's Disease,* P. Kahle and C. Haass, eds, Landes Bioscience, Georgetown, TX, 2003, pp. 1–32.

[21] D.W. Dickson, Tau and synuclein and their role in neuropathology, *Brain Pathol.* **9** (1999), 657–661.

[22] D.B. Fonseca, M.R.J. Sheehy, N. Blackman, P.M.J. Shelton and A.E. Prior, Reversal of a hallmark of brain ageing: lipofuscin accumulation, *Neurobiol. Aging* **26** (2005), 69–76.

[23] B.I. Giasson, J.E. Galvin, V.M.-Y. Lee and J.Q. Trojanowski, The cellular and molecular pathology of Parkinson's disease, in: *Neurodegenerative Dementias: Clinical Features and Pathological Mechanisms,* C.M. Clark and J.Q. Trojanowski, eds, McGraw Hill, New York, 2000, pp. 219–228.

[24] M. Goedert and M.G. Spillantini, Tauopathies and α-synucleinopathies, in: *Fatal Attractions: Protein Aggregates in Neurodegenerative Disorders,* V.M.Y. Lee, J.Q. Trojanowski, L. Buée and Y. Christen, eds, Springer, Berlin, 2000, pp. 66–86.

[25] D.A. Gray and J. Woulfe, Lipofuscin and aging: a matter of toxic waste, *Sci. Aging Knowledge Environ.* **2** (2005), 1–5.

[26] C. Hildebrand, S. Remahl, H. Persson and C. Bjartmar, Myelinated nerve fibres in the CNS, *Prog. Neurobiol.* **40** (1993), 319–384.

[27] P.R. Hof, K. Cox, W.G. Young, M.R. Celio, J. Rogers and J.H. Morrison, Parvalbumin-immunoreactive neurons in the neocortex are resistant to degeneration in Alzheimer's disease, *J. Neuropathol. Exp. Neurol.* **50** (1991), 451–462.

[28] P.R. Hof, E.A. Nimchinsky, M.R. Celio, C. Bouras and J.H. Morrison, Calretinin-immunoreactive neocortical interneurons are unaffected in Alzheimer's disease, *Neurosci. Lett.* **152** (1993), 145–149.

[29] B.T. Hyman and T. Goméz-Isla, Alzheimer's disease is a laminar, regional, and neural system specific disease, not a global brain disease, *Neurobiol. Aging* **15** (1994), 353–354.

[30] P. Jenner, Oxidative stress in Parkinson's disease, *Ann. Neurol.* **53**(suppl. 3) (2003), 26–38.

[31] P. Jenner and C.W. Olanow, Oxidative stress and the pathogenesis of Parkinson's disease, *Neurology* **47** (1996), 161–170.

[32] J.P. Kapfhammer and M.E. Schwab, Inverse patterns of myelination and GAP-43 expression in the adult CNS: neurite growth inhibitors as regulators of neuronal plasticity, *J. Comp. Neurol.* **340** (1994), 194–206.

[33] M. Marin-Padilla, Ontogenesis of the pyramidal cell of the mammalian neocortex and developmental cytoarchitectonics: A unifying theory, *J. Comp. Neurol.* **321** (1992), 223–240.

[34] M.M. Mesulam, From sensation to cognition, *Brain* **121** (1998), 1013–1052.

[35] V.M. Moceri, W.A. Kukull, I. Emanuel, G. van Belle and E.B. Larson, Early-life risk factors and the development of Alzheimer's disease, *Neurology* **54** (2000), 415–420.

[36] B.M. Morrison, P.R. Hof and J.H. Morrison, Determinants of neuronal vulnerability in neurodegenerative diseases, *Ann. Neurol.* **44**(suppl. 1) (1998), 32–44.

[37] R. Nieuwenhuys, The neocortex: an overview of its evolutionary development, structural organization and synaptology, *Anat. Embryol.* **190** (1994), 307–337.

[38] R. Nieuwenhuys, The greater limbic system, the emotional motor system and the brain, *Progr. Brain Res.* **107** (1996), 551–580.

[39] R. Nieuwenhuys, Structure and organization of fiber systems, in: *The Central Nervous System of Vertebrates,* (Vol. 1), R. Nieuwenhuys, H.J. Ten Donkelaar and C. Nicholson, eds, Springer, Berlin, 1999, pp. 113–157.

[40] S.I. Rapoport, Brain evolution and Alzheimer's disease, *Rev. Neurol. (Paris)* **144** (1988), 79–90.

[41] B. Reisberg, A. Pattschull-Furlan, E. Franssen, S.G. Sclan, A. Kluger, L. Dingcong and S.H. Ferris, Dementia of the Alzheimer type recapitulates ontogeny inversely on specific ordinal and temporal parameters, in: *Neurodevelopment, Aging and Cognition,* I. Kostovic, S. Knezevic, H.M. Wisniewski and G.J. Spillich, eds, Birkhäuser, Boston, 1992, pp. 345–369.

[42] B. Reisberg, E.H. Franssen, S.M. Hasan, I. Monteiro, I. Boksay, L.E.M. Souren, S. Kenowsky, S.R. Auer, S. Elahi and A. Kluger, Retrogenesis: clinical, physiologic, and pathologic mechanisms in brain aging, Alzheimer's and other dementing processes, *Eur. Arch. Psychiatry Clin. Neurosci.* **249**(suppl. 3) (2003), 28–36.

[43] R.S. Sohal, Oxidative stress hypothesis of aging, *Free Radical Biol. Med.* **33** (2002), 573–574.

[44] P.A. Szweda, M. Camouse, K.C. Lundberg, T.D. Oberley and L.I. Szweda LI, Aging, lipofuscin formation, and free radical-mediated inhibition of cellular proteolytic systems, *Aging Res. Rev.* **2** (2003), 383–405.

[45] M. Tolnay and A. Probst, Review: tau protein pathology in Alzheimer's disease and related disorders, *Neuropathol. Appl. Neurobiol.* **25** (1999), 171–187.

[46] J.Q. Trojanowski and V.M.Y. Lee, "Fatal attractions" of proteins. A comprehensive hypothetical mechanism underlying Alzheimer's disease and other neurodegenerative disorders, *Ann. N. Y. Acad. Sci.* **924** (2000), 62–67.

[47] M.S. van der Knaap and J. Valk, *Magnetic Resonance of Myelin, Myelination, and Myelin Disorders,* (2nd ed.), Springer, Berlin, 1995.

[48] M.S. van der Knaap, J. Valk, C.J. Bakker, M. Schooneveld, J.A.J. Faber, J. Willemse and P.H.J.M. Gooskens, Myelination as an expression of the functional maturity of the brain, *Dev. Med. Child Neurol.* **33** (1991), 849–857.

[49] P.I. Yakovlev and A.R. Lecours, The myelogenetic cycles of regional maturation of the brain, in: *Regional development of the brain in early life,* A. Minkowksi, ed., Blackwell, Oxford, 1967, pp. 3–70.

[50] K. Zilles, Architecture of the human cortex, in: *The Human Nervous System,* (2nd ed.), G. Paxinos and J.K. Mai, eds, Elsevier Academic Press, San Diego, London, 2004, pp. 997–1060.

Neurodegeneration and hereditary dementias: 40 years of learning

Bernardino Ghetti
Indiana University School of Medicine, Indianapolis, IN, USA
E-mail: bghetti@iupui.edu

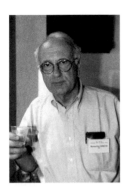

Abstract. The invitation to participate in the commemorative issue celebrating the 100th anniversary of Dr. Alois Alzheimer's report on the disease that would later bear his name has evoked memories of my early experiences in the study of dementia, my teachers, my role-models, my aspirations and my accomplishments. Early in my career, I was fascinated with the study of hereditary neurological disorders. The observation of families in which dementia was inherited in an autosomal dominant pattern excited my scientific curiosity. Three very different phenotypes in patients from three separate families have been the basis for novel scientific discovery, which has taken place over the past 30 years. This could not have taken place without the help of many generous patients and their families as well as wonderful colleagues for whom I am deeply grateful. Some of the original observations in these families have led to the discovery of genetic mutations in three genes that are among the most commonly affected in hereditary dementia. The work on these families has enriched the scientific community and our knowledge of dementing illnesses.

1. Introduction

The invitation to participate in the commemorative issue celebrating the 100th anniversary of Dr. Alois Alzheimer's first report on the disease that would later bear his name has evoked memories of my career [1].

I first became familiar with the concept of dementia when in high school I read the following in one of Juvenalis' (60–140 A.D.) satires: "... omni membrorum damno major dementia, quae nec nomina servorum nec vultum agnoscit amici, cum quo praeterita coenavit nocte, nec illos, quos genuit, quos eduxit"; "... worse still than all decay of limbs is memory's decay, which recalls neither his slaves' names nor the friend's features, with whom he supped but yesternight, nor those whom he begot and bred [46]." Only a few years later, a more complete picture of dementia started to unfold in front of me. As a medical student, I started an internship in the Institute of Psychiatry at the University of Pisa in 1963. The director of the institute at that time was Dr. Pietro Sarteschi, a neurologist and psychiatrist, whose father, also a psychiatrist, had written a paper in 1909 entitled "Contribution to the Pathologic Histology of Senile Dementia" [70]. It was Professor Sarteschi who directed me toward the study of neuropathology and eventually to Dr. Gian Carlo Guazzi's laboratory where I studied from 1968 to 1970 [10,11,22,26,44,67]. It was there that I was introduced to the wonderfully mysterious world of this discipline. During that time, I read a translation of Dr. Alzheimer's paper originally published in 1907, Dr. Van Bogaert's papers on familial Alzheimer disease, Dr. Terry's papers on the ultrastructure of plaques and neurofibrillary tangles and the proceedings of the CIBA symposium held in London on November 11th–13th 1969 [6,86,87,103,105]. By bringing together neurologists, pathologists, psychiatrists and biophysicists, the symposium organized by Dr. W.H. McMenemey encapsulated the multiple facets of Alzheimer disease and related disorders.

Following a letter written in 1969 by Dr. Guazzi, Dr. Robert Terry agreed to allow me to study in his laboratory provided I had my own funding and that I stayed at least two years. I was successful in obtaining a scholarship from the Italian National Research Council and in May 1970 I set sail for the Albert Einstein College of Medicine where I was to study axonal, synaptic and dendritic pathology as well as the modality of trans-synaptic degeneration in animal models [27, 28,41,67]. Upon my arrival, Dr. Henryk Wisniewski was assigned to be my mentor by Dr. Terry. I found working with Henry, to be exciting due to his wealth of ideas and high level of energy. The excitement reached a very high point when one afternoon while examining tissue from an aged monkey under an electron microscope, I observed paired helical filaments similar to those characteristic of Alzheimer's neurofibrillary tangles. I showed Henry my findings and within minutes Dr. Terry and several members of his team surrounded the electron microscope [104].

The intellectual atmosphere at the Albert Einstein College of Medicine was extraordinary. The faculty in neuropathology and neuroscience was composed by well-known scientists. In addition, lectures by visiting scholars were another source of wonder. It is still fresh in my memory, the long list of neuroscientists who were already classics in the literature or who would become such in the following few years. Among the lectures on dementia by many visiting speakers, I remember those by Drs. Corsellis, Sourander, Tomlinson, and Brion. Among the neuroscience lectures, one that stands out in my memory is that by Dr. Richard Sidman. I saw the potential for studying neurological mutant mice as a model of the neurodegenerative process. All of this influenced me to the point that by 1973 I had decided not to return to my alma mater.

After six years of studying at the Albert Einstein College of Medicine, the time came for me to move on even though the separation was very hard. Dr. Wolfgang Zeman invited me to become a member of his neuropathology team at the Indiana University School of Medicine. I accepted with great trepidation. During the time between my acceptance and my starting date, Dr. Zeman decided to leave Indiana University and we never worked together.

At Indiana University, I developed two lines of research. One was directed to the study of nerve cell degeneration in experimental models and the other was directed to the study of human hereditary dementia. I studied the process of nerve cell degeneration in New Zealand rabbits inoculated with various chemical agents and in neurological mutant mice. Using chemical agents that disrupt the cytoskeleton, I was able to observe how maytansine, maytanprine, nocodazole and other agents affected microtubules, induced neurofibrillary pathology and affected the axoplasmic transport [19–21,25,33,71]. Using metallic aluminum powder, a chronic intoxication was induced that led to the accumulation of neurofilaments and to nerve cell loss [7,25,31,89]. In spite of multiple attempts, the formation of the type of tangles that were characteristic of Alzheimer disease never took place. In the area of neurological mutant mice, numerous studies using the weaver mutant mice and Purkinje cell degeneration mice were carried out for over twenty years [24,32, 34,38–40,47,49–51,72,73,88,90–92,94,97–102]. One important finding was the discovery that the neurons of the substantia nigra in weaver mutant mice degenerate causing a severe dopamine deficiency in the nigrostriatal system [73]. These animal studies involved many people and I am particularly grateful to the following for their interactions: S. Bayer, S. Dlouhy, M.E. Hodes, M.J. Schmidt, L.C. Triarhou, T. Verina, and J. Wei.

My work on human hereditary dementia began in 1976 by studying the neuropathology of an autosomal dominant form of Alzheimer disease in a family that had been identified by Dr. Zeman. Over the subsequent 30 years, my work involved several forms of hereditary dementias and numerous families.

The approach has been that of studying carefully the main neuropathologic characteristics of any given genetically-determined dementing illness, identifying unique features of the disease process by classic neuropathology, and electron microscopy. As new techniques of immunohistochemistry, biochemistry, and molecular genetics became available to my laboratory, our approach widened to include the immunohistochemical and biochemical characterization of protein deposits as well as the genetic linkage analysis and DNA sequencing of candidate genes.

I was very fortunate that many investigators shared their enthusiasm and expertise in these research efforts. I am particularly grateful to the following people for their contributions in molecular genetic and biochemical studies: M. Benson, R.A. Crowther, S. Dlouhy, B. Frangione, M. Goedert, A. Klug, L. Miravalle, J. Murrell, P. Parchi, P. Piccardo, S. Prusiner, A. Roher, M.G. Spillantini, F. Tagliavini, R. Vidal and K. Young. I am equally grateful to the following individuals for their contributions in the neuropathologic studies: O. Bugiani, B. Crain, E. Cochran, M.B. Delisle, P. Gambetti, G. Giaccone, J. Ironside, S. Mirra, P.K. Panegyres, S. Spina, M. Takao and K. Yamaguchi. Also, the following people have contributed to clinical studies: B. Boeve, M. Farlow, D. Kareken, O. Rascol, C. Rentz and F. Unverzagt. There are many more people with whom I have collaborated and I have been fortunate to have been associated with, including those generous individuals who have shared cases with my laboratory. I am grateful to the NINDS and the NIA for providing financial support during the last three decades. I have also been blessed to have received support from many wonderful staff members including C. Alyea, L. Bailey, B. Dupree, F.R. Epperson, B.S. Glazier, and R. Richardson.

2. Familial Alzheimer disease

Upon my arrival at Indiana University in 1976, I started to analyze a brain biopsy and autopsy from an individual that Dr. Zeman studied in the late 1960s. The patient had been diagnosed with Alzheimer disease and several members of her family had been known to have developed dementia in their fifth decade of life. I discussed with members of the family about the possibility of continuing the studies initiated a few years earlier by Dr. Zeman. The sister of Dr. Zeman's patient died in 1980 in a mental institution and I was able to obtain the brain through the assistance of this patient's daughter. I am very grateful to her for her help in carrying on the analysis of this family. She continued to help me until she became affected along with other individuals from her generation.

This type of AD was peculiar. There was a very severe neurofibrillary pathology with paired helical filaments, but the plaques were not typical. In 1991, Jill Murrell, a graduate student in Dr. Merrill Benson's laboratory, found a V717F mutation in the $A\beta PP$ gene in affected individuals from two generations of this family [48,56]. This was the first mutation found to be associated with familial Alzheimer disease reported by a laboratory in the United States. Dr. Martin Farlow continues to follow members of the family from the clinical point of view [14,16].

Over the past fifteen years, numerous familial cases of AD have been studied clinically, neuropathologically, biochemically and genetically [8,53–55,69,95]. The multidisciplinary approach has allowed us to characterize the phenotypes associated with two $A\beta PP$ mutations, several *Presenilin 1* mutations and one *Presenilin 2* mutation (Table 1). In some instances, novel mutations have been identified (marked with an asterisk in Table 1) [17,57,68,82,83].

3. The Indiana Kindred

In 1977, Dr. Jans Muller who had succeeded Dr. Zeman as the Director of the Division of Neuropathology assigned to me a brain of a patient from an Indiana family that had been traced for many generations. There were numerous multicentric amyloid cores surrounded by a neuritic crown in the cerebral cortex. These plaques were quite different from those associated with Alzheimer disease in both size and shape. There were numerous neurofibrillary tangles throughout the cortex and subcortical nuclei. The cerebellum had large plaques in the molecular and granular cell layer. In 1978, the brother passed away and a brain autopsy was carried out. I found that this individual's brain contained the same pathologic lesions. We debated on the nature of the disease. In 1985, these two cases were finally published with the title "Cerebellar plaques in familial Alzheimer's disease (Gerstmann-Sträussler-Scheinker Variant?)" [2]. Shortly after, using antibodies against the prion protein it was then clear that the core of the plaque was immunoreactive for the prion protein and not for the $A\beta$ protein of Alzheimer disease; therefore, we realized that we were dealing with a novel pathologic phenotype of Gerstmann-Sträussler-Scheinker disease. We embarked on a study that was directed toward understanding the clinical and neuropathologic aspects of the disease as well as the biochemical pathology of the prion protein and the molecular genetics [13,15, 23,35–37,42,43,45,93,107–109]. With the help of Dr. Fabrizio Tagliavini, who at the time was a part of Dr. Blas Frangione's laboratory, it was possible to uncover the nature of the prion protein amyloid within the core of the plaques. The main molecular component of the core was a fragment of the prion protein. At the same time, a linkage analysis, carried out by Dr. Stephen Dlouhy, revealed that the disease in the Indiana Kindred was linked to chromosome 20 and a molecular genetic analysis carried out by Dr. Karen Hsiao in Dr. Stanley Prusiner's laboratory identified the F198S mutation in the *Prion Protein* gene in affected members of this family [13,45].

Over the past fifteen years, we have studied several additional hereditary prion diseases, identified novel mutations (marked with an asterisk in Table 2), and characterized several pathologic phenotypes [60–66, 77–80,85]. One of the most unexpected findings was the prion protein amyloid angiopathy, which is characterized by deposition of PrP amyloid at the level of cerebral blood vessels and the presence of severe tau pathology in neurons [34].

Table 1
Alzheimer disease

Gene	Mutations
Amyloid β Protein Precursor gene	V717F*, V717L*
Presenilin 1 gene	A79V, F105L, Y115C, M139V, I143T, M146L, L166P*, S169L, G217D*, K239E, A260V, V261F, V261I, P264L, R269G, C410Y, A426P, A431E*, del exon 9
Presenilin 2 gene	N141I

Table 2
Prion disease

Disease	Mutations
GSS	P102L, A117V, G131V, H187R, F198S*, D202N*, Q212P*, Q217R
PrP-CAA	Y145 Stop
fCJD	E200K, V210I

Table 3
FTDP-17

Gene	Mutations
Tau gene	N279K, P301L, P301S*, S305N, Exon 10 +3*, Exon 10 +16, G389R*, R406W

Table 4
Other dementias

Gene	Mutations
Neuroserpin gene	S52R
Ferritin Light Polypeptide gene	498-499insTC

4. Multiple System Tauopathy with Presenile Dementia (MSTD) Family

One of the pivotal moments of my scientific work was when in 1993 I initiated the studies of the neuropathology of cases from a family with a mysterious autosomal dominant disease. After twenty five years in neuropathology, I had not seen anything like what I saw in the proband of the MSTD family. Using antibodies to tau, I saw a landscape that was not familiar to me. Tau deposits in neurons and glia, in the gray and white matter, throughout the central nervous system. Dr. Jill Murrell carried out a linkage analysis and found that MSTD is linked to a three cM region on chromosome 17q21–22 [58]. Biochemical studies carried in collaboration with Dr. Maria Grazia Spillantini and Dr. Michel Goedert revealed that abnormal filaments from the brain of the affected individuals consists of tau isoforms with four repeats [74,75]. Molecular genetic analysis carried out by Dr. Spillantini and Dr. Murrell revealed the presence of a mutation in the third nucleotide of the intron following exon 10 of the Tau gene [76]. The neuropathologic study of additional familial cases of dementia associated with severe tau pathology and in some instances Pick bodies led to the identification of mutations in the Tau gene, some being novel (marked with an asterisk in Table 3) [5,9,12,18,29,52,59].

5. Other neurodegenerative dementias

Neurodegenerative dementias with protein deposits continue to be revealed through the careful neuropathologic examination followed by biochemical and molecular genetic analyses [81,84,96]. Recently, we have studied diseases that are characterized by the accumulation of neuroserpin in neurons and ferritin in neurons and glia (Table 4). Dr. Benson and Dr. Murrell have found the mutation in the neuroserpin protein and Neuroserpin gene respectively [81,106]. Dr. Vidal has characterized a hereditary ferritinopathy associated with severe deposition of ferritin peptides throughout the central nervous system and tc duplications in Ferritin Light Polypeptide gene [96].

As Alois Alzheimer stated in the closing of his 1907 paper, the same words are still true today. His words were "On the whole, it is evident that we are dealing with a peculiar, little known disease process. In recent years, these particular disease-processes have been detected in great numbers. This fact should stimulate us to further study and analysis of this particular disease. We must *not be satisfied to force it into the existing group of well-known disease patterns*. It is clear that there exists many more mental diseases than our text books indicate. In many such cases, a further histological examination must be effected to determine the characteristics of each single case. We must reach the stage in which the vast well-known disease groups must be subdivided into many smaller groups, each one with its own clinical and anatomical characteristics."

References

[1] A. Alzheimer, Über eine eigenartige Erkrankung der Hirnrinde, *Allg Z Psychiatrie Psychisch-Gerichtl Med.* **64** (1907), 146–148.

[2] B. Azzarelli, J. Muller, B. Ghetti, M. Dyken and P.M. Conneally, Cerebellar plaques in familial Alzheimer's disease (Gerstmann-Sträussler-Scheinker Variant?), *Acta Neuropathol. (Berl)* **65** (1985), 235–246.

[3] S.A. Bayer, K.V. Wills, L.C. Triarhou, T. Verina, J.D. Thomas and B. Ghetti, Selective vulnerability of late-generated dopaminergic neurons of the substantia nigra in weaver mutant mice, *Proc. Natl. Acad. Sci. USA* **92** (1995), 9237–9140.

[4] S.A. Bayer, K.V. Wills, J. Wei, Y. Feng, S. Dlouhy, M.E. Hodes, T. Verina and B. Ghetti, Phenotypic effects of the weaver gene are evident in the embryonic cerebellum but not in the ventral midbrain, *Develop. Brain Res.* **96** (1996), 130–137.

[5] B. Boeve, I.W. Tremont-Lukats, A.J. Waclawik, J.R. Murrell, B. Hermann, C.R. Jack, M.M. Shiung, G.E. Smith, D.S. Knopman, A.R. Nair, N. Lindor, V. Koppikar and B. Ghetti, Longitudinal Characterization of Two Siblings with frontotemporal dementia associated with the S305N *Tau* mutation, *Brain* **128** (2005), 752–772.

[6] L. Van Bogaert, M. Maert and E. De Smedt, Sur les formes familiaires precoces de la maladie d' Alzheimer, *Monatschr. Psychiatrie* **102** (1940), 249.

[7] O. Bugiani and B. Ghetti, Progressing encephalomyelopathy with muscular atrophy, induced by aluminum powder, *Neurobiol. Aging* **3** (1982), 209–222.

[8] O. Bugiani, G. Giaccone, B. Frangione, B. Ghetti and F. Tagliavini, Alzheimer patients: preamyloid deposits are more widely distributed than senile plaques throughout the central nervous system, *Neurosci. Lett.* **103** (1989), 263–268.

[9] O. Bugiani, J.R. Murrell, G. Giaccone, M. Hasegawa, G. Ghigo, M. Tabaton, M. Morbin, A. Primavera, F. Carella, C. Solaro, M. Grisoli, M. Savoiardo, M.G. Spillantini, F. Tagliavini, M. Goedert and B. Ghetti, Frontotemporal dementia and corticobasal degeneration in a family with a Pro301Ser mutation in tau, *J. Neuropathol Exp Neurol* **58** (1999), 667–677.

[10] G.B. Cassano, B. Ghetti, E. Gliozzi and E. Hansson, Autoradiographic distribution study of "Short-Acting" and "Long-Acting" barbiturates: S35-Thiopentone and C14-Phenobarbitone, *Br. J. Anaesthesia* **39** (1967), 11–20.

[11] G.B. Cassano, P.L. Viola, B. Ghetti and L. Amaducci, The distribution of inhaled mercury (Hg203) vapors in the brain of rats and mice, *J. Neuropathol. Exp. Neurol.* **28** (1969), 308–320.

[12] M.-B. Delisle, J. Murrell, R. Richardson, J.A. Trofatter, O. Rascol, X. Soulages, M. Mohr, P. Calvas and B. Ghetti, A mutation at codon 279 (N279K) in exon 10 of the tau gene causes a tauopathy with dementia and supranuclear palsy, *Acta Neuropathol.* **98** (1999), 62–77.

[13] S.R. Dlouhy, K. Hsiao, M.R. Farlow, T. Foroud, P.M. Conneally, P. Johnson, S.B. Prusiner, M.E. Hodes and B. Ghetti, Linkage of the Indiana kindred of Gerstmann-Sträussler-Scheinker disease to the prion protein gene, *Nature Genet.* **1** (1992), 64–67.

[14] M.R. Farlow, B. Ghetti, M.D. Benson, J.S. Farrow, W.E. Van Nostrand and S.L. Wagner, Low cerebrospinal-fluid concentrations of soluble amyloid ß-protein precursor in hereditary Alzheimer's disease, *The Lancet.* **340** (1992), 453–454.

[15] M.R. Farlow, B. Ghetti, S.R. Dlouhy, G. Giaccone, O. Bugiani, F. Tagliavini and S. Wagner, Cerebrospinal fluid levels of amyloid ß-protein precursor are low in Gerstmann-Sträussler-Scheinker, Indiana kindred, *Neurology*, **44** (1994), 1508–1510.

[16] M.R. Farlow, J. Murrell, B. Ghetti, F. Unverzagt, S. Zeldenrust and M.D. Benson, Clinical characteristics in a kindred with early onset Alzheimer's disease and their linkage to a G to T change at position 2149 of the amyloid-precursor protein gene, *Neurology* **44** (1994), 105–111.

[17] M.R. Farlow, J.R. Murrell, F.W. Unverzagt, M. Phillips, M. Takao, C. Hulette and B. Ghetti, Familial Alzheimer's Disease with Spastic Paraparesis Associated with a Mutation at Codon 261 of the Presenilin 1 Gene, in: *Alzheimer's Disease: Advances in Etiology, Pathogenesis and Therapeutics*, K. Iqbal, S.S. Sisodia and B. Winblad, eds, John Wiley and Sons Ltd., Chichester, England, 2001, pp. 53–60.

[18] A. Gemignani, P. Pietrini, J.R. Murrell, B.S. Glazier, P. Zolo, M. Guazzelli and B. Ghetti, Slow wave and REM sleep mechanisms are differently altered in hereditary Pick disease associated with the *Tau* G389R mutation, *Arch. Italiennes de Biologie* **143** (2005), 65–79.

[19] B. Ghetti, Induction of neurofibrillary degeneration following treatment with maytansine *in vivo*, *Brain Res.* **163** (1979), 9–19.

[20] B. Ghetti, Experimental studies on neurofibrillary degeneration, in: *Aging of the Brain and Dementia, Aging*, (Vol. 13), L. Amaducci, A.N. Davison and P. Antuono, eds, Raven Press, New York, NY, 1980, pp. 183–198.

[21] B. Ghetti, C. Alyea, J. Norton and S. Ochs, Effects of vinblastine on microtubule density in relation to axoplasmic transport, in: *Axoplasmic Transport*, D. Weiss, ed., Springer-Verlag, New York, Wien, 1982, pp. 322–327.

[22] B. Ghetti, A. Amati, M.V. Turra, A. Pacini, M. Del Vecchio and G.C. Guazzi, Werdnig-Hoffmann-Wohlfart-Kugelberg-Welander disease: nosological unity and clinical variability in intrafamilial cases, *Acta Geneticae Medicae et Gemellologiae* **20** (1971), 43–58.

[23] B. Ghetti, S.R. Dlouhy, G. Giaccone, O. Bugiani, B. Frangione, M.R. Farlow and F. Tagliavini, Gerstmann-Sträussler-Scheinker disease and the Indiana Kindred, *Brain Pathol.* **5** (1995), 61–75.

[24] B. Ghetti, R.W. Fuller, B.D. Sawyer, S.K. Hemrick-Luecke and M.J. Schmidt, Purkinje cell loss and the noradrenergic system in the cerebellum of pcd mutant mice, *Brain Res. Bull.* **7** (1981), 711–714.

[25] B. Ghetti and P. Gambetti, Comparative immunocytochemical characterization of neurofibrillary tangles in experimental maytansine and aluminum encephalopathies, *Brain Res.* **277** (1983), 388–393.

[26] B. Ghetti, G.C. Guazzi, R.V. De Masi and A. Cecio, Epilessia mioclonica giovanile con macchia rosso-ciliegia al fordo dell'occhio, Studio istologico ed ultrastrutturale della biopsia epatica, *Acta Neurol.* **25** (1970), 252–260.

[27] B. Ghetti, D.S. Horoupian and H.M. Wisniewski, Transsynaptic response of the lateral geniculate nucleus and the pattern of degeneration of the nerve terminals in the rhesus monkey after eye enucleation, *Brain Res.* **45** (1972), 31–48.

[28] B. Ghetti, D.S. Horoupian and H.M. Wisniewski, Acute and long-term transneuronal response of dendrites of lateral geniculate neurons following transection of the primary visual afferent pathway, in: *Physiology and Pathology of Dendrites, Advances in Neurology*, (Vol. 12), G.W. Kreutzberg, ed., Raven Press, New York, NY, 1975, pp. 401–424.

[29] B. Ghetti, M. Hutton and Z.K. Wszolek, Frontotemporal dementia and Parkinsonism linked to chromosome 17 associated with *Tau* gene mutations (FTDP-17*T*), in: *Neurodegeneration. The Molecular Pathology of Dementia and Movement Disorders*, D. Dickson, ed., ISN Neuropath Press, Basel, 2003, pp. 86–102.

[30] B. Ghetti, J. Murrell, M.D. Benson and M.R. Farlow, Spectrum of amyloid ß-protein immunoreactivity in hereditary Alzheimer disease with a guanine to thymine missense change at position 1,924 of the APP gene, *Brain Res.* **571** (1992), 133–139.

[31] B. Ghetti, M. Musicco, J. Norton and O. Bugiani, Nerve cell loss in the progressive encephalopathy induced by aluminum powder: A morphologic and semiquantitative study of the Purkinje cell, *Neuropathol. Appl. Neurobiol.* **11** (1985), 31–53.

[32] B. Ghetti, J. Norton and L.C. Triarhou, Nerve cell atrophy and loss in the inferior olivary complex of "Purkinje cell degeneration" (pcd) mutant mice, *J. Comp. Neurol.* **260** (1987), 409–422.

[33] B. Ghetti and S. Ochs, On the relation between microtubule density and axoplasmic transport in nerves treated with Maytansine *in vitro*, in: *Peripheral Neuropathies, Developments in Neurology*, (Vol. 1), N. Canal and G. Pozza, eds, Elsevier North Holland Biomedical Press, Amsterdam, 1978, pp. 177–186.

[34] B. Ghetti, P. Piccardo, M.G. Spillantini, Y. Ichimiya, M. Porro, F. Perini, T. Kitamoto, T. Tateishi, C. Seiler, B. Frangione, O. Bugiani, G. Giaccone, F. Prelli, M. Goedert, S.R. Dlouhy and F. Tagliavini, Vascular Variant of Prion Protein Cerebral Amyloidosis with τ-Positive Neurofibrillary Tangles: The Phenotype of the Stop Codon 145 Mutation in PRNP, *Proc. Natl. Acad. Sci. USA* **93** (1996), 744–748.

[35] B. Ghetti, P. Piccardo, B. Frangione, O. Bugiani, G. Giaccone, K. Young, F. Prelli, M.R. Farlow, S.R. Dlouhy and F. Tagliavini, Prion protein amyloidosis, *Brain Pathol.* **6** (1996), 127–145

[36] B. Ghetti, P. Piccardo, R. Frangione, R. Vidal and J. Ghiso, Neuropathology and genetics of prion protein and British cerebral amyloid angiopathies, in: *Cerebrovascular amyloidosis (CAA) in Alzheimer's Disease and Related Disorders*, M.M. Verbeek, R.M.W. de Waal and H.V. Vinters, eds, 2000, pp. 237–247.

[37] B. Ghetti, F. Tagliavini, C.L. Masters, K. Beyreuther, G. Giaccone, L. Verga, M.R. Farlow, P.M. Conneally, S.R. Dlouhy, B. Azzarelli and O. Bugiani, Gerstmann-Sträussler-Scheinker disease: II. Neurofibrillary tangles and plaques with PrP-amyloid coexist in an affected family, *Neurology* **39** (1989), 1453–1461.

[38] B. Ghetti, L.C. Triarhou, C.J. Alyea, S.R. Dlouhy and R.C. Karn, Unique cerebellar phenotype combining granule and Purkinje cell loss: morphological evidence for weaver*pcd double mutant mice, *J. Neurocytol.* **20** (1991), 27–38.

[39] B. Ghetti and L.C. Triarhou, The Purkinje cell degeneration mutant: a model to study the consequences of neuronal degeneration, in: *Cerebellar degenerations: clinical neurobiology*, A. Plaitakis, ed., Kluwer Academic Publishers, Boston, Mass., 1992, pp. 159–181.

[40] B. Ghetti, L. Truex, B. Sawyer, S. Strada and M.J. Schmidt, Exaggerated cyclic AMP accumulation and glial cell reaction in the cerebellum during Purkinje cell degeneration in pcd mutant mice, *J. Neurosci. Res.* **6** (1981), 789–801.

[41] B. Ghetti and H.M. Wisniewski, On degeneration of terminals in the cat striate cortex, *Brain Res.* **44** (1972), 630–635.

[42] G. Giaccone, F. Tagliavini, L. Verga, B. Frangione, M.R. Farlow, O. Bugiani and B. Ghetti, Neurofibrillary tangles of the Indiana kindred of Gerstmann-Sträussler-Scheinker disease share antigenic determinants with those of Alzheimer disease, *Brain Res.* **530** (1990), 325–329.

[43] G. Giaccone, L. Verga, O. Bugiani, B. Frangione, D. Serban, S.B. Prusiner, M.R. Farlow, B. Ghetti and F. Tagliavini, Prion protein preamyloid and amyloid deposits in Gerstmann-Sträussler-Scheinker disease, Indiana kindred, *Proc. Natl. Acad. Sci. USA* **89** (1992), 9349–9353.

[44] G.C. Guazzi, B. Ghetti, F. Barbieri, B. Frangione and A. Cecio, Myoclonus-epilepsy with cherry-red spot in adult: a peculiar form of mucopolysaccharidosis. A clinical, genetical, chemical and ultrastructural study, *Acta Neurol.* **28** (1973), 542–549.

[45] K. Hsiao, S.R. Dlouhy, M.R. Farlow, C. Cass, M. Da Costa, P.M. Conneally, M.E. Hodes, B. Ghetti and S.B. Prusiner, Mutant Prion Protein in Gerstmann-Sträussler-Scheinker disease with neurofibrillary tangles, *Nature Genet.* **1** (1992), 68–71.

[46] D. Iunii Iuvenalis, Satirae in M. Hendry (ed), http://www.curculio.org/Juvenal/s10.html, 2004.

[47] M. Kambouris, B. Ghetti, S.R. Dlouhy, L.C. Triarhou, L. Sangameswaran, F. Luo and M.E. Hodes, Novel cDNA clones obtained by antibody screening of a mouse cerebellar cDNA expression library, *Mol. Brain Res.* **25** (1994), 183–191.

[48] J.J. Liepnieks, B. Ghetti, M.R. Farlow, A.D. Roses and M.D. Benson, Characterization of amyloid fibril ß-peptide in familial Alzheimer's disease with APP 717 mutations, *Biochem. Biophys. Res. Comm.* **197** (1993), 386–392.

[49] A. Migheli, A. Attanasio, W.-H. Lee, S.A. Bayer and B. Ghetti, Detection of apoptosis in weaver cerebellum by electron microscopic in situ end-labeling of fragmented DNA, *Neurosci. Lett.* **199** (1995), 53–56.

[50] A. Migheli, R. Piva, J. Wei, A. Attanasio, S. Casolino, M.E. Hodes, S.R. Dlouhy, S. Bayer and B. Ghetti, Diverse cell death pathways result from a single missense mutation in weaver mouse, *Am. J. Pathol.* **151** (1997), 1629–1638.

[51] A. Migheli, R. Piva, S. Casolino, C. Atzori, S.R. Dlouhy and B. Ghetti, A cell cycle alteration precedes apoptosis of granule cell precursors in the weaver mouse cerebellum, *Am. J. Pathol.* **155** (1999), 365–373.

[52] S.S. Mirra, J.R. Murrell, M. Gearing, M.G. Spillantini, M. Goedert, R.A. Crowther, A.I. Levey, R. Jones, J. Green, J.M. Shoffner, B.H. Wainer, M.L. Schmidt, J.Q. Trojanowski and B. Ghetti, Tau pathology in a family with dementia and a P301L mutation in tau, *J. Neuropathol. Exp. Neurol.* **58** (1999), 335–345.

[53] T. Moehlmann, E. Winkler, X. Xuefeng, E. Edbauer, J. Murrell, A. Capell, C. Kaether, H. Zheng, B. Ghetti, C. Haass and H. Steiner, Presenilin-1 mutations of leucine 166 equally affect the generation of the Notch and APP intracellular domains independent of their effect on Aβ42 production, *Proc. Natl. Acad. Sci. USA* **99** (2002), 8025–8030.

[54] L. Miravalle, M. Calero, M. Takao, A.E. Roher, B. Ghetti and R. Vidal, Amino-terminally truncated Aβ peptide species are the main component of cotton wool plaques, *Biochemistry* **44** (2005), 10810–10821.

[55] J. Murrell, R.M. Evans, P.J. Boyer, P. Piccardo, J. Towfighi and B. Ghetti, Alzheimer disease with onset in adolescence due to a novel mutation in presenilin I (L166P), *J. Neuropathol. Exp. Neurol.* **59** (2000), 466.

[56] J. Murrell, M.R. Farlow, B. Ghetti and M.D. Benson, A mutation in the amyloid precursor protein (APP) associated

with hereditary Alzheimer's disease, *Science* **254** (1991), 97–99.

[57] J.R. Murrell, A.M. Hake, K.A. Quaid, M.R. Farlow and B. Ghetti, Early onset Alzheimer disease caused by a new mutation (V717L) in the APP gene, *Arch. Neurol.* **57** (2000), 885–887.

[58] J.R. Murrell, D. Koller, T. Foroud, M. Goedert, M.G. Spillantini, H.J. Edenberg, M.R. Farlow and B. Ghetti, Familial multiple-system tauopathy with presenile dementia localized to chromosome 17, *Am. J. Human Genet.* **61** (1997), 1131–1138.

[59] J.R. Murrell, M.G. Spillantini, P. Zolo, M. Guazzelli, M.J. Smith, M. Hasegawa, F. Redi, R.A. Crowther, P. Pietrini, B. Ghetti and M. Goedert, Tau gene mutation G389R causes a tauopathy with abundant Pick body-like inclusions and axonal deposits, *J. Neuropathol. Exp. Neurol.* **58** (1999), 1207–1226.

[60] P.K. Panegyres, K. Toufexis, B.A. Kakulas, P. Brown, B. Ghetti, P. Piccardo and S.R. Douhy, A new mutation [G131V] linked to Gerstmann-Sträussler-Scheinker disease, *Arch. Neurol.* **58** (2001), 1899–1902.

[61] P. Parchi, R. Castellani, S. Capellari, R.B. Petersen, K. Young, S.G. Chen, D.W. Dickson, A.A.F. Sima, J.Q. Trojanowski, M. Farlow, B. Ghetti and P. Gambetti, Molecular basis of phenotypic variability in sporadic Creutzeldt-Jakob disease: A novel classification, *Ann. Neurol.* **39** (1996), 767–778.

[62] P. Piccardo, S.R. Dlouhy, P.M.J. Lievens, K. Young, T.D. Bird, D. Nochlin, D.W. Dickson, H.V. Vinters, T.R. Zimmerman, I.R.A. Mackenzie, S.J. Kish, L.-C. Ang, C. De Carli, M. Pocchiari, P. Brown, C.J. Gibbs, D.C. Gajdusek, O. Bugiani, J. Ironside, F. Tagliavini and B. Ghetti, Phenotypic variability of Gerstmann-Sträussler-Scheinker disease is associated with prion protein heterogeneity, *J. Neuropathol. Exp. Neurol.* **57** (1998), 979–988.

[63] P. Piccardo, B. Ghetti, D.W. Dickson, H.V. Vinters, G. Giaccone, O. Bugiani, F. Tagliavini, K. Young, S.R. Dlouhy, C. Seiler, C. Jones, A. Lazzarini, L.I. Golbe, T.R. Zimmerman, S.L. Perlman, D.C. McLachlan, P.H. St George-Hyslop and A. Lennox, Gerstmann-Sträussler-Scheinker disease (P102L): amyloid deposits are best recognized by antibodies directed to epitopes in PrP region 90–165, *J. Neuropathol. Exp. Neurol.* **54** (1995), 790–801.

[64] P. Piccardo, J.P.M. Langeveld, A.F. Hill, S.R. Dlouhy, K. Young, G.A.H. Wells, G. Giaccone, G. Rossi, M. Bugiani, O. Bugiani, R.H. Meloen, J. Collinge, F. Tagliavini and B. Ghetti, An antibody raised against a conserved sequence of the prion protein recognizes pathologic isoforms in human and animal prion diseases, including vCJD and BSE, *Am. J. Pathol.* **152** (1998), 1415–1420.

[65] P. Piccardo, J.J. Liepnieks, A. William, S.R. Dlouhy, M.R. Farlow, K. Young, D. Nochlin, T.D. Bird, R.R. Nixon, M.J. Ball, C. DeCarli, O. Bugiani, F. Tagliavini, M.D. Benson and B. Ghetti, Prion proteins with different conformations accumulate in Gerstmann-Sträussler-Scheinker disease caused by A117V and F198S mutations, *Am. J. Pathol.* **158** (2001), 2201–2207.

[66] P. Piccardo, C. Seiler, S.R. Dlouhy, K. Young, M.R. Farlow, F. Prelli, B. Frangione, O. Bugiani, F. Tagliavini and B. Ghetti, Protease K resistant prion protein isoforms in Gerstmann-Sträussler-Scheinker Disease (Indiana kindred), *J. Neuropathol. Exp. Neurol.* **55** (1996), 1157–1163.

[67] C.S. Raine, B. Ghetti and M.L. Shelanski, On the association between microtubules and mitochondria within axons, *Brain Res.* **34** (1971), 389–393.

[68] J.M. Ringman, V. Jain, J. Murrell, B. Ghetti and E.J. Cochran, Human Gene Mutations: Gene Symbol: PSEN1, Disease: Alzheimer disease, *Human Genet.* **109** (2001), 242.

[69] A.E. Roher, T.A. Kokjohn, C. Esh, N. Weiss, J. Childress, W. Kalback, D.C. Luehrs, J. Lopez, D. Brune, Y.M. Kuo, M. Farlow, J. Murrell, R. Vidal and B. Ghetti, The human amyloid-beta precursor protein770 mutation V717F generates peptides longer than amyloid-beta-(40-42) and flocculent amyloid aggregates, *J. Biol. Chem.* **279** (2004), 5829–5836.

[70] U. Sarteschi, Contributo all' istologia patologica della presbiofrenia, *Rivista Sperim. Freniatria* **35** (1909), 464.

[71] Y. Sato, S.U. Kim and B. Ghetti, Induction of neurofibrillary tangles in cultured mouse neurons by maytanprine, *J. Neurol. Sci.* **68** (1985), 191–203.

[72] M.J. Schmidt and B. Ghetti, Exaggerated norepinephrine-stimulated ac-cumulation of cyclic AMP *in vitro* in cerebellar slices from pcd mutant mice following Purkinje cell loss, *J. Neural Transmission* **48** (1980), 49–56.

[73] M.J. Schmidt, B.D. Sawyer, K.W. Perry, R.W. Fuller, M.M. Foreman and B. Ghetti, Dopamine deficiency in the weaver mutant mouse, *J. Neurosci.* **2** (1982), 376–380.

[74] M.G. Spillantini, T.D. Bird and B. Ghetti, Frontotemporal dementia and Parkinsonism linked to chromosome 17: A new group of tauopathies, *Brain Pathol.* **8** (1998), 387–402.

[75] M.G. Spillantini, M. Goedert, R.A. Crowther, J.R. Murrell, M.R. Farlow and B. Ghetti, Familial multiple system tauopathy with presenile dementia: a disease with abundant neuronal and glial tau filaments, *Proc. Natl. Acad. Sci. USA* **94** (1997), 4113–4118.

[76] M.G. Spillantini, J.R. Murrell, M. Goedert, M.R. Farlow, A. Klug and B. Ghetti, Mutation in the tau gene in familial multiple system tauopathy with presenile dementia, *Proc. Natl. Acad. Sci. USA* **95** (1998), 7737–7741.

[77] F. Tagliavini, G. Giaccone, F. Prelli, L. Verga, M. Porro, J.Q. Trojanowski, M.R. Farlow, B. Frangione, B. Ghetti and O. Bugiani, A68 is a component of paired helical filaments of Gerstmann-Sträussler-Scheinker disease, Indiana kindred, *Brain Res.* **616** (1993), 325–328.

[78] F. Tagliavini, F. Prelli, J. Ghiso, O. Bugiani, D. Serban, S.B. Prusiner, M.R. Farlow, B. Ghetti and B. Frangione, The amyloid protein of Gerstmann-Sträussler-Scheinker disease (Indiana kindred) is an 11-Kd degradation product of PrP that starts at position 58 of the cDNA-deduced PrP sequence, *EMBO J.* **10** (1991), 513–519.

[79] F. Tagliavini, F. Prelli, L. Verga, G. Giaccone, R. Sarma, P. Gorevic, B. Ghetti, F. Passerini, E. Ghibaudi, G. Forloni, M. Salmona, O. Bugiani and B. Frangione, Synthetic peptides homologous to prion protein residues 106–147 form amyloid-like fibrils *in vitro*, *Proc. Natl. Acad. Sci. USA* **90** (1993), 9678–9682.

[80] F. Tagliavini, F. Prelli, M. Porro, G. Rossi, G. Giaccone, M.R. Farlow, S.R. Dlouhy, B. Ghetti, O. Bugiani and B. Frangione, Amyloid fibrils in Gerstmann-Sträussler-Scheinker disease (Indiana and Swedish Kindreds) express only PrP peptides encoded by the mutant allele, *Cell* **79** (1994), 95–703.

[81] M. Takao, M.D. Benson, J.R. Murrell, M. Yazaki, P. Piccardo, F.W. Unverzagt, R.L. Davis, P.D. Holohan, D.A. Lawrence, R. Richardson, M.R. Farlow and B. Ghetti, Neuroserpin mutation S52R causes neuroserpin accumulation in neurons and

is associated with progressive myoclonus epilepsy, *J. Neuropathol. Exp. Neurol.* **59** (2000), 1070–1086.

[82] M. Takao, B. Ghetti, I. Hayakawa, E. Ikeda, Y. Fukuuchi, L. Miravalle, P. Piccardo, J.R. Murrell, B.S. Glazier and A. Koto, A novel mutation (G217D) in the Presenilin 1 gene (PSEN1) in a Japanese family: presenile dementia and parkinsonism are associated with cotton wool plaques in the cortex and striatum, *Acta Neuropathol. (Berl)* **104** (2002), 155–170.

[83] M. Takao, B. Ghetti, J.R. Murrell, F.W. Unverzagt, G. Giaccone, F. Tagliavini, O. Bugiani, P. Piccardo, C. Hulette, B.J. Crain, M.R. Farlow and A. Heyman, Ectopic white matter neurons, a developmental abnormality that may be caused by the PSEN1 S169L mutation in a case of familial AD with myoclonus and seizures, *J. Neuropathol. Exp. Neurol.* **60** (2001), 1137–1152.

[84] M. Takao, B. Ghetti, H. Yoshida, P. Piccardo, Y. Narain, J.R. Murrell, R. Vidal, B.S. Glazier, R. Jakes, M. Tsutsui, M.G. Spillantini, R.A. Crowther, M. Goedert and A. Koto, Early-onset dementia with Lewy bodies, *Brain Pathol.* **14** (2004), 137–147.

[85] A.L. Taratuto, P. Piccardo, E.G. Reich, S.G. Chen, G. Sevlever, M. Schultz, A.A. Luzzi, M. Rugiero, G. Abecasis, M. Endelman, A.M. Garcia, S. Capellari, Z. Xie, E. Lugaresi, P. Gambetti, S.R. Dlouhy and B. Ghetti, Insomnia associated with thalamic involvement in E200K Creutzfeldt-Jakob disease, *Neurology* **58** (2002), 362–367.

[86] R.D. Terry, The fine structure of neurofibrillary tangles in Alzheimer's disease, *J. Neuropath. Exp. Neurol.* **22** (1963), 629–642.

[87] R.D. Terry, N.K. Gonatas and M. Weiss, Ultrastructural studies in Alzheimer's presenile dementia, *Am. J. Pathol.* **44** (1964), 269–297.

[88] L.C. Triarhou and B. Ghetti, The dendritic dopamine projection of the substantia nigra: phenotypic denominator of weaver gene action in hetero- and homozygosity, *Brain Res.* **501** (1989), 373–381.

[89] L.C. Triarhou, J. Norton, O. Bugiani and B. Ghetti, Ventral root axonopathy and its relation to the neurofibrillary degeneration of lower motor neurones in aluminum-induced encephalomyelopathy, *Neuropathol. Appl. Neurobiol.* **11** (1985), 407–430.

[90] L.C. Triarhou, J. Norton and B. Ghetti, Anterograde transsynaptic degeneration in the deep cerebellar nuclei of "Purkinje cell degeneration" (pcd) mutant mice, *Exp. Brain Res.* **66** (1987), 577–588.

[91] L.C. Triarhou, J. Norton and B. Ghetti, Mesencephalic dopamine cell deficit involves areas A8, A9 and A10 in weaver mutant mice, *Exp. Brain Res.* **70** (1988), 256–265.

[92] L.C. Triarhou, W.C. Low and B. Ghetti, Transplantation of ventral mesencephalic anlagen to hosts with genetic nigrostriatal dopamine deficiency, *Proc. Natl. Acad. Sci., USA* **83** (1986), 8789–8793.

[93] F.W. Unverzagt, M.R. Farlow, J. Norton, S.R. Dlouhy, K. Young and B. Ghetti, Neuropsychological function in patients with Gerstmann-Sträussler-Scheinker disease from the Indiana Kindred (F198S), *J. Internatl. Neuropsychol. Soc.* **3** (1997), 169–178.

[94] T. Verina, J. Norton, J. Sorbel, L. Triarhou, J. Richter, D. Laferty and B. Ghetti, Atrophy and loss of dopaminergic mesencephalic neurons in heterozygous weaver mice, *Exp. Brain Res.* **113** (1997), 5–12.

[95] R. Vidal, M. Calero, P. Piccardo, M.R. Farlow, F.W. Unverzagt, E. Mendez, A. Jimenez-Huete, R. Beavis, E. Gomez-Tortosa, J. Ghiso, B.T. Hyman, B. Frangione and B. Ghetti, Senile dementia associated with Aβ angiopathy and tau perivascular pathology but not neuritic plaques in patients homozygous for the APOE-ε4 allele, *Acta Neuropathol.* **100** (2000), 1–12.

[96] R. Vidal, B. Ghetti, M. Takao, C. Brefel-Courbon, E. Uro-Coste. B.S. Glazier, V. Siani, M.D. Benson, P. Calvas, L. Miravalle, O. Rascol and M.B. Delisle, Intracellular ferritin accumulation in neural and extraneural tissue characterizes a neurodegenerative disease associated with a mutation in the Ferritin Light Polypeptide gene, *J. Neuropathol. Exp. Neurol.* **63** (2004), 363–380.

[97] J. Wei, S.R. Dlouhy, S. Bayer, R. Piva, T. Verina, Y. Wang, F. Feng, M.E. Hodes, B. Dupree and B. Ghetti, In situ hybridization analysis of Girk2 expression in the developing CNS in normal and weaver mice, *J. Neuropathol. Exp. Neurol.* **56** (1997), 762–771.

[98] J. Wei, S.R. Dlouhy, J. Zhu, B. Ghetti and M.E. Hodes, Analysis of region-specific library constructed by sequence-independent amplification of microdissected fragments surrounding weaver (wv) gene on mouse chromosome 16, *Somatic Cell Mol. Genet.* **20** (1994), 401–408.

[99] J. Wei, S.R. Dlouhy, J. Zhu, Y. Wang, L. Fitzpatrick, B. Ghetti and M.E. Hodes, Linkage mapping of microdissected clones from distal mouse chromosome 16, *Somatic Cell nd Mol. Genet.* **22** (1996), 227–232.

[100] J. Wei, M.E. Hodes, R. Piva, Y. Feng, Y. Wang, B. Ghetti and S.R. Dlouhy, Characterization of murine Girk2 transcript isoforms: structure and differential expression, *Genomics* **51** (1998), 379–390.

[101] J. Wei, M.E. Hodes, Y. Wang, Y. Feng, B. Ghetti and S.R. Dlouhy, Direct cDNA selection with DNA microdissected from mouse chromosome 16: Isolation of novel clones and construction of a partial transcription map of the C3-C4 region, *Genome Res.* **6** (1996), 678–687.

[102] J. Wei, R.J. Hofstetter, S. Dlouhy, B. Ghetti, J. Nurnberger, Jr. and M.E. Hodes, Screening and isolating specific expressed mRNA from mouse cerebellum: subtractive hybridization, *Chinese J. Genet.* **18** (1991), 59–68.

[103] R.H. Wilkins and I.A. Brody, Alzheimer's disease, *Arch Neurol* **21** (1969), 109–110.

[104] H.M. Wisniewski, B. Ghetti and R.D. Terry, Neuritic (senile) plaques and filamentous changes in aged rhesus monkey, *J. Neuropath. Exp. Neurol.* **32** (1973), 566–584.

[105] G.E.W. Wolstenholme and M. O'Connor, *Alzheimer's disease and related conditions*, J&A Churchill, London, 1970.

[106] Yazaki, J.J. Liepnieks, J.R. Murrell, M. Takao, B. Guenther, P. Piccardo, M.R. Farlow, B. Ghetti and M.D. Benson, Biochemical characterization of a neuroserpin variant associated with hereditary dementia, *Am. J. Pathol.* **158** (2001), 227–233.

[107] R.D. Yee, M.R. Farlow, D.A. Suzuki, K.F. Betelak and B. Ghetti, Abnormal eye movements in Gerstmann-Sträussler-Scheinker disease, *Arch. Ophthalmol.* **110** (1992), 68–74.

[108] K. Young, H.B. Clark, P. Piccardo, S.R. Dlouhy and B. Ghetti, Gerstmann-Sträussler-Scheinker disease with the PRNP P102L mutation and valine at codon 129, *Mol. Brain Res.* **44** (1997), 147–150.

[109] K. Young, C.K. Jones, P. Piccardo, A. Lazzarini, L.I. Golbe, T.R. Zimmerman, D.W. Dickson, H. Vinters, M.E. Hodes, S. Dlouhy and B. Ghetti, Gerstmann-Sträussler-Scheinker disease with mutation at codon 102 and methionine at codon 129 of the PRNP in previously unreported patients, *Neurology*, **45** (1995), 1127–1134.

Topographic study of Alzheimer's neurofibrillary changes: A personal perspective

Asao Hirano* and Maki Iida

Division of Neuropathology, Department of Pathology, Montefiore Medical Center, Bronx, NY, USA

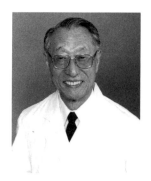

Abstract. Argentophilic neurofibrillary tangles were described in the cerebral cortex of Alzheimer's disease and later in the pigmented neurons in the brain stem of postencephalitic parkinsonism. In 1961, wide distribution of Alzheimer's neurofibrillary tangles in the central nervous system was observed in endemic fatal neurodegenerative diseases affecting the native Chamorro population on Guam: amyotrophic lateral sclerosis and parkinsonism-dementia complex on Guam. Abundant neurofibrillary tangles were found but no senile plaques. A topographic analysis of tangles in cases in Guam and at Montefiore were published in 1962 [23]. Thereafter, Alzheimer's neurofibrillary changes were documented in various areas of the nervous system of many other diseases. This communication is a brief review of the topographic investigation of Alzheimer's neurofibrillary changes. Occurrence of tangles in various conditions seems to indicate that various pathological agents can induce tangles. On the other hand, Alzheimer's neurofibrillary tangles, in general, show a rather striking predilection to affect particular neurons in the involved regions.

Keywords: Alzheimer's disease, Alzheimer's neurofibrillary changes, parkinsonism-dementia complex on Guam, topographic study

1. Introduction

As an author of one of the milestone studies in AD research [23], I was invited to participate in this issue to commemorate the Alzheimer Centennial. According to their planned format, we reviewed an earlier topographic study of Alzheimer's neurofibrillary changes and put it in the context of the following work.

2. Alzheimer's discovery of neurofibrillary changes in the cerebral cortex

In 1907 Alzheimer [2] first described neurofibrillary changes with the Bielschowsky silver method in the cerebral cortex of a 51-year-old woman who had had a 4 and half year history of progressive dementia. This was an epoch making discovery for the study of dementia. About a fourth to a third of all the neurons of the cerebral cortex revealed such changes. The distribution of this neuronal alteration was not specified further in this presentation. Later, in 1911 [3], Alzheimer clearly illustrated three stages of the fibrillary changes in pyramidal neurons. Dramatic alteration of affected ganglion cells with metallic impregnation was one of the most impressive findings in neuropathology and became the target of numerous investigations.

*Corresponding author: Asao Hirano, M.D., Division of Neuropathology, Department of Pathology, Montefiore Medical Center, 111 East 210th Street, Bronx, New York, 10467-2094 USA. Tel.: +1 718 920 4447; Fax: +1 718 653 3409; E-mail: ahirano@montefiore.org.

Analyzing 108 brains, including 48 with senile dementia, in 1911 Simchowicz [58] stressed the Ammon's horn as the area of predilection for neurofibrillary changes. He observed more of these alterations in the frontal and temporal cortexes and fewer in the occipital, motor and sensory cortex. He did not describe them in the brain stem but emphasized their absence in the cerebellum and spinal cord. As cases accumulated, topographic studies of Alzheimer's neurofibrillary changes, especially in the cerebral cortex were made by many investigators [23].

3. Neurofibrillary changes in the pigmented neurons of the brain stem in post-encephalitic parkinsonism

Neurofibrillary changes in the subcortical nuclei and brain stem were less conspicuous, and investigation of the neurofibrillary changes in published case reports was usually limited to the pyramidal neurons in the cerebral cortex. In 1953, Greenfield and Bosanquet reported special characteristics of these neurofibrillary changes in detail in the pigmented neurons of the brain stem in post-encephalitic parkinsonism [19] and reviewed previous reports on the observation of tangles by I. Fenyes in 1932 and J. Hallervorden in 1933. This paper attracted our attention for three reasons. First of all, clear and straightforward detailed histological pathology of Parkinson's disease was described. Basal ganglia were the target of neuropathological studies by many investigators. These studies, however, failed to reveal convincing results. In contrast, loss and alterations of the pigmented neurons in the substantia nigra were clearly described in this paper. Second, two characteristic neuronal inclusion bodies were observed in two different types of parkinsonism. Namely Lewy bodies were found in Parkinson's disease while neurofibrillary tangles were observed in postencephalitic parkinsonism. Accordingly, neuropathology contributed to diagnosis of two diseases. Third, there seemed to be a somewhat different configuration of neurofibrillary tangles in the brain stem from those found in Alzheimer's disease. Namely, neurofibrillary changes in the brain stem of the postencephalitic parkinsonism revealed, in general, globose-shaped tangles instead of flame-shaped tangles found in pyramidal neurons of the cerebral cortex in Alzheimer's disease. On the other hand, neither neurofibrillary changes nor Lewy bodies were found in their control cases.

4. Neurofibrillary changes in the nervous system among Chamorro natives of Guam

The island of Guam in the Pacific Ocean represents a geographic isolate with a phenomenally high incidence of fatal neurological diseases [24]. Best known of these ailments is amyotrophic lateral sclerosis (ALS) affecting the Chamorro population. ALS on Guam constituted approximately 5–10 percent of the adult deaths among the population. ALS on Guam was clinically and pathologically indistinguishable from ALS in any other part of the world. However, to our surprise, neurofibrillary tangles were consistently observed in certain areas of the central nervous system in all ALS cases on Guam [42]. They were found in the pyramidal neurons in the hippocampus, pigmented neurons in the brain stem as well as many other areas in the central nervous system.

During the course of ALS investigation on Guam, another fatal neurological disorder was discovered among the same population. The patients showed clinical features of parkinsonism and, in addition, to our surprise, many of them were associated with progressive dementia. Incidence of this disease was about equal to that of ALS. In addition some patients showed ALS syndrome. Family history was commonly found. A new term was coined to describe the clinical entity as parkinsonism-dementia complex (PDC) on Guam [24].

The brains of these PDC patients showed marked atrophy and severe depigmentation of the substantia nigra. Histological changes were characterized by neuronal loss and the presence of abundant neurofibrillary changes in the pigmented neurons of the brain stem and also in the pyramidal neurons in the hippocampus and certain specific areas in the central nervous system. The topography of Alzheimer's neurofibrillary changes was similar to the topography of those found in Guamanian ALS patients [25]. Initially postencephalitic parkinsonism was considered. A clinical history of encephalitis was, however, not obtained and oculogyric crises typical of postencephalitic parkinsonism were not observed in any of the patients.

Lewy bodies, the marker for Parkinson's disease, were, in general, not detected. Ten percent of 46 PDC cases examined revealed only a very small number of neurons with Lewy bodies in the brain stem but neurofibrillary tangle-bearing neurons were also found in the vicinity in all cases [26]. Furthermore neurons containing both Lewy bodies and tangles were observed in the midbrain of one case [26]. It is noteworthy that in spite of abundant neurofibrillary changes, senile plaques were usually absent in Guamanian cases unlike the cases in Alzheimer's disease.

5. Distribution of Alzheimer's neurofibrillary changes in cases in Guam [23,25]

In general, neurofibrillary changes were much more numerous in the PDC cases than in the ALS cases. However, in spite of the difference in the number of altered neurons, the distribution was essentially similar. Since neurofibrillary changes are so abundant and conspicuous without senile plaque formation in a wide area of the central nervous system we decided to investigate the topography of Alzheimer's neurofibrillary tangles in cases in Guam.

The distribution of the neurofibrillary changes in the parahippocampal gyrus and adjacent structures revealed that they were most abundant in the glomerular formation (entorhinal cortex). In the hippocampus, many neurons of the pyramidal cell layer as well as the end-plate showed these changes. They were most numerous in the Sommer's sector (CA 1) and subiculum. There was a rather abrupt decrease of these changes at the margin of Sommer's sector (CA2 and CA3). By contrast, not even a single neuron with neurofibrillary changes was seen in the lateral geniculate bodies. The frontal and temporal cortexes were always involved. On the other hand, these changes were quite rare in the visual cortex, especially in the calcarine region. Similarly, the pre- and post-Rolandic areas were usually spared these changes. They were practically absent from Betz cells.

The substantia innominata (nucleus basalis of Meynert), amygdaloid nucleus, adjacent temporal cortex and various hypothalamic nuclei were sites of severe involvement. Neurofibrillary changes were observed in the olfactory bulb in all seven cases examined. The subthalamic nuclei and globi pallidi contained occasional fibrillary changes, but they were rarely found in the putamen and caudate nuclei while the claustrum and adjacent insular cortex were commonly involved. They were relatively scant in the thalamus.

In the midbrain, the periaqueductal gray and midline structures were commonly involved. The neurones of the nucleus of the mesencephalic portion of the trigeminal nerve, however, were always free of fibrillary changes. These were present in the oculomotor nuclei. The substantia nigra was usually so severely damaged in the cases of PDC that neuronal loss was the most conspicuous feature, but neurofibrillary changes were always found in many of the remaining neurones. However, neurofibrillary changes were rarely found in the red nuclei.

In the pons and medulla, the locus caeruleus, the dorsal raphe nucleus, neurones in the midline structure and scattered neurons in reticular formation in the brain stem were always severely affected. On the other hand, hypoglossal nuclei and other motor nuclei only rarely contained these changes. Neurofibrillary changes were infrequently found in the neurones of the inferior olives and the dentate nuclei of the cerebellum.

Small numbers of neurones with tangles were observed in the spinal cord. On the other hand, these changes were not found in the Purkinje cells of the cerebellum in any of the cases.

Neurofibrillary tangles in the pyramidal cells are usually flame-shaped and tangles in the brain stem, hypothalamus, subcortical nuclei are, in general, globose-shaped in cases in Guam. The different configuration of tangles in these areas is based on the shape of neurons involved rather than the difference in the nature of the tangles.

In summary, neurofibrillary changes were found not only in cerebral cortex or pigmented neurons in the brain stem but they were distributed in certain specific neurons of the central nervous system. Certain neurons are prone to tangle formation. These are pyramidal cells in the Sommer's sector and glomerular formation, neurones in the nucleus basalis of Meynert, pigmented neurons in the brain stem and dorsal raphe nucleus, while others are infrequently affected, like Betz cells and the anterior horn cells in the spinal cord. No neurofibrillary changes are found in Purkinje cells. These findings are also, in general, applicable in various certain other diseases than ALS in Guam and PDC [23].

6. Further studies

6.1. Occurrence of Alzheimer's neurofibrillary changes

Since these studies, aged brains of Caucasians without known neurological disease have been shown to contain small numbers of Alzheimer's neurofibrillary tangles [23]. Furthermore, while usually fewer than in Guamanian ALS or PDC patients, the tangles were present and distributed in a similar manner in the Chamorros who died of other causes [4,26]. Numbers of affected neurons with neurofibrillary changes were more in Chamorros than Caucasians.

There have been other reports in which numerous Alzheimer's neurofibrillary changes have been found in wide distributions in the central nervous system.

These include subacute sclerosing panencephalitis [9, 41,43,44], Down's syndrome [8,45], brains of prizefighters [10,18,28,57], and progressive supranuclear palsy [61].

In addition, neurofibrillary changes have been recognized in the following diseases: certain lipidoses [33] especially Niemann-Pick disease type C [62], tuberous sclerosis [27], Salla disease [5], sclerosing angioma [40], meningoangiomatosis [21], Fukuyama congenital muscular dystrophy [64], Cockayne's syndrome [63], young adult form of dementia with neurofibrillary tangles and Lewy bodies [55], Hallervoden-Spatz disease [12,72], congenital hydrocephalus [14], normal pressure hydrocephalus [6,17], ganglioglioma [32,51,59], sudanophilic leukodystrophy [20], myotonic dystrophy [39,76], ipsilateral nuclei projecting to massive cerebral infarcts [16,35], retrograde development of Alzheimer's neurofibrillary tangles associated with necrotising encephalitis selectively involving the fornix and splenium [75], striatonigral degeneration [56], chronic alcoholics [11], verrucose dysplasia of the cerebral cortex [48], Ewing's sarcoma [53], corticobasal degeneration [15], frontotemporal dementia and parkinsonism linked to chromosome 17 (FTD-17) [60], diffuse neurofibrillary tangles with calcification [65], senile dementia of the neurofibrillary tangle type (tangle-only dementia) [73], among others [44, 72].

6.2. Topographical distribution of Alzheimer's neurofibrillary changes

Since a major histological hallmark and key diagnostic feature of Alzheimer's disease is the neurofibrillary changes [47], numerous intensive investigations of topographical distribution of the cerebral cortex have been reported. The topographic distribution of neurofibrillary changes in Alzheimer's disease was essentially similar to that found in cases in Guam. The most severe neurofibrillary changes were found in the entorhinal cortex, CA1 and the subiculum of the hippocampus, the amygdala and adjacent areas of temporal lobe, whereas the motor, somatic sensory, and primary visual areas were virtually unaffected [1,54]. In 1991, Braak and Braak reported that the progression of neurofibrillary changes followed a predictable pattern [7]. The first stage was marked by the transentorhinal region followed by the entorhinal region of the temporal cortex. The topographic distribution of Alzheimer's neurofibrillary changes in the cerebral cortex of Alzheimer's disease was concisely well documented by Mirra and Hyman in their chapter, Aging and dementia, in Greenfield's Neuropathology [47].

Interestingly, a striking difference was reported in the laminar distribution of neurofibrillary changes in parkinsonism-dementia complex on Guam and Alzheimer's disease by Hof et al. [31]. Guamanian cases demonstrated a preferential localization of neurofibrillary changes in superficial layers of the neocortex, whereas in Alzheimer's disease they predominated in the deep layers. Progressive supranuclear palsy case [30], postencephalitic parkinsonism [29], and dementia pugilistica cases [28] also demonstrated a preferential localization of neurofibrillary changes in layers II and III of the neocortex similar to Guamanian cases. Distribution of neurofibrillary changes in the hippocampal formation in these cases was similar to that observed in cases with Alzheimer's disease. However, distribution of neurofibrillary changes in a young boxer revealed neurofibrillary changes in all neocortical areas, but tangles were notably absent in the sites that are involved early in Alzheimer's disease: namely entorhinal cortex and hippocampal formation [18]. It was concluded that the mechanism of tangle formation induced by repetitive head trauma may be different from that in Alzheimer's disease.

Distributions of neurofibrillary changes in subcortical structures are similar to Guamanian cases but generally less pronounced. Among them, the nucleus basalis of Meynert deserve special attention for its selective and remarkable loss of cholinergic neurones [49,71]. Until now, no clear-cut evidence concerning cause(s) of Alzheimer's neurofibrillary tangles, except perhaps genetic factors, had been reported. We studied a case of massive cerebral infarct in the territory of the middle cerebral artery on one side of the brain. Many Alzheimer's neurofibrillary changes were observed in the nucleus basalis of Meynert, ipsilateral to the infarct [35]. Tangles were absent or rare in the opposite nucleus of the basalis of Meynert or in other areas of the brain. Considering the widespread projection of nucleus basalis of Meynert axons to the ipsilateral cerebral cortex, this suggests that formation of neurofibrillary tangles can occur as a retrograde reaction in nucleus basalis neurons secondary to massive, old cerebral infarction. Similar phenomena had been reported in other regions, such as the substantia nigra secondary to massive basal ganglia infarct [16] and subiculum secondary to necrotising encephalitis selectively involving the fornix and splenium [75].

During the study of the distribution of neurofibrillary changes, we found that limbic system seemed to be the site of predilection. Therefore we extended our study to the olfactory bulb and were surprised to find many Alzheimer's neurofibrillary tangles for the first time in all Guam cases examined [23]. There had been no confirmation reported on tangle formations in the olfactory bulb for 22 years after our observations. In 1984, Esiri and Wilcock described neurofibrillary tangles in the olfactory bulb in Alzheimer's disease [13]. Further extensive studies on olfactory involvement in neurodegenerative diseases have been reported thereafter [37,38,52,54]. The invariable observation of severe involvement of the olfactory regions in Alzheimer disease led Pearson et al. to suggest the possibility of the olfactory pathway as the site of initial involvement of the disease [54].

Neurofibrillary changes were also reported by Ishii [34] in Alzheimer's disease in the brain stem and hypothalamus although it was less intensively involved than Guamanian cases. Among these nuclei the dorsal raphe nucleus deserves special attention. Diffuse serotonergic fibers are presumed to project to the cerebral cortex from the nucleus raphe dorsalis of the midbrain in a manner similar to the cholinergic projections from the nucleus basalis of Meynert to the cerebral cortex. In Alzheimer's disease the dorsal raphe nucleus revealed 39 times more neurofibrillary tangles than those in the controls [74].

6.3. Immunohistochemical investigations of Alzheimer's neurofibrillary changes

During the past 25 years the advent of immunohistochemical techniques has made possible the evaluation of neurofibrillary tangles easier and much better than the modified Bielschowsky stain or other conventional silver impregnation techniques. For an example, we studied the topographic distribution and immunohistochemical characteristics of spinal cord neurofibrillary tangles in Guamanian cases, using antibodies to tau protein and ubiquitin [46]. The neurofibrillary tangles were immunoreactive with both antibodies, but staining for tau was more pronounced. As identified by this reactivity, all the Guamanian ALS and PDC cases examined showed spinal cord neurofibrillary tangles. The posterior horn had the most and the anterior horn, the least. In the posterior horn the neurofibrillary tangles were located mainly in the marginal areas. Large anterior horn cells disclosed few, if any, neurofibrillary tangles. In addition to perikaryal neurofibrillary tangles, tau-reactive neurites were found. Our results provided evidence that spinal cord neurofibrillary changes are not uncommon in Guamanian ALS and PDC and that they were more numerous than previously observed with conventional methods. Furthermore neuropil thread-like structures were demonstrated in spinal cord white matter in Guamanian ALS and PDC [66] and also in progressive supranuclear palsy [67] in addition to various areas of brain.

In addition to those areas described above, some other structures were reported to disclose Alzheimer's neurofibrillary tangles. The indusium griseum is a thin layer of gray substance on the dorsal aspect of the corpus callosum. It is also called supracallosal gyrus and is part of the structures of the limbic system. Neurofibrillary tangles were observed, for the first time, in the indusium griseum of patients with Alzheimer's disease [68]. Neurofibrillary tangles had not been thus far reported in neurons of the peripheral nervous system. In 1987 Kawasaki et al. [36] described the presence of many neurofibrillary tangles in the neurons of the upper cervical sympathetic ganglia in an elderly Japanese, non-demented patient. Occurrence of tangles was reported in the celiac ganglia of an aged individual [69], in the neurons of the spinal dorsal root ganglia of two of five patients with progressive supranuclear palsy [50] and in the sympathetic ganglia in two elderly individuals without Alzheimer pathology [70]. On the other hand, no neurofibrillary tangles were detected in the sympathetic or spinal ganglia in Alzheimer's disease and in progressive supranuclear palsy in the study of Wakabayashi et al. [70]. After reviewing 10 autopsy cases with neurofibrillary tangles in the sympathetic ganglia, Wakabayashi et al. concluded that neurofibrillary tangles in the peripheral ganglia are uncommon and develop independently of the neurofibrillary pathology that occurs in the central nervous system.

Along with the application of various advanced techniques further involvement of neuronal processes and synaptic terminals were recognized in various diseases manifested in neuropil threads and grains in addition to perikaryal tangles. Furthermore tau positive abnormal tangles were discovered not only in neurons but also in glial cells in certain diseases. These discoveries led to the concept of tauopathy. Original discovery of constricted form of neurofibrillary tangles in Alzheimer's disease with the electron microscope stimulated active fine structural investigations of tangles and along with immunohistochemical application of various antibodies for neurofibrillary tangles, vast amounts of information have been elucidated during the past century [22].

References

[1] S.E. Arnold, B.T. Hyman, J. Flory, A.R. Damasio and G.W. Van Hoesen, The topographical and neuroanatomical distribution of neurofibrillary tangles and neuritic plaques in the cerebral cortex of patients with Alzheimer's disease, *Cerebral cortex* **10** (1991), 103–116.

[2] A. Alzheimer, über eine eigenartige Erkrankung der Hirunrinde, *Zbl Nervenheik Psychiat* **30** (1907), 177–179.

[3] A. Alzheimer, Über eigenartige Krankheitsfalle des späteren Alters, *Z Ges Neurol Psychiat* **4** (1911), 356–385.

[4] F.H. Anderson, E.P. Richardson, Jr., H. Okazaki and J.A. Brody, Neurofibrillary degeneration on Guam. Frequency in Chamorros and non-Chamorros with no known neurological disease, *Brain* **192** (1979), 65–77.

[5] H. Autio-Harmainen, A. Oldfors, P. Saurander, M. Renlund, K. Dammert and S. Sinuila, Neuropathology of Salla disease, *Acta Neurolopathol* **75** (1988), 481–490.

[6] M.J. Ball, Neurofibrillary tangles in the dementia of "normal pressure" hydrocephalus, *Can J Neurol Sci* **3** (1976), 227–235.

[7] H. Braak and E. Braak, Neuropathological staging of Alzheimer-related changes, *Acta Neuropathol* **82** (1991), 239–259.

[8] P. Burger and F.S. Vogel, The development of the pathologic changes of Alzheimer's disease and senile dementia in patients with Down's syndrome, *Am J Pathol* **73** (1973), 457–468.

[9] J.A.N. Corsellis, Subacute sclerosing leukoencephalitis: clinical and pathological report of 2 cases, *J Mental Sci* **95** (1951), 570–583.

[10] J.A.N. Corsellis, C.J. Bruton and D. Freeman-Browne, The aftermath of boxing, *Psychol Med* **3** (1973), 270–303.

[11] K.M. Cullen and G.M. Halliday, Neurofibrillary tangles in chronic alcoholics, *Neuropathol Applied Neurobiol* **21** (1995), 312–318.

[12] D. Eidelberg, A. Sotrel, C. Joachim, D. Selkoe, A. Forman, W.W. Pendlebury and D.P. Perl, Adult onset Hallervorden-Spatz disease with neurofibrillary pathology: a discrete clinicopathological entity, *Brain* **110** (1987), 993–1013.

[13] M.M. Esiri and G.K. Wilcock, The olfactory bulbs in Alzheimer's disease, *J Neurol Neurosurg Psychiatry* **47** (1984), 56–60.

[14] K.J. Fan and G. Pezeshkpour, Neurofibrillary tangles in association with congenital hydrocephalus, *J Natl Med Assoc* **79** (1987), 1001–1004.

[15] M.B. Feany and D.W. Dickson, Widespread cytoskeletal pathology characterizes corticobasal degeneration, *Am J Pathol* **146** (1995), 1388–1396.

[16] L.S. Forno, Reaction of the substantia nigra to massive basal ganglia infarction, *Acta Neuropathol* **62** (1983), 96–102.

[17] S. Forno, P.J. Barbour and R I. Norville, Presenile dementia with Lewy bodies and neurofibrillary tangles, *Arch Neurol* **35** (1978), 818–822.

[18] J.F. Geddes, G.H. Vowles, S.F.D. Robinson and C. Sutcliffe, Neurofibrillary tangles, but not Alzheimer-type pathology, in a young boxer, *Neuropathology Appl Neurobiol* **22** (1996), 12–16.

[19] J.G. Greenfield and F.D. Bosanquet, The brain-stem lesions in parkinsonism, *Neurol Neurosurg Psychitry* **231** (1953), 213–226.

[20] K. Harada, W. Krucke, J.L. Mancardi and T.I. Mandybur, Alzheimer's tangles in sudanophilic leukodystrophy, *Neurology* **38** (1988), 55–59.

[21] J. Harper, B.W. Scheithauer, H. Okazaki and E.R. Laws, Jr., Meningo-angiomatosis: a report of six cases with special reference to the occurrence of neurofibrillary tangles, *J Neuropathol Exp Neurol* **45** (1986), 426–446.

[22] A. Hirano and H. Tomiyasu, *A guide to neuropathology*, Igaku-Shoin, Tokyo, 2003.

[23] A. Hirano and H.M. Zimmerman, Alzheimer's neurofibrillary changes. A topographic study, *Arch Neurol* **7** (1962), 227–224.

[24] A. Hirano, L.T. Kurland, R.S. Krooth and S. Lessell, Parkinsonism-dementia complex, an endemic disease on the island of Guam: 1. Clinical features, *Brain* **84** (1961), 642–661.

[25] A. Hirano, N. Malamud and L.T. Kurland, Parkinsonism-dementia complex, an endemic disease on the island of Guam: 2. Pathological features, *Brain* **84** (1961), 662–679.

[26] A. Hirano, N. Malamud, T.S. Elizan and L.T. Kurland, Amyotrophic lateral sclerosis and parkinsonism-dementia complex on Guam. Further pathological studies, *Arch Neurol* **15** (1966), 35–51.

[27] A. Hirano, R. Tuazon and H.M. Zimmerman, Neurofibrillary tangles, granulovacuolar bodies and argentophilic globules observed in tuberous sclerosis, *Acta Neuropathol* **11** (1968), 257–261.

[28] P.R. Hof, C. Bouras, L. Buée, A. Delacourte, D.P. Perl and J.H. Morrison, Differential distribution of neurofibrillary tangles in the cerebral cortex of dementia pugilistica and Alzheimer's disease cases, *Acta Neuropathol* **85** (1992), 23–30.

[29] P.R. Hof, A. Charpiot, A. Delacourte, L. Buée, D. Purohit, D.P. Perl and C. Bouras, Distribution of neurofibrillary tangles and senile plaques in the cerebral cortex in postencephalitic parkinsonism, *Neurosci Lett* **139** (1992), 10–14.

[30] P.R. Hof, A. Delacourte and C. Bouras, Distribution of cortical neurofibrillary tangles in progressive supranuclear palsy: a quantitative analysis of six cases, *Acta Neuropathol* **84** (1992), 45–51.

[31] P.R. Hof, D.P. Perl, A.L. Loerzel and J.H. Morrison, Neurofibrillary tangle distribution in the cerebral cortex of parkinsonism-dementia cases from Guam: differences with Alzheimer's disease, *Brain Res* **564** (1991), 306–313.

[32] A. Hori, R. Weiss and T. Schaake, Ganglioglioma containing osseous tissue and neurofibrillary tangles, *Arch Pathol Lab Med* **122** (1988), 653–655.

[33] D.S. Horoupian and S. S. Yang, Paired helical filaments in neurovisceral lipidoses (Juvenile dystrophic lipidoses), *Ann Neurol* **4** (1978), 404-411.

[34] T. Ishii, Distribution of Alzheimer's neurofibrillary changes in the brain stem and hypothalamus of senile dementia, *Acta Neuropathol* **6** (1966), 181–187.

[35] T. Kato, A. Hirano, T. Katagiri, H. Sasaki and S. Yamada, Neurofibrillary tangle formation in the nucleus basalis of Meynert ipsilateral to a massive cerebral infarct, *Ann Neurol* **23** (1988), 620–623.

[36] H. Kawasaki, S. Murayama, M. Tomonaga, N. Izumiyama and H. Shimada, Neurofibrillary tangles inhuman upper cervical ganglia: morphological study with immunohistochemistry and electron microscopy, *Acta Neuropathol* **75** (1987), 156–159.

[37] T. Kovács, N.J. Cairns and P.L.Lantos, β-amyloid deposition and neurofibrillary tangle formation in the olfactory bulb in aging and Alzheimer's disease, *Neuropathol Appl Neurobiol* **25** (1999), 481–491.

[38] T. Kovacs, N.J. Cairns and P.L. Lantos, Olfactory Centers in Alzheimer's disease: olfactory bulb is involved in early Braak's stages, *Neuroreport* **12** (2001), 285–288.

[39] S. Kuroda, Y. Ihara and R. Namba, Neurofibrillary changes in the brains of two siblings with myotonic muscular dystrophy, *Neuropathology* **9** (1988), 43–48.

[40] L. Liss, K. Ebner and D. Couri, Neurofibrillary tangles induced by sclerosing angioma, *Hum Pathol* **10** (1979), 104–108.

[41] N. Malamud, W. Haymaker and H. Pinkerton, Inclusion encephalitis with a clinicopathological report of three cases, *Amer J Pathol* **26** (1950), 133–153.

[42] N. Malamud, A. Hirano and L.T. Kurland, Pathoanatomic changes in amyotrophic lateral sclerosis with special references to the occurrence of neurofibrillary changes, *Arch Neurol* **5** (1961), 401–415.

[43] T.I. Mandybur, The distribution of Alzheimer's neurofibrillary tangles and gliosis in chronic subacute sclerosing panencephalitis, *Acta Neuropathol* **80** (1990), 307–310.

[44] T.I. Mandybur, A.S. Nagpaul, Z. Pappas and W.J. Niklowitz, Alzheimer neurofibrillary change in subacute sclerosing panencephalitis, *Ann Neurol* **1** (1977), 103–107.

[45] D.M.A. Mann, P.O. Yates and B. Marcyniuk, The topography of plaques and tangles in Down's syndrome patients of different ages, *Neuropathol Appl Neurobiol* **12** (1986), 447–457.

[46] S. Matsumoto, A. Hirano and S. Goto, Spinal cord neurofibrillary tangles of Guamanian amyotrophic lateral sclerosis and parkinsonism-dementia complex: An immunohistochemical study, *Neurology* **40** (1990), 975–979.

[47] S.S. Mirra and B. Hyman, Aging and dementia, in: *Greenfield's neuropathology*, (Vol. 2), D.I. Graham and P.L. Lantos, eds, Arnold, London 2002, pp. 195–271.

[48] M.A. Moran, A. Probst, C. Navarro and P. Gomez-Ramos, Alzheimer disease type neurofibrillary degeneration in verrucose dysplasias of the cerebral cortex, *Acta Neuropathol* **90** (1995), 356–365.

[49] I. Nakano and A. Hirano, Parkinson's disease: Neuron loss in the nucleus basalis without concomitant Alzheimer's disease, *Ann Neurol* **15** (1984), 415–418.

[50] M. Nishimura, Y. Namba, K. Ikeda, I. Akiguchi and M. Oda, Neurofibrillary tangles in the neurons of spinal dorsal root ganglia of patients with progressive supranuclear palsy, *Acta Neuropathol* **85** (1993), 453–457.

[51] M.A. Oberc-Greenwood, P.E. McKeever, P.L. Kornblith and B.H. Smith, A human ganglioglioma containing paired helical filaments, *Hum Pathol* **15** (1984), 834–838.

[52] T.G. Ohm and H. Braak, Olfactory bulb changes in Alzheimer's disease, *Acta Neuropathol* **73** (1987), 365–369.

[53] R. Okeda, A. Kanazawa, M. Yamada, Y. Ohkawa, K. Kawabata, M.A. Yoshida and T.A. Ikeuchi, 14-year-old patient with Ewing's sarcoma presenting at autopsy with multiple neurofibrillary tangles and Lewy bodies in addition to hemiatrophy of the central nervous system, *Clin Neuropathol* **16** (1997), 77–84.

[54] R.C.A. Pearson, M.M. Esiri, R.W. Hiorns, G.K. Wilcock and T.P.S. Powell, Anatomical correlates of the distribution of the pathological changes in the neocortex in Alzheimer disease, *Proc Natl Acad Sci USA* **82** (1985), 4531–4534.

[55] E.R. Popovich, H.M. Wisniewski, M.A. Kaufman, I. Grundke-Iqbal and G.Y. Wen, Young adult-form of dementia with neurofibrillary changes and Lewy bodies, *Acta Neuropathol* **74** (1987), 97–104.

[56] K. Renkawek and M.W.I.M. Horstink, Striatonigral degeneration with neurofibrillary tangles, *Acta Neuropathol* **86** (1993), 405–410.

[57] G.W. Roberts, D. Allsop and C. Bruton, The occult aftermath of boxing, *J Neurol Neurosurg Psychiatry* **53** (1990), 373–378.

[58] T. Simchowicz, Histologische Studien uber die senille Demenz, in: *Histologische und Histopathologische Arbeiten über die Grosshirnrinde mit besonderer Berucksichtiung der pathologischen Anatomie der Geisteskrankenheiten*, (Vol. 4), F. Nissl and A. Alzheimer, eds, Jena, Germany, Gustav Fischer Verlag, 1911, pp. 267–444.

[59] D. Soffer, F. Umansky and J.E. Goldman, Ganglioglioma with neurofibrillary tangles (NFTs): neoplastic NFTs of Alzheimer's disease, *Acta Neuropathol* **89** (1995), 451–453.

[60] M.G. Spillantini, T.D. Bird and B. Ghetti, Frontotemporal dementia and parkinsonism linked to chromosome 17: A new group of tauopathies, *Brain Pathology* **8** (1998), 387–402.

[61] J.C. Steel, J.C. Richardson and J. Olszewski, Progressive supranuclear palsy: a heterogeneous degeneration involving the brain stem, basal ganglia and cerebellum with vertical gaze and pseudobulbar palsy, nuchal dystonia and dementia, *Arch Neurol* **10** (1964), 333–359.

[62] K. Suzuki, C.C. Parker, P.G. Penchev, D. Katz, B. Ghetti, A.N. D'Agostino and E.D. Carstea, Neurofibrillary tangles in Niemann-Pick disease type C, *Acta Neuropathol* **89** (1995), 227–238.

[63] K. Takada and L.E. Becker, Cockayne's syndrome: report of two autopsy cases associated neurofibrillary tangles, *Clin Neuropathol* **5** (1986), 64–68.

[64] K. Takada, Y.-S. Rin, K. Sasagi, K. Sato, H. Nakamura and J. Tanaka, Long survival in Fukuyama congenital muscular dystrophy: occurrence of neurofibrillary tangles in the Nucleus basalis of Maynert and locus ceruleus, *Acta Neuropathol* **71** (1986), 228–232.

[65] K. Tsuchiya, H. Nakayama, S. Iritani, T. Arai, K. Niizato, C. Haggai, M. Matsushima and K. Ikeda, Distribution of basal ganglia lesions in diffuse Neurofibrillary tangles with calcification: a clinicopathological study of five autopsy cases, *Acta Neuropathol* **103** (2002), 555–564.

[66] T. Umahara, A. Hirano, S. Kato, N. Shibata and S.-H. Yen, Demonstration of neurofibrillary tangles and neuropil thread-like structures in spinal cord white matter in parkinsonism-dementia complex on Guam and in Guamanian amyotrophic lateral sclerosis, *Acta Neuropathol* **88** (1994), 180–184.

[67] T. Umahara, A. Hirano, S. Kato, N. Shibata and S.-H. Yen, Demonstration of neuropil thread-like structures in the spinal cord white matter in progressive supranuclear palsy: An immunohistochemical investigation, *Neuropathology* **15** (1995), 103–107.

[68] T. Umahara, A. Hirano, N. Shibata, S. Kato and T. Kawanami, Demonstration of neurofibrillary tangles in the indusium griseum and axonal disturbances in sagittal sulcal lesions of the corpus callosum: An immunohistochemical investigation, *Neuropathology* **16** (1996), 10–14.

[69] K. Wakabayashi, A. Furuta, H. Takahashi and F. Ikuta, Occurrence of neurofibrillary tangles in celiac ganglia, *Acta Neuropathol* **78** (1989), 448.

[70] K. Wakabayashi, S. Hayashi, T. Morita, Y. Shibasaki, Y. Watanabe and H. Takahashi, Neurofibrillary tangles in the peripheral sympathetic ganglia of non-Alzheimer elderly individuals, *Clin Neuropathol* **18** (1999), 171–175.

[71] P.J. Whitehouse, D.L. Price, A.W. Clark, J.T. Coyle and M.R. De Long, Alzheimer disease: evidence for selective loss of cholinergic neurons in the nucleus basalis, *Ann. Neurol* **10** (1981), 122–126.

[72] K. Wisniewski, G.A. Jervis, R.C. Moretz and H.M. Wisniewski, Alzheimer neurofibrillary tangles in diseases other than senile and presenile dementia, *Ann Neurol* **5** (1979), 288–294.

[73] M. Yamada, Senile dementia of the neurofibrillary tangle type (tangle-only dementia): Neuropathological criteria and clinical guidelines for diagnosis, *Neuropathology* **23** (2003), 311–317.

[74] T. Yamamoto and A. Hirano, Nucleus raphe dorsalis in Alzheimer's disease: Neurofibrillary tangles and loss of large neurons, *Ann Neurol* **17** (1985), 573–577.

[75] T. Yamamoto, H. Kurobe, J. Kawamura, S. Hashimoto and M. Nakamura, Subacute dementia with necrotising encephalitis selectively involving the fornix and splenium: retrograde development of Alzheimer's neurofibrillary tangles in subiculum, *J Neurol Sci* **96** (1990), 159–172.

[76] N. Yoshimura, M. Otake, K. Igarashi, M. Matsunaga, K. Takebe and H. Kudo, Topography of Alzheimer's neurofibrillary change distribution in myotonic dystrophy, *Clin Neuropathol* **9** (1990), 234–239.

Clinicopathological analysis of dementia disorders in the elderly – An update

Kurt A. Jellinger
Institute of Clinical Neurobiology, Kenyongasse 18, A-1070 Vienna, Austria
Tel.: +43 1 5266534; Fax: +43 1 5238634; E-mail: kurt.jellinger@univie.ac.at

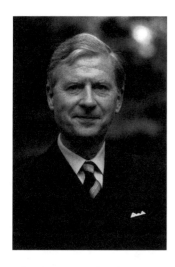

Abstract. A retrospective clinico-pathological study of a consecutive autopsy series of 1050 elderly demented individuals (mean age 83.4 ± 6.0 years; MMSE < 20) was performed. Clinical diagnoses were probable or possible Alzheimer disease (62.9%), nonspecific degenerative dementia (10.4%), vascular dementia (10%), Parkinson disease with dementia (9.5%), 1.5% mixed dementia, and 5.7% other disorders. At autopsy, 86% revealed Alzheimer-related pathology, but only 42.8% showed "pure" Alzheimer disease, with additional cerebrovascular lesions in 22.6% and Lewy body pathology in 10.8%, while among 660 cases of clinically suspected Alzheimer disease, Alzheimer pathology was seen in 93%, only 44.7% in "pure" form, and additional vascular lesions and Lewy bodies in 27.7 and 10%, respectively. The non-Alzheimer cases included Huntington and Creutzfeldt-Jakob disease, frontotemporal dementias, and others. These and other recent data indicate that in patients with the clinical diagnosis of Alzheimer disease its combination with cerebrovascular lesions and Lewy body pathologies is rather frequent. Comparison of clinical and postmortem diagnoses revealed postmortem confirmation of Alzheimer disease in 93%, of mixed and vascular dementia in 60 and 52.3%, respectively. 78% of clinically suspected degenerative dementias were pathologically definite Alzheimer disease, while in the clinical Parkinson + dementia group dementia with Lewy bodies accounted for 35%, Parkinson+Alzheimer disease, and "pure" Alzheimer disease for 29%, each. A sample of 207 prospectively studied elderly showed significant negative correlation between the preterminal psychostatus assessed by MMSE and the neuritic Braak stages, with a broad "gray" zone of Alzheimer lesions in mildly to moderately demented subjects. Similar relations between CDR and Braak stages were seen in very old subjects. The present study and the results of other recent series indicate increasing agreement between clinical and autopsy diagnoses in demented aged individuals with variable accuracy rates for different forms of dementia disorders.

Keywords: Dementia disorders, Alzheimer disease, clinico-pathological correlations, diagnostic accuracy rates

1. Introduction

In 1990, the relative incidence of major types of dementia disorders and the agreement rates between clinical and neuropathological diagnosis were analysed in a consecutive autopsy series of 675 elderly subjects in Vienna, Austria (mean age 79.5, SD 9.6 years). Clinical diagnosis of probable or possible Alzheimer disease (AD) was made in 59.2%, of vascular dementia (VaD) in 21.7%, of mixed AD+VaD dementia in 3.1%, of Parkinson's disease (PD) and other dementing disorders in 16%. At autopsy, 76.7% fulfilled the histological criteria for Alzheimer disease, but only 60% were "pure" forms, while 8.2% showed additional features of Parkinsonism and 7.9% coexisting cerebrovascular lesions indicating mixed AD+VaD. 15.7% were VaD with no or only very little AD pathology, 7.4% other central nervous system (CNS) disorders, and 0.3% of the brains showed nothing abnormal beyond age-related changes. The overall coincidence rates for the clinical and pathological diagnosis of AD were 85.2%, for VaD and mixed dementia 60.5–62%, respectively, but only 51% for PD/PD+AD [29]. These data and the results of other recent studies showing clinicopathological accuracy rates for AD ranging from 49 to 100% with a realistic mean of 81% and a mean specifity of the diagnosis of probable AD of 70% with a range of 47 to 100% (see [39]), emphasized the need for more appropriate clinical and neuropathological criteria in the diagnosis of dementias.

In the meantime, a number of guidelines for the clinical and neuropathological diagnosis of AD – e.g. the Consortium to Establish a Registry for Alzheimer Disease/CERAD [48], the Braak staging of neuritic AD changes [9], the Washington University quantitative criteria [5,6,44], and the guidelines of the National Institute for Aging (NIA) and the Ronald and Nancy Reagan Institute of the Alzheimer's Association (RI) for making the postmortem diagnosis of AD [27] have been established and the evaluation of the latter criteria, combining both CERAD and Braak scores, demonstrated fairly good correlations with the clinical dementia and good agreements with pathological methods, their easy and rapid use in AD and nondemented subjects, but much less reliability for other dementing disorders. Comparison of these criteria with clinical scores identified almost all cases with severe dementia, but often failed in mild to moderate dementias. Most nondemented cases were assigned to the low or intermediate categories, but several studies in those with no or only mild cognitive impairment showed a wide range of AD-related pathology, and even the combined use of all available criteria often could not distinguish between questionable and definite dementia (see Table 1). Although the sensitivity and specificity of the above algorithm are suggested to be around 90%, only 40 to 50% of the brains of patients with the clinical diagnosis of probable or possible AD show "pure" AD pathology, thus reducing their predictive value to 38–44% [8].

For dementia with Lewy bodies (DLB), a relatively new term for a progressive dementia syndrome, associated clinically with the core neuropsychiatric features of fluctuating cognition, visual hallucinations, and parkinsonian features, clinical consensus criteria are well established [45,46], but the pathological guidelines, based on scoring the numbers and distribution of Lewy bodies in the cerebral cortex and subcortical areas, did not provide definitive diagnostic criteria. Since they were formulated prior to the introduction of the specific alpha-synuclein immunohistochemistry for the detection of LBs [22], classification of most earlier cases appears questionable. The validity and reliability of consensus criteria for DLB is still variable, with a sensitivity and specificity ranging from 0 (!) to 100%, and positive and negative prediction values also between 0 and 100 (see [46]).

Among other dementing disorders, several recent consensus criteria for clinical and postmortem diagnosis of frontotemporal dementias (FTD), and other tauopathies, both sporadic and familial, have been proposed [51,59], but, due to continuous detection of new mutations, undergo frequent changes.

A particular problem are dementias associated with cerebrovascular disease, referred to as vascular dementia (VaD), vascular-ischemic dementia (VID) or vascular cognitive disorder/impairment (VCD/VCI). The currently used clinical diagnostic criteria – IDC 10; DSM-IV, SCANDDTC [11], and NINDS-AIREN criteria [57] – show variable sensitivity (average 50%) and specificity (range 65–98% [20,38,49,56], while the recent Mayo clinical criteria (temporal relationship between stroke and dementia or worsening of cognition or bilateral infarction in specific regions) were reported to have 76% sensitivity and 81% specificity for autopsy-proven VaD [38]. However, generally accepted and validated neuropathological criteria for VaD have not been established so far. Hence, the postmortem diagnosis of VaD/CVI currently is a subjective one and a matter of discussion (see [36]).

The same is true for so-called mixed type dementia (MD) characterized by combined pathologies of both AD and VaD or other dementing disorders, and the relationship between these conditions is controversial. Here again, generally accepted and validated histological criteria for the diagnosis of MD are not available, and its frequency is unknown, prevalence rates in autopsy series ranging from 2 to 56% in prospective studies and from 9 to 54% in retrospective studies with means around 15% [23,31,39,41]. Criteria for AD and VaD are of limited value for the diagnosis of MD, and more distinct criteria based on prospective clinico-pathological studies for this category are necessary. It should further be born in mind that all additional pathologies that frequently occur in the aged brain, may interact with the above changes in inducing cognitive impairment. Hence, the combination of two or more

Table 1
Likelihood of dementia (in percent) due to AD according to NIA-R-Institute criteria in various autopsy series

Disorder CERAD/Braak:	Low A/0–II	Interm. B/III–IV	High C/V/VI	Mean age (years)
Cochran et al. (1998)				
Demented ($n = 17$)	47	41	12	?
Non demented ($n = 40$)	72.5	22.5	5	?
Newell et al. (1999)				
AD ($n = 33$)	0	3	97	83
DLB ($n = 15$)	48	26	26	81
PSP ($n = 12$)	75	17	8	68
Controls ($n = 17$)	76	24	0	77
Harding et al. (1998)				
AD ($n = 31/22$-no LB) (CDR 1–3)	26/13	20/27	54/60	77
DLB, neocort. ($n = 11$)	73	18	9	76
PD ($n = 7$) (CDR 0–0.5)	83	17	0	79
Controls ($n = 18$) (CDR 0–0.5)	83	17	0	79
Davis et al. (1999)				
Controls ($n = 57$, MMSE 27–29)	88	–	12	84
McKee et al. (2002)				
AD ($n = 12$) (CDR 1–3)	0	17	83	81
Cogn. normal ($n = 23$) (CDR 0)	62	38	0	83
Jellinger (2003 [in Iqbal-Winblad])				
AD ($n = 100$) (MMSE 0–17)	0	24	76	85
DLB ($n = 36$) (MMSE 0–20)	25	33	42	77
PSP ($n = 10$)	70	20	10	72
PD dem. ($n = 20$, MMSE 0–20)	25	50	25	83
PD non dem. ($n = 17$, MMSE >20)	70	30	0	72
Controls ($n = 20$, MMSE 28–30)	100	0	0	81

pathological processes may influence the manifestation and severity of cognitive deficits and represents another major diagnostic challenge.

Given these preclusions and limits, we tried to evaluate the relative incidence of different typs of dementia disorders in a consecutive autopsy series of aged demented individuals.

2. Material and methods

The sample included 1050 consecutive autopsy cases of elderly subject in Vienna, Austria, derived from two large general hospitals with chronic care facilities in a 15-years' period (1989 to end of 2004). There were 665 female and 385 males aged at death 55 to 103 years (mean 82.4 ± 6.0 SD years). Retrospective evaluation of the hospital chards and autopsy assignments was blinded without knowledge of the neuropathological diagnoses. They all fulfilled the clinical criteria of at least moderate dementia according to ICD 10 and DSM IV with a Mini-Mental-Score (MMSE) below 20. Around 250 of these patients had been in the Vienna Prospective Dementia study [4], with regular clinical, neuropsychological and neuroimaging examinations, including MMSE evaluation, no longer than 6 months prior to death. From this series, 660 cases with the clinical diagnosis of probable or possible AD according to DSM-IV, CERAD, and NINCDS-ADRDA Work Group criteria [47] were evaluated separately. The remaining group of 390 autopsy cases had clinical diagnoses other than AD, senile dementia (10.7%), not specified ($n = 110$), VaD ($n = 106$), PDD ($n = 100$), Creutzfeldt-Jakob ($n = 21$) and Huntington's disease ($n = 17$), FTD ($n = 8$), and others ($n = 15$).

In all cases, a full post-mortem evaluation was performed (see [3,35]). All brains were examined according to an established protocol, and histological examination was performd on multiple paraffin blocks of frontal, cingulate, temporal, parietal, frontobasal, and occipital cortices, hippocampus with adjacent entorhinal cortex and amygdala, basal ganglia, brainstem and cerebellum, using routine stains, modified Bielschowsky, and occasionally Gallyas silver impregnations, and immunohistochemistry for tau-protein (antibody AT-8, Innogenetics, Ghent, Belgium), α-synuclein (Chemicon, Hofheim, Germany), GFAP (Daco, Gilstrup, Denmark), and Aβ amyloid peptide (clone 4G8, Signet Laboratories, Dedham, Ma, USA). Diagnosis of AD followed the CERAD criteria [48], Braak staging [9], and the NIA-Reagan Institute criteria [27]. Diagnosis of the other neurodegenerative disorders was made according to current guidelines (see above), that of VaD/VCI and mixed dementia followed recently published criteria (see [36]).

3. Results

In the current autopsy cohort of over 1000 elderly demented individuals with a mean age of 83.4 ± 6.0 years, collected in a 15-year period from two large general hospitals with chronic (geriatric) care facilities, retrospective evaluation of major clinical diagnosis revealed 62.9% possible or probable AD, 10.0% VAD, 9.5% PD with dementia (PDD), and 1.5% mixed dementia, while 10.4% were classified "degenerative dementias", and 5.7% were considered other dementing disorders, including Creutzfeldt-Jakob and Huntington's disease, frontotemporal dementias, and others.

At autopsy, among the total series, 86% revealed AD-related pathology, but only 42.8% showed "pure" AD of the classical plaque and tangle type and 7.4% had other or atypical AD forms, e.g. plaques"-only type, limbic AD (Braak stages up to 4), or neurofibrillary predominant type of senile dementia (NFT/SD), with neurofibrillary pathology mainly in the limbic system with no or very little amyloid deposits (see [32]). In the rest of cases, AD pathology was associated with various forms of cerebrovascular pathology (lacunar state, recent or old infarcts, hippocampal sclerosis) – 22.6%, Lewy body pathology (either DLB or AD plus PD, nigral lesions or so-called incidental Lewy body disease) – 10.8%, while 3.1% fulfilled current criteria of mixed dementia (AD plus severe lacunar state or multiple small or larger infarcts totalling up to 50 ml). 14% of the demented cohort revealed other pathologies: 7.3% showed different types of cerebrovascular pathology without AD lesions surmounting age-related limits – multiple infarct encephalopathy (MIE), subcortical atherosclerotic encephalopathy (SAE) or strategic infarct encephalopathy (SID), while 5.7% were other disorders associated with dementia (Creutzfeldt-Jakob and Huntington disease, FTD, chronic alcoholism, etc.). In one percent, the morphological basis of dementia was not detected even with extensive neuropathological and immunohistochemical investigations; they all had senile plaques but no isocortical neuritic AD lesions, with Braak stages below 3 and no further abnormalities (Table 2A).

Similar results were seen in the group of 660 clinically suspected AD patients. They showed AD pathology in 93%, which, however, was "pure" in only 44.7%,
while additional minor to moderate cerebrovascular lesions not fitting the criteria of "mixed" dementia were present in 27.7% and additional LB pathology in 10.1% (4.5% with criteria of DLB and 6.1% of PDD, i.e. combination of AD+PD), AD with nigral lesions and/or incidental Lewy body pathology, 1.8% each, corresponded to mixed dementia or showed AD plus other pathologies (multiple sclerosis, multisystem atrophy, tumors, etc.). Among the 6.8% non-AD cases, 2.4% showing "pure" vascular pathology without essential AD lesions were diagnosed VaD, while 3.8% represented other degenerative disorders associated with dementia. This group of clinically suspected AD included the following pathologies: FTD/Pick's disease ($n = 12$), CJD and brain tumor ($n = 3$ each), corticobasal degeneration ($n = 2$), and single cases of PSP, HIV-encephalitis, Huntington's disease, familial insomnia, and intravascular non-Hodgkins lymphoma ($n = 1$ each). 0.6% of this sample showed nothing abnormal beyond normal aging (Table 2B).

These data indicate that, although "pure" VaD and "mixed" dementia in large autopsy series of aged demented individuals are less frequent than previously suggested, combination of cerebrovascular lesions with AD pathology is rather frequent [3,28,35,62].

Comparison of clinical and postmortem diagnoses gave the following results (see Table 2B, Fig. 1): Among 660 patients with the clinical diagnosis of possible or probable AD, postmortem confirmation was achieved in 93%, with PD+AD and DLB in 10.6%, VaD and mixed dementia in 2.4 and 1.8%, respectively, while 3.8% revealed other disorders, and 0.6% revealed nothing abnormal beyond age-related changes. In the group of patients with the clinical diagnosis of "non-specific/degenerative dementias" ($n = 109$), around 78% were pathologically definite AD, less than 8% VAD, 6.7% mixed dementia, and the rest other dementing disorders (e.g. single cases of posttraumatic encephalopathy, atypical encephalitis, or Wernicke encephalopathy), with three negative cases. The clinical diagnosis of VAD ($N = 105$) was confirmed in 52.3%, while 32.4% morphologically revealed AD with or without lacunar states and/or mild cerebrovascular lesions, and 15.3% represented mixed dementia, i.e. definite AD (Braak stages 5 or 6) combined with severe lacunar state, multiple cortical and/or subcortical microinfarcts or larger cortical infarcts. In the clinical PDD group ($n = 100$) DLB and PD+AD accounted for 35 and 29%, respectively, "pure" AD without subcortical LB pathology was seen in 29% and "pure" PD (usually Braak PD stages 4 and 5) [10] without further

Table 2
Morphological diagnosis in consecutive Vienna autopsy series (1989–2004) (A) of demented individuals, 385 males, 665 females, age 50–103 (mean 83.3 ± 6.0) years; and (B) of patients with clinical diagnosis of probable or possible AD (mean age 81.3 ± 6.0 years)

Morphological diagnosis	(A)		(B)	
	n	%	n	%
"Pure" AD (CERAD pos., Braak V–VI)	400	38.1	280	42.4
Alzheimer type pathol. (plaque type 27/11, limbic AD 27/9, NFT/SD 25/23)	78	7.4	43	6.5
AD+CVD (lacun. state 140/123, infarcts old 53/38, infarcts recent 32/15, AH-sclerosis 12/17)	277	22.6	183	27.7
AD+cerebral hemorrhage (CAA)	28	2.7	15	2.3
Lewy body variant AD (27/22), Diff. Lewy body disease (28/8)	55	5.2	30	4.5
AD + Parkinson pathol. 27/18, +nigral lesions 24/12, +subcort. LBs 17/10 (incidental LBD)	58	5.6	40	6.1
MIX type dementia (AD+MIE 23/19, +SAE 8/2, +SID 2/1)	33	3.1	12	1.8
AD+other pathologies (tumors, MS, MSA, etc.)	14	1.3	12	1.8
Alzheimer pathology total	903	86.0	615	93.1
Vascular dementia (MIE 22/3, SAE 37/7, SID 16/4, AhScl 2/2)	77	7.3	16	2.4
Other disorders (Huntington disease, FTD, CJD, others)	60	5.7	25	3.8
Nothing abnormal beyond age	10	1.0	4	0.6
Non-Alzheimer pathologies	147	14.0	45	6.8
Total	1050	100.0	660	100.0

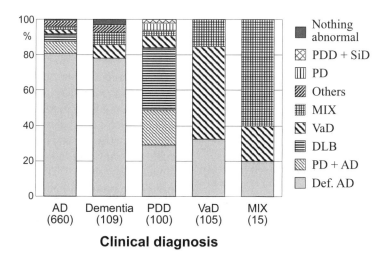

Fig. 1. Correlation between clinical and neuropathological diagnosis in 1050 consecutive autopsy cases of elderly individuals.

pathologies in only 4 percent; 7% showed predominantly cerebrovascular lesions without LB pathologies and were morphologically classified subcortical arteriosclerotic or strategic infarct encephalopathies (SIE), while 2 cases showed PD plus SIE, 3% were mixed dementias. Within the group of other dementing disorders ($n = 60$), Huntington's disease ($n = 17$) and FTDs ($n = 8$) had been diagnosed clinically in 90–100%, CJD ($n = 20$) only in 70%, the remainder showing the morphological pictures of AD or DLB, while other dementias were associated with Wernicke's or posttraumatic encephalopathies.

In the sample of 207 elderly individuals from the Vienna Prospective dementia Study with a mean age of 81.7 ± 8.6 years who had been examined clinically and neuropsychologically [4] no longer than 6 months prior to death, the final psychostatus assessed by the MMSE score was compared with the neuritic Braak stages of AD pathology (Fig. 2). In elderly patients without associated pathologies, there was a highly significant negative correlation between the MMSE score and Braak stages. Neocortical Braak stages 5 and 6 were mainly, but not exclusively, seen in severely demented, often no longer testable patients, while non-demented individuals or those with mild cognitive impairment (MCI), i.e. MMSE scores between 28 and 30, showed no or only very mild AD pathologies (negative or entorhinal Braak stages 0–2). Patients with mild to moderate dementia (MMSE 12–26) showed a wide range of neuritic AD pathology between Braak stages 0 to 5. Similar correlations have been observed in both younger individuals [13,14,19,26] and very old sub-

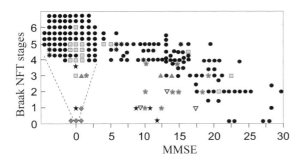

Fig. 2. Relationship between Mini Mental State Examination (MMSE) and Braak neuritic AD stages in 207 consecutive autopsies of aged individuals (mean age at death 81.4 ± 8.6 years).

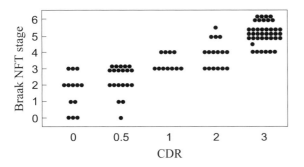

Fig. 3. Column scatter plot of Braak stages vs. Clinical Dementia Rating (CDR) scores in 100 oldest-old people (mean age at death 92.5 ± 2.5 years).

jects [17,21,30], indicating a broad "gray zone" of mild to moderate dementia showing a wide range of neuritic AD lesions (Fig. 3). The majority of demented DLB cases and of those with mixed dementia (AD + vascular encephalopathy) in the Vienna cohort also showed high neuritic Braak stages, with only a few brains showing Braak score 3, while the different types of VaD with low MMSE scores revealed only mild or even negative neuritic Braak stages (Fig. 2).

4. Discussion

Several recent prospective and retrospective clinico-patholgical studies of elderly demented subjects found average diagnostic accuracy rates between 43 and 100% (see [29,39]). However, the incidence of major types of cerebral disorders causing cognitive decline showed considerable variation, with considerable deviations between clinical and autopsy findings [1,7,18, 29,33,37,44,54]. The combination of the "possible" and "probable" categories of AD had higher sensitivity but lower specificity compared to the "probable" AD category alone which suggests that neuropathologically definite AD has a more pleomorphic clinical picture than previously suggested. Because AD with coexistent pathology is common, specificity improves when the pathological diagnosis of AD is broadened, to allow the diagnosis of AD to be made in the presence of other pathologies. This is clearly illustrated in the recent study, showing that the incidence of AD pathology in patients with the clinical diagnosis of possible and probable AD was 93%, but only less than 45% showed "pure" AD pathology, wheras the rest was associated with other pathologies, in particular cerebrovascular lesions and Lewy body changes. In the CERAD study, 85% of the clinically diagnosed AD cases met the histological criteria for AD, but only 43% were histologically "pure" forms, while additional PD markers or cerebrovascular lesions were present in 18 and 27%, respectively [48].

In most instances in routine clinical practice, the diagnostic criteria of the NINCDS-ADRDA workgroup, the DSM-IV, and others, yielded an accurate view of the diagnosis of AD accounting around 63% as compared to the pathological diagnosis of AD of about 86%.

In comparison to autopsy, considered the diagnostic "gold standard", the most important deficiencies in the clinical dignosis are (1) the failure to recognize that AD is the principal diagnosis in the setting of alternative medical or neurological diagnoses, and (2) failing to recognize relevant coexisting pathologies when most of the clinical picture looks into typical AD [39]. The agreement rate of 93% between the clinical diagnosis of possible/probable AD and its histopathological confirmation in the present cohort was similar or even higher than in other retrospective studies using similar clinical and morphological criteria [1,7,37,54], and was comparable to that in several recent prospective case control studies [44,58]. Only in small cohorts, using very highly selected populations, two research groups achieved a diagnostic accuracy for AD of 100% [42,50] which, however, appears not to be representative for the general AD and dementia population as a whole, since in one of these prospective studies of 31 autopsy cases using explicit clinical inclusion and exclusion criteria to idenify AD, additional histological features of PD and cerebral infarcts were present in 38 and 35% of the cases, respectively. Hence, the histological features of "pure" AD were present in only 33% of this cohort, while additional brain pathologies were observed in two-thirds of the cases that might have contributed to dementia [50]. A similar incidence of coexisting pathologies was seen in a recent cohort of 149 demented elderly subjects of the University of Washington group: Morphologically, "pure" AD was seen in only 57%, AD with other pathologies in 18%, PD, DLB with or without other coexistent pathologies in almost 10%, and "pure" VaD and no primary diagnosis in 0.7%, each [44]. In the Nun study patients with autopsy-confirmed AD plus cerebrovascular lesions had a higher prevalence of dementia than those without infarcts [55]. In a population-based study in the UK among 209 autopsies of elderly subjects, 48% being demented, 78% with cerebrovascular lesions and 70% with AD pathology, the proportion of multiple vascular pathology was higher in the demented group [52], while only 21% showed "pure" AD [16]. In a health maintenance organization study dementia registry, only 36% of patients had AD and not other findings, while 45% had pathologically definite AD plus coexistent vascular lesions, 22% plus DLB features [40]. Among 333 autopsied men in the Honolulu-Asian Aging Study (120 demented, 115 marginal, 96 with normal cognition), 24% of the dementias were linked with vascular lesions, and dementia frequency more than doubled with coexistent cerebrovascular lesions (45 vs 20%) [54]. Hence, the majority of demented elderly patients, often clinically suggested as AD, in fact show combined pathologies, most frequently with associated vascular or Lewy body pathologies. In the group of cases clinically diagnosed as "nonspecific degenerative dementia", 78% showed AD pathology, VaD and mixed dementia accounted for 7.6 and 6.7%, respectively, while 4.6% showed other disorders, and 2.9% nothing abnormal beyond age-related lesions.

Compared to AD, in the present cohort, the accuracy rates between clinical and neuropathological classification were lower in the VAD group and for mixed dementias which were 52.3 and 60%, respectively, while between 20 and 32% of these patients showed "pure" AD pathology. These accuracy data were similar to those in our previous cohort (60.5 and 61.9%, respectively), but were higher than in other autopsy series of demented patients, where the sensitivity for VaD ranged from 25 to 44.4%, and that of mixed dementia was around 31% [60,61]. In the group of PDD cases, 35% showed the pathology of DLB, 20% of combined PD plus AD, while 29% revealed AD pathology with our without minor coexisting cerebrovascular lesions; 4.6% showed other pathologies, e.g. multisystem degeneration or PSP, and 2.9% had nothing abnormel. In general, non-demented PD patients have AD pathology largely restricted to the limbic system, corresponding to Braak stages 4 or less, whereas PPD cases often have severe neuritic AD lesions [14]. Some studies suggested diffuse or transitional DLB with mild to moderate AD pathology as the major pathological substrate of PDD [2]; others revealed significant correlations between cognitive impairment and widespread neuritic AD pathology [31]. In general, the main changes underlying dementia in PD seem to be Lewy body pathology in the cerebral cortex and limbic system, and frequent co-existence of neuritic AD pathology [15], with particular involvement of the limbic system, suggesting that both pathologies independently or synergistically contribute to dementia [25].

In addition to the major groups of dementing disorders, 60 cases showed other pathologies, the majority were CDJ and Huntington disease cases, which had been diagnosed clinically in 95 and 50%, respectively. Correct clinical diagnoses had been made in 6/8 FTD patients and 2/3 DLB cases, while those with dementia related to chronic alcoholism ($n = 9$) showed chronic Wernicke encephalopathy and posttraumatic lesions in 5 cases, AD and VaD in one case each.

The present study and the results of other recent series indicate increasing agreement between clinical and autopsy diagnosis in prospective and retrospective evaluation of case series of demented aged individuals when following standardized classification and consensus criteria. However, current data document variable accuracy and sensitivity rates for the morphological confirmation of the major clinical dementia groups. The presented data and the results of other recent clinico-pathological studies, indicate the need for more sophisticated and validated clinical and neuropathological critieria for an appropriate classification of dementing disorders in the elderly, in order to improve the diagnostic reliability as a major factor of early detection and effective management of dementias.

Acknowledgements

The author tahnks the clinicians of Lainz Hospital and of Otto Wagner Hospital, Vienna, Austria, for the clinical data, Mrs. V. Rappelsberger for excellent laboratory work, and E-Mitter-Ferstl, PhD, for secretarial and computer work. The study was partly supported by the Society for Support of Research in Experimental Neurology, Vienna, Austria.

References

[1] I. Alafuzoff, K. Iqbal, H. Friden, R. Adolfsson and B. Winblad, Histopathological criteria for progressive dementia disorders: clinical-pathological correlation and classification by multivariate data analysis, *Acta Neuropathol (Berl)* 74 (1987) 209-225.

[2] H. Apaydin, J.E. Ahlskog, J.E. Parisi, B.F. Boeve and D.W. Dickson, Parkinson disease neuropathology: later-developing dementia and loss of the levodopa response, *Arch Neurol* 59 (2002), 102–112.

[3] J. Attems, F. Lintner and K.A. Jellinger, Amyloid beta peptide 1-42 highly correlates with capillary cerebral amyloid angiopathy and Alzheimer disease pathology, *Acta Neuropathol (Berl)* 107 (2004), 283–291.

[4] C. Bancher, K. Jellinger, H. Lassmann, P. Fischer and F. Leblhuber, Correlations between mental state and quantitative neuropathology in the Vienna Longitudinal Study on Dementia, *Eur Arch Psychiatry Clin Neurosci* 246 (1996), 137–146.

[5] L. Berg, D.W. McKeel Jr., J.P. Miller, J. Baty and J.C. Morris, Neuropathological indexes of Alzheimer's disease in demented and nondemented persons aged 80 years and older, *Arch Neurol* 50 (1993), 349–358.

[6] L. Berg, D.W. McKeel Jr., J.P. Miller, M. Storandt, E.H. Rubin, J.C. Morris, J. Baty, M. Coats, J. Norton, A.M. Goate, J.L. Price, M. Gearing, S.S. Mirra and A.M. Saunders, Clinicopathologic studies in cognitively healthy aging and Alzheimer's disease: relation of histologic markers to dementia severity, age, sex, and apolipoprotein E genotype, *Arch Neurol* 55 (1998), 326–335.

[7] F. Boller, O.L. Lopez and J. Moossy, Diagnosis of dementia: clinicopathologic correlations, *Neurology* 39 (1989), 76–79.

[8] J.V. Bowler, D.G. Munoz, H. Merskey and V. Hachinski, Fallacies in the pathological confirmation of the diagnosis of Alzheimer's disease, *J Neurol Neurosurg Psychiatry* 64 (1998), 18–24.

[9] H. Braak and E. Braak, Neuropathological stageing of Alzheimer-related changes, *Acta Neuropathol (Berl)* 82 (1991), 239–259.

[10] H. Braak, K. Del Tredici, U. Rub, R.A. de Vos, E.N. Jansen Steur and E. Braak, Staging of brain pathology related to sporadic Parkinson's disease, *Neurobiol Aging* 24 (2003), 197–211.

[11] H.C. Chui, J.I. Victoroff, D. Margolin, W. Jagust, R. Shankle, and R. Katzman, Criteria for the diagnosis of ischemic vascular dementia proposed by the State of California Alzheimer's Disease Diagnostic and Treatment Centers, *Neurology* 42 (1992), 473–480.

[12] E.J. Cochran, J.A. Schneider, D.A. Bennett et al., Application of NIA/Reagan Institute Working Group Criteria for diagnosis of Alzheimer's disease to members of the Religious Orders Study (abstr.), *J Neuropathol Exp Neurol* 57 (1998), 508.

[13] D.G. Davis, F.A. Schmitt, D.R. Wekstein and W.R. Markesbery, Alzheimer neuropathologic alterations in aged cognitively normal subjects, *J Neuropathol Exp Neurol* 58 (1999), 376–388.

[14] A. Delacourte, J.P. David, N. Sergeant, L. Buee, A. Wattez, P. Vermersch, F. Ghozali, C. Fallet-Bianco, F. Pasquier, F. Lebert, H. Petit and C. Di Menza, The biochemical pathway of neurofibrillary degeneration in aging and Alzheimer's disease, *Neurology* 52 (1999), 1158–1165.

[15] M. Emre, Dementia associated with Parkinson's disease, *Lancet Neurol* 2 (2003), 229–237.

[16] M.S. Fernando and P.G. Ince, Vascular pathologies and cognition in a population-based cohort of elderly people, *J Neurol Sci* 226 (2004), 13–17.

[17] F. Garcia-Sierra, J.J. Hauw, C. Duyckaerts, C.M. Wischik, J. Luna-Munoz and R. Mena, The extent of neurofibrillary pathology in perforant pathway neurons is the key determinant of dementia in the very old, *Acta Neuropathol (Berl)* 100 (2000), 29–35.

[18] M. Gearing, S.S. Mirra, J.C. Hedreen, S.M. Sumi, L.A. Hansen and A. Heyman, The Consortium to Establish a Registry for Alzheimer's Disease (CERAD), Part X: Neuropathology confirmation of the clinical diagnosis of Alzheimer's disease, *Neurology* 45 (1995), 461–466.

[19] H.J. Gertz, J. Xuereb, F. Huppert, C. Brayne, M.A. McGee, E. Paykel, C. Harrington, E. Mukaetova-Ladinska, T. Arendt and C.M. Wischik, Examination of the validity of the hierarchical model of neuropathological staging in normal aging and Alzheimer's disease, *Acta Neuropathol (Berl)* 95 (1998), 154–158.

[20] G. Gold, P. Giannakopoulos, C. Montes-Paixao Junior, F.R. Herrmann, R. Mulligan, J.P. Michel and C. Bouras, Sensitivity and specificity of newly proposed clinical criteria for possible vascular dementia, *Neurology* 49 (1997), 690–694.

[21] G. Gold, C. Bouras, E. Kovari, A. Canuto, B.G. Glaria, A. Malky, P.R. Hof, J.P. Michel and P. Giannakopoulos, Clinical validity of Braak neuropathological staging in the oldest-old, *Acta Neuropathol (Berl)* 99 (2000), 579–582.

[22] E. Gomez-Tortosa, I. Gonzalo, S. Fanjul, M.J. Sainz, S. Cantarero, C. Cemillan, J.G. Yebenes and T. del Ser, Cerebrospinal fluid markers in dementia with Lewy bodies compared with Alzheimer disease, *Arch Neurol* 60 (2003), 1218–1222.

[23] J. Gunstad and J. Browndyke, Understanding incidence and prevalence rates in mixed dementia, in: *Vascular Dementia: Cerebrovascular Mechanisms and Clinical Management*, R.H. Paul, R. Cohen, B.R. Ott and S. Salloway, eds, Human Press Inc., Totowa, NJ, 2005, pp. 245–255.

[24] A.J. Harding and G.M. Halliday, Simplified neuropathological diagnosis of dementia with Lewy bodies, *Neuropathol Appl Neurobiol* 24 (1998), 195–201.

[25] A.J. Harding and G.M. Halliday, Cortical Lewy body pathology in the diagnosis of dementia, *Acta Neuropathol (Berl)* 102 (2001), 355–363.

[26] V. Haroutunian, D.P. Perl, D.P. Purohit, D. Marin, K. Khan, M. Lantz, K.L. Davis and R.C. Mohs, Regional distribution of neuritic plaques in the nondemented elderly and subjects with very mild Alzheimer disease, *Arch Neurol* 55 (1998), 1185–1191.

[27] B.T. Hyman and J.Q. Trojanowski, Consensus recommendations for the postmortem diagnosis of Alzheimer disease from the National Institute on Aging and the Reagan Institute Working Group on diagnostic criteria for the neuropathological assessment of Alzheimer disease, *J Neuropathol Exp Neurol* 56 (1997), 1095–1097.

[28] P.G. Ince, F.K. McArthur, E. Bjertness, A. Torvik, J.M. Candy and J.A. Edwardson, Neuropathological diagnoses in elderly patients in Oslo: Alzheimer's disease, Lewy body disease, vascular lesions, *Dementia* 6 (1995), 162–168.

[29] K. Jellinger, W. Danielczyk, P. Fischer and E. Gabriel, Clinicopathological analysis of dementia disorders in the elderly, *J Neurol Sci* 95 (1990), 239–258.

[30] K.A. Jellinger, Clinical validity of Braak staging in the oldest-old, *Acta Neuropathol* 99 (2000), 583–584.

[31] K.A. Jellinger, The pathology of ischemic-vascular dementia: an update, *J Neurol Sci* **203–204** (2002), 153–157.

[32] K.A. Jellinger, Plaque-predominant and tangle-predominant variants of Alzheimer's disease, in: *Neurodegeneration: The Molecular Pathology of Dementia and Movement Disorders*, D.W. Dickson, ed., ISN Neuropath Press, Basel, 2003, pp. 66–68.

[33] K.A. Jellinger, Is Alzheimer's disease a vascular disorder? *J Alzheimers Dis* **5** (2003), 247–250; discussion 251–262.

[34] K.A. Jellinger, Neuropathology of Alzheimer disease and clinical relevance, in: *Alzheimer's Disease and Related Disorders: Research Advances*, K. Iqbal and B. Winblad, eds, Ana Aslan Intl. Acad. of Aging, Bucharest, Romania, 2003, pp. 152–169.

[35] K.A. Jellinger and E. Mitter-Ferstl, The impact of cerebrovascular lesions in Alzheimer disease. A comparative autopsy study, *J Neurol* **250** (2003), 1050–1055.

[36] K.A. Jellinger, The neuropathologic substrates of vascular-ischemic dementia, in: *Current Clinical Neurology. Vascular Dementia: Cerebrovascular Mechanisms and Clinical Management*, R.H. Paul, R. Cohen, B.R. Ott and S. Salloway, eds, Humana Press, Totowa, NJ, 2005, pp. 23–57.

[37] C.L. Joachim, J.H. Morris and D.J. Selkoe, Clinically diagnosed Alzheimer's disease: autopsy results in 150 cases, *Ann Neurol* **24** (1988), 50–56.

[38] D.S. Knopman, W.A. Rocca, R.H. Cha, S.D. Edland and E. Kokmen, Incidence of vascular dementia in Rochester, Minn, 1985-1989, *Arch Neurol* **59** (2002), 1605–1610.

[39] D.S. Knopman, Alzheimer type dementia, in: *Neurodegeneration. The Molecular Pathology of Dementia and Movement Disorders*, D.W. Dickson, ed., ISN Neuropath Press, Basel, 2003, pp. 24–39.

[40] A. Lim, D. Tsuang, W. Kukull, D. Nochlin, J. Leverenz, W. McCormick, J. Bowen, L. Teri, J. Thompson, E. R. Peskind, M. Raskind and E.B. Larson, Clinico-neuropathological correlation of Alzheimer's disease in a community-based case series, *J Am Geriatr Soc* **47** (1999), 564–569.

[41] W.R. Markesbery, Vascular dementia, in: *Neuropathology of Dementing Disorders*, W. Markesbery, ed., Arnold Publishers, London, 1998, pp. 293–311.

[42] E.M. Martin, R.S. Wilson, R.D. Penn, J.H. Fox, R.A. Clasen and S.M. Savoy, Cortical biopsy results in Alzheimer's disease: correlation with cognitive deficits, *Neurology* **37** (1987), 1201–1204.

[43] A.C. McKee, N.W. Kowall, R. Au et al., Topography of neurofibrillary tangles distinguishes aging from Alzheimer disease (abstr.), *J Neuropathol Exp Neurol* **61** (2002), 488.

[44] D.W. McKeel, J.L. Price, J.P. Miller, E.A. Grant, C. Xiong, L. Berg and J.C. Morris, Neuropathologic criteria for diagnosing Alzheimer disease in persons with pure dementia of Alzheimer type, *J Neuropathol Exp Neurol* **63** (2004), 1028–1037.

[45] I.G. McKeith, D. Galasko, K. Kosaka, E.K. Perry, D.W. Dickson, L.A. Hansen, D.P. Salmon, J. Lowe, S.S. Mirra, E.J. Byrne, G. Lennox, N.P. Quinn, J.A. Edwardson, P.G. Ince, C. Bergeron, A. Burns, B.L. Miller, S. Lovestone, D. Collerton, E.N. Jansen, C. Ballard, R.A. de Vos, G.K. Wilcock, K.A. Jellinger and R.H. Perry, Consensus guidelines for the clinical and pathologic diagnosis of dementia with Lewy bodies (DLB): report of the consortium on DLB international workshop, *Neurology* **47** (1996), 1113–1124.

[46] I.G. McKeith, J. Mintzer, D. Aarsland, D. Burn, H. Chiu, J. Cohen-Mansfield, D. Dickson, B. Dubois, J.E. Duda, H. Feldman, S. Gauthier, G. Halliday, B. Lawlor, C. Lippa, O.L. Lopez, J. Carlos Machado, J. O'Brien, J. Playfer and W. Reid, Dementia with Lewy bodies, *Lancet Neurol* **3** (2004), 19–28.

[47] G. McKhann, D. Drachman, M. Folstein, R. Katzman, D. Price and E.M. Stadlan, Clinical diagnosis of Alzheimer's disease: report of the NINCDS-ADRDA Work Group under the auspices of Department of Health and Human Services Task Force on Alzheimer's Disease, *Neurology* **34** (1984), 939–944.

[48] S.S. Mirra, A. Heyman, D. McKeel, S.M. Sumi, B.J. Crain, L. M. Brownlee, F.S. Vogel, J.P. Hughes, G. van Belle and L. Berg, The Consortium to Establish a Registry for Alzheimer's Disease (CERAD). Part II. Standardization of the neuropathologic assessment of Alzheimer's disease, *Neurology* **41** (1991), 479–486.

[49] J.T. Moroney, E. Bagiella, D.W. Desmond, V.C. Hachinski, P.K. Molsa, L. Gustafson, A. Brun, P. Fischer, T. Erkinjuntti, W. Rosen, M.C. Paik and T.K. Tatemichi, Meta-analysis of the Hachinski Ischemic Score in pathologically verified dementias, *Neurology* **49** (1997), 1096–1105.

[50] J.C. Morris, D.W. McKeel Jr., K. Fulling, R.M. Torack and L. Berg, Validation of clinical diagnostic criteria for Alzheimer's disease, *Ann Neurol* **24** (1988), 17–22.

[51] D.G. Munoz, D.W. Dickson, C. Bergeron, I.R. Mackenzie, A. Delacourte and V. Zhukareva, The neuropathology and biochemistry of frontotemporal dementia, *Ann Neurol* **54**(Suppl 5) (2003), S24–S28.

[52] Neuropathology-Group, Pathological correlates of late-onset dementia in a multicentre, community-based population in England and Wales. Neuropathology Group of the Medical Research Council Cognitive Function and Ageing Study (MRC CFAS), *Lancet* **357** (2001), 169–175.

[53] K.L. Newell, B.T. Hyman, J.H. Growdon and E.T. Hedley-Whyte, Application of the National Institute on Aging (NIA)-Reagan Institute criteria for the neuropathological diagnosis of Alzheimer disease, *J Neuropathol Exp Neurol* **58** (1999), 1147–1155.

[54] H. Petrovitch, L.R. White, G.W. Ross, S.C. Steinhorn, C.Y. Li, K.H. Masaki, D.G. Davis, J. Nelson, J. Hardman, J.D. Curb, P.L. Blanchette, L.J. Launer, K. Yano and W.R. Markesbery, Accuracy of clinical criteria for AD in the Honolulu-Asia Aging Study, a population-based study, *Neurology* **57** (2001), 226–234.

[55] K.P. Riley, D.A. Snowdon and W.R. Markesbery, Alzheimer's neurofibrillary pathology and the spectrum of cognitive function: findings from the Nun Study, *Ann Neurol* **51** (2002), 567–577.

[56] W.A. Rocca and D.S. Knopman, Prevalence and incidence patterns of vascular dementia, in: *Vascular Cognitive Impairment. Preventable Dementia*, in: J.V. Bowler and V. Hachinski, eds, Oxford Univ. Press, Oxford, 2003, pp. 21–32.

[57] G.C. Román, T.K. Tatemichi, T. Erkinjuntti, J.L. Cummings, J.C. Masdeu, J.H. Garcia, L. Amaducci, J.M. Orgogozo, A. Brun, A. Hofman et al., Vascular dementia: diagnostic criteria for research studies. Report of the NINDS-AIREN International Workshop, *Neurology* **43** (1993), 250–260.

[58] R. Sulkava, T. Erkinjuntti, M. Haltia, A. Paetau, J. Palo and J. Wikström, Non-Alzheimer dementias fulfilling the NINCDS-ADRDA criteria for probable Alzheimer's disease, in: *Aging of the Brain and Dementia: Ten Years later*, L. Amaducci, ed., Abstract Book, Florence, 1989, pp. 125.

[59] J.Q. Trojanowski and D. Dickson, Update on the neuropathological diagnosis of frontotemporal dementias, *J Neuropathol Exp Neurol* **60** (2001), 1123–1126.

[60] J.P. Wade, T.R. Mirsen, V.C. Hachinski, M. Fisman, C. Lau and H. Merskey, The clinical diagnosis of Alzheimer's disease, *Arch Neurol* **44** (1987), 24–29.

[61] B. Winblad, W. Wallace, J. Hardy, C. Fowler, G. Bucht, I. Alafuzoff and R. Adolfson, Neurochemical, genetic and clinical aspects of Alzheimer's disease, in: *Dimensions in Aging,* M. Bergener, M. Ermini and H.B. Stähelin, eds, Academic Press, London, 1986, pp. 183–203.

[62] D. Zekry, C. Duyckaerts, J. Belmin, C. Geoffre, F. Herrmann, R. Moulias and J.J. Hauw, The vascular lesions in vascular and mixed dementia: the weight of functional neuroanatomy, *Neurobiol Aging* **24** (2003), 213–219.

The history of the paired helical filaments

Michael Kidd*

Department of Basic Medical Sciences, St George's, University of London, Cranmer Terrace, Tooting, London SW17 0RE, UK

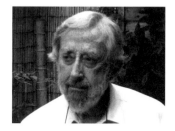

Abstract. The original recognition of the paired helical filaments is discussed and amplified. The original description of what are now the neuropil threads is mentioned. The ensuing importance of both these structures is emphasised and a morphology-based hypothesis of the development of the disease from the original stimuli is offered.

Keywords: Paired helical filaments, Alzheimer disease, neuropil threads, tau

1. Introduction

One hundred years ago Alois Alzheimer described neurofibrillary tangles in neocortical neurons in the dementing disease which now bears his name [2]. In 1961 when I set out to examine neocortical biopsies from Alzheimer's disease patients with the electron microscope I expected, like most people, that the neurofibrillary tangles would be composed of large numbers of normal, or maybe thickened neurofilaments. Neurofilaments had been well described using the the electron microscope by my old friend and teacher George Gray with Rainer Guillery [7]. I was therefore surprised and puzzled to find that the filaments of the tangle were not neurofilaments but a new type of filament which I called a 'paired helical filament' (PHF) [10].

It is necessary here to go into some detail on the subject of the recognition of cellular structures in the electron microscope because of the subsequent disputes as to the interpretation of the ultrastructural images of these unusual filaments. In general, tissues of almost any kind at some level of magnification show orientation of their constituents, including their cells. Below a certain size limit, however this orientation is often lost and is also often not possible with human cortical biopsies. It follows therefore that the ultrastructure of some features must be deduced on the assumption that they are observed in many different random orientations, and that these different images must be synthesised into a conceptual whole. The margins of these structures were more dense than the centre of the pair which at first sight made them paired filaments with some intervening material, but they appeared to be variable in oblique sections.

It took me some time to realise that these varying profiles were simply different views of the same filaments depending on the angle at which they sloped obliquely through the thickness of the section, especially if the section was rather too thick. I will show how I found this, as at the time of my Nature letter in 1963 [10] I was not able to present the geometrical arguments graphically; so that some authors did not seem to understand my description. The accompanying diagram (Fig. 1) shows how observing paired helical filaments from different sloping angles gives strange cycloidal profiles when seen with the electron microscope. I wished to avoid the term 'double helix', which would suggest that these helices had anything to do with the DNA helix, which they clearly had not. It then seemed

---

*Address for correspondence: Dr. M. Kidd, Anatomy, Department of Basic Medical Sciences, St George's, University of London, Cranmer Terrace, Tooting, London SW17 0RE, UK. Tel.: +44 0 20 8725 5207; Fax: +44 0 20 8725 3326; E-mail: mkidd@sgul.ac.uk.

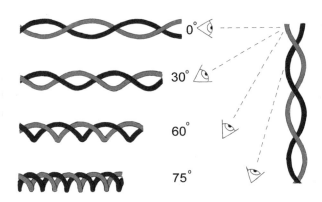

Fig. 1. Diagram showing the provenance of the irregular profiles seen in the EM when a PHF is viewed at various oblique angles, giving the views drawn on the left panel of the diagram. The conventional eyeballs and broken lines represent different possible viewpoints at the indicated angles of view. The observed projected images result from viewing one strand more transversely and the other more longitudinally. (From a computer program).

that Dr Robert Terry and co-workers [25,26] thought I was referring to all neurofilaments and not simply the tangle filaments (which I immediately had recognised were not neurofilaments); and both those publications recorded that the tangle filaments were 'not different from normal neurofilaments' in appearance – these authors did not then make a simultaneous identification of PHFs or of 'twisted tubules' or that they recognised these filaments as being structurally abnormal at that time. Some authors have referred to [26] as the first description of PHFs, but that publication clearly disagrees with this model. In [26] (published when my results were already known) Dr Terry and his colleagues referred to two different 'neurofilament' types, one constricted (or twisted) at intervals (without giving measurement of any periodicity) and the other untwisted. These were both referred to as normal neurofilaments, and no distinction was made between these and the tangle filaments. Tubules with fixed regularly-spaced twists would not show the structures seen in transverse or near-transverse sections seen in Fig. 7 of my publication [11], showing the dot-curve or double curve profiles described in the Nature letter [10]; explained in Figs 2a and 2b here. Curiously, in [26] Terry et al. show nearly identical profiles in their Fig. 12, but instead interpret them as 'circlets and triple density curved elements' and not as described by myself in [11], and they cite them as evidence of tubules with intermittent constrictions. Such a structure is difficult to visualise either as a macroscopic model or on the molecular scale we are dealing with here. In 1970 I showed the first images of negatively-stained PHFs, some of which showed flattening of the helix onto the

formvar film substrate [12] (Fig. 3). In 1968 Hirano and colleagues [9] described straight filaments in tangles in Alzheimer's cases and also in Guam-Parkinson dementia, and these did not appear to be neurofilaments. It was established by immunocytochemistry in 1987 [21] that these straight tangle filaments were tau-positive.

Thirteen years later, with co-authors Wisniewski and Narang [30] Terry agreed that these were paired helical filaments by using a high-angle electron microscope tilting stage; a method which showed by rotating the filament pair around its axis that the cross-over points move along the filament pair, as with a helix.

There has been a number of publications since then on the architecture of these unique features, using other physical methods of analysis of filamentous structures and deducing a variety of models of these structures. For example Polanen and his colleagues [22] published results using the atomic force microscope which seemed to suggest a flattened quasi-helical structure. However this model implies that in sections of solid material there would be images of regularly constricted ribbons with variable diameters, (since they would be randomly rotated in relation to the electron beam) and only those ribbons arranged at right angles to the electron beam would show the same appearance as that shown when on a flat substrate. Perhaps their observations show the effect of a flattening process when the grids were prepared and also a lack of resolving power in the atomic force microscope – although they did attempt to make corrections for the shape of the scanning tip.

Using image-averaging computer techniques on negatively-stained PHFs [28] Wischik in a group with

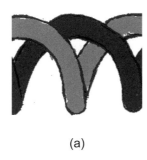 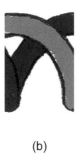

(a)   (b)

Fig. 2. These diagrams are derived from Fig. 1, and show the two main types of profile seen when an obliquely-sectioned PHF lies in a thin section.

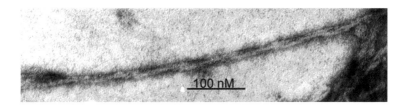

Fig. 3. Electron micrograph of a PHF in a preparation from a macerated formalin-fixed post-mortem brain from a case of Alzheimer's disease. This shows a paired filamentous structure with intervening material, with some evidence of flattening from a true helical form.

Aaron Klug confirmed that these are paired helical filaments, and that the individual filaments of the pair are L-shaped in transverse section. Crowther [5] also found that the so-called straight filaments [9] consist of the same two strands, but arranged differently so that they appear to be a single filament at usual electron microscopical resolutions.

In any event these abnormal structures are uniquely twisted, and this serves to distinguish certain brain diseases from others, for example helps to distinguish Alzheimer tangles from those in experimental aluminium myelo-encephalopathy [27]. The observations reported in my 1963 letter to Nature [10] also showed that these structures are present in neurites coursing through the neuropil. These were later named 'neuropil threads' by Braak et al. [4], where they amplified my observations and found an effective histological silver staining method for these neurites. My 1964 Brain paper [11] also showed that these filaments are present in neurites in the periphery of the the senile plaque. It should be emphasised that none of these observations could have been made if the PHFs were not recognisably different from normal neurofilaments. For example, the later identification of these tangle filaments as an abnormal form of tau – a microtubule-associated protein – could not have been made. I need not discuss at length the further observations which derived from my two publications since other papers in this volume will cover this evidence.

I admit that I was disappointed when I became convinced by the ample literature that the PHFs are essentially tau protein with some form of abnormal phosphorylation [6,8,15,18,29,31]. It may be remembered that, with some colleagues I suggested that the tangle protein and $A4\beta$ protein were the same [13]. As far as I was concerned this was mainly on grounds of 'scientific economy', how could there be 'two different amyloids in one head'? Well it seems that there are two since 'amyloid' at the histological level seems to be any filamentous protein that stains with Congo red to give birefringence (usually in a beta-pleated sheet form). This subject has been reviewed by Landon et al. [17].

2. Hypothesis

Those helices in scattered neurites in the neuropil consist of a more complete molecule than those of the cell body and are therefore probably earlier in date [16]. It is also interesting that the studies of the 1970s which showed tangles in remote places such as the basal nucleus of Meynert [1] and in some of the fourth ventricle nuclei [20] all suggest that the PHF material or influence travels centripetally from axon ending to perikaryon. In this context Braak & Braak [3] (using conventional histological methods) suggest that this process, whatever it is, starts chronologically in the entorhinal area and spreads outwards from there, and Ohm and Braak [19] show that this process also passes from the prepiriform cortex to the olfactory bulb. Prusiner [23] has proposed that the scrapie agent, chemically a normal protein, may exist as a non-functional abnormal structure, and that this configuration also converts normal molecules to the abnormal structure by some kind of non-DNA copying process. Could this be true of of the abnormal form of tau? The spread through and from the rhinencephalon is similar to that of some pathogens. Of course, I am not saying that abnormal tau is identical with prions, but perhaps it behaves like them. Such a process would necessarily involve phosphorylytic reactions unlike the prion copying process, perhaps the conformational change exposes phosphorylation sites.

In summary: I identified the tangle filaments as special, I identified them as twisted (= helical) but also I found them in the neuropil and in the periphery of the senile plaques.

Acknowledgements

I thank Dr. M.S. Pollanen and Dr. R.A. Crowther for original photographs.

References

[1] S.E. Arnold, B.T. Hyman, J. Flory, A.R. Damasio and G.W. Van Hoesen, The topographical and neuroanatomical distribution of neurofibrillary tangles and neuritic plaques in the cerebral cortex of patients with Alzheimer's disease, *Cereb Cortex* **1** (1991), 103–116.

[2] A. Alzheimer, *Neurol. Zentbl* **25** (1906), 1134.

[3] H. Braak and E. Braak, Neuropathological stageing of Alzheimer-related changes, *Acta Neuropathol (Berl)* **82**(4) (1991), 239–259.

[4] H. Braak, E. Braak, I. Grundke-Iqbal and K. Iqbal, Occurrence of neuropil threads in the senile human brain and in Alzheimer's disease: a third location of paired helical filaments outside of neurofibrillary tangles and neuritic plaques, *Neurosci Lett* **24** (1986), 351–355.

[5] R.A. Crowther, Straight and paired helical filaments in Alzheimer disease have a common structural unit, *Proc Nat Acad Sci USA* **88** (1991), 2288–2292.

[6] A. Delacourte and A. Defossez, Alzheimer's disease: Tau proteins, the promoting factors of microtubule assembly, are major components of paired helical filaments, *J Neurol Sci* **76**(2–3) (Dec. 1986), 173–186.

[7] E.G. Gray and R.W. Guillery, *J, Physiol (Lond)* **157** (1961), 581.

[8] I. Grundke-Iqbal, K. Iqbal, M. Quinlan, Y.C. Tung, M.S. Zaidi and H.M. Wisniewski, Microtubule-associated protein tau. A component of Alzheimer paired helical filaments, *J Biol Chem* **261** (1986), 6084–6089.

[9] A. Hirano, H.M. Dembitzer, L.T. Kurland and H.M. Zimmerman, Fine structure of some intraganglionic inclusions, *J Neuropathol and Exp Neurol* **27** (1968), 167–182.

[10] M. Kidd, Paired helical filaments in electron microscopy of Alzheimer's disease, *Nature (Lond)* **197** (1963), (4863) 192–193.

[11] M. Kidd, Alzheimer's disease: an electron microscopical study, *Brain* **87** (1964), 307–320.

[12] M. Kidd, Fig 1 in Discussion of paper by Hirano A in Alzheimer's Disease Wolstenholme G E W & O'Connor M eds, Churchill (Lond) (1970), 203.

[13] M. Kidd, D. Allsop and M. Landon, Senile plaque amyloid, paired helical filaments, and cerebrovascular amyloid in Alzheimer's disease are all deposits of the same protein, *Lancet* **1**(8423) (1985), 278–278.

[14] S.R. Korey, L. Scheinberg, R.D. Terry and A. Stern, *Trans Amer Neurol Assoc* **86** (1961), 90.

[15] K.S. Kosik, C.L. Joachim and D.J. Selkoe, Microtubule-associated protein tau is a major antigenic component of paired helical filaments in Alzheimer disease, *Proc Natl Acad Sci USA* **83** (1986), 4044–4048.

[16] M.A. Kurt, D.C. Davies and M. Kidd, Paired helical filament morphology varies with intracellular location in Alzheimer's disease brain, *Neuroscience Letters* **239** (1997), 41–44.

[17] M. Landon, M. Kidd and D. Allsop, Amyloidosis with particular reference to cerebral amyloid in Alzheimer's disease and the transmissible subacute encephalopathies, *Reviews in the Neurosciences* **1** (1987), 101–126.

[18] N. Nukina and Y. Ihara, One of the antigenic determinants of paired helical filaments is related to tau protein, *J Biochem (Tokyo)* **99** (1986), 1541–1554.

[19] T.G. Ohm and H. Braak, Olfactory bulb changes in Alzheimer's disease, *Acta Neuropathol* **72** (1987), 365–369.

[20] R.C.A. Pearson, K.C. Gatter and T.P.S. Powell, The cortical relationships of certain basal ganglia and the cholinergic basal forebrain nuclei, *Brain Research* **26** (1983), 327–330.

[21] G. Perry, P. Mulvihill, V. Manetto, I. Autillio-Gambetti and P. Gambetti, Immunocytochemical properties of Alzheimer straight filaments, *J Neuroscience* **7** (1987), 3736–3738.

[22] M.S. Pollanen, P. Marliewicz, M.C. Goh and C. Bergeron, Alzheimer paired helical filaments: a comparison with the twisted ribbon model, *Acta Neuropathologica* **90**(2) (1995), 194–197.

[23] S.B. Prusiner, Prions, *Sci Am* **251** (1984), 50–59.

[24] R.D. Terry, *Meeting of Amer Neuropathol Assoc* (June, 1963).

[25] R.D. Terry, The fine structure of neurofibrillary tangles in Alzheimer's disease, *J Neuropathol Exp Neurol* **22** (1963), 629–641.

[26] R.D. Terry, N.K. Gonatas and M. Weiss, Ultrastructural studies in Alzheimer's presenile dementia, *Am J Pathol* **44** (1964), 269–287.

[27] R.D. Terry and C. Pena, Experimental production of neurofibrillary degeneration. 2. Electron microscopy, phosphatase histochemistry and electron probe analysis, *J Neuropathol Exp Neurol* **24** (1965), 200–210.

[28] C.M. Wischik, R.A. Crowther, M. Stewart and M. Roth, Subunit structure of paired helical filaments in Alzheimer's disease, *J Cell Biol* **100** (1985), 1905–1912.

[29] C.M. Wischik, M. Novak, H.C. Thorgersen, P.C. Edwards, M.J. Runswick, R. Jakes, J.E. Walker, C. Milstein, M. Roth and A. Klug, Isolation of a fragment of tau derived from the core of the paired helical filament of Alzheimer disease, *Proc Nat Acad Sci USA (USA)* **85**(12) (1988), 4506–4510.

[30] H.M. Wisniewski, H.K. Narang and R.D. Terry, Neurofibrillary tangles of paired helical filaments, *J Neurol Sci* **27** (1976), 173–181.

[31] J.G. Wood, S.S. Mirra, N.J. Pollock and L.I. Binder, Neurofibrillary tangles of Alzheimer disease share antigenic determinants with the axonal microtubule-associated protein tau, *Proc Natl Acad Sci USA* **83** (1986), 4040–4043.

Synaptic Changes

Vulnerability to Alzheimer's pathology in neocortex: The roles of plasticity and columnar organization

M.M. Esiri[a,b,*] and S.A. Chance[a]
[a]*Department of Clinical Neurology, University of Oxford, Oxford, UK*
[b]*Department of Neuropathology, Oxford Radcliffe NHS Trust, Oxford, UK*

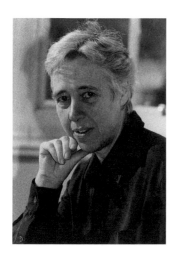

Abstract. Two principal findings in the Pearson et al. paper [73] are commented on here. The first is the regional selectivity within the cerebrum of neurofibrillary tangle (NFT) formation in Alzheimer's disease (AD) which targets association cortex and the primary olfactory cortex alone among regions of primary sensory cortex. The second finding is the clustering of NFT in columns of supra- and infra-granular layers of association cortex. We review recent evidence confirming these findings and comment on their possible significance. We consider that the most attractive hypothesis to explain the vulnerability of the olfactory system and association cortex is the persistent neural plasticity of these regions. On this basis there would be no need to postulate a progressive spreading process. The columnar distribution of clustered NFT can be well understood in the context of recent concepts of columnar organization of the cerebral cortex. The original interpretation that this distribution of NFT reflects pathology in neurons subserving cortico-cortical and cortico-subcortical connections seems to us to have stood the test of time.

Keywords: Alzheimer's disease, olfactory system, neocortex, cortical minicolumns, neural plasticity

1. Introduction

The Pearson et al. (1985) paper [73] was the outcome of collaboration in Oxford between two neuroanatomists (R.C.A. Pearson, T.P.S. Powell), a neuropathologist (M.M. Esiri), a geriatrician (G.K. Wilcock) and a statistician (R.W. Hiorns). A few years previous, Drs. Wilcock and Esiri teamed up to try to determine the feature of Alzheimer's disease (AD) pathology that most closely correlates with the *in vivo* cognitive deficit. This work had pointed decisively to neurofibrillary tangle (NFT) as that feature [96], a finding which has been repeatedly confirmed [10,11,68]. It therefore became logical to try to understand better the distribution of NFT in the hope that this enhanced understanding would lead to pathogenetic clues and potential preventive or therapeutic intervention for AD.

The neuroanatomical expertise of Carl Pearson and Tom Powell was crucial to our efforts. The late Tom Powell, who was one of the most distinguished neuroanatomists of his time [56], had spent decades undertaking meticulous experiments in animals tracing con-

---

*Address for correspondence: Department of Neuropathology, Radcliffe Infirmary, Oxford OX2 6HE, UK. Tel.: +44 1865 224403; Fax: +44 1865 224508; E-mail: Margaret.esiri@clneuro.ox.ac.uk.

nections between one part of the cerebral cortex and another and connections between the cerebral cortex and various subcortical nuclei. It was particularly satisfying to him that as he neared retirement he found that the knowledge gained from these experimental studies, undertaken in the spirit of pure intellectual enquiry, might inform a practical understanding of a condition that was increasingly being recognized as the major cause of dementia in humans.

The main findings of the Pearson et al. [73] paper were 1) that in AD, within the temporal, parietal, occipital and frontal lobes, it was the cortical association areas that were targeted for NFT formation while primary motor and sensory (exemplified here by visual) cortex, often in close proximity, were almost totally spared. A subsequent study of ours confirmed that this sparing was also true of primary auditory cortex [32]. The exception to this rule was the heavy involvement of the primary olfactory sensory cortex with NFT; 2) NFT occurred in clusters and involved predominantly pyramidal neurons within supra and infragranular layers with the clustering in these layers often being in register with each other. This clustering of NFT in cortical neurons presumptively giving rise to cortico-cortical (layer II and III) and cortico-subcortical (layer V) projections was closely reminiscent of the known origin of such projections from columns of neurons in experimental studies; 3) in all areas examined except the occipital association cortex NFT were more numerous in layer V than in layer III of association cortex; 4) cortical plaques had quite a different distribution even though this overlapped the distribution of NFT. Plaques occurred predominantly in layers II and III of association cortex and showed a random distribution with no clear clustering in these layers. This distribution was thought to be consistent with plaques occurring at axonal terminations. In brief, our paper clarified the anatomical connectional basis of the pathology of AD in cerebral cortex, in this way complementing work by Hyman et al. [51] published the previous year on the anatomical connectional basis of the hippocampal and entorhinal pathology in AD and the work by Arendt et al. [4] on the anatomical basis of nucleus basalis neuron loss and involvement of anatomically connected regions of cerebral cortex in plaque formation in AD.

The aspects of this work that we comment on below are the differential involvement of olfactory, in contrast to other, primary sensory cortex, and the columnar clustering of NFT.

2. The olfactory connection in AD

The olfactory connection emphasized in Pearson et al. [73] built on our earlier study of the olfactory bulbs in AD [31] in which we showed that the anterior olfactory nuclei regularly harbor NFT. Subsequent studies of this region have repeatedly confirmed this and shown the presence here of plaques and neuron loss as well [20,24,35,50,58,59,61,82,83,86,92]. Clinical impairment of the sense of smell, reflecting this pathology and pathology at central olfactory connections, has also become well recognized in AD [33,66,89]. Moving peripherally, the olfactory mucosa itself has been described as showing distinctive AD pathology or oxidative damage in AD [38,76,87,88,91] and biopsy of the olfactory mucosa was briefly considered to have potential diagnostic value. The olfactory system is now also recognized both clinically and pathologically to be involved in the pathology of Parkinson's disease [27, 45,60,63,98].

The observation contrasting with the olfactory system involvement in AD is the lack of involvement of other primary sensory systems as highlighted in [73]. This observation has been frequently noted [14,25,30, 39,74,79] but we still lack clear understanding of why it is. One explanation for the contrast between the fates of olfactory and other sensory systems in AD that has been considered is the possibility that an environmental factor that favors NFT formation may reach the brain along the readily accessible olfactory route and extend to the hippocampus and from thence to association but not primary sensory cortex. Possible factors that have been put forward are Herpes simplex virus (HSV) [41, 53,55,80], zinc [77] and aluminum [75]. HSV is readily transported across synapses and can be shown experimentally to extend via the olfactory pathways as well as trigeminal pathways to the brain [90]. Acute HSV encephalitis in humans has a distribution of damage closely corresponding to the areas most severely affected in AD [29]. On account of its wide distribution in humans, its capacity to establish latent infection in neurons [94] and its ability *in vitro* to promote amyloid-β fibril formation [22] HSV represents a plausible, if controversial, environmental factor to consider. In its favor are studies suggesting that HSV in the presence of ApoE ε4 genotype is a risk factor for AD [53].

Metal ions display a limited but still potentially significant ability to extend across synapses after entry to the brain via the olfactory system [77]. Zinc and aluminum have been investigated for possible cofactor roles in AD pathogenesis [75,77].

3. Relationship of neuronal plasticity to regional pathology in AD

Ease of entry of an environmental factor posing a risk of AD is not the only possible explanation for why the olfactory system damage is more severe in comparison to other sensory systems in AD. Another important property of the olfactory system, as of the hippocampus, that has become more apparent over the last 20 years is a high degree of local synaptic plasticity. Before discussing the relevance of this we need to consider broader views about the etiology of AD.

Much research on AD during the last 15 or so years has been based on the widely accepted amyloid cascade hypothesis [43,44,85] which considers that the initial step leading to the full-blown pathology of AD and its clinical consequences is an accumulation of amyloid-β as insoluble deposits in the extracellular space in a wide distribution in the brain, particularly the cerebral cortex. Fibrillary amyloid-β, or a precursor form of it, is considered to be toxic to neurons and capable of inducing NFT formation, although the exact mechanism by which amyloid-β causes NFT formation remains unclear. The amyloid hypothesis is based on the demonstration that mutations in the gene coding for amyloid-β protein precursor (AβPP) cause AD [40]. Further credence was provided by the recognition that other gene mutations that cause AD also influence the metabolism of AβPP. However, cases of AD caused by such mutations constitute only a tiny proportion of all AD cases and the pathogenetic route to the final common AD pathology may, in sporadic cases, be different and, indeed, varied. Recent work in transgenic animals engineered to contain both amyloid-promoting and NFT-promoting mutations gives credence to the pathogenetic sequence predicted by the amyloid hypothesis. Thus, removing the amyloid-β by immune clearance at a stage when hyperphosphylated tau had not accumulated prevented its accumulation. Conversely, allowing the amyloid-β plaques to re-form promoted hyperphosphorylated tau accumulation [12,71].

One problem with the amyloid cascade hypothesis, and one that is particularly pertinent to this review, is that it does not readily provide an explanation for the regionally selective distribution of NFT observed in AD. In some ways it might be easier to explain the widespread distribution of amyloid-β as secondary to NFT formation which, occurring initially in the transentorhinal regional and hippocampus [13] could give rise to widespread plaques if these were related to the axon terminals of NFT-bearing neurons; however, this would put the tangle cart in front of the amyloid-β horse. This brings us back to the idea that synaptic plasticity is a possible basis for explaining the vulnerability of medial temporal lobe structures, including the olfactory cortex, for NFT formation.

There is regional variation in the potential for neuroplasticity in the adult brain. Age-related dendritic growth is most pronounced in limbic cortical areas, while the primary sensory and motor cortex show either dendritic stability or regression [2,3,5,6]. An intermediate degree of dendritic remodeling occurs in association cortex. These results are mirrored by regional differences in growth associated protein (GAP-43) expression – greatest in limbic areas and lowest in motor and sensory areas.

Several aspects of neuroplasticity are evident in the adult CNS, including, alterations of dendritic ramifications, synaptic remodeling, long-term potentiation (LTP), axonal sprouting, neurite extension, synaptogenesis, and neurogenesis [64]. Simple behavioral challenges such as learning new associations, will induce these plastic processes in adult experimental animals. Neuronal death may also cause increased dendritic branching among remaining neurons [1]. Maintenance of synapse number is likely to require reactive synaptogenesis as existing synapses breakdown over time and must be replaced [64]. It is suggested that regions exhibiting high neuroplasticity are meeting a regional demand and that factors increasing the propensity to AD are those which make neurons work harder to meet those demands [64]. Increasing age is one such potent factor as free radical damage to cell membranes makes synapse maintenance more demanding. The resulting compensatory upregulation of neuroplastic activity may lead to the development of AD pathology. As more is discovered about molecular and metabolic aspects of neurogenesis and synaptic plasticity the more intricately enmeshed with AD these features seem to become.

Adaptive neuroplastic changes in synapses involve reversible phosphorylation including phosphorylation of tau similar to that seen in AD. Arendt [3] suggests that a modest increase in tau phosphorylation may protect neurons from apoptosis by stabilizing tau during periods of 'torpor states'. In an experimental setting such a state that has been investigated is hibernation in which brain (and body) metabolism and function are greatly reduced. Reversible tau phosphorylation in these conditions may mark sites where synapses are required to be re-established on arousal and represent a physiological adaptation to preserve synapses at times of reduced neuronal activity. One is tempted to wonder if some of the episodes of ill health or anesthesia that anecdotally often precede onset of initial symptoms of AD in humans may bear some similarity to such 'torpor states' and represent an opportunity for failure of reversal of tau phosphorylation and establishment of paired helical filaments (PHF) in the most plastic neurons. Kinases that phosphorylate tau in a PHF-like manner, and phosphatases that de-phosphorylate it, are all associated with the cell division cycle (see below).

Immature neurons at sites of neurogenesis, not surprisingly, undergo cell division cycle events. Molecules involved in the cell division cycle are, more unexpectedly, expressed in neurons in the human brain in aging and AD [2,3,62,69,70,72,93]. Loss of synapses exposes neurons to the risk of dedifferentiation and re-entry into the cell division cycle. The olfactory system in experimental animals is one where there is a remarkably high turnover of neurons even in adults. In rodents 1% of total olfactory bulb interneurons are added each day [26]. When neurons die their input to the next order neurons are deprived of their synaptic influence at least until newly formed, or already existing, neurons replace it. Re-entry into the cell division cycle may be reversible in the G1 phase but is irreversible in the G2 phase. Faced with an inability to divide a neuron in G2 may either die as a result of an apoptotic-like process, if cell death-promoting enzymes are active, or develop NFT under the influence of enzymes activated to prepare the cell for division. Significantly, cell cycle re-entry involves interconnected neurons in regions of vulnerability to NFT formation in AD and upregulation of amyloidogenic metabolic pathways of AβPP metabolism.

4. Other contributory factors

There have been a number of other factors that have been suggested to underlie vulnerability of brain regions to NFT formation.

4.1. Degree of myelination

A link between regional pathology distribution and regional vulnerability has also been proposed to be due to differential myelination. The majority of NFT-containing nuclei in AD (cholinergic basal forebrain neurons, locus ceruleus and the raphe nuclei) have cortical projections that are poorly myelinated. Other cortical projection neurons with few tangles, such as thalamic nuclei, have more myelination.

4.2. Influence of attenuated cholinergic innervation

A striking loss of cortical cholinergic innervation occurs in AD. Neurons of the basal nucleus of Meynert, which provide the main cholinergic innervation of the cortical mantle, are among the first cells to exhibit hyperphosphorylated tau and NFTs [64]. Normally, limbic areas, including the hippocampus and amygdala, contain the highest density of cholinergic axons. Association cortex exhibits an intermediate density, and primary visual cortex contains the lowest density of fibers [37]. The loss of cholinergic axons in AD also shows regional variation. The greatest loss is in the temporal lobe including entorhinal cortex and the hippocampus. Intermediate loss occurs in frontal and parietal association areas, as well as in the insula cortex and temporal pole. Primary motor, somatosensory and visual cortex, and the anterior cingulate undergo only a mild loss [37].

4.3. Calcium flux in neurons

Regulation of calcium flux within neurons is of great importance for synaptic plasticity. CaM kinase II is enriched in neurons susceptible to NFT formation. Some cortical neurons containing the calcium binding protein calbindin are enriched in normal aging but reduced in AD. Outside the cortex, primate nucleus basalis neurons in which calbindin is normally present in high amounts show reduced levels with aging which, if a similar reduction occurs in humans, may render them more susceptible to NFT formation in AD. Parvalbumin-containing neurons are well represented in monkey brain stem nuclei which, in humans, are resistant to NFT formation whereas calbindin neurons are well represented in nuclei that are vulnerable to NFT formation. This calcium binding protein variability with respect to vulnerability of neurons to NFT formation is important but does not on its own fully explain regional NFT distribution in cortex.

5. Clustering and columns in dementia

Subsequent to the Pearson et al. paper [73] it was found that NFT clustering is highly correlated with symptoms: "high numbers of NFTs restricted to small areas are more important in disturbing function than NFTs in a widespread distribution (with the same mean values)" [67]. In addition to the evidence that tangles are selectively distributed across cortical regions and their distribution is linked to symptom progression, this lends weight to the significance of tangle clustering. Although plaques also appear to show a degree of clustering [7] between dendritic clusters [57], the proximity of symptoms to pathology distribution is less striking than it is for tangles. The finding that NFTs are clustered coincidentally across supragranular and infragranular layers provides an important component of the argument that the pathology is distributed to some degree in a columnar fashion.

During embryonic development of the cerebral cortex the cells of the brain migrate towards the surface and form columns of cells. Our understanding of the functional role of these mini-columns is incomplete (see Fig. 1 for a structural description). They appear to be grouped into larger macro-columns, which form the basis of the mapping of functions across the brain's surface. Mini-columns are structurally disorganized in association cortex in AD [15]. Furthermore, the clustering of tangles is positively correlated with the degree of mini-column disruption [15]. A study of Down's syndrome brains suggests that children with the disorder exhibit early adult-like neuronal mini-column spacing [16]. This may relate to the apparently accelerated aging and early onset of AD in Down's syndrome.

Subsequently, the issue of columnar organization and clustering has been pursued with respect to other pathological structures. Disruption of the columnar organization of glial processes has been reported for AD [21]. Lewy bodies and Pick bodies [8,9] also exhibit clustered distributions. The potency of a link between pathology that clusters and mini-column abnormality is also borne out by the finding that mini-columns were disrupted even in the absence of an overall loss of neurons, in a group of patients with Lewy body dementia [15]. In AD, the finding of NFT clustering may offer some insight into the roles that plasticity and connectivity play in the spread of pathology.

6. Columns and connectivity

It is possible that the modular organization of the cortex from mini-columns, to macro-columns, to surface regions, determines the pattern of pathological spread in Alzheimer's disease and, consequently, the pattern of function loss. The progression of pathological changes through anatomically connected regions in AD is consistent with the concept of the disease exploiting the brain's modular organization at the regional level. The macro-column is a smaller anatomical module, which has a diameter reflecting the tangential spread of afferent projections to the cortex of approximately 500–800 microns [84]. Smaller still, at 50–90 microns, is the mini-column. NFT clustering occurs at a similar scale to that of macro-column size. In a follow-up to the 1985 paper Hiorns et al. [47] observed that the distribution of the cells of origin of ipsilateral cortico-cortical projections to a given cortical area were clustered in bands of a similar size to macro-columns and a distribution comparable to that of NFTs in AD.

Casanova [17] has anticipated that "the spread of neurofibrillary tangles (NFT) preferentially to corticopetal neurons causes clustering of the neurodegenerative changes which reflect modular structure".

The cells of a macro-column are selectively interconnected with those of other macro-columns which share a similar stimulus sensitivity. The development of NFT in neurons of layers III and V is consistent with the spatial coincidence of supragranular and infragranular NFT clusters due to shared connectivity of cells in the same macro-column. Consequently NFT clustering may reflect the selective grouping of connections which is fundamental to columnar organization (Fig. 2). However, the formation of columns also depends on the segregation of competing inputs and this requires neuronal plasticity.

7. Columns and neuronal plasticity

The most common macro-columns investigated are the ocular dominance and orientation preference columns of visual cortex. This columnar organization is dependent on excitatory competition and cell plasticity. Glutamate (NMDAR1) receptor function is required for the development of orientation selectivity [81] and manipulation of GABAergic inhibition perturbs the development of columnar architecture [46]. Markers of dendritic arborization also reflect macro-column organization during development [34]. SMI32 neurofilament protein is absent at ocular dominance column borders and as a result of monocular stimulus deprivation its distribution is altered. In monocular deprived dominance columns MAP2 is reduced, concomitant with a reduction in size of the deprived columns. When age related dendritic remodeling occurs, as the demand for plasticity increases again late in life, the association between macro-column size and MAP2 expression may be informative.

Myelin staining also varies in distribution according to macro-columnar organization during development.

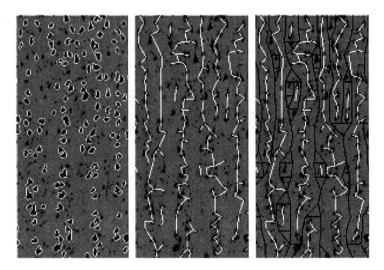

Fig. 1. (Left) Large pyramidal cells (outlined in white), can be used by minicolumn detection software (see ref. 16) to identify areas of high cell concentration. (Middle) White lines depict the geometric minimum distance trees defining the cores of the minicolumns. (Right) Black lines depict the boundaries of the areas of high cell concentration, used to compute minicolumn width and spacing.

It is more intense in ocular dominance column centers compared to the column borders and becomes darker and wider in columns dominant due to monocular stimulus deprivation. If myelination is linked to pathological susceptibility in AD, one may expect that the myelin sparse macro-column borders will show greater vulnerability. It is not clear how macro-columns are affected in AD, but age-related cortical shrinkage and the disruption of mini-columns suggests that macro-columns may become smaller and less defined. A smaller myelinated core and greater disruption of the periphery would exaggerate this process.

Regional variation in the extent of remodeling seems to reflect the hierarchy of dendrite complexity, with greater remodeling occurring in areas containing more complex and more spinous processes. The demand for remodeling to integrate associations in an aging network may be most intense in these regions. Just as the dendritic complexity of pyramidal neurons in association cortex tends to be greater than that of neurons in the primary sensory regions [28] so too mini-column number and spacing reflect the hierarchical relationship between primary and association auditory cortex, with wider mini-columns in the association cortex [19].

8. Columns and cortical cholinergic innervation

One of the first groups of cells to be lost in Alzheimer's disease are cholinergic neurons in the nucleus basalis of Meynert and other nuclei such as the diagonal band and medial septum that normally project to the hippocampus and mesial temporal region [37, 99].

The cholinergic system stimulates both muscarinic and nicotinic receptors. Several of the normal actions of activating these receptors may render cells that lose their cholinergic innervation vulnerable to Alzheimer's pathology. Protein kinase C is a common second messenger coupled to both M1 and M3 muscarinic receptors. One of its actions is to enhance α-secretase which cleaves the AβPP molecule and inhibits formation of amyloid protein. It also inhibits glycogen synthase kinase-3 (GSK3) which phosphorylates tau. Muscarinic agonists therefore increase non-amyloidogenic metabolism of AβPP and reduce tau phosphorylation [36,65]. The nicotinic α7 receptor is the receptor for amyloid. Amyloid binding to the receptor may stimulate pathology in AD, including tau phosphorylation [95].

Acetylcholine projections are known to innervate the cerebral cortex in a modular distribution, spanning macro-columns, and are believed to contribute to relevant stimulus detection by excitation of the stimulus-sensitive column and inhibition of the surrounding columns. Cholinergic innervation of macro-columns can be altered by behavioral conditioning in animals [97]. Auditory cortex is particularly densely innervated by cholinergic projections, and this may contribute to this region's comparative resistance to pathology. It may also confer sensitivity to the effect of anticholinesterase medication on this region since

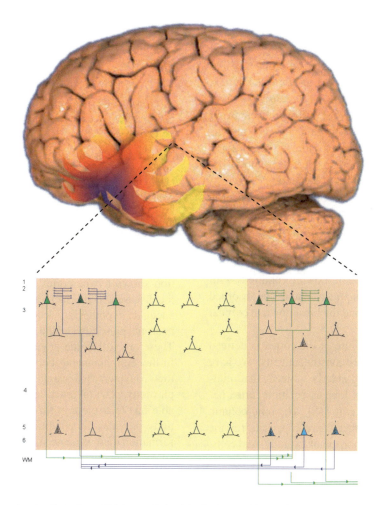

Fig. 2. (Top) The purple, red and yellow glow of high neural plasticity is shown with its origin in olfactory areas of the medial and anterior temporal cortex. Its spread seems to reflect the spread of AD pathology. (Bottom) The columnar organisation of connections and tangle distribution in a cross-section of superior temporal association cortex is illustrated schematically. Layer III pyramidal cells sending feedforward connections through the white matter (WM) are green, layer V pyramidal cells sending feedback connections are blue. Pink and yellow zones are macrocolumns demonstrating selective connectivity to each other (pink connects to pink). Tangles (black filled cells) cluster in macrocolumns.

conditioning-related responses in auditory cortex can be manipulated in humans by altering levels of acetylcholine.

9. Columns and inhibitory neurons

Acetylcholine projections from the Basal nucleus innervate a proportion of inhibitory interneurons. The innervation of nicotinic receptors on inhibitory cells in layer V excites the vertical axons of inhibitory cells to upper layers, therefore, enhancing columnar inhibition. Many of the inhibitory neurons in receipt of cholinergic projections have the columnar dendritic morphology and electrophysiological properties of double bouquet cells [100]. This is a major class of calbindin-containing interneurons. We have found calbindin-cell size is larger in subjects with larger minicolumns. High immunoreactivity to calbindin is also found (in layers III and IV) at the borders of macro-columns and it is thought to be associated with synaptic competition on excitatory neurons [34]. Calbindin in neurons appears to be relatively protective in aging, but may be lost as AD advances [42,52]. Therefore an interaction between acetylcholine, calbindin cell inhibition, and columnar organization in AD is plausible.

10. Columns and normal aging

In normal aging a distributed synaptic loss may be absorbed as cortical shrinkage with only a subtle effect on cognitive performance. Degeneration of terminal dendrites is prominent in Layer 1 in prefrontal cortex, with a 30–60% reduction of synapse density per unit volume, in aging monkeys [78]. A 46% decrease in spine number and density has been reported in humans over 50 years old [54]. However, a threshold appears to be reached that marks the boundary between normal decline with aging and the onset of dementia. The transition involves additional synaptic loss as well as neuron loss and the development of plaques and tangles that are the pathological hallmarks of AD. In AD, synapse loss exceeds that which can be accounted for by neuron loss through NFT formation [49] and is likely to be an early event in degeneration showing continuity with normal aging. Further synaptic loss cannot be absorbed by the neuronal network and the breakdown in cortical structure becomes focal.

The mini-column structure of the cortex is defined by the contacts between its constituent cells. We have shown, in work on normal elderly subjects, that mini-column width in temporal lobe association cortex becomes less with normal aging [18]. The mini-column represents a larger unit that can compensate for the lost connections of a proportion of its individual cells. However, as more synapses and dendrites are lost the column structure will begin to break down. In monkeys, mini-columns in the frontal cortex become more disorganized with increasing age and this disorganization is correlated with age-related cognitive decline [23]. The apparently greater deficit of plasticity in association cortex reflects regional differences in the effect of aging on minicolumn structure. In normal human aging, there is mini-column narrowing in middle temporal and superior temporal auditory association cortex, while the normally more narrowly spaced mini-columns of primary auditory cortex show little change [18] (Fig. 3). A threshold will be reached sooner in areas of cortex with minimal redundancy, such as the serially connected entorhinal-hippocampal pathway [48]. At this point the benefit of columnar organization is lost and the coordinated connectivity of mini-columnar units reveals its double-edged nature as it provides a basis for the focal clustering of pathological features with the result that the clustering of tangles is positively correlated with the degree of mini-column disruption [15].

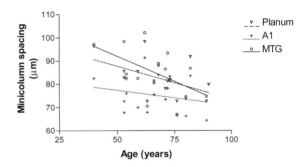

Fig. 3. Scatterplot with best fit regression lines. Columns become thinner with increasing age in temporal lobe association cortex of the MTG (middle temporal gyrus) ($r - 0.53$, $p < 0.05$) and Planum temporale (BA 22) ($r - 0.49$, $p < 0.05$) but the correlation does not hold for primary auditory cortex (A1) ($r - 0.21$, $p = 0.44$).

11. Conclusion

The regional selectivity with respect to NFT formation shown by the cortex in AD is a core feature of the disease and still lacks a full explanation. The most adequate hypothesis to account for it is, in our opinion, neuronal plasticity and the mechanisms that underlie it. These are still in the process of being elucidated and further enlightenment about AD can be expected to follow from increased insights into the nature of neuronal plasticity. The hibernation model seems to us a valuable one to explore in this context. If neuronal plasticity provides the conditions needed to support NFT formation there is no need to postulate any progressive spread of an etiological 'agent'.

The columnar distribution of NFT in association cortex in AD reflects the fate of mini- and macro-columns with their integral contribution to cortical organization. Methods of study that are sensitive to this organization have more to contribute to an understanding both of neuronal plasticity and of brain aging and AD.

The thinking behind the Pearson et al. paper [73] was that neuroanatomical knowledge has much to contribute to an understanding of AD. In the intervening years neuroanatomists have continued to provide significant insights about the disease. Are such contributions still relevant today? We think they are. Transgenic animal models of AD show a non-uniform anatomical distribution of pathology that needs interpretation in the light of neuroanatomical knowledge. Neural plasticity, which we have suggested may have an important role to play in the etiology of the disease, is regionally restricted and reflects neuroanatomical reality. And the dismantling of specific cortico-cortical connections, which determines the phenotypic expression of the disease, can only be understood on the basis of neuroanatomical knowledge. Long may the neuroanatomical-neuropathological connection flourish in AD research.

References

[1] L.F. Agnati, F. Benfenati, V. Solfrini, G. Biagini, K. Fuxe, D. Guidolin, C. Carani and I. Zini, Brain aging and neuronal plasticity, *Ann N Y Acad Sci* **673** (1992), 180–186.

[2] T. Arendt, Synaptic plasticity and cell cycle activation in neurons are alternative effector pathways: the Dr. Jekyll and Mr. Hyde concept of Alzheimer's disease or the yin and yang of neuroplasticity, *Prog Neurobiol* **71** (2003), 83–248.

[3] T. Arendt, Neurodegeneration and plasticity, *Int J Dev Neurosci* **22** (2004), 507–514.

[4] T. Arendt, V. Bigl, A. Tennstedt and A. Arendt, Neuronal loss in different parts of the nucleus basalis is related to neuritic plaque formation in cortical target areas in Alzheimer's disease, *Neuroscience* **14** (1985), 1–14.

[5] T. Arendt, M.K. Bruckner, H.J. Gertz and L. Marcova, Cortical distribution of neurofibrillary tangles in Alzheimer's disease matches the pattern of neurons that retain their capacity of plastic remodelling in the adult brain, *Neuroscience* **83** (1998), 991–1002.

[6] T. Arendt, C. Schindler, M.K. Bruckner, K. Eschrich, V. Bigl, D. Zedlick and L. Marcova, Plastic neuronal remodeling is impaired in patients with Alzheimer's disease carrying apolipoprotein epsilon 4 allele, *J Neurosci* **17** (1997), 516–529.

[7] R.A. Armstrong, Is the clustering of beta-amyloid (A beta) deposits in the frontal cortex of Alzheimer patients determined by blood vessels? *Neurosci Lett* **195** (1995), 121–124.

[8] R.A. Armstrong, N.J. Cairns and P.L. Lantos, Dementia with Lewy bodies: clustering of Lewy bodies in human patients, *Neurosci Lett* **224** (1997), 41–44.

[9] R.A. Armstrong, N.J. Cairns and P.L. Lantos, Clustering of Pick bodies in patients with Pick's disease, *Neurosci Lett* **242** (1998), 81–84.

[10] P.V. Arriagada, J.H. Growdon, E.T. Hedley-Whyte and B.T. Hyman, Neurofibrillary tangles but not senile plaques parallel duration and severity of Alzheimer's disease, *Neurology* **42** (1992), 631–639.

[11] L.M. Bierer, P.R. Hof, D.P. Purohit, L. Carlin, J. Schmeidler, K.L. Davis and D.P. Perl, Neocortical neurofibrillary tangles correlate with dementia severity in Alzheimer's disease, *Arch Neurol* **52** (1995), 81–88.

[12] L.M. Billings, S. Oddo, K.N. Green, J.L. McGaugh and F.M. Laferla, Intraneuronal Abeta causes the onset of early Alzheimer's disease-related cognitive deficits in transgenic mice, *Neuron* **45** (2005), 675–688.

[13] H. Braak and E. Braak, Neuropathological stageing of Alzheimer-related changes, *Acta Neuropathol (Berl)* **82** (1991), 239–259.

[14] A. Brun and E. Englund, Regional pattern of degeneration in Alzheimer's disease: neuronal loss and histopathological grading, *Histopathology* **5** (1981), 549–564.

[15] S.V. Buldyrev, L. Cruz, T. Gomez-Isla, E. Gomez-Tortosa, S. Havlin, R. Le, H.E. Stanley, B. Urbanc and B.T. Hyman, Description of microcolumnar ensembles in association cortex and their disruption in Alzheimer and Lewy body dementias, *Proc Natl Acad Sci USA* **97** (2000), 5039–5043.

[16] D. Buxhoeveden, A. Fobbs, E. Roy and M. Casanova, Quantitative comparison of radial cell columns in children with Down's syndrome and controls, *J Intellect Disabil Res* **46** (2002), 76–81.

[17] M.F. Casanova, Modular concepts of brain organization and the neuropathology of psychiatric conditions, *Psychiatry Res* **118** (2003), 101–102.

[18] S.A. Chance, M. Casanova, A.E. Switala, T.J. Crow and M.M. Esiri, Minicolumn thinning in temporal lobe association cortex but not primary auditory cortex in normal human ageing, *Acta Neuropathologica* (in press).

[19] S.A. Chance, The ageing human brain: regional hierarchy of subtle columnar changes, *Nutrition and Health* (in press).

[20] S. Christen-Zaech, R. Kraftsik, O. Pillevuit, M. Kiraly, R. Martins, K. Khalili and J. Miklossy, Early olfactory involvement in Alzheimer's disease, *Can J Neurol Sci* **30** (2003), 20–25.

[21] J.A. Colombo, B. Quinn and V. Puissant, Disruption of astroglial interlaminar processes in Alzheimer's disease, *Brain Res Bull* **58** (2002), 235–242.

[22] D.H. Cribbs, B.Y. Azizeh, C.W. Cotman and F.M. LaFerla, Fibril formation and neurotoxicity by a herpes simplex virus glycoprotein B fragment with homology to the Alzheimer's A beta peptide, *Biochemistry* **39** (2000), 5988–5994.

[23] L. Cruz, D.L. Roe, B. Urbanc, H. Cabral, H.E. Stanley and D.L. Rosene, Age-related reduction in microcolumnar structure in area 46 of the rhesus monkey correlates with behavioral decline, *Proc Natl Acad Sci USA* **101** (2004), 15846–15851.

[24] D.C. Davies, J.W. Brooks and D.A. Lewis, Axonal loss from the olfactory tracts in Alzheimer's disease, *Neurobiol Aging* **14** (1993), 353–357.

[25] M.C. De Lacoste and C.L. White, 3rd, The role of cortical connectivity in Alzheimer's disease pathogenesis: a review and model system, *Neurobiol Aging* **14** (1993), 1–16.

[26] F. Doetsch and R. Hen, Young and excitable: the function of new neurons in the adult mammalian brain, *Curr Opin Neurobiol* **15** (2005), 121–128.

[27] R.L. Doty, D.P. Perl, J.C. Steele, K.M. Chen, J.D. Pierce, Jr., P. Reyes and L.T. Kurland, Olfactory dysfunction in three neurodegenerative diseases, *Geriatrics* **46**(1) (1991), 47–51.

[28] G.N. Elston and M.G. Rosa, Pyramidal cells, patches, and cortical columns: a comparative study of infragranular neurons in TEO, TE, and the superior temporal polysensory area of the macaque monkey, *J Neurosci* **20** (2000), RC117.

[29] M.M. Esiri, Herpes simplex encephalitis. An immunohistological study of the distribution of viral antigen within the brain, *J Neurol Sci* **54** (1982), 209–226.

[30] M.M. Esiri, R.C. Pearson, J.E. Steele, D.M. Bowen and T.P. Powell, A quantitative study of the neurofibrillary tangles and the choline acetyltransferase activity in the cerebral cortex and the amygdala in Alzheimer's disease, *J Neurol Neurosurg Psychiatry* **53** (1990), 161–165.

[31] M.M. Esiri and G.K. Wilcock, The olfactory bulbs in Alzheimer's disease, *J Neurol Neurosurg Psychiatry* **47** (1984), 56–60.

[32] M.M. Esiri and G.K. Wilcock, Cerebral amyloid angiopathy in dementia and old age, *J Neurol Neurosurg Psychiatry* **49** (1986), 1221–1226.

[33] J.I. Feldman, C. Murphy, T.M. Davidson, A.A. Jalowayski and G.G. de Jaime, The rhinologic evaluation of Alzheimer's disease, *Laryngoscope* **101** (1991), 1198–1202.

[34] S.B. Fenstemaker, L. Kiorpes and J.A. Movshon, Effects of experimental strabismus on the architecture of macaque monkey striate cortex, *J Comp Neurol* **438** (2001), 300–317.

[35] H. Ferreyra-Moyano and E. Barragan, The olfactory system and Alzheimer's disease, *Int J Neurosci* **49** (1989), 157–197.

[36] O.V. Forlenza, J.M. Spink, R. Dayanandan, B.H. Anderton, O.F. Olesen and S. Lovestone, Muscarinic agonists reduce tau phosphorylation in non-neuronal cells via GSK-3beta inhibition and in neurons, *J Neural Transm* **107** (2000), 1201–1212.

[37] C. Geula, Abnormalities of neural circuitry in Alzheimer's disease: hippocampus and cortical cholinergic innervation, *Neurology* **51** (1998), S18–29; discussion S65–67.

[38] H.A. Ghanbari, K. Ghanbari, P.L. Harris, P.K. Jones, Z. Kubat, R.J. Castellani, B.L. Wolozin, M.A. Smith and G. Perry, Oxidative damage in cultured human olfactory neurons from Alzheimer's disease patients, *Aging Cell* **3** (2004), 41–44.

[39] P. Giannakopoulos, P.R. Hof and C. Bouras, Selective vulnerability of neocortical association areas in Alzheimer's disease, *Microsc Res Tech* **43** (1998), 16–23.

[40] A. Goate, M.C. Chartier-Harlin, M. Mullan, J. Brown, F. Crawford, L. Fidani, L. Giuffra, A. Haynes, N. Irving, L. James et al., Segregation of a missense mutation in the amyloid precursor protein gene with familial Alzheimer's disease, *Nature* **349** (1991), 704–706.

[41] W.B. Grant, A. Campbell, R.F. Itzhaki and J. Savory, The significance of environmental factors in the etiology of Alzheimer's disease, *J Alzheimers Dis* **4** (2002), 179–189.

[42] J.R. Greene, N. Radenahmad, G.K. Wilcock, J.W. Neal and R.C. Pearson, Accumulation of calbindin in cortical pyramidal cells with ageing; a putative protective mechanism which fails in Alzheimer's disease, *Neuropathol Appl Neurobiol* **27** (2001), 339–342.

[43] J. Hardy and D. Allsop, Amyloid deposition as the central event in the aetiology of Alzheimer's disease, *Trends Pharmacol Sci* **12** (1991), 383–388.

[44] J.A. Hardy and G.A. Higgins, Alzheimer's disease: the amyloid cascade hypothesis, *Science* **256** (1992), 184–185.

[45] P.J. Harrison and R.C. Pearson, Olfaction and psychiatry, *Br J Psychiatry* **155** (1989), 822–828.

[46] T.K. Hensch and M.P. Stryker, Columnar architecture sculpted by GABA circuits in developing cat visual cortex, *Science* **303** (2004), 1678–1681.

[47] R.W. Hiorns, J.W. Neal, R.C. Pearson and T.P. Powell, Clustering of ipsilateral cortico-cortical projection neurons to area 7 in the rhesus monkey, *Proc Biol Sci* **246** (1991), 1–9.

[48] P.R. Hof, T. Bussiere, G. Gold, E. Kovari, P. Giannakopoulos, C. Bouras, D.P. Perl and J.H. Morrison, Stereologic evidence for persistence of viable neurons in layer II of the entorhinal cortex and the CA1 field in Alzheimer disease, *J Neuropathol Exp Neurol* **62** (2003), 55–67.

[49] P.R. Hof and J.H. Morrison, The aging brain: morpho-molecular senescence of cortical circuits, *Trends Neurosci* **27** (2004), 607–613.

[50] B.T. Hyman, P.V. Arriagada and G.W. Van Hoesen, Pathologic changes in the olfactory system in aging and Alzheimer's disease, *Ann N Y Acad Sci* **640** (1991), 14–19.

[51] B.T. Hyman, G.W. Van Horsen, A.R. Damasio and C.L. Barnes, Alzheimer's disease: cell-specific pathology isolates the hippocampal formation, *Science* **225** (1984), 1168–1170.

[52] S. Iritani, K. Niizato and P.C. Emson, Relationship of calbindin D28K-immunoreactive cells and neuropathological changes in the hippocampal formation of Alzheimer's disease, *Neuropathology* **21** (2001), 162–167.

[53] R.F. Itzhaki, W.R. Lin, D. Shang, G.K. Wilcock, B. Faragher and G.A. Jamieson, Herpes simplex virus type 1 in brain and risk of Alzheimer's disease, *Lancet* **349** (1997), 241–244.

[54] B. Jacobs, L. Driscoll and M. Schall, Life-span dendritic and spine changes in areas 10 and 18 of human cortex: a quantitative Golgi study, *J Comp Neurol* **386** (1997), 661–680.

[55] G.A. Jamieson, N.J. Maitland, G.K. Wilcock, J. Craske and R.F. Itzhaki, Latent herpes simplex virus type 1 in normal and Alzheimer's disease brains, *J Med Virol* **33** (1991), 224–227.

[56] E.G. Jones, Making brain connections: neuroanatomy and the work of TPS Powell, 1923–1996, *Annu Rev Neurosci* **22** (1999), 49–103.

[57] K.S. Kosik, J. Rogers and N.W. Kowall, Senile plaques are located between apical dendritic clusters, *J Neuropathol Exp Neurol* **46** (1987), 1–11.

[58] T. Kovacs, N.J. Cairns and P.L. Lantos, beta-amyloid deposition and neurofibrillary tangle formation in the olfactory bulb in ageing and Alzheimer's disease, *Neuropathol Appl Neurobiol* **25** (1999), 481–491.

[59] T. Kovacs, N.J. Cairns and P.L. Lantos, Olfactory centres in Alzheimer's disease: olfactory bulb is involved in early Braak's stages, *Neuroreport* **12** (2001), 285–288.

[60] P. Liberini, S. Parola, P.F. Spano and L. Antonini, Olfaction in Parkinson's disease: methods of assessment and clinical relevance, *J Neurol* **247** (2000), 88–96.

[61] L.D. Loopuijt and J.B. Sebens, Loss of dopamine receptors in the olfactory bulb of patients with Alzheimer's disease, *Brain Res* **529** (1990), 239–244.

[62] A. McShea, P.L. Harris, K.R. Webster, A.F. Wahl and M.A. Smith, Abnormal expression of the cell cycle regulators P16 and CDK4 in Alzheimer's disease, *Am J Pathol* **150** (1997), 1933–1939.

[63] R.I. Mesholam, P.J. Moberg, R.N. Mahr and R.L. Doty, Olfaction in neurodegenerative disease: a meta-analysis of olfactory functioning in Alzheimer's and Parkinson's diseases, *Arch Neurol* **55** (1998), 84–90.

[64] M.M. Mesulam, Neuroplasticity failure in Alzheimer's disease: bridging the gap between plaques and tangles, *Neuron* **24** (1999), 521–529.

[65] D. Muller, H. Wiegmann, U. Langer, S. Moltzen-Lenz and R.M. Nitsch, Lu 25–109, a combined m1 agonist and m2 antagonist, modulates regulated processing of the amyloid precursor protein of Alzheimer's disease, *J Neural Transm* **105** (1998), 1029–1043.

[66] C. Murphy and S. Jinich, Olfactory dysfunction in Down's Syndrome, *Neurobiol Aging* **17** (1996), 631–637.

[67] Z. Nagy, M.M. Esiri, K.A. Jobst, J.H. Morris, E.M. King, B. McDonald, S. Litchfield and L. Barnetson, Clustering of pathological features in Alzheimer's disease: clinical and neuroanatomical aspects, *Dementia* **7** (1996), 121–127.

[68] Z. Nagy, M.M. Esiri, K.A. Jobst, J.H. Morris, E.M. King, B. McDonald, S. Litchfield, A. Smith, L. Barnetson and A.D. Smith, Relative roles of plaques and tangles in the dementia of Alzheimer's disease: correlations using three sets of neuropathological criteria, *Dementia* **6** (1995), 21–31.

[69] Z. Nagy, M.M. Esiri and A.D. Smith, Expression of cell division markers in the hippocampus in Alzheimer's disease and other neurodegenerative conditions, *Acta Neuropathol (Berl)* **93** (1997), 294–300.

[70] Z. Nagy, M.M. Esiri and A.D. Smith, The cell division cycle and the pathophysiology of Alzheimer's disease, *Neuroscience* **87** (1998), 731–739.

[71] S. Oddo, L. Billings, J.P. Kesslak, D.H. Cribbs and F.M. LaFerla, Abeta immunotherapy leads to clearance of early, but not late, hyperphosphorylated tau aggregates via the proteasome, *Neuron* **43** (2004), 321–332.

[72] O. Ogawa, X. Zhu, H.G. Lee, A. Raina, M.E. Obrenovich, R. Bowser, H.A. Ghanbari, R.J. Castellani, G. Perry and M.A. Smith, Ectopic localization of phosphorylated histone H3 in Alzheimer's disease: a mitotic catastrophe? *Acta Neuropathol (Berl)* **105** (2003), 524–528.

[73] R.C. Pearson, M.M. Esiri, R.W. Hiorns, G.K. Wilcock and T.P. Powell, Anatomical correlates of the distribution of the pathological changes in the neocortex in Alzheimer disease, *Proc Natl Acad Sci USA* **82** (1985), 4531–4534.

[74] R.C. Pearson and T.P. Powell, The neuroanatomy of Alzheimer's disease, *Rev Neurosci* **2** (1989), 101–122.

[75] D.P. Perl and P.F. Good, Aluminum, Alzheimer's disease, and the olfactory system, *Ann N Y Acad Sci* **640** (1991), 8–13.

[76] G. Perry, R.J. Castellani, M.A. Smith, P.L. Harris, Z. Kubat, K. Ghanbari, P.K. Jones, G. Cordone, M. Tabaton, B. Wolozin and H. Ghanbari, Oxidative damage in the olfactory system in Alzheimer's disease, *Acta Neuropathol (Berl)* **106** (2003), 552–556.

[77] E. Persson, J. Henriksson, J. Tallkvist, C. Rouleau and H. Tjalve, Transport and subcellular distribution of intranasally administered zinc in the olfactory system of rats and pikes, *Toxicology* **191** (2003), 97–108.

[78] A. Peters, C. Sethares and M.B. Moss, The effects of aging on layer 1 in area 46 of prefrontal cortex in the rhesus monkey, *Cereb Cortex* **8** (1998), 671–684.

[79] J.L. Price, P.B. Davis, J.C. Morris and D.L. White, The distribution of tangles, plaques and related immunohistochemical markers in healthy aging and Alzheimer's disease, *Neurobiol Aging* **12** (1991), 295–312.

[80] R.B. Pyles, The association of herpes simplex virus and Alzheimer's disease: a potential synthesis of genetic and environmental factors, *Herpes* **8** (2001), 64–68.

[81] A.S. Ramoa, A.F. Mower, D. Liao and S.I. Jafri, Suppression of cortical NMDA receptor function prevents development of orientation selectivity in the primary visual cortex, *J Neurosci* **21** (2001), 4299–4309.

[82] P.F. Reyes, D.A. Deems and M.G. Suarez, Olfactory-related changes in Alzheimer's disease: a quantitative neuropathologic study, *Brain Res Bull* **32** (1993), 1–5.

[83] P.F. Reyes, G.T. Golden, P.L. Fagel, R.G. Fariello, L. Katz and E. Carner, The prepiriform cortex in dementia of the Alzheimer type, *Arch Neurol* **44** (1987), 644–645.

[84] H.L. Seldon, Structure of human auditory cortex. II. Axon distributions and morphological correlates of speech perception, *Brain Res* **229** (1981), 295–310.

[85] D.J. Selkoe, Cell biology of the amyloid beta-protein precursor and the mechanism of Alzheimer's disease, *Annu Rev Cell Biol* **10** (1994), 373–403.

[86] R.G. Struble and H.B. Clark, Olfactory bulb lesions in Alzheimer's disease, *Neurobiol Aging* **13** (1992), 469–473.

[87] M. Tabaton, S. Cammarata, G.L. Mancardi, G. Cordone, G. Perry and C. Loeb, Abnormal tau-reactive filaments in olfactory mucosa in biopsy specimens of patients with probable Alzheimer's disease, *Neurology* **41** (1991), 391–394.

[88] B.R. Talamo, R. Rudel, K.S. Kosik, V.M. Lee, S. Neff, L. Adelman and J.S. Kauer, Pathological changes in olfactory neurons in patients with Alzheimer's disease, *Nature* **337** (1989), 736–739.

[89] M.D. Thompson, K. Knee and C.J. Golden, Olfaction in persons with Alzheimer's disease, *Neuropsychol Rev* **8** (1998), 11–23.

[90] A.H. Tomlinson and M.M. Esiri, Herpes simplex encephalitis. Immunohistological demonstration of spread of virus via olfactory pathways in mice, *J Neurol Sci* **60** (1983), 473–484.

[91] J.Q. Trojanowski, P.D. Newman, W.D. Hill and V.M. Lee, Human olfactory epithelium in normal aging, Alzheimer's disease, and other neurodegenerative disorders, *J Comp Neurol* **310** (1991), 365–376.

[92] Y. Tsuboi, Z.K. Wszolek, N.R. Graff-Radford, N. Cookson and D.W. Dickson, Tau pathology in the olfactory bulb correlates with Braak stage, Lewy body pathology and apolipoprotein epsilon4, *Neuropathol Appl Neurobiol* **29** (2003), 503–510.

[93] I. Vincent, M. Rosado and P. Davies, Mitotic mechanisms in Alzheimer's disease? *J Cell Biol* **132** (1996), 413–425.

[94] E.K. Wagner and D.C. Bloom, Experimental investigation of herpes simplex virus latency, *Clin Microbiol Rev* **10** (1997), 419–443.

[95] H.Y. Wang, D.H. Lee, C.B. Davis and R.P. Shank, Amyloid peptide Abeta(1–42) binds selectively and with picomolar affinity to alpha7 nicotinic acetylcholine receptors, *J Neurochem* **75** (2000), 1155–1161.

[96] G.K. Wilcock and M.M. Esiri, Plaques, tangles and dementia. A quantitative study, *J Neurol Sci* **56** (1982), 343–356.

[97] N.J. Woolf, Global and serial neurons form A hierarchically arranged interface proposed to underlie memory and cognition, *Neuroscience* **74** (1996), 625–651.

[98] Z.K. Wszolek and K. Markopoulou, Olfactory dysfunction in Parkinson's disease, *Clin Neurosci* **5** (1998), 94–101.

[99] Z.J. Wynn and J.L. Cummings, Cholinesterase inhibitor therapies and neuropsychiatric manifestations of Alzheimer's disease, *Dement Geriatr Cogn Disord* **17** (2004), 100–108.

[100] Z. Xiang, J.R. Huguenard and D.A. Prince, Cholinergic switching within neocortical inhibitory networks, *Science* **281** (1998), 985–988.

Synaptic remodeling during aging and in Alzheimer's disease

Eliezer Masliah[a,b,*], Leslie Crews[a] and Lawrence Hansen[a,b]
[a]*Department of Neurosciences, University of California, San Diego, La Jolla, California, USA*
[b]*Department of Pathology, University of California, San Diego, La Jolla, California, USA*

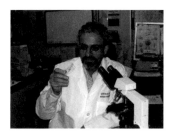

Abstract. Cognitive functioning is dependent on synapse density in the brain. Factors modulating synapse density might include the balance between synaptic pruning and sprouting. Loss of synapses during aging might explain cognitive decline and while previous reports have suggested a 10–15% synapse loss occurs during the normal aging process, more recent studies have found that decline in synaptic density only occurs after 65 years of age. In this context, the main objective of this manuscript is to discuss the findings of our 1993 study in light of more recent studies in aging, synapses and Alzheimer's disease.

Keywords: Alzheimer's disease, amyloid, synapse loss, synaptic plasticity, AβPP

1. Introduction

Since the seminal contribution by Alois Alzheimer in 1907 [2], considerable progress has been made in understanding the pathogenesis and etiology of this devastating neurological condition. Because familial Alzheimer's disease (AD) is associated with mutations within the amyloid β-protein precursor (AβPP) gene [32,39,104] or the β-secretase complex [101], a regulator of amyloid β protein (Aβ) production, most studies have focused at understanding the role of Aβ protein in the mechanisms of neuronal damage and neurodegeneration. However, several lines of evidence suggest that although the amyloid deposits and the plaques are useful diagnostic markers, they are not the best correlate to the neuronal damage and cognitive alterations. In fact, we, as well as several other groups, have found that synaptic damage is an early pathological hallmark of AD [19,38,47,59,65,79,80,91] and that it is the best correlate to the cognitive deficits in these patients [20,102,108]. Therefore the physical basis for the dementia in AD is the loss of synaptic contacts, although other AD-related pathologies might also participate [5].

These findings were brought about by the question as to what extent synapse loss in AD is part of the spectrum of synaptic remodeling during aging, or if it is an independent pathological process [87,109] (Fig. 1). In response to this query, in the early 90's we undertook a study to further understand the effects of aging on synapse loss in AD, as well as its relationship to amyloid deposition in non-demented controlled aged individuals [73]. For this purpose, sections from the frontal cortex of control (ages 16–98 years) and AD patients were double-labeled with antibodies against synaptophysin (a synaptic marker) and Aβ protein and analyzed by confocal microscopy. We found that individuals older than 60 years of age had an average 20% decrease in synapse density compared with individuals younger than 60 years of age. There were no significant correlations between the age and the number of

*Corresponding author: Dr. E. Masliah, Department of Neurosciences, University of California, San Diego, La Jolla, CA 92093-0624, USA. Tel.: 858 534 8992; Fax: 858 534 6232; E-mail: emasliah@ucsd.edu.

amyloid-positive plaques or between synaptic density and the number of amyloid plaques. Further analysis of the digitized serial optical images showed focal areas of synapse loss and distended synaptophysin-containing boutons in the mature plaques of the normal aged cases. However, we found no microscopic changes in the synaptic content inside and outside the diffuse plaques. Taken together, the data suggested that a loss of synaptic input in the neocortex is an age-dependent factor that contributes to the overall synaptic loss in AD, but that this might be largely independent of the amyloid deposits [73].

As part of this Alzheimer Anniversary Issue of the Journal, the main objective of this manuscript is to discuss the findings of our 1993 study in the context of more recent studies in aging, synapses and AD.

2. Synapse loss during the aging process

Mild decline of cognitive functions is a known occurrence during normal aging. Functions that decline include speed of learning, performance and name recall [89]. However, vocabulary, information storage and several other executive functions are not affected as is the case in AD patients [89]. The substrate of the cognitive decline during aging has long been a subject of controversy; initial studies focused at the potential role of neuronal loss. However, studies by Terry et al. [105] and Haug et al. [40] demonstrated that in human brains, total neuronal populations do not decline but rather shrink into a smaller size class. This suggested that reduction in the synapto-dendritic complexity might precede the changes in the neuronal cell body. In the 70's and 80's diverse ultrastructural studies in the aged human brain as well as Golgi impregnation studies showed a significant decrease in the hippocampal dentate gyrus and frontal cortex synapses [1,7,31,46]. Consistent with these studies, our group as well as others have shown that during normal aging there is a 10–15% loss of synapses in the frontal cortex, compared to the 25–50% loss observed in AD [60,73]. Since then, a few more studies in the aging human brain have been published, among them probably the most comprehensive is the one by Scheff et al. [94]. This study utilized short postmortem brain samples from neurologically control patients analyzed by electron microscopy and stereology. This study found that the total synapse density in the superior middle frontal cortex is not decreased in individuals older than 65 years of age, and suggests that the synapse loss in AD might be disease-related rather than part of the aging process [94]. Both studies in experimental animal models as well as in the aging human brain have shown some variability in the results and degree of synapse decline that might correlate with learning deficits [30,86]. Several technical factors might explain the variability observed among various groups, including age range and distribution of samples, homogeneity of brain regions, gender, sampling strategy and method to estimate synapse numbers [94]. However, it is likely that independently of the differences observed by these studies, subtle changes in synaptic functioning and morphology occur during aging that might account for the cognitive decline [73]. A promising direction to investigate such changes in real time is the recent development of transgenic (tg) animal models expressing green fluorescent protein (GFP) and GFP-tagged synaptic and dendritic molecules such as postsynaptic density protein-95 (PSD95), synaptophysin and others that allow imaging of synapses and spines over a period of time using two-photon microscopy laser technology. Recent reports in this direction using GFP-tagged neurons in mice have shown that a fraction of persistent spines grew gradually during development until adulthood. At 6 months of age spines turn over more slowly, possibly reflecting differences in capacity for experience-dependent plasticity [44].

The functional and structural stability of the CNS microcircuitries during aging depends on the stability of the circuitries [42] and on the neuronal capacity to exchange information across the synaptic junction [24]. Neurons generate complex patterns of synaptic interconnectivity that exhibit a remarkable plasticity both during development and adulthood [85]. Synaptic functioning depends on the patterns of synaptic plasticity and density. Synaptic density might depend on synaptic pruning, synaptogenesis, synapse remodeling and spine dynamics, among others [42]. Furthermore, synapse density might depend on the balance between factors promoting synapse pruning and sprouting. During the aging process, decline in spine activity, decreased synaptosomal membrane fluidity [15], increased synapse pruning and reduced expression, and oxidative alterations in cytoskeletal, signaling and vesicle molecules might be responsible for the decreased synaptic function. Other factors mediating synapse and spine stability include expression and activity of calcium dependent proteolytic enzymes such as calpain. On the other hand, decreased activity of regulatory mechanisms involved in remodeling and sprouting, including deficient expression of growth factors, signaling pathways involved or molecules such

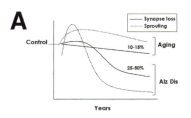 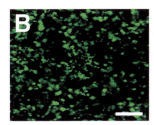 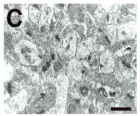

Fig. 1. Synaptic loss and sprouting during aging and in AD. (A) Diagrammatic representation of trends in synapse populations during aging and AD. (B) Presynaptic boutons in aged brain identified by laser scanning confocal microscopy of synaptophysin-labeled sections. (C) Synapses in aged brain visualized by electron microscopy. Bar = 35 μm (B), 15 μm (C).

as growth associated protein-43 (GAP43) might also play a role. Elucidating the mechanisms involved in regulating synaptic density, plasticity and regeneration in the adult CNS has long been an area of intense investigation for both basic neurobiologists and for those interested in developing novel treatments for AD and other neurodegenerative disorders.

3. Synaptic pathology in Alzheimer's disease

Alzheimer's disease is the most common neurodegenerative dementing illness affecting the elderly [27, 50,51]. AD is characterized clinically by progressive cognitive decline and neuropathologically by early loss of synapses (Fig. 2A–D), formation of neurofibrillary tangles (NFTs), and neuritic plaques (NPs) composed of aggregated Aβ in the neocortex and limbic system [28,75,107]. The pathogenesis of the synaptic damage in AD can be divided into two phases: 1) in the early stages, the disease is characterized by synaptic dysfunction (initiation phase; loss of plasticity) and 2) in a second phase, cycles of aberrant sprouting and neuritic disorganization eventually result in neurodegeneration (propagation phase; degeneration).

The progression of the neuropathological lesions including synapse loss in these disorders and their relationship with the cognitive deficits are central to the understanding of the mechanisms involved in dementia [67]. In this regard, studies conducted in patients with early stages of AD suggest that the neurodegenerative process initiates in the entorhinal cortex (EC) resulting in denervation of the hippocampus with loss of synapses in the molecular layer of the dentate gyrus (DG), followed by degeneration of the neocortex and nucleus basalis of Meynert (NbM) [10,11,63,68,72]. Plaque formation, development of NFTs and gliosis accompany this process. Of these pathological changes, early loss of synapses and tangle formation are the strongest correlates to the severity of the dementia [5,

20,108]. This sequence of events is consistent with experimental studies in the aged macaque [61] and in tg models of AD where synaptic loss and memory deficits precede amyloid deposition and plaque formation, but are associated with increased production of Aβ_{1-42} in the limbic system [63,84].

Thus, the dementia in AD is associated with the disruption of neuritic substructure and loss of synaptic contacts in specific cortical and subcortical areas [41]. The damage to these circuitries in early stages of AD results in memory loss followed by attention deficits, judgment impairments, mood changes, confusion and inability to maintain purposeful thinking [76]. Cases displaying clinical and neuropathological features of early or incipient AD showed a significant 20% loss of synapses in the outer molecular layer of the hippocampal DG [90,112]. Cases presenting with more severe disease showed a progressively more significant loss of synapses in the neocortex, as well as in the outer molecular layer of the hippocampal DG [62]. Further supporting these findings, measurements by electron microscopy and immunohistochemistry have both shown very strong correlations between synaptic numbers in the frontal cortex and tests of global cognition in AD [9,20,57,114]. These findings have been confirmed by immunochemical quantification of various synaptic proteins [114,118]. For example, the levels of the synaptic-like marker EP10 in all cortical areas and the hippocampus were correlated ($p < 0.05 - 0.01$) with the Blessed test, but not with the Object Memory Examination [21]. The concomitant atrophy and loss of dendritic spines in AD also contributes to the severity of dementia [3,8].

Ultrastructural analyses have shown a highly significant AD-related decline in synaptic numbers in lamina III and V in both superior and middle temporal gyrus [92] and cingulate cortex [94]. There were no correlations between synaptic density and synaptic apposition length or density of senile plaques [92]. In contrast, in the EC no change in synaptic density was

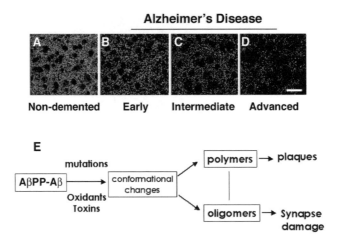

Fig. 2. Progressive synapse loss in AD. (A-D) Representative images of synaptic integrity in a non-demented control (A) and progressive synapse loss in early (B), intermediate (C) and advanced (D) AD. (E) Mechanisms involved in amyloid-mediated synapse loss in AD. Bar = 20 μm.

observed between control and AD, in either lamina III or V [93]. This preservation of synaptic numbers may be related to a plastic response that is greater in the entorhinal area than in other areas of the cortex [92]. In advanced stages of the disease, decline in synapse density is often accompanied by increased synapse size representing a compensatory response. In more advanced AD cases, as well as in cases with DLB, there is an approximate 30 to 50% loss of synapses in the frontal, parietal and temporal cortex [19,38,69,78,80,112]. In addition, ultrastructural studies have shown that in AD the synapses are swollen and abnormally accumulate cytoskeletal proteins, vesicles and lysosomes [33,34, 65]. For a comprehensive review on synapse loss and pathology the reader is advised to consult Jones and Harris [48] and Scheff and Price [95].

In addition to the extensive synapse loss observed in AD, there is abundant formation of dystrophic neurites, some scattered in the neuropil and others associated with amyloid fibrils and glial cells constituting neuritic plaques [22,77,106]. At the present time a controversy still exists as to the significance and origin of the neuritic components of the plaque. While some groups postulate that they represent degenerating processes, others suggest that at least a subpopulation of them might be aberrant sprouting neurites [18,29,71] based on the presence of GAP43 [71,100]. Previous studies in the aged monkey [16,17], as well as in the cortex in AD and DLB [4,57], have shown that the abnormal neuritic elements in the plaque contain several synaptic and axonal specific proteins including AβPP, GAP43, chromogranin, synaptophysin, EP10 antigen, SV-2, p65, synapsin, tau, and phosphorylated neurofilaments (detected by monoclonal antibody SMI312) [66, 112]. These studies support the possibility that plaque formation might start with synaptic and neuritic alterations accompanied by the accumulation of AβPP in the altered neurites, followed by amyloid deposition. AβPP, a molecule suggested to be centrally involved in AD [53,97], has been demonstrated to be transported in the axon to the presynaptic site [54] where it might play a role in synaptic plasticity.

4. Mechanisms of synapse loss in AD

The molecular mechanisms involved in mediating synapse loss and aberrant sprouting in AD are currently under investigation. However, most evidence points to excess accumulation of products of the AβPP β-secretory pathway (Fig. 2E). Supporting this view, several lines of investigation have shown that AβPP and its proteolytic fragments play a role in guiding growing neurites in the fetal brain [70,110], and *in vitro* studies have suggested that, depending on the concentration, AβPP and its fragments could be neurotoxic or neurotrophic [115]. Furthermore, AβPP is transported by fast axonal transport to the nerve terminals where it concentrates and plays a role in modulating memory formation [49,83] and glutamate levels at the synaptic cleft [74]. More recent studies have shown that of the products of the β-secretory pathway, soluble Aβ$_{1-42}$ stimulates sprouting of cholinergic fibers [64]. In contrast, aggregated Aβ interacts with the integrin leading to signaling though the focal adhesion pathway [35]. The resulting sprouting neurites eventually degenerate into dystrophic neurites similar to the ones observed in the mature plaques of AD patients. Taken together, these studies suggest that altered neuritic outgrowth and synapse formation in AD might be associated with abnormal processing of AβPP.

The mechanisms leading to synaptotoxicity and neurodegeneration in AD are currently under intense investigation. While several studies support the contention that early accumulation of Aβ oligomers plays a major role [52,56,96] (Fig. 2E); others have suggested that axonal transport and cytoskeletal alterations associated with tau phosphorylation might be important players in AD pathogenesis [6]. Both scenarios involve alterations in common and divergent signaling pathways that otherwise are critical mediators of synaptic functioning, neuronal survival and cell death. In familial forms of AD, mutations that increase or disturb the production of A$β_{1-42}$ have been shown to be involved in triggering the development of AD [13,23,32,97,117]. More recently, the role of Aβ in synaptic pathology in AD has been further investigated in synaptosomal preparations, where increased Aβ accumulation was associated with decreased PSD95 expression [36]. An excellent commentary on the subject by Dr. G. Perry accompanies the manuscript [58].

However, in sporadic AD it is less clear why Aβ accumulates. It has been proposed that while in some patients [e.g., those with Apolipoprotein E4 (apoE4) genotype], deficient Aβ clearance might be responsible, in others a shift in AβPP processing resulting from increased activity of proteolytic enzymes might be an important contributor [37]. Cleavage of AβPP by β-secretase results in the secretion of a large N-terminal ectodomain. In an alternative pathway, AβPP is also cleaved by β-secretase to generate a soluble NH$_2$-terminal fragment (AβPPs) and a 12-kDa COOH-terminal fragment (C99), which remains membrane bound. C99 is further cleaved by γ-secretase, resulting in the production of Aβ peptides, which vary in length [25]. The β-site AβPP-cleaving enzyme (BACE1) or β-amyloid-converting enzyme 1, has been identified as a membrane-bound aspartic protease and is now considered to carry out the major β-secretase activity *in vivo* [98,99,111]. Interestingly, recent studies have shown that in the brains of patients with sporadic AD, the levels of BACE1 expression are increased and AβPP C-terminus fragments are elevated [26,43,45, 88]. Thus, increased BACE1 activity might accelerate or augment AD-like pathology.

Although it appears clear that abnormal accumulation of products of the AβPP β-secretory pathway (e.g.: Aβ, C100) plays an important role in the pathogenesis of AD, it is less clear which are the precise cellular and molecular mechanisms involved. Several possibilities have been postulated, among them, some studies suggest that increased lysosomal leakage, increased intracellular trafficking of calcium, accumulation of intracellular Aβ in the synapse [103], reduced synaptic vesicle trafficking [12,116], deficient axonal transport, abnormal activation of signaling pathways and activation of caspases at the synapse terminal [81,82] might play a role in the mechanisms of synapse loss mediated by Aβ oligomerization. More recently, several lines of investigation have provided additional data suggesting that Aβ oligomers rather than fibrils [113] might directly damage synapses probably via activation of Fyn [14] and alterations in the expression of the synaptic plasticity associated molecule the activity-regulated cytoskeletal-associated protein (Arc) [55].

In conclusion, it is likely that either in combination or by themselves, these mechanisms might play an important role at the various stages of the neurodegenerative process in AD and they might represent attractive targets for future drug development.

Acknowledgments

This work was supported by NIH Grants AG18440, AG5131 and AG022074.

References

[1] I. Adams and D. Jones, Effects of normal and pathological aging on brain morphology: Neurons and synapses, in: *Current topics in research on synapses*, (Vol. 4), D. Jones and Alan R. Liss, eds, Inc., New York, 1987, pp. 16–17.
[2] A. Alzheimer, Uber eine eigenartige Erkrankung der Hirnrinde, *Algemeine Zeitschrift fur Psychiatric* **64** (1907), 146–148.
[3] B. Anderson, Dendritic correlates of dementia severity in Alzheimer's disease, *Med. Sci. Res.* **23** (1995), 597–599.
[4] H. Arai, M. Schmidt, V.-Y. Lee, H. Hurtig, B. Greenberg, C. Adler and J. Trojanowski, Epitope analysis of senile plaque components in the hippocampus of patients with Parkinson's disease, *Neurology* **42** (1992), 1315–1322.
[5] P. Arriagada, J. Growdon, E. Hedley-Whyte and B. Hyman, Neurofibrillary tangles but not senile plaques parallel duration and severity of Alzheimer's disease, *Neurology* **42** (1992), 631–639.
[6] J. Avila, F. Lim, F. Moreno, C. Belmonte and A.C. Cuello, Tau function and dysfunction in neurons: its role in neurodegenerative disorders, *Mol Neurobiol* **25** (2002), 213–231.
[7] C. Bertoni-Freddari, P. Fattoretti, T. Casoli, F. Masera, W. Meier-Ruge and J. Ulrich, Computer-assisted morphometry of synaptic plasticity during aging and dementia, *Path. Res. Pract.* **185** (1989), 799–802.

[8] C. Bertoni-Freddari, P. Fattoretti, A. Delfino, M. Solazzi, B. Giorgetti, J. Ulrich and W. Meier-Ruge, Deafferentative synaptopathology in physiological aging and Alzheimer's disease, *Ann N Y Acad Sci* **977** (2002), 322–326.

[9] K. Blennow, N. Bogdanovic, I. Alafuzoff, R. Ekman and P. Davidsson, Synaptic pathology in Alzheimer's disease: Relation to severity of dementia, but not to senile plaques, neurofibrillary tangles, or the ApoE4 allele, *J. Neural Transm.* **103** (1996), 603–618.

[10] E. Braak, H. Braak and E. Mandelkow, A sequence of cytoskeleton changes related to the formation of neurofibrillary tangles and neuropil threads, *Acta Neuropathol. (Berl)* **87** (1994), 554–567.

[11] H. Braak and E. Braak, Neuropathological stageing of Alzheimer-related changes, *Acta Neuropathol* **82** (1991), 239–259.

[12] S.L. Chan, K. Furukawa and M.P. Mattson, Presenilins and APP in neuritic and synaptic plasticity: implications for the pathogenesis of Alzheimer's disease, *Neuromolecular Med* **2** (2002), 167–196.

[13] M.-C. Chartier-Harlin, F. Crawford, H. Houlden, A. Warren, D. Hughes, L. Fidani, A. Goate, M. Rossor, P. Roques, J. Hardy and M. Mullan, Early-onset Alzheimer's disease caused by mutations at codon 717 of the β-amyloid precursor protein gene, *Nature* **353** (1991), 844–846.

[14] J. Chin, J.J. Palop, G.Q. Yu, N. Kojima, E. Masliah and L. Mucke, Fyn kinase modulates synaptotoxicity, but not aberrant sprouting, in human amyloid precursor protein transgenic mice, *J Neurosci* **24** (2004), 4692–4697.

[15] J.H. Choi and B.P. Yu, Brain synaptosomal aging: free radicals and membrane fluidity, *Free Radic Biol Med* **18** (1995), 133–139.

[16] L. Cork, C. Masters, K. Beyreuther and D. Price, Development of senile plaques. Relationships of neuronal abnormalities and amyloid deposits, *Am. J. Pathol.* **137** (1990), 1383–1392.

[17] L. Cork and D. Price, Relationships of abnormal neuronal processes and amyloid in plaques in aged monkeys, *J. Neuropathol. Exp. Neurol.* **49** (1990), 309.

[18] B. Cummings, J. Su, J. Geddes, W. Van Norstrand, S. Wagner, D. Cunningham and C. Cotman, Aggregation of the amyloid precursor protein within degenerating neurons and dystrophic neurites in Alzheimer's disease, *Neurosci* **48** (1992), 763–777.

[19] C. Davies, D. Mann, P. Sumpter and P. Yates, A quantitative morphometric analysis of the neuronal and synaptic content of the frontal and temporal cortex in patients with Alzheimer's disease, *J. Neurol. Sci.* **78** (1987), 151–164.

[20] S. DeKosky and S. Scheff, Synapse loss in frontal cortex biopsies in Alzheimer's disease: correlation with cognitive severity, *Ann. Neurol.* **27** (1990), 457–464.

[21] D. Dickson, H. Crystal, C. Bevona, W. Honer, I. Vincent and P. Davies, Correlations of synaptic and pathological markers with cognition of the elderly, *Neurobiol. Aging* **16** (1995), 285–304.

[22] D. Dickson, J. Farlo, P. Davies, H. Crystal, P. Fuld and S. Yen, Alzheimer disease. A double immunohistochemical study of senile plaques, *Am. J. Pathol.* **132** (1988), 86–101.

[23] K. Duff, C. Eckman, C. Zehr, X. Yu, C. Prada, J. Perez-Tur, M. Hutton, L. Buee, Y. Harigaya, D. Yager, D. Morgan, M. Gordon, L. Holcomb, L. Refolo, B. Zenk, J. Hardy and S. Younkin, Increased amyloid-β42(43) in brains of mice expressing mutant presenilin 1, *Nature* **383** (1996), 710–713.

[24] J. Eccles, The cerebral neocortex: a theory of its operation, in: *Cerebral Cortex*, (Vol. 2), Functional properties of cortical cells, E. Jones and A. Peters, eds, Plenum Press, New York, 1984, pp. 1–38.

[25] W.P. Esler and M.S. Wolfe, A portrait of Alzheimer secretases–new features and familiar faces, *Science* **293** (2001), 1449–1454.

[26] H. Fukumoto, B.S. Cheung, B.T. Hyman and M.C. Irizarry, β-secretase protein and activity are increased in the neocortex in Alzheimer disease, *Arch Neurol* **59** (2002), 1381–1389.

[27] D. Galasko, L. Hansen, R. Katzman, W. Wiederholt, E. Masliah, R. Terry, L. Hill, P. Lessin and L. Thal, Clinical-neuropathological correlations in Alzheimer's disease and related dementias, *Arch. Neurol.* **51** (1994), 888–895.

[28] M. Gearing, S. Mirra, J. Hedreen, S. Sumi, L. Hansen and A. Heyman, Neuropathology confirmation of the clinical diagnosis of Alzheimer's disease: CERAD. Part X, *Neurology* **45** (1995), 461–466.

[29] J. Geddes, K. Anderson and C. Cotman, Senile plaques as aberrant sprout stimulating structures, *Exp. Neurol.* **94** (1986), 767–776.

[30] Y. Geinisman, O. Ganeshina, R. Yoshida, R. W. Berry, J. F. Disterhoft and M. Gallagher, Aging, spatial learning, and total synapse number in the rat CA1 stratum radiatum, *Neurobiol Aging* **25** (2004), 407–416.

[31] P. Gibson, EM study of the number of cortical synapses in the brains of ageing people and people with Alzheimer-type dementia, *Acta Neuropathol. Berl* **62** (1983), 127–133.

[32] A. Goate, M.-C. Chartier-Harlin, M. Mullan, J. Brown, F. Crawford, L. Fidani, L. Guiffra, A. Haynes, N. Irving, L. James, R. Mant, P. Newton, K. Rooke, P. Roques, C. Talbot, R. Williamson, M. Rossor, M. Owen and J. Hardy, Segregation of a missense mutation in the amyloid precursor protein gene with familial Alzheimer's disease, *Nature* **349** (1991), 704.

[33] N. Gonatas, W. Anderson and I. Evangelista, The contribution of altered synapses in the senile plaque: an electron microscopic study in Alzheimer's disease, *J. Neuropathol. Exp. Neurol.* **26** (1967), 25–39.

[34] N. Gonatas and P. Gambetti, The pathology of the synapse in: *Alzheimer's disease. Ciba Foundation Symposium on Alzheimer's disease and related conditions*, G. Wolstenholme and O. London, eds, J & A Churchill, 1970.

[35] E.A. Grace, C.A. Rabiner and J. Busciglio, Characterization of neuronal dystrophy induced by fibrillar amyloid β: implications for Alzheimer's disease, *Neuroscience* **114** (2002), 265–273.

[36] K.H. Gylys, J.A. Fein, F. Yang, D.J. Wiley, C.A. Miller and G.M. Cole, Synaptic changes in Alzheimer's disease: increased amyloid-β and gliosis in surviving terminals is accompanied by decreased PSD-95 fluorescence, *Am J Pathol* **165** (2004), 1809–1817.

[37] C. Haas, A.Y. Hung, M. Citron, D.B. Teplow and D.J. Selkoe, β-Amyloid, protein processing and Alzheimer's disease, *Arzneimittelforschung* **45** (1995), 398–402.

[38] J. Hamos, L. DeGennaro and D. Drachman, Synaptic loss in Alzheimer's disease and other dementias, *Neurology* **39** (1989), 355–361.

[39] J. Hardy and A. Israel, Alzheimer's disease. In search of γ-secretase, *Nature* **398** (1999), 466–467.

[40] H. Haug, S. Kuhl, E. Mecke, N. Sass and K. Wasner, The significance of morphometric procedures in the investigation of age changes in cytoarchitectonic structures of human brain, *J. Hirnforsch.* **25** (1984), 353–374.

[41] P. Hof and J. Morrison, The cellular basis of cortical disconnection in Alzheimer disease and related dementing conditions, in: *Alzheimer disease*, R. Terry, R. Katzman and K. Bick, eds, Raven Press, New York, 1994, pp. 197–230.

[42] P.R. Hof and J.H. Morrison, The aging brain: morphomolecular senescence of cortical circuits, *Trends Neurosci* **27** (2004), 607–613.

[43] R.M. Holsinger, C.A. McLean, K. Beyreuther, C.L. Masters and G. Evin, Increased expression of the amyloid precursor β-secretase in Alzheimer's disease, *Ann Neurol* **51** (2002), 783–786.

[44] A.J. Holtmaat, J.T. Trachtenberg, L. Wilbrecht, G.M. Shepherd, X. Zhang, G.W. Knott and K. Svoboda, Transient and persistent dendritic spines in the neocortex in vivo, *Neuron* **45** (2005), 279–291.

[45] J.T. Huse, K. Liu, D.S. Pijak, D. Carlin, V.M. Lee and R.W. Doms, β-secretase processing in the trans-Golgi network preferentially generates truncated amyloid species that accumulate in Alzheimer's disease brain, *J Biol Chem* **277** (2002), 16278–16284.

[46] P. Huttenlocher, Synaptic density in human frontal cortex – developmental changes and effects of aging, *Brain Res* **163** (1979), 195–205.

[47] B. Hyman, G. Van Hoesen, L. Kromer and A. Damasio, Perforant pathway changes in the memory impairment of Alzheimer's disease, *Ann. Neurol.* **20** (1986), 472–481.

[48] D. Jones and R. Harris, An analysis of contemporary morphological concepts of synaptic remodelling in the CNS: Perforated synapses revisited, *Rev. Neurosci.* **6** (1995), 177–219.

[49] F. Kamenetz, T. Tomita, H. Hsieh, G. Seabrook, D. Borchelt, T. Iwatsubo, S. Sisodia and R. Malinow, APP Processing and synaptic function, *Neuron* **37** (2003), 925–937.

[50] R. Katzman, Alzheimer's disease is a degenerative disorder, *Neurobiol. Aging* **10** (1989), 581–582–588–590.

[51] Z. Khachaturian, Diagnosis of Alzheimer's disease, *Arch. Neurol.* **42** (1985), 1097–1105.

[52] W.L. Klein, Aβ toxicity in Alzheimer's disease: globular oligomers (ADDLs) as new vaccine and drug targets, *Neurochem Int* **41** (2002), 345–352.

[53] E. Koo, P.J. Lansbury and J. Kelly, Amyloid diseases: Abnormal protein aggregation in neurodegeneration, *Proc. Natl. Acad. Sci. USA* **96** (1999), 9989–9990.

[54] E. Koo, L. Park and D. Selkoe, Amyloid β-protein as a substrate interacts with extracellular matrix to promote neurite outgrowth, *Proc. Natl. Acad. Sci. USA* **90** (1993), 4749–4752.

[55] P.N. Lacor, M.C. Buniel, L. Chang, S.J. Fernandez, Y. Gong, K.L. Viola, M.P. Lambert, P.T. Velasco, E.H. Bigio, C.E. Finch, G.A. Krafft and W.L. Klein, Synaptic targeting by Alzheimer's-related amyloid β oligomers, *J Neurosci* **24** (2004), 10191–10200.

[56] H.A. Lashuel, D.M. Hartley, B.M. Petre, J.S. Wall, M.N. Simon, T. Walz and P.T. Lansbury, Jr., Mixtures of wild-type and a pathogenic (E22G) form of Aβ40 in vitro accumulate protofibrils, including amyloid pores, *J Mol Biol* **332** (2003), 795–808.

[57] H. Lassmann, R. Weiler, P. Fischer, C. Bancher, K. Jellinger, E. Floor, W. Danielczyk, F. Seitelberger and H. Winkler, Synaptic pathology in Alzheimer's disease: immunological data for markers of synaptic and large dense-core vesicles, *Neurosci* **46** (1992), 1–8.

[58] H.G. Lee, P.I. Moreira, X. Zhu, M.A. Smith and G. Perry, Staying connected: synapses in Alzheimer disease, *Am J Pathol* **165** (2004), 1461–1464.

[59] C. Lippa, J. Hamos, D. Pulaski-Salo, L. DeGennaro and D. Drachman, Alzheimer's disease and aging: Effects on perforant pathway perikarya and synapses, *Neurobiol. Aging* **13** (1992), 405–411.

[60] X. Liu, C. Erikson and A. Brun, Cortical synaptic changes and gliosis in normal aging, Alzheimer's disease and frontal lobe degeneration, *Dementia* **7** (1996), 128–134.

[61] L. Martin, C. Pardo, L. Cork and D. Price, Synaptic pathology and glial reponses to neuronal injury precede the formation of senile plaques and amyloid deposits in the aging cerebral cortex, *Am. J. Pathol.* **145** (1994), 1358–1381.

[62] E. Masliah, Mechanisms of synaptic pathology in Alzheimer's disease, *J. Neural. Transm.* **53** (Suppl) (1998), 147–158.

[63] E. Masliah, The natural evolution of the neurodegenerative alterations in Alzheimer's disease, *Neurobiol. Aging* **16** (1995), 280–282.

[64] E. Masliah, M. Alford, A. Adame, E. Rockenstein, D. Galasko, D. Salmon, L.A. Hansen and L.J. Thal, Aβ1–42 promotes cholinergic sprouting in patients with AD and Lewy body variant of AD, *Neurology* **61** (2003), 206–211.

[65] E. Masliah, L. Hansen, T. Albright, M. Mallory and R. Terry, Immunoelectron microscopic study of synaptic pathology in Alzheimer disease, *Acta Neuropathol* **81** (1991), 428–433.

[66] E. Masliah, W. Honer, M. Mallory, M. Voigt, P. Kushner and R. Terry, Topographical distribution of synaptic-associated proteins in the neuritic plaques of Alzheimer disease hippocampus, *Acta Neuropathol* **87** (1994), 135–142.

[67] E. Masliah and F. LiCastro, Neuronal and synaptic loss, reactive gliosis, microglial response, and induction of the complement cascade in Alzheimer's disease, in: *Neurodegenerative dementias*, C. Clark and J. Trojanowski, eds, McGraw-Hill, New York, NY, 2000, pp. 131–146.

[68] E. Masliah, M. Mallory, M. Alford, R. DeTeresa, L.A. Hansen, D.W. McKeel, Jr. and J.C. Morris, Altered expression of synaptic proteins occurs early during progression of Alzheimer's disease, *Neurology* **56** (2001), 127–129.

[69] E. Masliah, M. Mallory, R. DeTeresa, M. Alford and L. Hansen, Differing patterns of aberrant neuronal sprouting in Alzheimer's disease with and without Lewy bodies, *Brain Res* **617** (1993), 258–266.

[70] E. Masliah, M. Mallory, N. Ge and T. Saitoh, Amyloid precursor protein is localized in growing neurites of neonatal rat brain, *Brain Res* **593** (1992), 323–328.

[71] E. Masliah, M. Mallory, L. Hansen, M. Alford, T. Albright, R. DeTeresa, R. Terry, J. Baudier and T. Saitoh, Patterns of aberrant sprouting in Alzheimer disease, *Neuron* **6** (1991), 729–739.

[72] E. Masliah, M. Mallory, L. Hansen, R. DeTeresa, M. Alford and R. Terry, Synaptic and neuritic alterations during the progression of Alzheimer's disease, *Neurosci. Lett.* **174** (1994), 67–72.

[73] E. Masliah, M. Mallory, L. Hansen, R. DeTeresa and R. Terry, Quantitative synaptic alterations in the human neocortex during normal aging, *Neurology* **43** (1993), 192–197.

[74] E. Masliah, J. Raber, M. Alford, M. Mallory, M. Mattson, C. Westland and L. Mucke, Regulation of excitatory amino acid transporters by amyloid protein precursor (APP) and its relations to neuroprotective APP effects in transgenic mice, *J. Biol. Chem.* (1997).

[75] E. Masliah, E. Rockenstein, I. Veinbergs, Y. Sagara, M. Mallory, M. Hashimoto and L. Mucke, b amyloid peptides enhance a-synuclein accumulation and neuronal deficits in a

[76] E. Masliah and D. Salmon, Neuropathological correlates of dementia in Alzheimer's disease, in: *Cerebral Cortex. Neurodegenerative and age-related changes in structure and function of cerebral cortex*, (Vol. 14), A. Peters and J. Morrison, eds, Plenum Publishers, New York, NY, 1999, pp. 513–551.

[75] transgenic mouse model likning Alzheimer's and Parkinson's disease, *Proc Natl Acad Sci USA* **98** (2001), 12245–12250.

[77] E. Masliah, A. Sisk, M. Mallory, L. Mucke, D. Schenk and D. Games, Comparison of neurodegenerative pathology in transgenic mice overexpressing V717F b-amyloid precursor protein and Alzheimer's disease, *J. Neurosci.* **16** (1996), 5795–5811.

[78] E. Masliah and R. Terry, The role of synaptic pathology in the mechanisms of dementia in Alzheimer's disease, *Clin. Neurosci.* **1** (1994), 192–198.

[79] E. Masliah, R. Terry, M. Alford, R. DeTeresa and L. Hansen, Cortical and subcortical patterns of synaptophysin-like immunoreactivity in Alzheimer disease, *Am. J. Pathol.* **138** (1991), 235–246.

[80] E. Masliah, R. Terry, R. DeTeresa and L. Hansen, Immunohistochemical quantification of the synapse-related protein synaptophysin in Alzheimer disease, *Neurosci. Lett.* **103** (1989), 234–239.

[81] M.P. Mattson, Apoptosis in neurodegenerative disorders, *Nat. Rev. Mol. Cell. Biol.* **1** (2000), 120–129.

[82] M.P. Mattson, Oxidative stress, perturbed calcium homeostasis, and immune dysfunction in Alzheimer's disease, *J Neurovirol* **8** (2002), 539–550.

[83] R. Mileusnic, C.L. Lancashire, A.N. Johnston and S.P. Rose, APP is required during an early phase of memory formation, *Eur J Neurosci* **12** (2000), 4487–4495.

[84] L. Mucke, E. Masliah, G. Q. Yu, M. Mallory, E. M. Rockenstein, G. Tatsuno, K. Hu, D. Kholodenko, K. Johnson-Wood and L. McConlogue, High-level neuronal expression of Aβ 1–42 in wild-type human amyloid protein precursor transgenic mice: synaptotoxicity without plaque formation, *J Neurosci* **20** (2000), 4050–4058.

[85] P. Patterson, Process outgrowth and the specificity of connections, in: *An introduction to molecular neurobiology*, Z. Hall, ed., Sinauer Associates, Inc, Sunderland, Massachusetts, 1992, pp. 388–427.

[86] A. Peters, C. Sethares and M.B. Moss, The effects of aging on layer 1 in area 46 of prefrontal cortex in the rhesus monkey, *Cereb Cortex* **8** (1998), 671–684.

[87] J.L. Price, D.W. McKeel, Jr. and J.C. Morris, Synaptic loss and pathological change in older adults–aging versus disease? *Neurobiol Aging* **22** (2001), 351–352.

[88] S. Rossner, J. Apelt, R. Schliebs, J. R. Perez-Polo and V. Bigl, Neuronal and glial β-secretase (BACE) protein expression in transgenic Tg2576 mice with amyloid plaque pathology, *J Neurosci Res* **64** (2001), 437–446.

[89] D. Salmon, L. Thal, N. Butters and W. Heindel, Longitudinal evaluation of dementia of the Alzheimer type: a comparison of 3 standarized mental status examinations, *Neurology* **40** (1990), 1225–1230.

[90] W. Samuel, E. Masliah and R. Terry, Hippocampal connectivity and Alzheimer's dementia: effects of pathology in a two-component model, *Neurology* **44** (1994), 2081–2088.

[91] S. Scheff, S. DeKosky and D. Price, Quantitative assessment of cortical synaptic density in Alzheimer's disease, *Neurobiol. Aging* **11** (1990), 29–37.

[92] S. Scheff and D. Price, Synapse loss in the temporal lobe in Alzheimer's disease, *Ann. Neurol.* **33** (1993), 190–199.

[93] S. Scheff, D. Sparks and D. Price, Quantitative assessment of synaptic density in the entorhinal cortex in Alzheimer's disease, *Ann. Neurol.* **34** (1993), 356–361.

[94] S.W. Scheff and D.A. Price, Alzheimer's disease-related synapse loss in the cingulate cortex, *J Alzheimers Dis* **3** (2001), 495–505.

[95] S.W. Scheff and D.A. Price, Synaptic pathology in Alzheimer's disease: a review of ultrastructural studies, *Neurobiol Aging* **24** (2003), 1029–1046.

[96] D.J. Selkoe, Alzheimer's disease is a synaptic failure, *Science* **298** (2002), 789–791.

[97] D.J. Selkoe, T. Yamazaki, M. Citron, M.B. Podlisny, E.H. Koo, D.B. Teplow and C. Haass, The role of APP processing and trafficking pathways in the formation of amyloid β-protein, *Ann N Y Acad Sci* **777** (1996), 57–64.

[98] S. Sinha, J. Anderson, V. John, L. McConlogue, G. Basi, E. Thorsett and D. Schenk, Recent advances in the understanding of the processing of APP to β amyloid peptide, *Ann N Y Acad Sci* **920** (2000), 206–208.

[99] S. Sinha, J.P. Anderson, R. Barbour, G.S. Basi, R. Caccavello, D. Davis, M. Doan, H.F. Dovey, N. Frigon, J. Hong, K. Jacobson-Croak, N. Jewett, P. Keim, J. Knops, I. Lieberburg, M. Power, H. Tan, G. Tatsuno, J. Tung, D. Schenk, P. Seubert, S.M. Suomensaari, S. Wang, D. Walker, V. John et al., Purification and cloning of amyloid precursor protein β-secretase from human brain, *Nature* **402** (1999), 537–540.

[100] J. Six, U. Lubke, M.-B. Lenders, M. Vandermeeren, M. Mercken, M. Villanova, A. Van de Voorde, J. Gheuenst, J.-J. Martin and P. Cras, Neurite sprouting and cytoskeletal pathology in Alzheimer's disease: a comparative study with monoclonal antibodies to growth-associated protein B-50 (GAP43) and paired helical filaments, *Neurodegeneration* **1** (1992), 247–255.

[101] P.H. St George-Hyslop and A. Petit, Molecular biology and genetics of Alzheimer's disease, *C R Biol* **328** (2005), 119–130.

[102] C.I. Sze, J.C. Troncoso, C. Kawas, P. Mouton, D.L. Price and L.J. Martin, Loss of the presynaptic vesicle protein synaptophysin in hippocampus correlates with cognitive decline in Alzheimer disease, *J. Neuropathol. Exp. Neurol.* **56** (1997), 933–944.

[103] R.H. Takahashi, T.A. Milner, F. Li, E.E. Nam, M.A. Edgar, H. Yamaguchi, M.F. Beal, H. Xu, P. Greengard and G.K. Gouras, Intraneuronal Alzheimer Aβ42 accumulates in multivesicular bodies and is associated with synaptic pathology, *Am J Pathol* **161** (2002), 1869–1879.

[104] R. Tanzi, J. Gusella, P. Watkins, G. Bruns, P. St.George-Hyslop, M. van Keuren, D. Patterson, S. Pagan, D. Kurnik and R. Neve, Amyloid β protein gene: cDNA, mRNA distribution and genetic linkage near the Alzheimer locus, *Science* **235** (1987), 880–884.

[105] R. Terry, R. DeTeresa and L. Hansen, Neocortical cell counts in normal human adult aging, *Ann. Neurol.* **21** (1987), 530–539.

[106] R. Terry, N. Gonatas and M. Weiss, Ultrastructural studies in Alzheimer's presenile dementia, *Am. J. Pathol.* **44** (1964), 269–297.

[107] R. Terry, L. Hansen and E. Masliah, Structural basis of the cognitive alterations in Alzheimer disease, in: *Alzheimer disease*, R. Terry and R. Katzman, eds, Raven Press, New York, 1994, pp. 179–196.

[108] R. Terry, E. Masliah, D. Salmon, N. Butters, R. DeTeresa, R. Hill, L. Hansen and R. Katzman, Physical basis of cognitive alterations in Alzheimer disease: synapse loss is the major

correlate of cognitive impairment, *Ann. Neurol.* **30** (1991), 572–580.

[109] R.D. Terry and R. Katzman, Life span and synapses: will there be a primary senile dementia? *Neurobiol Aging* **22** (2001), 347–348; discussion 353–354.

[110] B. Trapp, P. Hauer, C. Haney and D. Wirak, APP is expressed in fetal brain and is associated with neuronal development, *J. Neuropathol. Exp. Neurol.* **51** (1992), 358.

[111] R. Vassar, B.D. Bennett, S. Babu-Khan, S. Kahn, E.A. Mendiaz, P. Denis, D.B. Teplow, S. Ross, P. Amarante, R. Loeloff, Y. Luo, S. Fisher, J. Fuller, S. Edenson, J. Lile, M.A. Jarosinski, A.L. Biere, E. Curran, T. Burgess, J.C. Louis, F. Collins, J. Treanor, G. Rogers and M. Citron, β-secretase cleavage of Alzheimer's amyloid precursor protein by the transmembrane aspartic protease BACE, *Science* **286** (1999), 735–741.

[112] K. Wakabayashi, W. Honer and E. Masliah, Synapse alterations in the hippocampal-entorhinal formation in Alzheimer's disease with and without Lewy body disease, *Brain Res* **667** (1994), 24–32.

[113] D.M. Walsh, I. Klyubin, J.V. Fadeeva, M.J. Rowan and D.J. Selkoe, Amyloid-β oligomers: their production, toxicity and therapeutic inhibition, *Biochem Soc Trans* **30** (2002), 552–557.

[114] R. Weiler, H. Lassmann, P. Fischer, K. Jellinger and H. Winkler, A high ratio of chromogranin A to synaptin/synaptophysin is a common feature of brains in Alzheimer and Pick disease, *FEBS Lett* **263** (1990), 337–339.

[115] B. Yankner, L. Duffy and D. Kirschner, Neurotrophic and neurotoxic effects of amyloid b protein: reversal by tachykinin neuropeptides, *Science* **250** (1990), 279–282.

[116] P.J. Yao, M. Zhu, E.I. Pyun, A.I. Brooks, S. Therianos, V.E. Meyers and P.D. Coleman, Defects in expression of genes related to synaptic vesicle traffickingin frontal cortex of Alzheimer's disease, *Neurobiol Dis* **12** (2003), 97–109.

[117] S.G. Younkin, The AAP and PS1/2 mutations linked to early onset familial Alzheimer's disease increase the extracellular concentration and Aβ 1–42 (43), *Rinsho Shinkeigaku* **37** (1997), 1099.

[118] S. Zhan, K. Beyreuther and H. Schmitt, Quantitative assessment of the synaptophysin immuno-reactivity of the cortical neuropil in various neurodegenerative disorders with dementia, *Dementia* **4** (1993), 66–74.

Alzheimer's disease-related alterations in synaptic density: Neocortex and hippocampus

Stephen W. Scheff* and Douglas A. Price
Sanders-Brown Center on Aging, University of Kentucky College of Medicine, Lexington, KY 40536-0230, USA

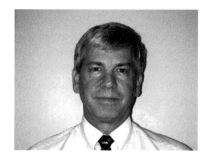

Abstract. Alzheimer's disease (AD) is a progressive disorder that is characterized by the accumulation of neuropathologic lesions and neurochemical alterations. Ultrastructural investigations in many association regions of the neocortex and the hippocampal dentate gyrus have demonstrated a disease-related decline in numerical synaptic density. This decline in brain connectivity occurs early in the disease process and strongly correlates with the cognitive decline observed in AD. The synapse loss does not appear to be an inevitable consequence of the aging process. This article reviews the ultrastructural studies assessing AD-related synaptic loss and the possible compensatory changes in the synaptic complex that occur as a result of the loss in brain connectivity.

Keywords: Plasticity, limbic, cognition, synapse, ultrastructure

1. Introduction

The prevalence of neuropathology such as senile plaques (SP) and neurofibrillary tangles (NFT) not only in the neocortex but also the hippocampus and other limbic structures has been the driving force for a plethora of research in AD. The progressive decline in cognitive function has been strongly associated with the presence of increased incidence of this neuropathology beginning with the original work by Blessed et al. [8] and the excellent work by Braak and Braak [9–12]. Numerous studies have now shown that non-demented elderly individuals can manifest significant numbers of these neuropathologic lesions in the cerebral cortex, suggesting that SP and NFT may be a feature of normal brain aging [4,16,18,28,39,43,44,65,75,91]. What differentiates AD from normal aging is the early subtle impairment in cognitive function. These individuals lose their ability to store recent information, which subsequently has devastating consequences for every day living. There is now accumulating evidence that the reason for the progressive cognitive decline is a loss of synapses resulting in a disruption of corticocortical connectivity. The present review examines the ultrastructural studies that support the synaptic loss hypothesis of AD.

2. Age-related synaptic change

Most neurobiology text dealing with age-related changes in the central nervous system include a section describing neuronal and synapse decline in neocortical and subcortical structures. These discussions usually rely upon older literature that was initially fueled by the dramatic pictures of "wind swept neurons" published by the Scheibels [87–90]. The ad-

*Corresponding author: Stephen W. Scheff, Sanders-Brown Center on Aging, Room 101 Sanders-Brown, University of Kentucky, Lexington, KY 40536-0230, USA. Tel.: +1 859 257 1412 ext 270; Fax: +1 859 323 2866; E-mail: sscheff@email.uky.edu.

vent of the new stereology [30,31,95] and unbiased sampling techniques have begun to challenge the older views of the aged CNS by demonstrating patterns of minimal neuronal loss in individuals without significant neuropathology [68]. Recent studies of the entorhinal cortex, an area believed to be an early site of AD-related pathology, shows no significant change in total neuron number as a function of aging [46,74]. Most notably there does appear to be a significant age-related loss of white matter, suggesting a loss of brain connectivity indicative of a loss of synapses. The loss of such brain connectivity is important since several studies have now demonstrated a good correlation between synaptic numbers and cognitive ability [19,96,97].

Issues concerning inevitable age-related changes in synaptic connectivity are complicated since the methods for identifying and quantifying synapses in human tissue are either indirect (immunohistochemical, ELISA) or labor intensive (electron microscopy). Early studies reported significant age-related loss of synapses in the frontal region (Brodmann areas 9, 10, 46) [53, 54,57], inferior parietal (Brodmann area 39, 40) [54], inferior temporal (Brodmann area 20) [54] and posterior cingulate cortex (Brodmann area 23) [54] using immunohistochemical (IHC) synaptophysin analysis. Individuals over the age of 60 show less synapses compared to younger individuals. Two ultrastructural studies [1,27] also reported age-related loss of synapses in neocortex. Gibson reported a decline in the superior frontal region while Adams [1] demonstrated an age-related change in the pre-central cortex (Brodmann area 4). In this latter study no age-related change was observed in the post-central gyrus (Brodmann area 3), an area that is primary sensory cortex. An ELISA and immunoblotting study with synaptophysin [37] failed to detect any age-related differences in the occipital cortex (Brodmann area 17), superior temporal cortex (Brodmann area 22), or hippocampus, suggesting that different regions of the neocortex age differently.

Unlike most of the previous assessments of age-related changes in synaptic numbers, we used an ultrastructural approach and sampled two different laminae (III & V) of Brodmann area 9 [84]. Stereological methods were employed in an attempt to obtain an unbiased estimate of the synaptic packing density. Constraints on tissue acquisition at the time of autopsy precluded estimating total synaptic numbers. Detailed measurements were of cortical thickness and careful evaluations were made for possible influences related to neuropathologic lesions. This study is unique in that at least five short post mortem (PMI < 11 h; mean 5.5, SD 2.2) cases were obtained for each decade of life and all were believed to be from individuals who were considered neurologically normal and without cognitive impairment. Ages for the subjects ranged from 20–89 years. Most of the individuals 65 years of age and older had been cognitively tested within 1 yr prior to death. Almost all of the cases were from well educated individuals (mean 16.1 years, SD 2.1) and each age group had almost equal numbers of males and females. A previous study has shown that gender of the individual is an important factor in predicting neocortical neuron number and can account for as much as 21% of the variance [68]. It required almost eight years to collect these autopsy samples since younger individuals (20–50 years of age) who expire without CNS involvement are typically not autopsied within an acceptable PMI for this study at the university hospital.

In addition to the above cases we obtained 5 cases from individuals older than 89 who also met the PMI, education and neurologically intact, criterion. These additional five cases were not included in the initial analysis because they represented individuals that could have been considered "survivors" since they were considered to be outside of the normal human life expectancy [3]. The results of the entire group are shown in Fig. 1. Neither lamina 3 or 5 showed any significant correlation with age indicating that the packing density of synapses in this Brodmann area remains stable. In addition there were no significant gender effects indicating that both males and females had equivalent packing densities. An interesting change was observed when comparing individuals in the ninth decade of life with those of the second and third decade. In both laminae, the older group was significantly lower, suggesting that whatever mechanism is used to maintain synaptic numbers, it begins to wane in the oldest old. Similar aging results have been observed by other groups [21, 22]. These results are important because they support the idea that neocortical regions in cognitively normal individuals can maintain constant synaptic numbers throughout the normal life expectancy. Surprisingly, individuals greater than 89 show a precipitous drop in synaptic numbers yet did not show significant cognitive decline. It is tempting to categorize this as a case of cognitive reserve. Numerous studies have reported AD-related loss of synapses in the frontal cortex [17, 19,58–60,69,79,97,105]. Our results suggest that age-related synaptic loss in the frontal cortex does not appear to be a contributing factor in the AD dementia.

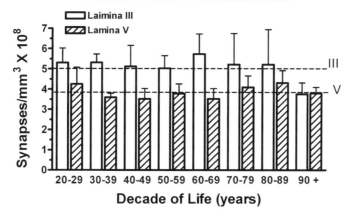

Fig. 1. Numerical synaptic density in the superior frontal cortex, Brodmann area 9, was determined for subjects of different age at the time of death. A minimum of five subjects were evaluated for each decade of life beginning at age 20. All subjects are believed to have been cognitively normal prior to death. Synaptic density was determined in both lamina III and V of the cortex using transmission electron microscopy. Dashed lines indicate the overall mean for each lamina. Bars represent group mean and standard deviation. (see [84] for details).

3. AD-related synaptic alterations in neocortex

The laboratory had the opportunity to assess possible changes in synaptic numbers in numerous areas of the neocortex in both AD and non-demented control subjects. One of the earliest studies utilized conventional transmission electron microscopy (EM) to examine the frontal cortex [79]. In that particular study, and in many of our subsequent investigations, two different laminae (III and V) were evaluated. Previous work in the laboratory [20] demonstrated significant changes in cholinergic circuitry in the frontal cortex of AD subjects. The greatest changes in choline acetyltransferase (ChAT) activity were observed in laminae III and V. These same laminae also contained substantial AD-related neuropathology and were relatively easy to identify with the light microscope when preparing samples for ultrastructural analysis. We hypothesized that if there was a significant change in synaptic numbers in AD they would most likely be detected in these two laminae. In order to make comparisons with other areas of the neocortex more standardized, we continued to study these two laminae throughout almost all of our ultrastructural investigations. While one could argue that different laminae may be more important for different areas, it was the above logic that guided us throughout our experiments.

These initial experiments were challenging in that specific criterion had to be met. Since our Alzheimer's Disease Research Center (ADRC) was not tracking large numbers of non-demented control subjects at that time. From previous human synapse studies it was obvious that not only did the tissue need to come from short PMI subjects, but also that the groups needed to be matched in terms of age. All of the AD subjects had been closely followed in the clinic and met the NINCDS-NIA clinical criteria for probable AD [63] and pathological criteria for tissue diagnosis of AD as well [45]. All of the AD subjects were considered to be "end-stage" with an average illness duration of 8 years. The control subjects were obtained from the normal autopsy service at the university hospital and retrospective review of medical charts were gleaned to determine whether or not there was any clinical history of neurological or psychiatric disease. As the ADRC began to expand its patient base to include non-demented elderly individuals, relevant clinical neurological data was available. Since we limited the PMI to a maximum of 13 h, and the average PMI was 7–8 hours, the quality of the tissue was quite good and the identification of synapses with transmission EM was acceptable (Fig. 2).

Although the same individuals acquired tissue at each of the autopsies, the number of samples taken from any given region was limited and certainly didn't represent the entire Brodmann region. This is important because consequently we could not apply all the rules of unbiased stereology. A minimum of three tissue blocks per region were taken from each subject and 15 disectors were evaluated from this tissue. From these samples the number of synapses per mm^3 was calculated. The findings from this initial set of experiments were better than expected. The detailed analysis revealed a highly significant 42% loss of synapses in lamina III

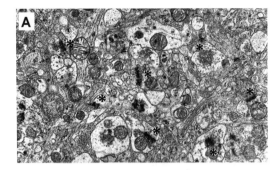

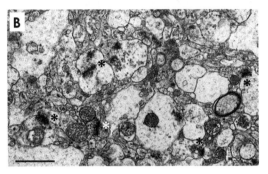

Fig. 2. Electron micrographs of human middle temporal gyrus (lamina III) 8 h postmortem are shown. Micrograph A is from one of the non-demented control subjects and the micrograph in B is from an end-stage Alzheimer subject that is age-matched. Asterisks indicate some of the synaptic complexes that are clearly visible in these samples and demonstrate the quality of the tissue that was routinely used in the ultrastructural studies. Calibration bar = 1 μm.

and a 29% loss in laminae V, very similar to results reported earlier [17]. We failed to detect any age-related change in synaptic density in either the non-demented control group or the AD group similar to the findings from our more extensive normal aging study [84]. A regression analysis also failed to show any relationship between the laminar width and the synaptic density ruling out atrophy as a mechanism to increase packing density in the control subjects. The significant AD-related synaptic decline observed in both laminae supported the previously published IHC reports, although the overall magnitude of the decline appeared to be greater with the synaptophysin antibody [58]. Nevertheless, the ultrastructural studies and the IHC results agreed that during the course of the disease, the frontal cortex failed to maintain the normal compliment of synapses.

One question that was heavily discussed in our group concerned how early in the course of the disease was the cortical circuitry altered as a result of a loss of significant synaptic numbers and was the decline in synapses responsible for the progressive cognitive decline that was the behavioral hallmark of the disease. We were

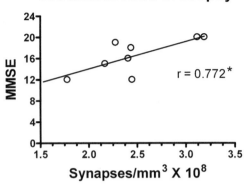

Fig. 3. Individuals were administered a test of overall cognitive function, Mini-Mental Status Exam (MMSE), shortly before undergoing a biopsy of the superior frontal cortex. The results showed a significant ($r = +0.772$) correlation with the synaptic packing density observed in lamina III of the superior frontal cortex (Brodmann area 9). The results suggest that loss of synaptic connectivity in this region is reflected by lower scores on the MMSE, indicative of a decline in cognitive function. The open circles represent individual patient scores and synaptic density. $^*p < 0.01$.

fortunate enough to be able to shed some light on this question. A large study was in progress to assess the benefit of intracerebroventricular bethanechol chloride infusion in AD subjects as a means of enhancing the cholinergic circuitry [34]. Patients in an early stage of the disease were selected for biopsy according to the NINCDS criteria [63] and only admitted if their mini-mental state examination (MMSE) scores were between 10 and 24 and their global deterioration rating (GDS) was 4–5 [76]. Tissue was obtained from Brodmann area 9 on the right side and immediately processed for ultrastructural analysis. The quality of this tissue was far superior to any of the autopsy tissue that we had been working with and synaptic profiles were much easier to detect. We were concerned that this might influence the counting especially since we did not have any "normal" biopsy control tissue. Our investigation concentrated on lamina III, which showed the greatest loss in the autopsy tissue. Synaptic values were significantly higher in the biopsy group when compared to the autopsy AD subjects but showed a dramatic 35% loss of synapses compared to age-matched autopsy control subjects. These subjects also had a significant loss of ChAT activity [19]. Since these subjects had completed an MMSE just prior to biopsy, it was possible to compare their scores with the individual synaptic volume density.

Results of this analysis are shown in Fig. 3 and demonstrated a highly significant correlation ($r = 0.772$, $p < 0.01$) indicating that as the number synapses in the superior frontal cortex declined so did the individuals cognitive status of the individual. These results also indicated that synaptic loss may be an early event in progression of AD. Davies et al. [17] suggested a similar scenario in their more limited biopsy study of frontal cortex. Rather than suggest that the specific loss of synapses in the frontal cortex was the cause for the cognitive decline, we considered the synaptic decline as indication that many regions of the neocortex may be involved early in the disease process. There was also the possibility that some type of plasticity may be dysfunctional in the neocortex despite the fact that some indication of synaptogenesis may be active in the AD brain [23,77]. Terry and colleagues [97] have also presented strong multivariate analysis indicating that loss of neocortical synapses is functionally very important in the cognitive decline associated with AD.

At the time of tissue acquisition for the frontal cortex study, we had the foresight to collect samples from several other areas as well. Retrospectively it would have been advantageous to collect tissue from as many different areas as possible, but because of the labor intensiveness of processing tissue for EM analysis and the lack of being able to predict which areas would subsequently be important, we limited our acquisitions to the frontal, superior and middle temporal, and entorhinal cortex (ERC). The ERC tissue was more difficult to obtain than the other areas because it is a small area and in demand by the neuropathologist. Early on we reported a somewhat surprising finding. Following a careful analysis of both lamina III and V in 10 AD and aged-matched controls, we were unable to detect a significant change in ERC synaptic density [85]. These results were somewhat controversial since this limbic cortical area performs an important role as a relay between the hippocampal formation and other neocortical regions. Information from various regions of the brain converges on the ERC, which subsequently provides an excitatory input by way of the perforant path to the outer molecular layer of the dentate gyrus. It was already known that the ERC was affected early in the disease process [9,33,40,99]. This cortical area is somewhat problematic to work with because the cytoarchitectonics varies greatly. Consequently, the analysis was confined to the more caudal aspects of the cortical structure. The major pathology in the ERC is concentrated to lamina II and the upper aspects of lamina III, consisting of numerous neurons with neurofibrillary tangles and a concomitant loss of neurons in this region. We speculated that the maintenance of synaptic numbers might be the result of a synaptic compensatory response resulting from a loss of afferents to this region [98]. It is important to consider that a simple maintenance of synaptic numbers does not necessarily indicate normal functional quality or if the synapses utilize the same neurotransmitter. It is interesting to note that IHC studies have failed to demonstrate a decline in synaptophysin ERC staining when compared to appropriate control material [32,59].

We were interested in determining if the synaptic decline observed in the frontal region was isolated to that region or part of a cortical pattern and the ERC was more of an exception. Numerous studies concerning the distribution of neuropathological lesions in AD implicated the temporal lobe as a region that was significantly affected in the disease process. Several IHC studies reported significant loss of synaptophysin staining in both the superior and middle temporal lobes [58, 59,97]. Our results demonstrated a 23–33% loss of synapses in the temporal lobe [80]. As with area 9, both laminae III and V in both the middle (Brodmann area 21) and superior (Brodmann area 22) temporal lobe areas were significantly affected (Fig. 4). Again, these reports supported an initial speculation that early in the disease process the synaptic numbers in the temporal lobe were affected [17]. Curiously, the magnitude of synapse loss was not as robust as that observed with IHC. Both temporal lobe regions showed similar declines in synaptic density.

Many of the same subjects used in our first autopsy study of area 9 were also assigned to this investigation and afforded us the opportunity to test for possible correlations between cortical regions. Our cross correlation analysis was somewhat interesting. When we combined all the data from both the AD and control subjects, there emerged a very strong correlation between area 9 and both areas 21 and 22 for both laminae III and V. As shown in Fig. 5, both regions of the temporal lobe appeared to correlate to the synaptic density in area 9 to the same degree. However, when we analyzed the AD subjects separately there was virtually no indication that the two regions responded the same. Loss of synapses in the frontal cortex did not predict temporal lobe changes. The strongest correlations within the AD group, although not very robust, were between the two temporal lobe regions. The disease process most likely affects regions of the association cortex in a different temporal manner perhaps based upon different corticocortical connectivity [10,12]. Other variables that need to be considered are the relatively small sample size and the fact that the AD cases used in these studies are "end-stage" and most likely reflect the greatest amount of synaptic decline for these regions.

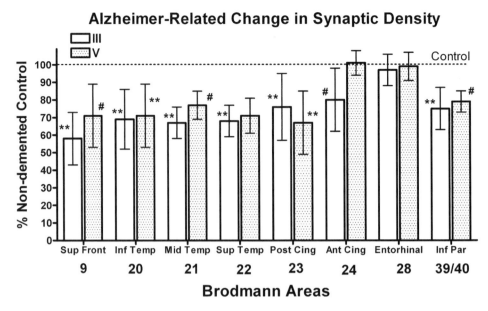

Fig. 4. Alzheimer related changes in the density of synapses in various regions of the neocortex. Values are plotted as a percent change of the mean value of age- and PMI-matched control group. All tissue was obtained within 13 h postmortem and represents end-stage of the disease. The entorhinal cortex (Brodmann area 28) failed to show any significant loss for either lamina III or V. Lamina V of the anterior cingulated region (Brodmann area 24) also failed to show any disease-related loss of synaptic density. Open bars represent lamina III and shaded bars represent lamina V. Bars represent group means with standard deviation and was calculated from a minimum of 9 Alzheimer subjects. # $p < 0.05$,** $p < 0.01$.

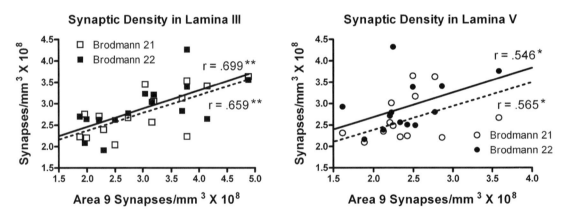

Fig. 5. Many of the same subjects analyzed for possible changes in synaptic numbers in the superior frontal cortex (Brodmann area 9) were also assessed for possible changes in the middle temporal (Brodmann 21) and superior temporal (Brodmann 22) cortical regions. When both non-demented control subjects and AD subjects are combined, both cortical regions show a strong correlation with the values obtained in Area 9. In A the results are shown for lamina III and in B the results for lamina V are displayed. For both cortical regions the relationship with Area 9 is almost identical. However, when only the AD cases are analyzed the correlation is no longer significant. Each of the symbols represents an individuals synaptic density for each area. ** $p < 0.01$.

Many areas of the neocortex appear to be affected in AD and the progression appears to follow a course involving specific brain regions early in the disease process [10,11,41,75]. The cingulate gyrus, consisting of both the anterior (Brodmann area 24) and posterior (Brodmann area 23) cingulate cortex has recently been identified as an area that may play an important role in the early progression of the disease [38,50,64,103]. The anterior cingulate plays a prominent role connecting the frontal lobe and various subcortical structures, while the posterior cingulate is involved in a variety of memory and spatial orientation functions [100].

As with previous investigations, both AD and non-demented control groups were age and PMI-matched with the AD subjects having an average of 9 year illness duration indicative of "end-stage" of the disease. Most of the control cases were from individuals that had been followed by the UK-ADRC and were recently cognitively tested. The brains of the AD subjects contained abundant SP and NFT in the hippocampus and neocortical regions. Cortical samples were taken from both the anterior and posterior regions of the cingulate in each subject and great care was used to ensure that the same region was assessed between subjects and groups. As we discovered later, this was a fortunate decision since we were unaware of the heterogeneity of this brain region and its diverse connectivity. Laminae III and V were examined in order that the results could be compared and contrasted with previous results. Both the anterior and posterior cingulated cortex demonstrated significant loss of synaptic numbers in AD [81]. The posterior cingulate gyrus demonstrated greater loss in both lamina III (24%) and lamina V (33%) compared to the anterior cingulate in the AD group. Surprisingly, the anterior cingulate region only showed a loss in lamina III (20%) and no decline in lamina V (Fig. 4). This lack of synaptic loss in area 24 was extremely puzzling and we initially attributed it to a possible basic difference in afferents to this area [101, 102]. We subsequently learned that the portion of the cingulate gyrus used in this investigation, the caudal anterior cingulate, connects to several supplemental motor regions and plays a role in motor activities. Numerous morphological studies have demonstrated that both motor and primary sensory areas are the least affected in AD and the involvement of area 24 in this motor system may be directly related to the maintenance of synapses. Synaptophysin IHC has also demonstrated a loss in the posterior cingulate with values considerably greater than we obtained [54]. A chemical analysis of synapsin I levels, a neuron-specific synaptic vesicle phosphoprotein, failed to show any AD-related change in the cingulated cortex [70]. Correlations between the two cingulate areas were similar to that found in the temporal lobe. While there was a positive trend in the data, neither region could be used to predict the response of the other.

Several early studies had reported significant loss of synaptophysin staining (44–57%) in the inferior parietal cortex (Brodmann area 39–40) [54,58,59,97]. This neocortical region is known to be heavily involved in AD and has been implicated in significant oxidative damage [15,49]. The inferior parietal region is a multimodal association area intimately involved in language comprehension rather than language expression. Deficits in tasks related to verbal fluency, such as those observed in AD, are affected by disruption of the circuitry in this region. Tissue samples from individuals with illness duration similar to those used for the other cortical regions was obtained at autopsy and processed as before for transmission EM. Both lamina III and V was analyzed for possible AD-related changes. As shown in Fig. 6, we observed a significant (25%) decline in synapses in lamina III and a 21% decline in lamina V. We also began to sample the inferior temporal gyrus (Brodmann are 20). This region is intricately connected to the parahippocampal gyrus and a region affected early in the disease [5,24–26]. It is a tertiary association area that plays an important role in higher visual function and believed to provide part of the anatomical substrate for the perception and memory of shapes and objects. Some of the same subjects used to study the inferior parietal region were also sampled in this study. We again observed a significant decline (31%) in synaptic numbers in lamina III and a similar (29%) decline in lamina V. The declines observed were very similar to those previously obtained for the superior and middle temporal gyrus. For the AD subjects, there was a very high correlation ($r = 0.882$) between the two lamina in this cortical region suggesting that the two laminae are affected at the same time and to the same degree.

4. AD-related synaptic alterations in the hippocampus

Early studies of morphological substrates underlying the progressive AD dementia involved the hippocampal formation and specifically the molecular layer of the hippocampal dentate gyrus. As noted above, the granule cell dendrites in the outer molecular layer (OML) of the dentate gyrus receive a very significant input from the ipsilateral entorhinal cortex, an area that is noted for its abundance of NFT containing cells in AD. Many of the early IHC studies concentrated on this region and reported significant declines in staining [13,29,32, 35,37,51,59,104,105]. A previous ultrastructural study also reported a loss of synapses in this region of the dentate gyrus [6]. The laboratory felt it was important to directly visualize synaptic numbers within the hippocampus since the magnitude of the loss reported in the IHC studies varied considerably between laboratories and the previous ultrastructural study only examined the supragranular region of the dentate gyrus.

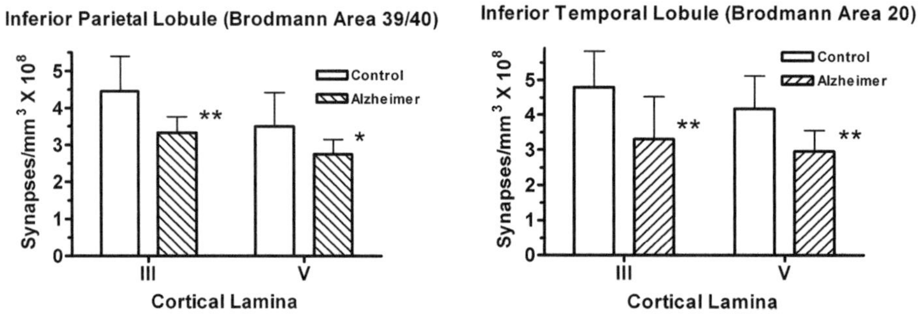

Fig. 6. Synaptic density measurements determined by quantitative ultrastructural analysis in the inferior parietal lobule (Brodmann area 39/40) and the inferior temporal lobule (Brodmann area 20). Both laminae III and V in each of the two cortical regions of the Alzheimer group (stripped bars) showed a significant decline in synaptic numbers compared to age- and postmortem-matched non-demented controls (open bars). Bars represent group means with standard deviation * $p < 0.05$; ** $p < 0.01$.

Although the primary afferents to the OML arise from the entorhinal cortex, and these neurons are known to be affected early in the disease, we speculated that a compensatory plasticity response in the OML of AD subjects, similar to that observed in experimental animal [78] and also reported in AD [23], might alter the synaptic circuitry. Ten short PMI (< 8 h) non-demented control subjects were compared to age and PMI-matched AD subjects that had an illness duration of approximately 9 years indicative of end-stage in the disease. A stereological sampling scheme was used to estimate the packing density of synapses in the OML. We found a significant 21% loss of synapses in the OML [86] and a 15% decline in the inner molecular layer (IML) as shown in Fig. 7 [82]. Coupled with these findings was a significant (26%) decline in the width of the dentate gyrus molecular layer in the AD group that could significantly impact upon the packing density and result in an underestimation of the total synaptic loss.

We interpreted the synaptic decline in the OML as a reduction in plasticity in this region that occurs in the end-stage of the disease. It is unknown whether or not synaptic numbers in this region are affected early in the disease. If this region is vulnerable and fails to maintain a normal compliment of synapses, it might explain some of the memory changes observed in individuals with mild cognitive impairment [73]. In all of the cases used in these investigations, the diagnosis of AD was based upon not only neuropathological findings of the autopsy tissue, but also according to NINCDS-NIA clinical criteria. These criterion are important when interpreting possible AD-related changes especially when the variance within groups is quite large. Two previous studies reporting changes in hippocampal IHC stated that many of their AD subjects had either

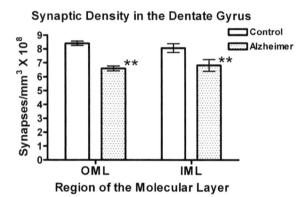

Fig. 7. The molecular layer of the hippocampal dentate gyrus was evaluated in short post mortem tissue from Alzheimer's disease subjects with a long duration illness. Age- and PMI-matched non-demented subjects were also evaluated. Both the outer 2/3 (OML) and inner 1/3 (IML) of the molecular layer were evaluated separately. The greatest loss was observed in the OML but a significant decline in synaptic density was also observed for the IML suggesting that whatever mechanism is responsible for the synaptic decline it may affect not only afferents but also target neurons. Bars represent group means and standard deviation. ** $p < 0.01$.

no change in staining or only very mild changes [29, 51].

The more interesting finding from our hippocampal studies was the significant decline in the IML. This region of the dentate gyrus differs from the OML in that it does not receive input from the ERC. Like the OML, this synaptic zone receives cholinergic afferents originating in the septal region, fibers originating from the dentate polymorph cells, along with fibers originating from the thalamus, hypothalamus and brainstem nuclei [42]. Our studies of the dentate gyrus also monitored changes in the packing density of granule cells in both the AD and control groups and allowed us to calculate a synapse to granule cell ratio for this region. We observed a significant decline in this ratio for both the IML (27%) and the OML (29%). The decrement indicates that reasons for the loss of synapses are a global problem probably affecting both afferents and target cells.

5. Changes in apposition size

Early in our work on synaptic decline in AD we observed that the size of the synaptic contacts in the AD tissue was substantially larger compared to the non-demented controls [79]. Studies in both human and animal work had reported similar findings and suggested it might be part of a compensatory mechanism [2,7,14, 17,36,52]. As shown in Fig. 8, we observed a significant inverse correlation in almost all of the neocortical regions we studied [79–82,86], suggesting that this is a common response throughout the neocortex and hippocampus. As the number of synapses declined in a given region, the size of the residual synapses increased. Initially we thought this change in synaptic size may be a response found only in end-stage AD subjects. Our studies clearly show that this compensatory response not only occurs in control subjects but also can be observed early in the course of the disease [19].

To test the hypothesis that the change in synapse size in the AD material might be the result of a preferential loss of small synapses from the neuropil, we constructed frequency histograms of the size of over 8,000 synapses in both the middle and superior temporal gyrus [80]. While the shape of the histograms was very similar between both the AD and control subjects, the distribution of synapses for the AD samples was skewed to the right, indicative of clear shift in the central location of synapse size. This suggests that the change occurred throughout the entire distribution of synapses and that the loss was not targeted towards smaller synapses. Since the AD and non-demented controls were both age and PMI-matched, the overall increase in apposition size in the AD group is most likely disease related. Other than a change in the size of the apposition length, the synapses in both the AD and non-demented control tissue appeared identical with approximately the same packing density of synaptic vesicles. Although we did not specifically quantify the total number of perforated and non-perforated synapses, the frequency did not appear to differentiate the two groups.

Possible functional importance of this change in synapse size has been a topic of speculation with our group from the very first study [79]. We used the synaptic measurements to determine the total synaptic contact area (TSCA) in each of the regions that were investigated and subsequently compared the AD and non-demented control groups. The results of the analysis were surprising. For many of the areas, the increase in the synaptic size off set the significant loss of synapses in terms of the TSCA (Table 1). Only two areas that manifested a significant increase in synaptic size (area 9 lamina III; area 22 lamina III) was their a failure to restore TSCA. In two other areas (Brodmann 20 and 39/40) there was no significant change in synaptic size and consequently the TSCA was significantly reduced. This may indicate that these neocortical areas have lost a significant amount of their plasticity potential during the progressive course of the disease. The failure to completely restore TSCA in area 9 in end-stage subjects is in contrast to the biopsy data from early AD subjects that does demonstrate a restoration of TSCA.

We have previously proposed a model that might help to interpret the importance of the synaptic enlargement and TSCA in AD [83]. In this model, target neurons strive to maintain a set level of contacts and they do so by monitoring the overall level of synaptic contact. As inputs decline, the target neurons signal the need for new afferents to replace those lost. As part of the compensatory process, remaining afferents enlarge and subsequently reduce the strength of the signal of the target neuron. Maximal denervation would generate the strongest signal in an attempt to attract synaptic contact. In end-stage of the disease process, some areas of the AD brain are more involved than others. In these regions one would expect to see preserved TSCA perhaps early in the disease and subsequently a failure to maintain TSCA later, such as in area 9. As the disease progresses not only do the target neurons fail to initiate and maintain a strong attracting signal, but afferents also fail to launch a compensatory response (increase in synapse size). The overall effect is a loss of synaptic density coupled with a decline in baseline TSCA. It is extremely interesting that the two regions that demonstrated a failed compensatory response were areas known to be affected early in the disease and areas with the smallest synapses of all the regions investigated.

6. Possible basis for synaptic decline in AD

The amyloid cascade hypothesis states that amyloid β protein precursor (AβPP) and presenilin (PS) mutations combine to promote the formation of a highly

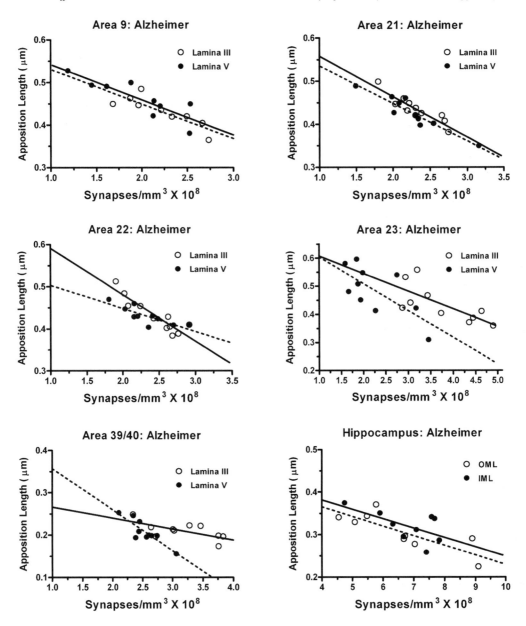

Fig. 8. Relationship between synaptic apposition length and the numerical density of synapses in different regions of the neocortex and hippocampus is displayed. Graphs are representative of the findings in both lamina III (o) and V (•) for the Alzheimer group. As the density of synapses in the different cortical regions declined, the size of the apposition length of the residual synapses enlarged. This may be a compensatory mechanism used by the different cortical structures to maintain total synaptic contact area. Lines represent simple regression analysis.

insoluble amyloid-β (Aβ) and that the progressive accumulation of Aβ triggers neuronal and synaptic abnormalities associated with AD. The key biochemical component of the AD plaque is fibrillar amyloid beta protein that is an end product of the processing of the AβPP, a protein that may play an important role in synaptic activity and cell adhesion. Early in our investigations of synaptic change in AD we stained tissue adjacent to that used for ultrastructural study and subsequently counted the number of SP and attempted to correlate it to the synaptic counts. Individual counts were made for both lamina III and V. In every area studied the number of plaques was significantly greater than in the non-demented controls. However, the number of plaques failed to demonstrate any significant relationship to synaptic numbers in either lamina [79,80,84].

Table 1
Change in total synaptic contact area (TSCA) in Alzheimer's disease

Region studied	% Synaptic change	% Apposition change	% TSCA change
Area 9			
Lamina III	− 42	+ 23	− 11
Lamina III (Biopsy)	− 35	+ 28	+ 5
Lamina V	− 29	+ 20	+ 2
Area 20			
Lamina III	− 31	+ 5	− 26
Lamina V	− 29	+ 3	− 17
Area 21			
Lamina III	− 33	+ 22	+ 3
Lamina V	− 23	+ 15	0
Area 22			
Lamina III	− 32	+ 16	− 9
Lamina V	− 29	+ 19	+ 5
Area 23			
Lamina III	− 23	+ 17	+ 7
Lamina V	− 33	+ 23	− 1
Area 24			
Lamina III	− 20	+ 29	+ 28
Lamina V	+ 3	+ 2	+ 10
Area 39/40			
Lamina III	− 25	− 4	− 27
Lamina V	− 30	− 1	− 30
Hippocampus			
OML	− 21	+ 18	+ 4
IML	− 15	+ 12	+ 4

It is unclear, however, if amyloid load correlates with changes in synaptic numbers. There is now mounting evidence that a soluble from of Aβ (sAβ) is also found in brain tissue of both normal and AD patients [47,48] and may be correlated with synaptic loss [55,66].

As a further test of the significance of amyloid deposits and synaptic decline we studied individuals who had a 75% or greater stenosis of at least one major epicardial artery at the time of death. These nondemented individuals have a very high incidence of diffuse agryophyilic plaques equivalent to that found in AD subjects [93,94]. Synaptic numbers in the frontal, middle temporal, and superior temporal (only areas studied) from heart disease subjects were equivalent to those in our previous tissue from non-demented controls and significantly higher than the AD subjects [83]. The NFT in these subjects with heart disease was at the same density as that found in our non-demented controls without heart disease.

There is also increasing evidence that oxidative stress and damage are fundamentally involved in the pathogenesis of AD [56,71,72] although the exact role in the progression of the disease is still controversial [92]. Oxidative damage is one of the earliest events in AD with some evidence that levels diminish with duration of the disease [67]. We tested whether or not measures of oxidative stress/damage might correlate with synaptic numbers in two regions (inferior parietal and inferior temporal) of the AD tissue. Tissue adjacent to that used for ultrastructural analysis was frozen in liquid nitrogen at the time of autopsy and subsequently evaluated. Both of these areas demonstrated significant declines in the end-stage AD tissue (Fig. 6). While none of the correlations were significant, probably because of the long PMI and disease duration, there was a trend in the direction of the correlations. Measures of increased oxidative damage (4-hydroxynonenal) were higher in individuals with lower synaptic counts [83] as were markers of antioxidants (superoxide dismutase; glutathione). The analysis of oxidative stress/damage was determined for the entire cortical region while the synaptic counts were carried out in specific lamina. Nevertheless, we are encouraged by these findings and new experiments are underway to further explore the relationship.

7. Conclusion and summary

Synaptic connectivity lies at the very essence of brain function and requires that a multitude of cellular machinery work in concert to maintain this connectivity. Synapses are certainly not permanent structures within the CNS and many experimental studies have documented the loss and reacquisition of these morphological structures under conditions as "simple" as hormonal change, stress, and learning [61,62]. Aging in the nervous system does not necessary result in a loss of neurons or neuronal connectivity as evidenced by our results assessing synaptic density in the frontal cortex. These results amplify the devastating consequences observed in AD. Even early in the disease process the frontal association cortex is significantly altered and must contribute to the decline in the individual's cognitive ability. The ability to attend to a stimulus and subsequently determine the merit of that stimulus requires that multiple associational areas of the cortex work in concert. The ability to store important information and to recall that information also requires that multiple regions of the brain work together. The progressive cognitive decline observed in AD most likely reflects an anatomical disruption in the cooperation of various regions of the CNS. Our ultrastructural studies over the last decade and a half have documented the decline of cortical connectivity in multiple association regions of the neocortex and portions of the hippocampus. Clearly the nervous system tries to respond to the impending loss of the connectivity but the compensatory response appears to ultimately fail with progression of the disease. The challenge is to isolate the mechanism(s) underlying this loss of connectivity early in the disease process and to mount a therapeutic regime that halts the synaptic loss and encourages synaptogenesis. Even with a replacement of synaptic numbers it is unclear that the most appropriate connectivity will be made and that the ravished nervous system will be able to incorporate an altered circuitry to carry out its complicated tasks. It is important that we attempt to make headway in this regard and probe the underlying resilience of the nervous system.

Acknowledgements

This research was supported by the National Institute of Health grants AG05144, AG05119, AG12138, AG12986 and AG14449, and the Alzheimer's Association.

References

[1] I. Adams, Comparison of synaptic changes in the precentral and postcentral cerebral cortex of aging humans: a quantitative ultrastructural study, *Neurobiol Aging* **8** (1987), 203–212.

[2] I. Adams, Plasticity of the synaptic contact zone following loss of synapses in the cerebral cortex of aging humans, *Brain Res* **424** (1987), 343–351.

[3] E. Arias, United States life tables, 2002, *Natl Vital Stat Rep* **53** (2004), 1–38.

[4] P.V. Arriagada, K. Marzloff and B.T. Hyman, Distribution of Alzheimer-type pathologic changes in nondemented elderly individuals matches the pattern in Alzheimer's disease, *Neurology* **42** (1992), 1681–1688.

[5] T.G. Beach, W.G. Honer and L.H. Hughes, Cholinergic fibre loss associated with diffuse plaques in the non-demented elderly: the preclinical stage of Alzheimer's disease? *Acta Neuropathol (Berl)* **93** (1997), 146–153.

[6] C. Bertoni-Freddari and P. Fattoretti, Computer-assisted morphometry of synaptic plasticity during aging and dementia, *Path Res Pract* **185** (1989), 799–802.

[7] C. Bertoni-Freddari, P. Fattoretti, T. Casoli, W. Meier-Ruge and J. Ulrich, Morphological adaptive response of the synaptic junctional zones in the human dentate gyrus during aging and Alzheimer's disease, *Brain Res* **517** (1990), 69–75.

[8] G. Blessed, B. Tomlinson and M. Roth, The association between quantitatiave measures of dementia and of senile changes in cerebral grey matter of elderly subjects, *Br J Psychiatry* **114** (1968), 797–811.

[9] H. Braak and E. Braak, Neurofibrillary changes confined to the entorhinal region and an abundance of cortical amyloid in cases of presinile and senile dementia, *Acta Neuropathol* **80** (1990), 479–486.

[10] H. Braak and E. Braak, Neuropathological stageing of Alzheimer-related changes, *Acta Neuropathol* **82** (1991), 239–259.

[11] H. Braak and E. Braak, Pathology of Alzheimer's disease. in: *Neurodegenerative Diseases,* D.B. Calne, ed., Vol., W.B. Saunders, Co., Philadelphia, 1994, pp. 585–613.

[12] H. Braak, E. Braak and J. Bohl, Staging of Alzheimer-related cortical destruction, *Euro Neurol* **33** (1993), 403–408.

[13] L.M. Cabalka, B.T. Hyman, C.R. Goodlett, T.C. Ritchie and G.W. Van Hoesen, Alteration in the pattern of nerve terminal protein immunoreactivity in the perforant pathway in Alzheimer's disease and in rats after entorhinal lesions, *Neurobiol Aging* **13** (1992), 283–291.

[14] R.K. Carlin and P. Siekevitz, Plasticity in the central nervous system: do synapses divide? *Proc Natl Acad Sci USA* **80** (1983), 3517–3521.

[15] A. Castegna, M. Aksenov, V. Thongboonkerd, J.B. Klein, W.M. Pierce, R. Booze, W.R. Markesbery and D.A. Butterfield, Proteomic identification of oxidatively modified proteins in Alzheimer's disease brain. Part II: dihydropyrimidinase-related protein 2, alpha-enolase and heat shock cognate 71, *J Neurochem* **82** (2002), 1524–1532.

[16] H. Crystal, D. Dickson, P. Fuld, D. Masur, R. Scott, M. Mehler, J. Masdeu, C. Kawas, M. Aronson and L. Wolfson, Clinico-pathologic studies in dementia: nondemented subjects with pathologically confirmed Alzheimer's disease, *Neurology* **38** (1988), 1682–1687.

[17] C.A. Davies, D.M.A. Mann, P.W. Sumpter and P.O. Yates, A quantitative morphometric analysis of the neuronal and synaptic content of the frontal and temporal cortex in patients with Alzheimer's disease, *J Neurol Sci* **78** (1987), 151–164.

[18] A.D. Dayan, Quantitative histological studies on the aged human brain. I. Senile plaques and neurofibrillary tangles in "normal" patients, *Acta Neuropathol (Berl)* **16** (1970), 85–94.

[19] S.T. DeKosky and S.W. Scheff, Synapse loss in frontal cortex biopsies in Alzheimer's disease: correlation with cognitive severity, *Ann Neurol* **27** (1990), 457–464.

[20] S.T. DeKosky, S.W. Scheff and W.R. Markesbery, Laminar organization of cholinergic circuits in human frontal cortex in Alzheimer's disease, *Neurol* **35** (1985), 1425–1431.

[21] D.G. Flood, S.J. Buell, C.H. Defiore, G.J. Horwitz and P.D. Coleman, Age-related dendritic growth in dentate gyrus of human brain is followed by regression in the 'oldest old', *Brain Res* **345** (1985), 366–368.

[22] D.G. Flood, S.J. Buell, G.J. Horwitz and P.D. Coleman, Dendritic extent in human dentate gyrus granule cells in normal aging and senile dementia, *Brain Res* **402** (1987), 205–216.

[23] J. Geddes, D. Monahan, C. Cotman, I.T. Lott, R. Kim and H. Chui, Plasticity of hippocampal circuitry in Alzheimer's disease, *Science* **230** (1985), 1179–1181.

[24] P. Giannakopoulos, P.R. Hof and C. Bouras, Selective vulnerability of neocortical association areas in Alzheimer's disease, *Microsc Res Tech* **43** (1998), 16–23.

[25] P. Giannakopoulos, P.R. Hof, A.S. Giannakopoulos, F.R. Herrmann, J.P. Michel and C. Bouras, Regional distribution of neurofibrillary tangles and senile plaques in the cerebral cortex of very old patients, *Arch Neurol* **52** (1995), 1150–1159.

[26] P. Giannakopoulos, P.R. Hof, J.P. Michel, J. Guimon and C. Bouras, Cerebral cortex pathology in aging and Alzheimer's disease: a quantitative survey of large hospital-based geriatric and psychiatric cohorts, *Brain Res Rev* **25** (1997), 217–245.

[27] P.H. Gibson, EM study of the numbers of cortical synapses in the brains of aging people and people with Alzheimer-type dementia, *Acta Neuropathol (Berl)* **62** (1983), 127–133.

[28] W.P. Goldman, J.L. Price, M. Storandt, E.A. Grant, D.W. McKeel, Jr., E.H. Rubin and J.C. Morris, Absence of cognitive impairment or decline in preclinical Alzheimer's disease, *Neurology* **56** (2001), 361–367.

[29] S. Goto and A. Hirano, Neuronal inputs to hippocampal formation in Alzheimer's disease and in parkinsonism-dementia complex on Guam, *Acta Neuropathol* **79** (1990), 545–550.

[30] H.J. Gundersen, T.F. Bendtsen, L. Korbo, N. Marcussen, A. Moller, K. Nielsen, J.R. Nyengaard, B. Pakkenberg, F.B. Sorensen, A. Vesterby et al., Some new, simple and efficient stereological methods and their use in pathological research and diagnosis, *APMIS* **96** (1988), 379–394.

[31] H.J.G. Gundersen, P. Bagger, T.F. Bendtsen, S.M. Evans, L. Korbo, N. Marcussen, A. Moller, K. Nielsen, J.R. Nyengaard, B. Pakkenberg, F.B. Sorensen, A. Vesterby and M.J. West, The new stereological tools: disector, fractionator, nucleator and point sampled intercepts and their use in pathological research and diagnosis, *APMIS* **96** (1988), 857–881.

[32] J. Hamos, L. DeGennaro and D. Drachman, Synaptic loss in Alzheimer's disease and other dementias, *Neurology* **39** (1989), 355–361.

[33] L.A. Hansen, E. Masliah, S. Quijada-Fawcett and D. Rexin, Entorhinal neurofibrillary tangles in Alzheimer disease with Lewy bodies, *Neurosci Lett* **129** (1991), 269–272.

[34] R.E. Harbaugh, T.M. Reeder and H.J. Senter, Intracerebroventricular bethanechol chloride infusion in Alzheimer's disease: results of a collaborative, double-blind study, *J Neurosurg* **71** (1989), 481–486.

[35] O. Heinonen, H. Soininen, H. Sorvari, O. Kosunen, L. Paljarvi, E. Koivisto and P.J. Riekkinen, Loss of synaptophysin-like immunoreactivity in the hippocampal formation is an early phenomenon in Alzheimer's disease, *Neuroscience* **64** (1995), 375–384.

[36] D.E. Hillman and S. Chen, Plasticity of synaptic size with constancy of total synaptic contact area on Purkinje cells in the cerebellum, *Prog Clin Biol Res* **59A** (1981), 229–245.

[37] W.G. Honer, D.W. Dickson, J. Gleeson and P. Davies, Regional synaptic pathology in Alzheimer's disease, *Neurobiol Aging* **13** (1992), 375–382.

[38] C. Huang, L.O. Wahlund, L. Svensson, B. Winblad and P. Julin, Cingulate cortex hypoperfusion predicts Alzheimer's disease in mild cognitive impairment, *BMC Neurol* **2** (2002), 9.

[39] B.M. Hubbard, G.W. Fenton and J.M. Anderson, A quantitative histological study of early clinical and preclinical Alzheimer's disease, *Neuropathol Appl Neurobiol* **16** (1990), 111–121.

[40] B. Hyman, G. Van Hoesen, L. Kromer and A. Damasio, Perforant pathway changes and memory impairment of Alzheimer's disease, *Ann Neurol* **20** (1986), 472–481.

[41] B.T. Hyman, G.W. Van Hoesen and A.R. Damasio, Memory-related neural systems in Alzheimer's disease: an anatomic study, *Neurology* **40** (1990), 1721–1730.

[42] R. Insausti and D.G. Amaral, Hippocampal formation, in: *The Human Nervous System*, G. Paxinos and J.K. Mai, eds, Vol., Elsevier, San Diego, 2004, pp. 871–914.

[43] R. Katzman, R. Terry, R. DeTeresa, T. Brown, P. Davies, P. Fuld, X. Renbing and A. Peck, Clinical, pathological, and neurochemical changes in dementia: a subgroup with preserved mental status and numerous neocortical plaques, *Ann Neurol* **23** (1988), 138–144.

[44] A.M. Kazee and E.M. Johnson, Alzheimer's disease pathology in not-demented elderly, *J Alz Dis* **1** (1998), 81–89.

[45] Z.D. Khachaturian, Diagnosis of Alzheimer's disease, *Arch Neurol* **42** (1985), 1097–1105.

[46] J.H. Kordower, Y. Chu, G.T. Stebbins, S.T. DeKosky, E.J. Cochran, D. Bennett and E.J. Mufson, Loss and atrophy of layer II entorhinal cortex neurons in elderly people with mild cognitive impairment, *Ann Neurol* **49** (2001), 202–213.

[47] A. Koudinov, E. Matsubara, B. Frangione and J. Ghiso, The soluble form of Alzheimer's amyloid beta protein is complexed to high density lipoprotein 3 and very high density lipoprotein in normal human plasma, *Biochem Biophys Res Commun* **205** (1994), 1164–1171.

[48] A.R. Koudinov, N.V. Koudinova, A. Kumar, R.C. Beavis and J. Ghiso, Biochemical characterization of Alzheimer's soluble amyloid beta protein in human cerebrospinal fluid: association with high density lipoproteins, *Biochem Biophys Res Commun* **223** (1996), 592–597.

[49] C.M. Lauderback, J.M. Hackett, F.F. Huang, J.N. Keller, L.I. Szweda, W.R. Markesbery and D.A. Butterfield, The glial glutamate transporter, GLT-1, is oxidatively modified by 4-hydroxy-2-nonenal in the Alzheimer's disease brain: the role of Abeta1-42, *J Neurochem* **78** (2001), 413–416.

[50] Y.C. Liao, R.S. Liu, Y.C. Lee, C.M. Sun, C.Y. Liu, P.S. Wang, P.N. Wang and H.C. Liu, Selective hypoperfusion of anterior cingulate gyrus in depressed AD patients: a brain SPECT finding by statistical parametric mapping, *Dement Geriatr Cogn Disord* **16** (2003), 238–244.

[51] C.F. Lippa, J.E. Hamos, D. Pulaski-Salo, L.J. Degennaro and D.A. Drachman, Alzheimer's disease and aging: effects on perforant pathway perikarya and synapses, *Neurobiol Aging* **13** (1992), 405–411.

[52] J.E. Lisman and K.M. Harris, Quantal analysis and synaptic anatomy – integrating two views of hippocampal plasticity, *Trends Neurosci* **16** (1993), 141–147.

[53] X. Liu and A. Brun, Synaptophysin immunoreactivity is stable 36 h postmortem, *Dementia* **6** (1995), 211–217.

[54] X. Liu, C. Erikson and A. Brun, Cortical synaptic changes and gliosis in normal aging, Alzheimer's disease and frontal lobe degeneration, *Dementia* **7** (1996), 128–134.

[55] L.F. Lue, Y.M. Kuo, A.E. Roher, L. Brachova, Y. Shen, L. Sue, T. Beach, J.H. Kurth, R.E. Rydel and J. Rogers, Soluble amyloid beta peptide concentration as a predictor of synaptic change in Alzheimer's disease, *Am J Pathol* **155** (1999), 853–862.

[56] W.R. Markesbery and J.M. Carney, Oxidative alterations in Alzheimer's disease, *Brain Pathol* **9** (1999), 133–146.

[57] E. Masliah, M. Mallory, L. Hansen, R. DeTeresa and R.D. Terry, Quantitative synaptic alterations in the human neocortex during normal aging, *Neurology* **43** (1993), 192–197.

[58] E. Masliah, R. Terry, R. DeTeresa and L. Hansen, Immunohistochemical quantification of the synapse-related protein synaptophysin in Alzheimer disease, *Neurosci Lett* **103** (1989), 234–239.

[59] E. Masliah, R.D. Terry, M. Alford, R. DeTeresa and L.A. Hansen, Cortical and subcortical patterns of synaptophysin-like immunoreactivity in Alzheimer's disease, *Am J Pathol* **138** (1991), 235–246.

[60] E. Masliah, R.D. Terry, M. Mallory, M. Alford and L.A. Hansen, Diffuse plaques do not accentuate synapse loss in Alzheimer's disease, *Am J Pathol* **137** (1990), 1293–1297.

[61] B. McEwen, K. Akama, S. Alves, W.G. Brake, K. Bulloch, S. Lee, C. Li, G. Yuen and T.A. Milner, Tracking the estrogen receptor in neurons: implications for estrogen-induced synapse formation, *Proc Natl Acad Sci USA* **98** (2001), 7093–7100.

[62] B.S. McEwen and A.M. Magarinos, Stress and hippocampal plasticity: implications for the pathophysiology of affective disorders, *Hum Psychopharmacol* **16** (2001), S7–S19.

[63] G. McKhann, D. Drachman, M. Folstein and D. Katzman, Clinical diagnosis of Alzheimer's disease, *Neurology* **34** (1984), 939–944.

[64] S. Minoshima, B. Giordani, S. Berent, K.A. Frey, N.L. Foster and D.E. Kuhl, Metabolic reduction in the posterior cingulate cortex in very early Alzheimer's disease, *Ann Neurol* **42** (1997), 85–94.

[65] J.C. Morris, M. Storandt, S.W. McKeel, E.H. Rubin, J.L. Price, E.A. Grant and L. Berg, Cerebral amyloid deposition and diffuse plaques in "normal" aging: Evidence for presymptomatic and very mild Alzheimer's disease, *Neurology* **46** (1996), 707–719.

[66] L. Mucke, E. Masliah, G.Q. Yu, M. Mallory, E.M. Rockenstein, G. Tatsuno, K. Hu, D. Kholodenko, K. Johnson-Wood and L. McConlogue, High-level neuronal expression of A beta 1–42 in wild-type human amyloid protein precursor transgenic mice: synaptotoxicity without plaque formation, *J Neurosci* **20** (2000), 4050–4058.

[67] A. Nunomura, G. Perry, G. Aliev, K. Hirai, A. Takeda, E.K. Balraj, P.K. Jones, H. Ghanbari, T. Wataya, S. Shimohama, S. Chiba, C.S. Atwood, R.B. Petersen and M.A. Smith, Oxidative damage is the earliest event in Alzheimer disease, *J Neuropathol Exp Neurol* **60** (2001), 759–767.

[68] B. Pakkenberg and J.G. Gundersen, Neocortical neuron number in humans: effect of sex and age, *J Comp Neurol* **384** (1997), 312–320.

[69] M.M. Paula-Barbosa, A. Saraiva, M.A. Tavares, M.M. Borges and R.W.H. Verwer, Alzheimer's disease: maintenance of neuronal and synaptic densities in frontal cortical layers II and III, *Acta Neurol Scand* **74** (1986), 404–408.

[70] E. Perdahl, R. Adolfsson, I. Alafuzoff, K.A. Albert, E.J. Nestler, P. Greengard and B. Winblad, Synapsin I (protein I) in different brain regions in senile dementia of Alzheimer type and in multiinfarct dementia, *J Neural Trans* **60** (1984), 133–141.

[71] G. Perry, A.D. Cash and M.A. Smith, Alzheimer Disease and Oxidative Stress, *J Biomed Biotechnol* **2** (2002), 120–123.

[72] G. Perry, M.A. Taddco, A. Nunomura, X. Zhu, T. Zenteno-Savin, K.L. Drew, S. Shimohama, J. Avila, R.J. Castellani and M.A. Smith, Comparative biology and pathology of oxidative stress in Alzheimer and other neurodegenerative diseases: beyond damage and response, *Comp Biochem Physiol C Toxicol Pharmacol* **133** (2002), 507–513.

[73] R.C. Petersen, R. Doody, A. Kurz, R.C. Mohs, J.C. Morris, P.V. Rabins, K. Ritchie, M. Rossor, L. Thal and B. Winblad, Current concepts in mild cognitive impairment, *Arch Neurol* **58** (2001), 1985–1992.

[74] J.L. Price, A.I. Ko, M.J. Wade, S.K. Tsou, D.W. McKeel and J.C. Morris, Neuron number in the entorhinal cortex and CA1 in preclinical Alzheimer disease, *Arch Neurol* **58** (2001), 1395–1402.

[75] L.J. Price, P.B. Davis, J.C. Morris and D.L. White, The distribution of tangles, plaques and related immunohistochemical markers in health aging and Alzheimer's disease, *Neurobiol Aging* **12** (1991), 295–312.

[76] B. Reisberg, S.H. Ferris, M.J. de Leon and T. Crook, The Global Deterioration Scale for assessment of primary degenerative dementia, *Am J Psychiatry* **139** (1982), 1136–1139.

[77] A. Represa, C. Duychaerts, E. Tremblay, J.J. Hauw and Y. Ben-Ari, Is senile dementia of the Alzheimer type associated with hippocampal plasticity, *Brain Res* **457** (1988), 355-359.

[78] S.W. Scheff, Synaptic reorganization after injury: the hippocampus as a model system, in: *Neural Regeneration and Transplantation,* F.J. Seil, ed., Vol., Alan R. Liss, New York, 1989, pp. 137–156.

[79] S.W. Scheff, S.T. DeKosky and D.A. Price, Quantitative assessment of cortical synaptic density in Alzheimer's disease, *Neurobiol Aging* **11** (1990), 29–37.

[80] S.W. Scheff and D. Price, Synapse loss in the temporal lobe in Alzheimer's disease, *Ann Neurol* **33** (1993), 190–199.

[81] S.W. Scheff and D.A. Price, Alzheimer's disease-related synapse loss in the cingulate cortex, *J Alz Dis* **3** (2001), 495–505.

[82] S.W. Scheff and D.A. Price, Synaptic density in the inner molecular layer of the hippocampal dentate gyrus in Alzheimer disease, *J Neuropathol Exp Neurol* **57** (1998), 1146–1153.

[83] S.W. Scheff and D.A. Price, Synaptic pathology in Alzheimer's disease: a review of ultrastructural studies, *Neurobiol Aging* **24** (2003), 1029–1046.

[84] S.W. Scheff, D.A. Price and D.L. Sparks, Quantitative assessment of possible age-related change in synaptic numbers in the human frontal cortex, *Neurobiol Aging* **22** (2001), 355–365.

[85] S.W. Scheff, D.L. Sparks and D.A. Price, Quantitative assessment of synaptic density in the entorhinal cortex in Alzheimer's disease, *Ann Neurol* **34** (1993), 356–361.

[86] S.W. Scheff, D.L. Sparks and D.A. Price, Quantitative assessment of synaptic density in the outer molecular layer of the

hippocampal dentate gyrus in Alzheimer's disease, *Dementia* **7** (1996), 213–220.
[87] M.E. Scheibel, R.D. Lindsay, U. Tomiyasu and A.B. Scheibel, Progressive dendritic changes in aging human cortex, *Exp Neurol* **47** (1975), 392–403.
[88] M.E. Scheibel, R.D. Lindsay, U. Tomiyasu and A.B. Scheibel, Progressive dendritic changes in the aging human limbic system, *Exp Neurol* **53** (1976), 420–430.
[89] M.E. Scheibel, U. Tomiyasu and A.B. Scheibel, The aging human Betz cell, *Exp Neurol* **56** (1977), 598–609.
[90] M.E. Scheibel, U. Tomiyasu and A.B. Scheibel, Dendritic changes in the aging human rhinencephalon, *Trans Am Neurol Assoc* **101** (1976), 23–26.
[91] F.A. Schmitt, D.G. Davis, D.R. Wekstein, C.D. Smith, J.W. Ashford and W.R. Markesbery, "Preclinical" AD revisited: neuropathology of cognitively normal older adults, *Neurology* **55** (2000), 370–376.
[92] M.A. Smith, C.A. Rottkamp, A. Nunomura, A.K. Raina and G. Perry, Oxidative stress in Alzheimer's disease, *Biochim Biophys Acta* **1502** (2000), 139–144.
[93] D.L. Sparks, L. Huaichen, S.W. Scheff, C.M. Coyne and J.C. Hunsaker, Temporal sequence of plaque formation in the cerebral cortex of non-demented individuals, *J Neuropath Exp Neurol* **52** (1993), 135–142.
[94] D.L. Sparks, J.C. Hunsaker, S.W. Scheff, R.J. Kryscio, J.L. Henson and W.R. Markesbery, Cortical senile plaques in coronary artery disease, aging and Alzheimer's disease, *Neurobiol Aging* **11** (1990), 601–607.
[95] D.C. Sterio, The unbiased estimation of number and sizes of arbitrary particles using the disector, *J Microsc* **134** (1984), 127–136.
[96] C.I. Sze, J.C. Troncoso, C. Kawas, P. Mouton, D.L. Price and L.J. Martin, Loss of the presynaptic vesicle protein synaptophysin in hippocampus correlates with cognitive decline in Alzheimer disease, *J Neuropathol Exp Neurol* **56** (1997), 933–944.
[97] R.D. Terry, E. Masliah, D.P. Salmon, N. Butters, R. DeTeresa, R. Hill, L.A. Hansen and R. Katzman, Physical basis of cognitive alterations in Alzheimer's disease: synapse loss is the major correlate of cognitive impairment, *Ann Neurol* **30** (1991), 572–580.
[98] G.W. Van Hoesen, The parahippocampal gyrus: new observations regarding its cortical connections in the monkey, *Trends Neurosci* (1982), 345–350.
[99] G.W. Van Hoesen, B.T. Hyman and A.R. Damasio, Entorhinal cortex pathology in Alzheimer's disease, *Hippocampus* **1** (1991), 1–8.
[100] B.A. Vogt, F.D. M. and O.C. R., Functional Heterogeneity in Cingulate Cortex: The Anterior Executive and Posterior Evaluative Regions, *Cerebral Cortex* **443** (1992), 1047–3211.
[101] B.A. Vogt and P.D. N., Cingulate Cortex of the Rhesus Monkey: II. Cortical Afferents, *J Comp Neurol* **262** (1987), 271–289.
[102] B.A. Vogt, P.D. N. and R. D., Cingulate Cortex of the Rhesus Monkey: I. Cytoarchitecture and Thalamic Afferents, *J Comp Neurol* **262** (1987), 256–270.
[103] B.A. Vogt, G.W. Van Hoesen and L.J. Vogt, Laminar distribution of neuron degeneration in posterior cingulate cortex in Alzheimer's disease, *Acta Neuropath* **80** (1990), 581–589.
[104] K. Wakabayaski, W.G. Honer and E. Masliah, Synapse alterations in the hippocampal-entorhinal function in Alzheimer's disease with and without Lewy body disease, *Brain Res* **667** (1994), 24–32.
[105] S.-S. Zhan, K. Beyreuther and H.P. Schmitt, Quantitative assessment of the synaptophysin immuno-reactivity of the cortical neuropil in various neurodegenerative disorders with dementia, *Dementia* **4** (1993), 66–74.

My own experience in early research on Alzheimer disease

Robert D. Terry
Department of Neurosciences, University of California San Diego, USA
E-mail: rterry@ucsd.edu

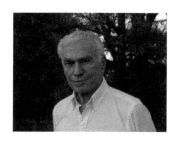

Abstract. This brief paper reviews the work on dementia by the Neuropathology group at the Einstein College of Medicine and later at the University of California, San Diego, from the time of our first approaches to Alzheimer Disease in 1959. The electron microscope studies concerned the tangle (got it wrong) and then the plaque (got it right). Lysosomes and active microglia were noted in the plaques. Axoplasmic transport was suggested to be abnormal. We studied the plaques in old dogs and old monkeys, and then went on to use image analysis to count neurons in the neocortex of Alzheimer cases and in examples of normal aging. Later in San Diego we quantified presynaptic boutons and recognized their loss as the major direct cause of dementia. Many collaborators including Henry Wisniewski participated in these early attempts to understand the disease.

In 1959 I moved from Montefiore Hospital where I had been nominally in charge of Neuropathology (Dr. Harry Zimmerman was still very active) to the Albert Einstein College of Medicine across the Bronx to form a new neuropathology section in the Department of Pathology but, very significantly, with space in Neurology of which Saul Korey was Chair. Saul and I immediately began discussions about possible collaborative research on human disease. He was a neurochemist and I an electron microscopist having learned the technique in Paris a few years previously.

We settled on Tay Sachs disease and Alzheimer disease (AD) because both were distributed diffusely in the neocortex, microscopically identifiable and fatal. Cortical biopsies were to be performed by Leo Davidoff, a superb senior neurosurgeon.

Tay Sachs specimens yielded spectacular pictures [20], but AD was more durable in terms of lasting interest and complexity. We knew of no one else working in the field. Of course, we, like everyone else, had no idea of the real prevalence of the disorder. Within a few years it became apparent that the most common form of senile dementia was in most aspects identical to the very rare presenile AD, and then the real size of the affected population began to dawn on us. But it was not until 1976 that my colleague Robert Katzman's brief publication [6] brought the attention of clinicians and government to bear on the problem.

Davidoff's frontal biopsies were carefully excised and excellently preserved, and readily revealed the first EM (Siemens) images of the neurofibrillary tangle. I think that ours at Montefiore had been the first electron microscope in a neuropath lab in 1954, but the new Siemens apparatus in the Einstein lab was vastly more effective. The only previous ultrastructural work on the normal central neuron had been published by Palay [12], but the microtubules were not very clear in the published images. On that basis I thought that the tangle was made up of twisted microtubules [15], but Kidd proved correct in identifying the fibers as paired helical filaments (PHF) [7]. My own micrographs had displayed numerous circular profiles, so I persisted with the twisted tubule notion until Wisniewski, Narang & I presented a scale model which when sectioned to scale perfectly reproduced the EM images of PHF, and explained the circular profiles on the basis of section thickness [23].

Meanwhile the plaque proved more difficult to elucidate. It was only after studying EM sections from no fewer than 150 blocks, that I finally felt confident to publish [17]. We identified the amyloid, the neurites, the microglia and the astrocytes. Others published soon thereafter, but Luse [9] apparently did not notice the amyloid, and Kidd [8], even after trans-Atlantic consultations, essentially confirmed all we had already written. Suzuki and I applied the acid phosphatase technique to the sections proving that the dense bodies common in the dystrophic neurites were lysosomes [14]. We also suggested in that paper the possibility that axoplasmic transport was reduced in the affected neurons because of the diminished and twisted microtubules, and that this might be relevant to the dystrophic neurites.

Silver stains were slow, expensive and of variable quality, so I turned to thioflavin S following the work of P. Schwartz [13] who had used thioflavin T to demonstrate senile amyloid in aged organs other than the brain. With an excitation filter bluer than the usual FITC filter, the images were brilliant and the technique was sensitive, simple, quick and inexpensive. Manual counting of plaques and tangles was feasible, but our correlations with *in vivo* psychologic tests never came up to the levels reported by Blessed et al. [1].

I managed to acquire an image analysis apparatus (the first in a US neuropath lab) thanks to a generous grant from the Kresge Foundation, and we began cell counting utilizing the new editing capacity to separate contiguous cells, eliminate blood vessels and artifacts, and, also important, to measure the cross-section area of the neuronal somata [19]. Neuron counts were statistically low in AD but did not correlate with cognition with the expected strength. Later counting cortical neurons in normal aging (in specimens mostly provided by Joe Rogers, PhD) produced surprising results which were at strong variance from the classical data. We found that there was little or no loss of neurons in normal aging, but significant shrinkage of the large neuronal somata [16]. It is important to note that while stereologic methods have recently replaced and even condemned image analysis, careful results do not differ from those we had reported [4,19]!

Meanwhile, in collaboration with Henry Wisniewski, Dino Ghetti and others, we examined by EM the brains of old dogs [22] and old monkeys [21]. We reported that both species had typical plaques with amyloid, but no PHF and no tangles.

In about 1976, Peter Davies, working in Edinborough, reported that choline acetyl transferase (ChAT) was significantly depressed in Alzheimer cortex [2]. Peter was readily persuaded to join us in New York, where we pursued the cholinergic aspects and other chemical abnormalities including the deficiency of somatostatin [3].

The cholinergic findings opened the field to the pharmacologists and neuro biologists.

It was a few years later, now at UCSD, that Eliezer Masliah and I developed a technique for staining synapses with anti-synaptophysin and for quantifying their population density, first by image analysis [10]. The confocal microscope (I think ours was the first in a neuropath lab) enabled even more precise, semi-automated synapse counts [11]. Here, finally, we found the sort of strong clinico-pathologic correlations with tests of cognition that were entirely convincing of a rational causal mechanism of dementia [18].

During those first 15 or 20 years, I was most fortunate to have in the lab for a year or more Kinuko Suzuki, Nick Gonatas, Mike Shelanski, Henryk Wisniewski, Dino Ghetti, Mauro Dal Canto, Dick Horoupian, Roy Weller, Jan Leestma, Fernando Aleu, Cedric Raine, John Prineas, Peter Davies, Khalid Iqbal, Jim Powers, Jim Goldman, Sue Yen, Dennis Dickson and several other excellent people. I hesitate to say that I trained them, because what I really did was simply to provide the environment and leave them pretty much alone to develop. Their collaboration and their individual work played a major role in all our thinking and in whatever we accomplished.

Indeed, I've been very lucky.

References

[1] G. Blessed, B.E. Tomlinson and M. Roth, The association between quantitative measures of dementia and of senile changes in the cerebral gray matter of elderly subjects, *Brit. J. Psych.* **114** (1968), 797–811.

[2] P. Davies and A. Maloney, Selective loss of central cholinergic neurons in Alzheimer's disease, *Lancet* **2** (1976), 1403.

[3] P. Davies and R.D. Terry, Cortical somatostatin-like immunoreactivity in cases of Alzheimer's disease and senile dementia of the Alzheimer type, *Neurobiology of Aging* **2** (1981), 9–14.

[4] I.P. Everall, R. DeTeresa, R.D. Terry and E. Masliah, Comparison of two quantitative methods for the evaluation of neuronal number in the frontal cortex in Alzheimer disease, *J. Neuropath. & Expmt. Neurol.* **56** (1997), 1202–1206.

[5] T. Gomez-Isla, R. Hollister, H. West, S. Mui, J.H. Growden, R.C. Petersen, J.E. Parisi and B.T. Hyman, Neuronal loss correlates with but exceeds neurofibrillary tangles in Alzheimer's disease, *Ann. Neurol.* **41** (1997), 17–24.

[6] R. Katzman, The prevalence and malignancy of Alzheimer's disease: A major killer, *Arch. Neurol.* **33** (1976), 217–218.

[7] M. Kidd, Paired helical filaments in electron microscopy in Alzheimer's disease, *Nature* **197** (1963), 192–193.

[8] M. Kidd, Alzheimer's disease:an electron microscopic study, *Brain* **87** (1964), 307–320.

[9] S.A. Luse, The ultrastructure of senile plaques, *Am. J. Path.* **44** (1964), 553–563.

[10] E. Masliah, R.D. Terry, R. DeTeresa and L.A. Hansen, Immunohistochemical quantification of the synapse- related protein synaptophysin in Alzheimer disease, *Neurosci. Letters* **103** (1989), 234–239.

[11] E. Masliah, R.D. Terry, M. Mallory, M. Alford and L.A. Hansen, Diffuse plaques do not accentuate synapse loss in Alzheimer's disease, *Am. J. Path.* **137** (1990), 1293–1297.

[12] S.L. Palay and G.E. Palade, The fine structure of neurons, *J. Biophys. and Biochem. Cytology* **1** (1955), 69–88.

[13] P. Schwarz, Amyloid degeneration and tuberculosis in the aged, *Gerontologia* **18** (1972), 321–362.

[14] K. Suzuki and R.D. Terry, Fine structural localization of acid phosphatase in senile plaques in Alzheimer's presenile dementia, *Acta Neuropathologica* **8** (1967), 276–284.

[15] R.D. Terry, The fine structure of neurofibrillary tangles in Alzheimer's disease, *J. Neuropath. & Expmt. Neurol.* **22** (1963), 629–642.

[16] R.D. Terry, R. DeTeresa and L.A. Hansen, Neocortical cell counts in normal human adult aging, *Ann. Neurol.* **21** (1987), 530–539.

[17] R.D.Terry, N.K. Gonatas and M. Weiss, Ultrastructural studies in Alzheimer's presenile dementia, *Am. J. Path.* **44** (1964), 269–297.

[18] R.D. Terry, E. Masliah, D.P. Salmon, N. Butters, R. DeTeresa, R. Hill, L.A. Hansen and R. Katzman, Physical basis of cognitive alterations in Alzheimer disease: synapse loss is the major correlate of cognitive impairment, *Ann. Neurol.* **30** (1991), 572–580.

[19] R.D.Terry, A. Peck, R. DeTeresa, R. Schechter and D.S. Horoupian, Some morpho-metric aspects of the brain in senile dementia of the Alzheimer type, *Ann. Neurol.* **10** (1981), 184–192.

[20] R.D. Terry and M. Weiss, Studies in Tay Sachs disease. II Ultrastructure of the cerebrum J, *Neuropath. & Expmt. Neurol.* **22** (1963), 18–55.

[21] H.M. Wisniewski, B. Ghetti and R.D. Terry, Neuritic (senile) plaques and filamentous changes in aged rhesus monkeys, *J. Neuropath. & Expmt. Neurol.* **32** (1973), 566–584.

[22] H.M. Wisniewski, A.B. Johnson, C.S. Raine, W.J. Kay and R.D. Terry, Senile plaques and cerebral amyloidosis in aged dogs. A histochemical and ultrastructural study, *Lab. Invest.* **23** (1970), 287–296.

[23] H.M. Wisniewski, H.K. Narang and R.D. Terry, Neurofibrillary tangles of paired helical filaments, *J. Neural. Sci.* **27** (1976), 173–181.

Amyloid

Molecular basis of memory loss in the Tg2576 mouse model of Alzheimer's disease

Karen H. Ashe*

Departments of Neurology, Neuroscience and Graduate Program in Neuroscience, University of Minnesota, Minneapolis, MN 55455, USA; Geriatric Research, Education and Clinical Center, Minneapolis Veterans Affairs Medical Center, Minneapolis, MN 55417, USA

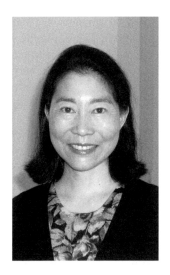

Abstract. Understanding the pathophysiology and treatment of Alzheimer's disease is vitally important. Alzheimer's disease threatens to affect currently at least 30% of all individuals currently alive in the 12 most financially developed countries, unless interventions are discovered to prevent or treat the disease. Although memory loss is the cardinal symptom of Alzheimer's disease, the pathophysiological mechanisms leading to cognitive deficits are poorly understood. It is difficult to address this problem in human studies, and impossible in cultured cells. Therefore, animal models are needed to elucidate the molecular mechanisms leading to dementia. A large number of animal models have focussed upon the role of amyloid plaques in the pathogenesis of Alzheimer's disease, because amyloid plaques are an essential diagnostic feature of the disease. However, the mechanism by which amyloid plaques or their principal molecular constituent, the amyloid-β protein (Aβ), disrupt cognitive function is not well understood. Herein, I describe my perspective on what we have learned about how Aβ impairs memory from research on Alzheimer's disease in mice and rats.

Keywords: Memory, transgenic, mice, rats, Morris water maze, operant behavioral task, Aβ oligomers

1. Natural history of Alzheimer's disease

To appreciate the context in which animal models have helped us understand the pathophysiology of memory loss, it is important to delineate the natural history of Alzheimer's disease. Alzheimer's disease has a very insidious onset; we do not know precisely when neural dysfunction begins. The brains of patients dying with Alzheimer's disease are devastated by widespread plaques, tangles and neuron loss. In 1999 it became clear that there is a prodrome to Alzheimer's disease, which is frequently referred to as mild cognitive impairment [12]. These individuals have subjective complaints and mild clinical abnormalities on examination. The brains of individuals at this stage of illness have some plaques and tangles, but neuron loss is restricted to the entorhinal cortex [4,11].

Intriguingly, asymptomatic individuals at risk genetically for Alzheimer's disease have evidence of brain dysfunction in functional magnetic resonance imaging and positron emission tomography studies [2,13], suggesting that there may be a latent phase of Alzheimer's disease. Although we do not know what kind of brain pathology exists in these individuals, it is likely that they have rare plaques and tangles, because these neuropathological abnormalities appear in autopsy series

---

*Address for correspondence: Karen H. Ashe, MD, PhD, Department of Neurology, Mayo Mail Code 295, 420 Delaware Street, SE, Minneapolis, MN 55455, USA. Tel.: +1 612 626 0652; Fax: +1 612 626 2639; E-mail: hsiao005@umn.edu.

of cognitively intact individuals after the age of 40 [9]. However, neuron numbers in asymptomatic individuals are normal [11]. Thus, pre-clinical individuals at high risk for Alzheimer's disease have no neuronal loss but may have subtle abnormalities in brain function.

2. Memory function in APP transgenic mouse models of Alzheimer's disease

When I began research on Alzheimer's disease 1 year ago, the role of structural changes in the pathogenesis of the cognitive dysfunction, such as amyloid plaques, neurofibrillary tangles, synaptic degeneration and neuron loss, dominated the field, and still governs the conduct of much of the research today. In 1995 I began to doubt the primacy of these structural abnormalities when the first transgenic mice expressing the amyloid β protein precursor (AβPP) created in my laboratory at the University of Minnesota developed age-related neurological deficits in the absence of plaques or neurodegenerative changes [6]. It became clear that focusing on brain dysfunction, in addition to structural brain pathology, was crucial and indispensable to achieving a genuine and complete understanding of the pathogenesis of Alzheimer's disease. Thus, began an 11-year quest to determine the molecular basis of brain dysfunction in AβPP transgenic mice, which came to a successful conclusion earlier this year when my colleagues and I showed that a 56kDa soluble complex of Aβ, called Aβ*56 in the brains of the Tg2576 mouse model of Alzheimer's disease that disrupts cognitive function in the absence of amyloidosis or neuronal loss [5,10].

In Alzheimer's disease there is severe neurodegeneration, but in the Tg2576 model there is memory impairment without structural changes [5,8]. It is precisely because of this difference that I believe our discovery of Aβ*56 is so important. The identification and isolation of Aβ*56, a highly specific form of soluble Aβ which impairs memory in the absence of neurodegenerative changes, offers the potential for detecting its correlate in humans with pre-clinical Alzheimer's disease. If we are ever to develop truly effective treatments for Alzheimer's disease, we need to target the molecule which initiates brain dysfunction and abort the disease before permanent structural changes have developed. The discovery of Aβ*56 provides a specific answer to the central question of the nature of the molecular entity initiating brain dysfunction in a mouse model of Alzheimer's disease, with attendant therapeutic implications.

3. Intellectual and technical advances leading to the discovery of Aβ*56

Never before has the specific molecule causing brain dysfunction in cognitively impaired animals modelling a neurodegenerative disease been identified and isolated. In the effort to determine the molecular basis of memory loss in Alzheimer's disease, there were numerous technical and intellectual hurdles to overcome. The first major technical challenge was to create a transgenic mouse model amenable to memory testing. Drawing upon experience creating the first transgenic mouse model of neurodegenerative disease, an inherited form of prion disease [7], my colleagues and I created Tg2576 mice by expressing mutant AβPP at adequately high levels in the appropriate background strain of mice [5]. The second challenge was to develop memory tests for mice with sufficient sensitivity, specificity and dynamic range. Valuable discussions with Michela Gallagher at Johns Hopkins University led us to tailor the Morris water maze to suit mice in different background strains [14]. The third challenge was to separate brain proteins with high fidelity into fractions corresponding to relevant subcellular compartments. The secret to overcoming this problem involved a series of biochemical extractions of brain tissue meticulously designed by Sylvain Lesné, in my laboratory [10]. The fourth challenge was to develop a highly sensitive cognitive bioassay for soluble Aβ oligomers. James Cleary at the Minneapolis VA Medical Center and I developed a suitable rat operant behavioral paradigm that is at least one order of magnitude more sensitive than traditional rodent behavioral tests, such as the Morris water maze. In collaboration with Dennis Selkoe and Dominic Walsh at Harvard Medical School, we demonstrated adverse effects on cognitive function of 20 μl of picomolar solutions of Aβ oligomers injected into the cerebral ventricles of healthy, young rats [3]. Michela Gallagher and Ming Teng Koh then extended these studies to show that Aβ*56 injected into the lateral ventricles of young rats transiently disrupted spatial reference memory using a modified, highly sensitive version of the Morris water maze [10].

The main intellectual dilemma was appreciating that the solution to the enigma that the dramatic increase in all previously measured Aβ occurred at a time when memory deficits were unchanging implied the existence of a specific soluble complex of Aβ which disrupted memory in the absence of neuronal loss or Aβ amyloidosis, called Aβ* [1]. Another was recognizing that

ELISA assays, which have become the standard method for measuring Aβ, fail to detect Aβ*. A third was becoming aware that Tg2576 mice mimick pre-clinical Alzheimer's disease better than they resemble actual Alzheimer patients.

We surmounted the intellectual and technical obstacles along the road leading to the discovery of the 56 kDa soluble complex of Aβ because stimulating and fruitful collaborations both within and outside my laboratory and University. In addition to the individuals named above, Greg Cole at UCLA, Steven Younkin at Mayo Clinic Jacksonville and Brad Hyman at Harvard Medical School helped to perform the first molecular pathological and biochemical characterizations of the Tg2576 mouse. These individuals, along with George Carlson at the McLaughlin Research Institute and Paul Chapman at Cardiff University, helped formulate the Aβ* hypothesis.

4. Conclusion

Animal models are essential for elucidating the pathophysiological and molecular mechanisms leading to dementia in Alzheimer's disease. Transgenic mouse models expressing Aβ, the principle molecular component of amyloid plaques in Alzheimer's disease, have helped to determine the molecular and cellular processes involved in producing cognitive deficits. Soluble Aβ oligomers are the leading candidate for Aβ species responsible for disrupting memory in AβPP transgenic mice. Recently, we identified and isolated a soluble Aβ complex, called Aβ*56, causing memory deficits in the Tg2576 mouse model of Alzheimer's disease.

If Aβ*56 can be detected and successfully targeted in humans with pre-clinical Alzheimer's disease, then this would be likely to have a similar impact in the field of neurology as the early detection and treatment of high blood pressure and high cholesterol have had in the field of stroke and myocardial infarction prevention. Thus, the study of a mouse model of pre-clinical Alzheimer's disease has been a valuable endeavour because it may lead to therapies that will prevent the irreversible structural changes found in Alzheimer's disease. Although the Tg2576 model, created in my laboratory, is the most widely used model of Alzheimer's disease in the world, the majority of investigators using the model have yet to recognize that it more closely mimics individuals at high risk for developing Alzheimer's disease than it resembles actual Alzheimer patients. This knowledge, together with our discovery of Aβ*, places the Alzheimer's research community in the position of being able to develop interventions for treating Alzheimer's disease before significant structural changes have occurred.

References

[1] K.H. Ashe, Learning and memory in transgenic mice modeling Alzheimer's disease, *Learn. Mem.* **8** (2001), 301–308.
[2] S.Y. Bookheimer, M.H. Strojwas, M.S. Cohen, A.M. Saunders, M.A. Pericak-Vance, J.C. Mazziotta and G.W. Small, Patterns of brain activation in people at risk for Alzheimer's disease, *N. Engl. J. Med.* **343** (2000), 450–456.
[3] J.P. Cleary, D.M. Walsh, J.J. Hofmeister, G.M. Shankar, M.A. Kuskowski, D.J. Selkoe and K.H. Ashe, Natural oligomers of the amyloid-beta protein specifically disrupt cognitive function, *Nat. Neurosci.* **8** (2005), 79–84.
[4] T. Gómez-Isla, J.L. Price, J.D.W. McKeel, J.C. Morris, J.H. Growdon and B.T. Hyman, Profound loss of layer 2 entorhinal cortex neurons occurs in very mild Alzheimer's disease, *J. Neurosci.* **16** (1996), 4491–4500.
[5] K. Hsiao, P. Chapman, S. Nilsen, C. Eckman, Y. Harigaya, S. Younkin, F. Yang and G. Cole, Correlative memory deficits, Aβ elevation, and amyloid plaques in transgenic mice, *Science* **274** (1996), 99–102.
[6] K.K. Hsiao, D.R. Borchelt, K. Olson, R. Johannsdottir, C. Kitt, W. Yunis, S. Xu, C. Eckman, S. Younkin, D. Price, C. Iadecola, H.B. Clark and G. Carlson, Age-related CNS disorder and early death in transgenic FVB/N mice overexpressing Alzheimer amyloid precursor proteins, *Neuron* **15** (1995), 1203–1218.
[7] K.K. Hsiao, M. Scott, D. Foster, D.F. Groth, S.J. DeArmond and S.B. Prusiner, Spontaneous neurodegeneration in transgenic mice with mutant prion protein, *Science* **250** (1990), 1587–1590.
[8] M.C. Irizarry, M. McNamara, K. Fedorchak, K. Hsiao and B.T. Hyman, APPSw transgenic mice develop age-related A beta deposits and neuropil abnormalities, but no neuronal loss in CA1, *J. Neuropathol. Exp. Neurol.* **56** (1997), 965–973.
[9] D.S. Knopman, J.E. Parisi, A. Salviati, M. Floriach-Robert, B.F. Boeve, R.J. Ivnik, G.E. Smith, D.W. Dickson, K.A. Johnson, L.E. Petersen, W.C. McDonald, H. Braak and R.C. Petersen, Neuropathology of cognitively normal elderly, *J. Neuropathol. Exp. Neurol.* **62** (2003), 1087–1095.
[10] S. Lesné, M.T. Koh, L. Kotilinek, R. Kayed, C.G. Glabe, A. Yang, M. Gallagher and K.H. Ashe, A specific amyloid-β protein assembly in the brain impairs memory, *Nature* **440** (2006), 352–357.
[11] J.C. Morris and A.L. Price, Pathologic correlates of nondemented aging, mild cognitive impairment, and early-stage Alzheimer's disease, *J. Mol. Neurosci.* **17** (2001), 101–118.
[12] R.C. Petersen, G.E. Smith, S.C. Waring, R.J. Ivnik, E.G. Tangalos and E. Kokmen, Mild cognitive impairment: clinical characterization and outcome, *Arch. Neurol.* **56** (1999), 303–308.
[13] G.W. Small, L.M. Ercoli, D.H. Silverman, S.C. Huang, S. Komo, S.Y. Bookheimer, H. Lavretsky, K. Miller, P. Siddarth, N.L. Rasgon, J.C. Mazziotta, S. Saxena, H.M. Wu, M.S. Mega, J.L. Cummings, A.M. Saunders, M.A. Pericak-Vance, A.D. Roses, J.R. Barrio and M.E. Phelps, Cerebral metabolic and cognitive decline in persons at genetic risk for Alzheimer's disease, *Proc. Natl. Acad. Sci. USA* **97** (2000), 6037–6042.

[14] M.A. Westerman, D. Cooper-Blacketer, A. Mariash, L. Kotilinek, T. Kawarabayashi, L.H. Younkin, G.A. Carlson, S.G. Younkin and K.H. Ashe, The relationship between Abeta and memory in the Tg2576 mouse model of Alzheimer's disease, *J. Neurosci.* **22** (2002), 1858–1867.

Soluble amyloid-β in the brain: The scarlet pimpernel

Massimo Tabaton[a] and Pierluigi Gambetti[b]
[a]University of Genova, Institute of Neurology, Via De Toni 5, 16132 Genova, Italy
Tel.: +39 0 10 353 7064; Fax: +39 0 10 353 8639; E-mail: mtabaton@neurologia.unige.it
[b]Case Western Reserve University, 2085 Adelbert Road, Room 419, Cleveland, Ohio 44106, USA
Tel.: +1 216 368 0587; Fax: +1 216 368 4090; E-mail: Pierluigi.Gambetti@case.edu

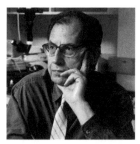
Pierluigi Gambetti

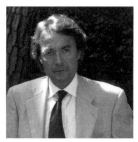
Massimo Tabaton

Abstract. Researchers since the 1990s have predominantly focused on the amyloid hypothesis and the formation of amyloid fibrils as the culprit behind AD when we began working on soluble Aβ (sAβ). Unexpectedly, this work produced several novel findings. First, we observed that N-terminal truncated peptides are the major components of soluble and insoluble Aβ in AD; secondly, that all sAβ species belong to the 42 form and the sAβ x-40 species is virtually absent in AD parenchyma; thirdly, that Aβ 42 in the soluble form is non-detectable by immunoblots in plaque-free, normal brains. The later observation that sAβ 42 species is present in amyloid β protein precursor (AβPP) over-expressing brains of patients with Down syndrome in prenatal and early postnatal development argued that sAβ is present in brain in abnormal conditions and that its appearance seeds Aβ aggregation and accumulation. Although the sAβ we described in intact brain tissue appeared to match the soluble Aβ oligomers detected in cell media, which were subsequently shown to be the most toxic form of Aβ, our research has been virtually ignored by the Alzheimer field. It continues nevertheless. Recently we demonstrated that the sAβ species present in physiologically aging brains are different from those present in brains with sporadic AD as the latter form oligomers more quickly, are more toxic to neurons, and produce more severe membrane damage than the Aβ species associated with normal brain aging. Furthermore, in familial AD, the composition of soluble Aβ appears to dictate distinctive features of the disease phenotype introducing the notion of Aβ strains, a concept well established in prion diseases.

1. Once upon a time there were insoluble fibrils

Amyloid fibrils and paired helical filaments... the veterans of Alzheimer research have been haggling with these terms for a long time. After the first description of their fine structure [25], amyloid and paired helical filaments (PHF) have been considered the main structural lesions of Alzheimer's disease (AD). But which of them is the real culprit? To answer this question, scientists in the early eighties examined correlations; they morphometrically assessed these two lesions at autopsy in subjects cognitively tested shortly before death. These quantitative studies, however, failed to identify the primary lesion.

The identification of β-protein, or A4 (later called amyloid-β) [Aβ], as the constituent of amyloid fibrils, and the cloning and positioning of its precursor protein (AβPP) gene, led to the amyloid, or cascade, hypothesis. This hypothesis was put forth when, besides the evidence of Down's syndrome, it was shown that AβPP mutations caused familial AD and also when it was demonstrated that amyloid fibrils killed neurons in culture [5,6,8,10,13,31]. By then, we were in the nineties and all researchers who believed in the amyloid hypothesis were focused on understanding how $A\beta$ could form amyloid fibrils. Other topics of interest were the chemical and physical properties of $A\beta$ and the length of its C-terminus. Primarily, however, researchers wanted to know how amyloid fibrils caused toxicity in neurons. The culprit turned out to be the insoluble fibrils; they were visible, rigid and sticky. These fibers had all the features of the Bad and the Ugly. In contrast, $A\beta$ by itself was the Good, since, as reported by Selkoe et al., $A\beta$, at low, non-forming fibril concentrations, actually promoted neuronal survival [29].

2. The concept of soluble amyloid-β

The idea of working on soluble $A\beta$ ($sA\beta$) came to us in 1991. By this time, the use of anti-$A\beta$ antibodies had led to the discovery of diffuse plaques and their amorphous non-fibrillary appearance [30]. We predicted that diffuse plaques were different from neuritic plaques in terms of $A\beta$ species and associated proteins, and we chose to examine the cerebellar cortex because it was the brain region that exclusively contained such diffuse plaques. The first study was carried out in AD brains using immunoblot to compare fractions extracted with various detergents from the cerebral cortex with similar fractions extracted from the cerebellum. Differences between the cerebral cortex and cerebellum were not found. Paradoxically, the use of detergents to extract $A\beta$ caused poor peptide resolution and a smear of reactivity that blurred the actual migration of the peptides; immunoblots were still developed with diaminobenzidine at the time.

In 1992, Steven Younkin and his group at the Institute of Pathology of Case Western Reserve University and Selkoe's group, independently, discovered that $A\beta$ is normally produced by cells, and that in the cell media $A\beta$ was present in a soluble, non-aggregated form [7, 21]. We were aware of the Younkin's finding prior to its publication as Steve worked on the same floor as we did and had informed our group of their results. The evidence that $sA\beta$ was produced under normal conditions triggered our decision to immediately search for $sA\beta$ in brain tissue of normal and AD subjects in order to answer two questions: First, whether $sA\beta$ was present in the soluble fraction of brain tissue from individuals who were not only cognitively intact but also free of amyloid, neuritic and diffuse plaques; secondly, whether soluble and insoluble $A\beta$ present in the AD brains had the same composition.

The project was straightforward. We analyzed water-soluble and insoluble fractions of the cerebral cortex and cerebellum from AD cases. As normal controls we used cerebral cortex and cerebellum from age matched, normal individuals that immunocytochemistry on sections obtained from the very same brain tissues used to generate the fractions excluded the presence of all types of AD plaques [22].

3. A novel pattern of $A\beta$ composition

The results were unexpected. Water-soluble $A\beta$, immunoprecipitated from AD brains, was loaded onto Tris-Tricine gels, and detected on blots using 4G8 antibody. Results revealed three sharp bands of 4.5 kDa, 4.0 kDa, and 3.3 kDa, respectively. Using monoclonal antibodies specific to different portions of $A\beta$ and to the C-termini 40 and 42 (provided by Drs. Seubert and Shenk, Elan Inc., and Takeda, Inc.), we were able to establish that the low MW bands corresponded to the N-terminal truncated $A\beta$ species and that all the $A\beta$ peptides belonged to the long "42" form. Moreover, the intermediate 4 kDa band was consistently the most prominent in all 20 AD cases examined. Insoluble $A\beta$, extracted from amyloid fractions with formic acid, showed an identical immunoblot pattern. We also ascertained that water-soluble $A\beta$ was not detectable with this particular method in the cerebral cortex that was free of plaques. Instead, immunoblots performed on the cerebrospinal fluid (CSF) from normal subjects demonstrated a single 4.5 kDa band corresponding to full-length $A\beta$ 1–40/42.

This study disclosed many novel findings that were further defined by us at a later date. It also included data that would be published by other investigators in the years following our original work. Firstly, our research established that N-terminal truncated peptides are the major components of soluble and insoluble $A\beta$ in AD. Secondly, we showed that all $A\beta$ species belong to the 42 form and the $A\beta$ x-40 species is virtually absent in AD parenchyma. Previous direct analysis of amyloid fractions yielded the wrong $A\beta$ composition, probably due to large parts of $A\beta$ species being lost by harsh extraction methods [14]. Hence, our method was the first to allow for the precise determination of the type of $A\beta$ species that accumulates in AD brains, as was confirmed in the following years [9,19]. Thirdly, our study demonstrated that Aβ 42 in the soluble form is non-detectable by immunoblots in plaque-free, normal brains. Advances in ECL sensitivity allowed us to ascertain eight years later that 1 ng is the threshold amount for Aβ 1–42 detection in immunoblots using 4G8. Concomitantly, a sandwich ELISA assay with a detection limit of 5 pg for Aβ 42 (IBL, Gumna) failed to detect Aβ 42 in soluble fractions obtained from normal cerebral cortex from 40–60 year-old, plaque-free individuals [23]. This finding implies that Aβ 42 does not exist in significant amounts in the normal brain, and that its appearance seeds Aβ aggregation. This, in turn, triggers the process of Aβ accumulation, which is the initial event in AD. These results also argue for the presence of a mechanism rapidly binding or breaking down Aβ 42, such as the complex system of extracellular proteases (neprylisin, IDE, plasmin, etc.) discovered in later years.

So, our first study had in its core many data that were subsequently shown to be critical in the understanding of AD pathogenesis. Nevertheless, the study [22] was almost ignored by the Alzheimer field. Why?

4. The reasons for an unsuccessful discovery

We failed to exploit the potential of our findings. We did not precisely characterize (with mass spectrometry) the composition of sAβ. We also failed to emphasize and quantitatively determine the predominance of the N-terminal truncated Aβ species over the full-length form, nor did we determine the state of aggregation of sAβ. This characterization was completed only in our follow-up studies. Perhaps the most important omission was that we did not bring to the forefront the concept of sAβ being absent in the normal brain. As we stated above, Aβ 42 species is virtually undetectable in soluble brain fractions from normal brain. That is the crucial point: the appearance of Aβ 42 in the soluble fraction of cerebral cortex and its detection in immunoblots mark the initial formation of soluble and diffusible Aβ aggregates. It is the first clear sign that the process of Aβ accumulation has started. Only recently, in an article revealing that Aβ is different in AD than in normal aging, we demonstrated that in the presence of diffuse plaques, sAβ constitutively exists in the brain in the form of small aggregates larger than 10 kDa and composed of a mixture of variable Aβ species. These aggregates separate under denaturing conditions into monomers and several SDS-resistant oligomers [15].

Thus, we were not effective in the presentation of our data, and our message was neither received nor understood. We also encountered an inexplicable, silent (in one instance public) opposition to our data and conclusions, which were systematically ignored or reproduced, at least in part, without sufficient acknowledgement. Perhaps, researchers who were influential at the time were unsympathetic to the idea that data from cell cultures showing the presence of Aβ under normal conditions might not be applicable to brain tissue *in situ*. Several groups claimed to have found sAβ in normal brains following ELISA quantification of "soluble" Aβ extracted with detergents or formic acid [11,20]. Unfortunately, most of these studies used the brains of cognitively-intact elderly people as controls. These brains almost invariably contain diffuse plaques, a sign that the process of Aβ accumulation has already occurred. The basic concept of sAβ, the native counterpart of the toxic diffusible oligomers, was still misunderstood.

5. Our studies on soluble Aβ go on... slowly

In 1992–1993, we planned the studies that we were going to carry out in the following years: direct analysis of sAβ species, timing of Aβ appearance and accumulation, and type and pattern of Aβ species in early-onset familial AD. The execution of this plan slowed down for logistical reasons (i.e., one of us went back to Italy to an unfinished lab). The studies were re-initiated in 1995 with an important contribution by Claudio Russo, a research associate from Italy, who came to Cleveland to work on these projects.

Our collaboration with Takaomi Saido, who generously provided antibodies specific for various Aβ N-termini, allowed for the initial characterization of the sAβ composition, which was later better defined with MALDI-TOF mass spectrometry (MS). Using epitope mapping, we determined that a) the Aβ forming the highest MW band on the immunoblot started with an aspartic acid at position 1; b) the peptide best represented in AD was Aβ 3–42, with the glutamate cyclized into pyroglutamate, and was the major part of the intermediate 4 kDa band; and c) Aβ pyroglutamate 11–42 migrates with the smaller 3.3 kDa band. Analyses with MS then demonstrated other Aβ species truncated at the N-terminus, including 2–42, 3–42 and 4–42, that were not detectable in all cases of AD. Results also showed that Aβ 1–40 was found only in AD cases with intense parenchymal amyloid angiopathy [17,18]. The timing of sAβ aggregation and accumulation was investigated by analyzing the brains of 22 cases of Down's syndrome spanning both prenatal and postnatal periods. Soluble Aβ 42 was detected in half of the fetal brains, and in all postnatal cases, even in the young cases (from 4 days up to 14 years old) where diffuse amyloid plaques had not yet formed. In the same study, we established that the pyroglutamate 3–42 peptide appeared later than the full-length form, and its appearance correlated with the formation of amyloid plaques. Soluble Aβ1–40 and Aβx-40 were not detected in any Down's syndrome case examined [24]. This study had two major implications: 1) the overproduction of total Aβ due to AβPP over expression in Down's syndrome, causes the seeding of only the Aβ 42 species; and 2) the initial seeding may begin more than a decade before amyloid fibrils are formed.

6. How are the soluble and diffusible Aβ oligomers *in vitro* related to the soluble Aβ aggregates in brain tissue?

In 1995, Podlisny et al. in Selkoe's group reported that sAβ secreted *in vitro* forms SDS-insoluble oligomers [16]. The same group reported in a series of articles written between 2000 and 2002 that Aβ oligomers secreted by cells cause neuronal dysfunction *in vivo* [26,28]. These findings revolutionized the concept of amyloid toxicity and changed the interpretation of AD pathogenesis. As was subsequently demonstrated, Aβ oligomers are more neurotoxic than Aβ fibrils [27]. This propensity for toxicity applies to other amyloid-forming peptides [1]. The soluble and diffusible Aβ oligomers were identified as the actual trigger of AD pathogenesis, and various hypotheses were put forward to explain how they caused neuronal dysfunction and degeneration [12]. This novel line of research was well received. The term "soluble Aβ" became a hot buzzword among researchers, and a large part of subsequent studies in the Alzheimer field focused on this issue.

We were surprised by the lack of acknowledgement of our study on brain sAβ. The soluble Aβ that we previously had described clearly looked like the native, diffusible aggregates that Selkoe et al. had found in the cell media and that were neurotoxic upon inoculation into mouse brain. Furthermore, our studies on Down's syndrome, that had demonstrated the existence of sAβ oligomers in the absence of amyloid, could further support the hypothesis that under special conditions, such as overproduction, soluble Aβ aggregates could exist in human brain in the absence of detectable amyloid. A possible explanation for the apparent discrepancy between Selkoe et al.'s data on cell culture and ours on intact brain tissue is that Aβ is indeed produced under normal conditions but in brain tissue it is immediately sequestered or rapidly catabolized, possibly with the participation of other tissue components. When this Aβ removal mechanism is overwhelmed by overproduction, as in Down's syndrome, or by impaired removal, Aβ deposition and plaque formation start. Later, we were even more surprised when several groups began to search for native, soluble Aβ oligomers in brain tissue using correct, albeit complicated, methods such as using antibodies specific for the conformation of Aβ small aggregates. These studies completely ignored the fact that almost ten years earlier we had shown that the presence of sAβ could be demonstrated with a simple immunoblot [4]. "Our" soluble Aβ seems to have disappeared from the literature, but, as we stated above, perhaps we were not vocal enough. So, the brain sAβ remained damned elusive... like the Scarlet Pimpernel, "we sought it here, we sought it there...".

7. The composition of soluble Aβ dictates the AD pathologic phenotype: The concept of "Aβ strains"

The study of the sAβ pattern in familial AD, planned in 1993, was carried out in 1999. The results demonstrated that the soluble and plaque-related Aβ species truncated at the N-terminus preferentially accumulated in the brains of subjects carrying presenilin-1 (PSEN1) mutations as compared to sporadic AD. This suggested that *PSEN1* not only affected the γ-secretase cleavage but also cleavage by β-secretase [18]. Furthermore, the over-representation of the Aβ N-terminus truncated species was associated with a more malignant phenotype of AD as determined by the earlier age of onset and the more rapid course.

We suspected the existence of a correlation between the molecular pattern of sAβ and the disease phenotype, and also that this correlation might reflect the type and degree of Aβ neurotoxicity. We pursued this idea in several different ways. One avenue was the comparative study of the sAβ species associated with physiological brain aging and with sporadic AD. Even in cognitively-intact individuals, aging of the brain is very often associated with Aβ deposition but not with NFT, suggesting that in these subjects Aβ accumulation does not produce neuronal damage [2]. When we compared plaque-containing, but NFT-free brains from cognitively-intact individuals against AD brains, the results were striking. We found that the species of sAβ present in physiologically aging brains was different from those present in brains with sporadic AD; the full-length 1–42 was the predominant Aβ species in brain aging, while in AD the N-terminus truncated pyroglutamate 3–42 Aβ species was the best represented. We also observed that the Aβ species associated with AD forms oligomers more quickly, are more toxic to neurons, and produce more severe membrane damage than the Aβ species associated with normal brain aging [15]. Hence, the two different patterns of soluble Aβ have specific properties of aggregation and toxicity that correspond to two quite different phenotypes: 1. "normal" brain aging, characterized by scarce neuronal pathology and normal mental status; 2. AD.

A second approach to the study was the correlation between disease phenotype and Aβ species, or Aβ strains, provided by a case study of an early-onset AD brain bearing a novel *PSEN1* mutation. The disease presented in the third decade with a cerebellar syndrome and myoclonus later followed by rapidly progressive dementia. The clinical diagnosis was atypical prion disease. The histopathological examination showed a novel pattern of Aβ deposition that was widespread and abundant and heavily involved in the cerebellar cortex, where diffuse amyloid plaques were associated with severe loss of the Purkinje cell arborization. This *PSEN1* mutation caused a novel pattern of Aβ secretion in *PSEN1* mutated cells characterized by a three-fold increase of both the 40 and 42 Aβ species. The combination of the soluble and insoluble Aβ species present in the brain tissue was also novel: About 90% of the accumulating Aβ, which included not only the 42 but also the 40 C-terminus species, was N-terminal truncated. These findings illustrate a similarity between the scrapie prion protein (PrP^{Sc}) of prion diseases and the Aβ protein of AD that is much closer than previously suspected. In prion diseases, different conformers of PrP^{Sc}, termed prion strains, dictate the phenotype, in terms of age at onset and duration of the clinical disease as well as distribution, severity, and timing of the brain alterations [3]. It is tempting to speculate that the combination of different Aβ species, determined by genetic and epigenetic factors, leads to differently conformed Aβ soluble aggregates that exhibit a large spectrum of toxicity. The term "Aβ strains" seems appropriate to label this novel concept. Perhaps with our contributions, and those of other laboratories, sAβ is becoming less elusive now.

Acknowledgements

We are grateful to Ms. Allison Marsh for her contribution to the manuscript. Supported by NIH grants AG14359, AG08012, CDC grant CCU 515004, the Britton Fund.

References

[1] M. Bucciantini, E. Giannoni, F. Chiti, F. Baroni, L. Formigli, J. Zurdo, N. Taddei, G. Ramponi, C.M. Dobson and M. Stefani, Inherent toxicity of aggregates implies a common mechanism for protein misfolding diseases, *Nature* **416** (2002), 507–511.

[2] D.W. Dickson, H.A. Crystal, L.A. Mattiace, D.M. Masur, A.D. Blau, P. Davies, S.H. Yen and M.K. Aronson, Identification of normal and pathological aging in prospectively studied nondemented elderly humans, *Neurobiol Aging* **13** (1992), 179–189.

[3] P. Gambetti, P. Parchi, S. Capellari, C. Russo, M. Tabaton, J.K. Teller and S.G. Chen, Mechanisms of phenotypic heterogeneity in prion, Alzheimer and other conformational diseases, *J Alzheimers Dis* **3** (2001), 87–95.

[4] C.G. Glabe, Conformation-dependent antibodies target diseases of protein misfolding, *Trends Biochem Sci* **29** (2004), 542–547.

[5] G.G. Glenner and C.W. Wong, Alzheimer's disease: initial report of the purification and characterization of a novel cerebrovascular amyloid protein, *Biochem Biophys Res Commun* **120** (1984), 885–890.

[6] A.M. Goate, A.R. Haynes, M.J. Owen, M. Farrall, L.A. James, L.Y. Lai, M.J. Mullan, P. Roques, M.N. Rossor, R. Williamson et al., Predisposing locus for Alzheimer's disease on chromosome 21, *Lancet* **1** (1989), 352–355.

[7] C. Haass, M.G. Schlossmacher, A.Y. Hung, C. Vigo-Pelfrey, A. Mellon, B.L. Ostaszewski, I. Lieburg, E.H. Koo, D. Schenk, D.B. Teplow et al., Amyloid beta-peptide is produced by cultured cells during normal metabolism, *Nature* **359** (1992), 322–325.

[8] J.A. Hardy and G.A. Higgins, Alzheimer's disease: the amyloid cascade hypothesis, *Science* **256** (1992), 184–185.

[9] J.T. Huse, K. Liu, D.S. Pijak, D. Carlin, V.M. Lee and R.W. Doms, Beta-secretase processing in the trans-Golgi network preferentially generates truncated amyloid species that accumulate in Alzheimer's disease brain, *J Biol Chem* **277** (2002), 16278–16284.

[10] J. Kang, H.G. Lemaire, A. Unterbeck, J.M. Salbaum, C.L. Masters, K.H. Grzeschik, G. Multhaup, K. Beyreuther and B. Muller-Hill, The precursor of Alzheimer's disease amyloid A4 protein resembles a cell-surface receptor, *Nature* **325** (1987), 733–736.

[11] T. Kawarabayashi, L.H. Younkin, T.C. Saido, M. Shoji, K.H. Ashe and S.G. Younkin, Age-dependent changes in brain, CSF, and plasma amyloid (beta) protein in the Tg2576 transgenic mouse model of Alzheimer's disease, *J Neurosci* **21** (2001), 372–381.

[12] H.A. Lashuel, D. Hartley, B.M. Petre, T. Walz and P.T. Lansbury, Jr., Neurodegenerative disease: amyloid pores from pathogenic mutations, *Nature* **418** (2002), 291.

[13] C.L. Masters, G. Simms, N.A. Weinman, G. Multhaup, B.L. McDonald and K. Beyreuther, Amyloid plaque core protein in Alzheimer disease and Down syndrome, *Proc Natl Acad Sci USA* **82** (1985), 4245–4249.

[14] H. Mori, K. Takio, M. Ogawara and D.J. Selkoe, Mass spectrometry of purified amyloid beta protein in Alzheimer's disease, *J Biol Chem* **267** (1992), 17082–17086.

[15] A. Piccini, C. Russo, A. Gliozzi, A. Relini, A. Vitali, R. Borghi, L. Giliberto, A. Armirotti, C. D'Arrigo, A. Bachi, A. Cattaneo, C. Canale, S. Torrassa, T.C. Saido, W. Markesbery, P. Gambetti and M. Tabaton, Beta amyloid is different in normal aging and in Alzheimer's disease, *J Biol Chem* **280** (2005), 34186–34192.

[16] M.B. Podlisny, B.L. Ostaszewski, S.L. Squazzo, E.H. Koo, R.E. Rydell, D.B. Teplow and D.J. Selkoe, Aggregation of secreted amyloid beta-protein into sodium dodecyl sulfate-stable oligomers in cell culture, *J Biol Chem* **270** (1995), 9564–9570.

[17] C. Russo, T.C. Saido, L.M. DeBusk, M. Tabaton, P. Gambetti and J.K. Teller, Heterogeneity of water-soluble amyloid beta-peptide in Alzheimer's disease and Down's syndrome brains, *FEBS Lett* **409** (1997), 411–416.

[18] C. Russo, G. Schettini, T.C. Saido, C. Hulette, C. Lippa, L. Lannfelt, B. Ghetti, P. Gambetti, M. Tabaton and J.K. Teller, Presenilin-1 mutations in Alzheimer's disease, *Nature* **405** (2000), 531–532.

[19] N. Sergeant, S. Bombois, A. Ghestem, H. Drobecq, V. Kostanjevecki, C. Missiaen, A. Wattez, J.P. David, E. Vanmechelen, C. Sergheraert and A. Delacourte, Truncated beta-amyloid peptide species in pre-clinical Alzheimer's disease as new targets for the vaccination approach, *J Neurochem* **85** (2003), 1581–1591.

[20] Y. Shinkai, M. Yoshimura, Y. Ito, A. Odaka, N. Suzuki, K. Yanagisawa and Y. Ihara, Amyloid beta-proteins 1–40 and 1–42(43) in the soluble fraction of extra- and intracranial blood vessels, *Ann Neurol* **38** (1995), 421–428.

[21] M. Shoji, T.E. Golde, J. Ghiso, T.T. Cheung, S. Estus, L.M. Shaffer, X.D. Cai, D.M. McKay, R. Tintner, B. Frangione et al., Production of the Alzheimer amyloid beta protein by normal proteolytic processing, *Science* **258** (1992), 126–129.

[22] M. Tabaton, M.G. Nunzi, R. Xue, M. Usiak, L. Autilio-Gambetti and P. Gambetti, Soluble amyloid beta-protein is a marker of Alzheimer amyloid in brain but not in cerebrospinal fluid, *Biochem Biophys Res Commun* **200** (1994), 1598–1603.

[23] M. Tabaton and A. Piccini, Role of water-soluble amyloid-beta in the pathogenesis of Alzheimer's disease, *Int J Exp Pathol* **86** (2005), 139–145.

[24] J.K. Teller, C. Russo, L.M. DeBusk, G. Angelini, D. Zaccheo, F. Dagna-Bricarelli, P. Scartezzini, S. Bertolini, D.M. Mann, M. Tabaton and P. Gambetti, Presence of soluble amyloid beta-peptide precedes amyloid plaque formation in Down's syndrome, *Nat Med* **2** (1996), 93–95.

[25] R.D. Terry, N.K. Gonatas and M. Weiss, Ultrastructural Studies In Alzheimer's Presenile Dementia, *Am J Pathol* **44** (1964), 269–297.

[26] D.M. Walsh, I. Klyubin, J.V. Fadeeva, W.K. Cullen, R. Anwyl, M.S. Wolfe, M.J. Rowan and D.J. Selkoe, Naturally secreted oligomers of amyloid beta protein potently inhibit hippocampal long-term potentiation *in vivo*, *Nature* **416** (2002), 535–539.

[27] D.M. Walsh, I. Klyubin, J.V. Fadeeva, M.J. Rowan and D.J. Selkoe, Amyloid-beta oligomers: their production, toxicity and therapeutic inhibition, *Biochem Soc Trans* **30** (2002), 552–557.

[28] D.M. Walsh, B.P. Tseng, R.E. Rydel, M.B. Podlisny and D.J. Selkoe, The oligomerization of amyloid beta-protein begins intracellularly in cells derived from human brain, *Biochemistry* **39** (2000), 10831–10839.

[29] J.S. Whitson, D.J. Selkoe and C.W. Cotman, Amyloid beta protein enhances the survival of hippocampal neurons *in vitro*, *Science* **243** (1989), 1488–1490.

[30] H. Yamaguchi, S. Hirai, M. Morimatsu, M. Shoji and Y. Harigaya, Diffuse type of senile plaques in the brains of Alzheimer-type dementia, *Acta Neuropathol* (*Berl*) **77** (1988), 113–119.

[31] B.A. Yankner, L.K. Duffy and D.A. Kirschner, Neurotrophic and neurotoxic effects of amyloid beta protein: reversal by tachykinin neuropeptides, *Science* **250** (1990), 279–282.

Mice as models: Transgenic approaches and Alzheimer's disease

Dora Games*, Manuel Buttini, Dione Kobayashi, Dale Schenk and Peter Seubert
Elan Pharmaceuticals, 800 Gateway Blvd., South San Francisco, CA 94080, USA

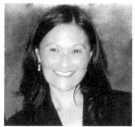
Dora Games

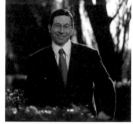
Dale Schenk

Abstract. Progress in understanding and treating Alzheimer's disease (AD) has been tremendously bolstered by the era of transgenic models of AD. The identification of disease-causing mutations in proteins such as amyloid-β precursor protein (βAPP) and presenilin1 (PS1), together with the discovery of other high risk factors (e.g., Apolipoprotein E4), as well as pathogenic mutations in the tau protein has led to the creation of several transgenic mice, including those expressing bi- and tri-genic constructs. Each model has unique pathologies that provide insights into disease mechanisms and interactive features of neuropathologic cascades. More importantly, therapeutic hypotheses are now testable in a manner unheard of less than 15 years ago. The wealth of new approaches currently in clinical and preclinical evaluations can be directly attributed to the impact of these animals on our ability to model relevant aspects of the disease. As a result, we may see containment or even the elimination of AD in the near future as a direct consequence of these advances.

Keywords: Transgenic mice, βAPP, amyloid-β, Alzheimer's disease, plaques, pathology, therapeutic, immunization

1. Introduction

One hundred years after Alzheimer's disease (AD) was first described in a demented female patient, transgenic mice have been engineered that express bits of human genetic material and develop neuropathologies that resemble her catastrophic disease. Today we take transgenic mouse models of AD for granted; however, a little over a decade ago they did not exist at all. These valuable animals are now extensively used for both mechanistic studies and the evaluation of previously untestable potential therapeutic interventions. The purpose of this commentary is to review a few illustrative examples of the applications to AD research and the subsequent advancements made possible since the first transgenic AD models were identified in the mid 1990s. Insights about the complex components of disease continue to emerge as the use of these mice and their descendents escalate in the AD field. This expedited progress in disease modeling offers real hope for the eventual treatment and cure of AD.

1.1. The first generation of transgenic mouse models of AD

Transgenic mice are produced by the introduction of a human gene sequence into the mouse genome, resulting in expression of a human protein. This is most commonly achieved by the microinjection of a complementary DNA construct, but genomic fragments complete with promoters, introns and exons have been used

---

*Corresponding author: Dora Games, Ph.D., 800 Gateway Blvd., South San Francisco, CA 94080, USA. Tel.: +1 650 877 7687; Fax: +1 650 877 7486; E-mail: dora.games@elan.com.

to express a single whole gene, while other methods manipulate endogenous genes to "knock in" a human sequence. Regardless of the tactic, the challenge of creating a mouse model of AD involves recapitulating a chronic, progressive disease that takes decades to develop in humans within the short lifespan (about two years) of a mouse.

In the early to mid-1990s several laboratories attempted to generate such mice by overexpressing a variety of human amyloid-β precursor protein (hβAPP) constructs and by using various promoters. At the time, our laboratories had tried for many years to develop any kind of *in vivo* model; not using only transgenic technology, but also grafts of transfected cells and infusions of amyloid-β peptide (Aβ) directly into the brain [33]. None of these early approaches produced anything that looked like an amyloid plaque or other recognizable AD-type pathology. The first report of amyloid deposition in a transgenic mouse was published in 1991 by Quon et al. [86]. This effect was produced by expressing wildtype βAPP751 under control of the NSE promoter. Although deposits meeting classic plaque criteria were very rare and infrequent, the mice did exhibit age-related cognitive deficits. At that time, the paucity of overt AD pathology made disease-related implications of the behavioral findings difficult to place, although recent behavioral studies support non-plaque, Aβ-related effects on cognition (see "Behavioral Abnormalities" below). The creation of a robust animal model of amyloid deposition remained elusive, and was an unyielding roadblock that blocked the assessment of therapeutic approaches.

At the heart of most attempts to create an βAPP transgenic mouse was the goal of expressing enough hβAPP in the CNS to produce amyloid deposits. After many years of searching for this signature trait, mice were created by Exemplar, Inc. that expressed high levels of hβAPP in the CNS. We examined the brains of mice that were a year old, reasoning that plaque pathology might take time to accumulate in mice as it does in humans. We were able to see numerous extracellular deposits of human Aβ in the cortex and hippocampus of the first brain we examined. We subsequently found that a number of these deposits were associated with dystrophic neurites and, as in human AD cases, activated astrocytes and microglia. We contacted Dr. Eliezer Masliah, who performed the first confocal analysis of these lesions and confirmed what we saw using standard light microscopy. We were very encouraged; it was possible, after all, to model a number of aspects of AD pathology in mice. This confirmed that endogenous enzymatic processes had cleaved human βAPP and produced Aβ that was appropriately deposited into plaques. Better yet, this meant that relevant biologic systems were in place that would support therapeutic target discovery for AD.

1.2. Common features of βAPP transgenic mice

We named the animal that we examined the "PDAPP" mouse, a shortened nomenclature for the PDGF-β chain promoter that was driving the "Indiana" mutation (βAPP V717F) associated with certain cases of familial AD [79] which increased the relative proportion of the more aggregation-prone Aβ isoform Aβ42 [96]. A minigene construct allowed for alternative splicing to overproduce all three major βAPP isoforms on a mixed triple background strain (C57bl6 XSWXDBA), resulting in a four to six fold increase in expression of hβAPP compared to endogenous mouse protein. In subsequent analyses [32] we found that similar to AD, diffuse and compacted plaque pathology developed over time. Regions of the brain that were first affected at around 6 months of age were the cingulate cortex and hippocampus, followed by an accelerated involvement of the remaining cortex and certain subcortical areas such as the striatum and thalamus, but not the cerebellum [52]. Dystrophic neurites were closely linked to the compacted plaques, as were the first waves of astrocytosis and microgliosis. Importantly synaptic loss was also identified in the cortex and hippocampus, accompanied by further gliosis. Cytoskeletal abnormalities, including the accumulation of phosphorylated neurofilaments and tau, have also been documented at the ultrastructural level [70]. Although the cytoskeletal alterations did not form the paired helical filaments typical of AD, the displacement of filaments from an axonal to somatic location, as well as their accumulation in dystrophic neurites resembled some aspects of early AD pathology. However, the severity and abundance of these cytoskeletal abnormalities were mild compared to the human disease. The development of more aggressive neurofibrillary (NFT) pathology would come later, with the creation of bigenic mice (See "NFT Pathology" below). Interestingly, synaptophysin immunoreactivity (used as a correlate measure of synaptic loss), was decreased in young transgenic mice prior to plaque deposition, but worsened with age. Could these early changes be due to the overexpression of βAPP or soluble (not deposited) Aβ. Answers to questions such as these would have to await the advent of Aβ-lowering agents that could be administered to the mice (See "Immunotherapy" below).

In 1996, Hsiao et al. described a transgenic mouse (Tg2576) that used the hamster prion promoter to express another disease-causing mutated form of βAPP (K670N/M671L, "βAPP Swedish", βAPPSwe) that increases total Aβ production. The Tg2576 mouse also deposited Aβ plaques, formed neuritic dystrophy and developed gliosis beginning at around 6–10 months, as well as progressive behavioral deficits [44]. The development of this mouse also underscored the interactive effects of background strain on pathology and survival, since early death affected the mice when bred to FVB/N or C57Blk6 strains, but not the C57Blk6/SJL combination. The confirmation of AD-type pathology in a second mouse line using a different promoter to drive a different mutation highlighted the reliability and power of the transgenic approach for modeling this chronic disease. The Tg2576 mouse has since become the most widely used transgenic mouse in the AD field, and has been crossed with several other transgenic mice, including those for bigenic studies (See "Genetic Manipulations" below).

The recapitulation of Aβ plaque and plaque-related pathologies was described by Sturchler-Pierrat et al. [94] in another line, the APP23 mice. The Thy1 promoter was employed to drive strong neuronal expression of hβAPP with the βAPP$_{Swe}$ mutation. In addition to the predominantly cortical and hippocampal Aβ and neuritic plaque pathologies, these mice were reported to have some neuronal loss in the hippocampal CA1 region, which correlated with plaque load (also see "Neuronal Loss" below). More recently, neocortical cell loss was also described in these mice, despite increased neuronal numbers at a young age [7]. An especially predominant feature of these animals was severe vascular amyloid pathology, or cerebral congophilic amyloid angiopathy (CAA) [107]. Indeed, the vascular damage was so pronounced as to model certain aspects of hemorrhagic stroke. The emerging picture became clearer: plaques, neuritic pathology (Fig. 1) and gliosis were common features of hβAPP transgenic mice, but certain other aspects of pathology (e.g. vascular amyloid) differed amongst models (Table 1). Among the myriad factors influencing pathology were background strain, promoter, hβAPP mutation, expression levels and ratios of Aβ40:Aβ42 production.

Other successful transgenic approaches involved the introduction of entire genomic copies of the hβAPP gene (R1.40 YAC [57,59]), expression of very effective combinations of mutations to increase Aβ levels and accelerate pathology (TgCRND8 [17]) and gene-targeting to produce Aβ deposition in the absence of hβAPP overexpression (βAPP$^{NLh/NLh}$/PS1$^{P262L/P264L}$ [30]).

1.3. Degenerative changes in transgenic mice

Despite difficulties with producing widespread neuronal loss in transgenic mice (Also see "Neuronal Loss" below), both hβAPP and presenilin 1 (PS1; a second gene linked to certain familial AD cases [92]) transgenic mice develop several anatomical deficits that should adversely affect neuronal function. Synaptic loss, a strong correlate to cognitive decline in AD, is evident in some [32,78] but not all [97] models. Importantly, this substrate of neuronal function can be modulated by altering Aβ levels (Fig. 2; See "Immunotherapy" below). A number of detrimental changes in the cholinergic system have also been reported in hβAPP and PS1 transgenic mice, including degeneration of choline acetyl transferase (ChAT)-positive fibers [68], an alteration of vesicular acetylcholine (VAChT)-immunoreactive bouton densities [45], reductions in cholinergic terminal density [2,35], as well as a reorganization of cortical terminals [109]. Fibrillar amyloid deposition is frequently associated with neuritic pathology (Fig. 1), and with synaptic abnormalities and breakage of neuronal branches [101], as well as the focal loss of neurons [102]. Evidence of altered brain metabolism including decreased glucose utilization [88,103] and N-acetylaspartate (NAA [105]) has also been reported. Others have reported deficiencies in long-term potentiation (LTP [62,100]) and other measures of synaptic transmission [29], as well as disturbances in sleep and circadian rhythms [46]. These impairments are likely due to a variety of factors, as deficits in pre-plaque-bearing mice have also been reported, including LTP transmission [36,82], corpus callosum length [38] dendritic structure [110] and dentate gyrus volume [87].

1.4. Behavioral abnormalities

In addition to the AD-like histopathological features of hβAPP and PS1 transgenic mice, these mouse models also demonstrate cognitive deficits that have been extensively examined (Table 2). Impairments in memory-based tasks have been described in several hβAPP transgenic models, including PDAPP, Tg2576, APP23, and TgCRND8 mice. The majority of these hβAPP transgenic mice have abnormalities in hippocampally-mediated spatial memory tasks such as

Table 1
Key Features of Representative Transgenic Mice

Mouse	Transgene	Strain	Promoter	Phenotype									Ref
				AP	INeur. Aβ	DN	VA	Gli	Syn Loss	NFT	NL	COG	
NSEAPP	βAPP 751	JU	NSE	+				+		−	−	++	[86]
PDAPP	βAPP$_{Indiana}$	B6/D2/SW	PDGF-b	+++	+	++	+	+++	++	−	−	++	[32]
Tg2576	βAPP$_{Swe}$	B6/SJL	PrP	++	+	+	++	++		−	−	++	[44]
APP23	βAPP$_{Swe}$	B6/D2	Thy1	+++		++	+++	+++		−	+	++	[94]
PSAPP	βAPP$_{Swe}$ PS1 M146L	B6/SW/D2	PDGF-b PrP	++++		+++	++	+++		−	−	++	[43]
APPDutch	βAPP E693Q	B6	Thy1	+			++++	+++					[41]
TGFβ1/APP	TGF-$_b$1βAPP$_{Swe}$ AP$_{Indiana}$	Balbc/SJL/ B6/D2	GFAP PDGF-b	+		+	+++	++					[112]
TAPP	Tau P301L βAPP$_{Swe}$	B6/D2/SW	PrP	++		+	++	++		++	+	NA	[64]
3XTG	PS1 M146V βAPP$_{Swe}$ Tau P301L	B6	Thy1.2	++	++++	+++		+++		++			[82]
APP-PS1	βAPP$_{Swe}$, βAPP$_{London}$ PS1M146L	B6/CBA	Thy-1 HMG	+++	++++	+++		+++		−	+++		[91]

Mouse strains: B6 = C7BL6; D2 = DBA2; SW = Swiss Webster
Phenotypes: AP = Amyloid Plaques; INeur. Aβ = Intraneuronal Aβ; DN = Dystrophic Neurites; VA = Vascular Amyloid;
Gli = Giosis; Syn Loss = Synaptic Loss; NFT = Neurofibrillary Tangle Pathology; NL = Neuronal Loss; Cog = Cognitive Deficits
Symbols: + = present; ++ = consistent feature; +++ = abundant; ++++ = very abundant; − = not present; blank square: not reported
NA: Not applicable due to other deficits
Table format modeled after Higgins et al. [42].

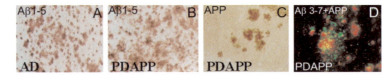

Fig. 1. Examples of Aβ plaque and related pathologies typical of transgenic mouse models of AD. Aβ plaques reacted with a human-specific Aβ antibody (3D6- recognizing the first 5 amino acids of Aβ), in sections of the neocortex from an (A) AD brain and (B) the PDAPP transgenic mouse. (C) Plaque associated dystrophic neurites, labeled with an antibody against human βAPP (8E5). (D) Confocal image of a compacted amyloid plaque (red) associated with dystrophic neurites (green) in a PDAPP mouse.

the water maze, the radial arm water maze, the circular holeboard maze, contextual fear conditioning, operant learning, passive avoidance, and the T- and Y-mazes [11,13,17,20,22,24,43,46,53,55,85,106]. In addition, hβAPP mice display impaired performance in a number of non-spatial memory tasks, including auditory startle, eyeblink conditioning, object recognition, and paired pulse inhibition [11,24,58,72,104]. While some aspects of all of these impairments are present before the appearance of Aβ deposits in singly-transgenic hβAPP mice, other deficits in working memory retention and acquisition in the water maze, the holeboard maze, and auditory startle tasks progressively worsen with age and parallel the appearance of cerebral plaques [11,13,53,106]. Transgenic hβAPP mice also have a wide range of non-memory sensorimotor perturbations, including hyperactivity, reductions in open field activity and disturbed sleep/wake patterns, which suggest a broad hβAPP phenotype that may include anxiety in addition to established memory impairments [1,11,24,58,104].

Examination of the types and onset of behavioral phenotypes in hβAPP and PS1 mice has served to strengthen the concept that excess Aβ production can drive cognitive loss. Correlations between the decrease in behavioral performance and the rise of insoluble pre-deposition amyloid assemblies such as oligomers and protofibrils have been reported [19,56], and may serve as harbingers of future pathology and further cognitive decline. Indeed, in doubly-transgenic models of AD which overexpress human mutant forms of βAPP and PS1 that drive more rapid accumulation of amyloid, the onset of water maze and Y-maze cognitive deficits is earlier relative to singly transgenic hβAPP animals [1, 22,43,56].

2. The manipulation of pathologies: Mechanistic insights and therapeutic potentials

The characterization of AD-type lesions in transgenic mice set the stage for the next compelling use of these animals: the manipulation of their phenotypes to either exacerbate or ameliorate the lesions. This valuable information could reveal either mechanistic insights or actual therapeutic approaches that may ultimately lead to disease modifying treatments for AD. The pathologies in hβAPP transgenic mice have been manipulated by two major methods: (1) genetically, by the co-expression of other genes and (2) by the administration of exogenous agents.

3. Genetic manipulations

3.1. Aβ plaque-related pathologies

The quest to reveal causal factors of Aβ deposition and modulate plaque formation began with the first confirmation of bona fide Aβ plaques in hβAPP mice, and continues to this day. These hallmarks of AD plaque pathology, despite controversy over their direct role in toxicity, still represent the principle gauge by which disease-relevant mechanisms and potential therapeutics are measured. Factors that enhance or deter the production, clearance or aggregation of plaques have all been examined in transgenic mouse models of AD.

Shortly after plaque pathology was produced in the PDAPP and Tg2576 mice, transgenic expression of disease-linked mutant PS1 was found to subtly elevate Aβ42 in the absence of extracellular plaque formation [25]. This effect was also further established by other investigators who produced several mutant PS1 lines that were cross-bred with wildtype hβAPP transgenic mice [18]. Remarkably, when mutant PS1 and Tg2576 mice were cross-bred, the resulting bigenic mice had greatly enhanced and accelerated plaque deposition compared to the original line of TG2576 mice [43]. Plaque acceleration was also demonstrated in another study of bigenic mice expressing another PS1 mutation (A246E), together with the βAPPSwe mutation, while it did not occur in bigenic mice expressing wildtype PS1 [8]. Intriguingly, these early observations suggested that exacerbated plaque pathology might result from shifting ratios of Aβ40:Aβ42.

Recently this notion was further substantiated by elegant and innovative experiments that directly examined the effects of altering Aβ40:Aβ42 ratios in various transgenic mouse lines. Interestingly many Aβ mutations do not reside at the β and γ secretase cleavage sites of βAPP, but occur more internally within the Aβ domain. These typically do not produce the full extent of parenchymal plaque pathology, but instead result in increased CAA. One such mutation in the Aβ sequence is E693Q (Aβ Dutch) [41]. Herzig et al. [41] developed several transgenic lines of mice that expressed either: (1) human wildtype βAPP, (2) Aβ Dutch or (3) Aβ Dutch and mutant PS1 (PS45 mice; G3848 mutation). In young mice prior to plaque deposition, these lines were characterized by differences in Aβ40:Aβ42 ratios, with Aβ Dutch> wildtype βAPP > bigenic AβDutch/PS45. The greater degree of Aβ40 production in the Aβ Dutch mice resulted in profound CAA formation, with the virtual absence of parenchymal plaques and concomitant vascular smooth muscle cell degeneration, hemorrhages and neuroinflammation. In contrast, wildtype βAPP mice, expressing similar levels of transgenic βAPP protein but with an Aβ40/Aβ42 ratio nearly half that of the Aβ Dutch, developed parenchymal plaques with very limited vascular deposits. Notably, it took on the order of 1.5 years to develop the respective wildtype βAPP and Aβ Dutch phenotypes. When the Aβ Dutch mice were crossed with the PS45 mice that carried a PS1 mutation known to increase Aβ42 production, their phenotype was dramatically altered. Instead of the typical vascular deposition pattern, parenchymal plaques became the dominant form of Aβ pathology; therefore, the pathologies were not simply additive, but shifted. These results imply that the different species of Aβ, although all neuronally produced, interact differently with separate extracellular environments and associated loci within the CNS. However, the complexity of these systems is demonstrated by the recent observations of Cheng et al. [14]. Mice transgenic for another mutation at the same Aβ site ("Arctic" mutation; E693G), as well as the βAPP Swe and βAPP Indiana mutations, developed aggressive parenchymal plaque deposition and associated neuritic pathology, despite a high Aβ40:42 ratio. However, no obvious increase in CAA was found. These mice also had an increased C99/hβAPP ratio (enhanced beta secretase cleavage) and accumulated shorter Aβ species in their brains. The myriad factors affecting the fate of Aβ moieties underscores the importance of considering the impact of potential therapeutics on Aβ homeostasis when the production or clearance of specific isoforms is differentially modified.

In support of the hypothesis that Aβ deposition may be differentially regulated in the CNS, plaque formation in βAPP transgenic mice has been modified by a number of co-expressed proteins. The E4 allele (apoE4) of the lipid carrier protein apolipoprotein E (ApoE) is well established as a risk factor for the development of sporadic AD [89,93], while the ApoE2 and ApoE3 isoforms are associated with lower risk [27]. Autopsy studies of AD brains reveal that a greater plaque load was more associated with the ApoE4 than the ApoE3 carriers [48,74]. In order to directly compare the differential effects of these alleles on plaque formation, several lines of bigenic PDAPP mice were created by knocking out endogenous mouse ApoE and replacing it with one of the three human ApoE alleles [26]. It emerged that, compared to mice with endogenous ApoE that was either left intact or knocked out, expression of the human Apo E3 and ApoE4 isoforms in bigenic mice actually delayed Aβ deposition, with ApoE3 having the greatest effect. It was also observed that only ApoE2 prevented the development of fibrillar plaques, and interestingly, the proportion of Aβ in the soluble pool of pre-plaque bearing mice differed with expression of the various ApoE isoforms. Intriguingly, and similar to the Herzig paper above, the two conditions (endogenous Apo E intact, Apo E knocked out) with the highest levels of Aβ42 (and therefore lowest Aβ40:42 ratios), had the greatest degree and most rapid development of parenchymal plaque formation. Conversely substantial CAA was reported to develop in TG2576/apoE4 "knock-in" bigenic mice and was associated with a higher Aβ40:42 ratio in brain [31]. Therefore, the modulation and ultimate deposition fate of specific isoforms of Aβ responsible for the parenchymal and CAA plaque pathologies are likely due to numerous interacting factors, some of which (like inflammatory processes) may be further induced or perpetuated by the disease process itself.

A robust inflammatory response has been documented in AD (for a review see [73]) and is generally believed to be detrimental. However, studies using bigenic mice by Wyss-Coray et al. [112] have demonstrated that under certain conditions, appropriately stimulated inflammatory responses may be beneficial. Plaque pathology was shown to be dramatically reduced by co-expression of the inflammatory mediator, transforming growth factor-β1 (TGF-β1), in astrocytes of hβAPP transgenic mice. The decrease in amyloid load was also associated with a reduction in compact plaque-associated neuritic dystrophy as visualized with a hyperphosphorylated tau antibody. Complicating the picture and reminiscent of the studies mentioned above, the decrease in parenchymal load was associated with an increased CAA burden and vascular degeneration [113]. This inverse correlation between plaque load and CAA was also observed in sections from AD brain, and a positive correlation was found in the human cases between TGF-β1 mRNA levels and CAA severity [112]. In an earlier study, it was shown that transgenic TGF-β1 expression was associated with a pronounced alteration of the extracellular matrix (ECM), including increased deposition of laminin, fibronectin and heparin sulphate proteoglycan [111]. The amount of Aβ42 did not appear to be altered in young bigenic mice. Instead, the expression of TGF-β1 in perivascular astroglial endfeet resulted in CAA formation in older animals, possibly due to the increase of perlecan and fibronectin in the vascular ECM beginning at a young age.

Since C3, a central component of the complement-mediated inflammatory cascade, was elevated in the brains of TGF-β1/βAPP bigenic mice, Wyss-Coray and his colleagues created another line of bigenic mice to determine the role of C3 in plaque deposition [114]. Complement-related receptor protein (Crry), an inhibitor of C3 convertases, inhibits the pro-inflammatory capability of C3. When soluble Crry was expressed in hβAPP mice, the resulting bigenic mice actually had a 2–3 fold increase in plaque load. An accumulation of electron dense neurons, loss of the neuronal marker Neu N and a decrease in MAP-2 positive dendrites in the bigenic mice suggested that degenerative cascades might also have been potentiated by C3 inhibition.

New insights regarding the regulation of amyloid processing continue to emerge using bigenic βAPP mice. An example comes from a recent study in which transgenic mice overexpressing the neuronal adaptor protein X11b were crossed with the Tg2576 transgenic mice [63]. X11b is a member of a family of adaptor proteins that can bind to the carboxyl terminus of βAPP. Plaque formation was markedly reduced in these older bigenic mice. Similar results were reported by this group after overexpression of a related protein, X11a, in TG2576 mice. Although the precise mechanisms underlying these effects remain unknown, it illustrates the potential of alternative Aβ-modulating approaches.

3.2. Neurodegenerative pathologies

As indicated above, βAPP transgenic mice have a number of deficits that indicate neuronal function is compromised. However these deteriorations, although significant, do not model the hallmark neurofibrillary tangles (NFTs) and widespread neocortical and limbic neuronal loss of AD, despite the abundant presence of amyloid plaque pathologies.

3.3. Neuronal loss

Until quite recently, modeling significant neuronal loss in hβAPP transgenic mice remained elusive. The first incidence of neuronal loss was reported in the hippocampus of βAPP 23 transgenic mice (Table 1), however the magnitude (∼15%) was considerably smaller than that found in AD, where up to ∼90% of neurons are lost in layer II of the entorhinal cortex [37]. Additional studies have documented focal, neuronal loss associated with large and dense Thio S-positive plaques in PS1βAPP mice [102]. The effect was too small to be identified by standard unbiased stereological methods which were previously used to examine other hβAPP mice [49]. It appeared that despite the pronounced overproduction of Aβ, extensive neuronal loss could not be modeled- a dilemma illustrating the difficulty of reproducing a chronic, progressive human disease in rodents. However, significant neuronal loss has been reported very recently in mice expressing hβAPP by introducing multiple mutations [91] or using knock-in methods [10]. Schmitz et al. [91] expressed βAPP751 with both βAPP$_{Swe}$ and βAPP V717I (βAPP$_{London}$ [12]) mutations driven by the Thy1 promoter in mice with C57Bl6/CBA background. These mice were then crossed with C57Bl6 mice harboring the PS1 M146L mutation driven by a HMG promoter. Unbiased stereologic methods revealed a significant (∼35%) loss of hippocampal neurons compared to controls. The loss was detected not only in the vicinity of plaques, but also at distant, non-plaque associated areas. Despite some caveats related to controls and other experimental considerations [21], this is the first transgenic AD mouse model to convincingly develop a substantial degree of neuronal loss. An important characteristic of this effect is likely to be early intraneuronal Aβ immunoreactivity, which was present by 3 months of age [108]. A second report by Casas et al. [10] knocked-in two presenilin mutations (M233T/L235P) into a mouse that as then bred to a Thy-I promoter driven, double hβAPP (βAPP$_{Swe}$, βAPP$_{London}$) mutant transgenic mouse, with a resultant high 42:40 ratio. Again, extensive neuronal loss (>50%) was reported in the hippocampus that correlated with the accumulation of intraneuronal Aβ. Intraneuronal Aβ, particularly Aβ42, has also been implicated as an early event in Downs syndrome pathology [40,77] and AD [39]. Another more recent study demonstrated that behavioral deficits were correlated with intraneuronal Aβ in the 3xTg transgenic mice [6]: Also see "NFT Pathology" below and Table 1). It appears that the production of substantial neuronal loss in rodents requires quite aggressive tactics-the creation of these "triple and quadruple" mutated animals are certainly different creatures from the first generation of hβAPP mice. Despite these accomplishments, no significant NFT pathology developed in mice expressing hβAPP and PS1 mutations. For years, it was not clear that rodents could ever develop tangle pathology, under any condition.

3.4. NFT pathology

This quandary has since been addressed by the creation of bigenic mice that express mutated forms of human βAPP and tau proteins. Transgenic tau mice (called JNPL3 mice) were first created that expressed a mutated form of tau (P301L), linked to human cases of frontotemporal dementia and Parkinsonism linked to chromosome 17 (FTDP-17) in which NFTs are a predominant feature [65]. These mice developed the elusive NFT pathology, being appropriately labeled with the classic Congo red, thioflavin and silver-based stains. Pick body-type and pre-tangle lesions (tau immunoreactive only) were also found. The NFTs were predominantly located in subcortical regions, while the pre-tangle pathology was noted in the cortex and hippocampus. Severe motor deficits were associated with axonal degeneration and loss of motor neurons in the spinal cord. Insoluble tau from the brain and spinal cord of the mice co-migrated with insoluble tau from AD and FTDP-17 brains. Ultrastructural analysis revealed intraneuronal accumulations of 15–20 nm straight and wavy filaments composed of tau [67]. Although the characteristic periodic twists typical of NFTs found in AD [54] were not seen in the mice, the morphology was similar to a number of other human tauopathies. In order to examine the effects of Aβ production on this NFT pathology, the P310L mice were crossed to Tg2576 mice (the bigenic progeny called TAPP mice) [64]. Although the extent of Aβ pathology was not affected in the TAPP mice, a striking alteration in the distribution of the NFTs occurred. In older female mice, they were found in the hippocampus, subiculum and cortex –regions that rarely or never formed NFTs in the JNPL3 animals. The increased NFT pathology developed in regions that were predominantly affected with plaque pathology. However, the close morphological association between plaque and NFT pathologies typically seen in AD was not observed, suggesting that other non-plaque but Aβ-related events were inducing the NFT pathology. The demonstration of Aβ-driven tau exacerbations provided tantalizing support for overlap in neurodegenerative cascades across disorders involving intraneuronal protein accumulation. This possibility was further supported by the characterization of triple transgenic mice (3XTg-AD) that expressed PS1 (M146V) and βAPPSwe mutations, as well as a tau (P301L) mutation [82]. Aβ accumulation preceded the development of tau pathology. Tau then accumulated in hippocampal and cortical regions, and progressively became hyperphosphorylated. More definitively, another series of experiments showed that clearance of Aβ by Aβ based immunotherapy led to a reduction in intraneuronal tau [81], as well as the rescue of early cognitive deficits [6]. Taken together these observations imply that impacting one feature of disease (i.e. Aβ production) may alter other aspects of a converging degenerative cascade (i.e. tau accumulation).

One of the most relevant pathological correlates to cognitive decline found in both AD and βAPP mice is the loss of neocortical and hippocampal synaptic terminals, which is associated with a decrease in synaptophysin protein [71,98]. Genetic manipulations that affect this degenerative pathology in βAPP transgenic mice have provided novel insights about the modulation of synaptic density under presumably toxic conditions associated with AD-type pathologies. The coexpression of additional genes in these mice reveals how other factors may interact in this environment to either exacerbate or rescue the deficit. For example, when bigenic βAPP mice harboring both the Indiana (V717F) and Swedish (K670N, M671L) mutations (βAPP$_{Swe, Ind}$) were crossed with Fyn kinase knockout mice, the loss of hippocampal synaptophysin was abolished, as was the correlation between synaptophysin density and Aβ levels [16]. Conversely, the overexpression of FYN in the transgenic mice exacerbated the synaptic loss, as well as induced a premature mortality. Interestingly, the aberrant sprouting of axonal terminals characteristic of the βAPP bigenic mice was not effected by the FYN kinase manipulations, suggesting that it was regulated by a separate pathway. Another example of effectors of synaptic integrity involves the apolipoproteins (ApoEs). Apolipoprotein E4 is a well-established risk factor for the development of AD [27,93]. In addition to the previously mentioned effects on plaque and cerebrovascular pathology, apolipoproteins appear to differentially modulate the age-dependent loss of synaptophysin in βAPP transgenic mice. For example, the expression of ApoE3 delayed the age-related loss of presynaptic terminals in hβAPP (βAPP$_{Swe, Ind}$)/Apo E-null mice, while this effect was not observed with ApoE4 expression. Notably, these effects appeared independent of plaque-deposition [9].

Postsynaptic deficits represent another important indicator of synaptic degeneration, and these have been identified in βAPP transgenic mice by different detection methods. An acceleration of the age-dependent loss of dendritic spines on hippocampal neurons in both TG2576 and PDAPP mice was identified by the classic Golgi silver staining method [61]. This deficit was reversed in TG2576 mice by the overexpression of Apo E2. Interestingly, the loss of spines in both lines of mice was found to occur before overt plaque deposition, raising the possibility that ApoE2 modulated the detrimental effects of a soluble Aβ moiety.

4. Therapeutic interventions

Aside from having utility in characterizing the progression and interdependencies of various AD-like pathologies, the overriding goal of these animal models of the disease is to employ them in identifying therapies for treating, and ideally preventing or reversing, the disease in man. Before transgenic models became available, trying to identify potential Alzheimer's disease modifying therapies was an extremely difficult proposition. One approach has been to conduct epidemiological searches of various patient databases to identify therapies that may impact the course or induction of AD. The results of these efforts remain in many cases controversial or not borne out in actual clinical trials and include investigations of anti-inflammatory drugs, vitamins, hormone replacement therapy, cholesterol lowering agents, and essentially all medicines commonly dosed into large populations of elderly subjects [115].

A number of trials to monitor AD progression with potential protective or preventative therapies have also been initiated based on various hypotheses, typically using medicines approved for other indications. Such studies serve to illustrate the huge cost, lengthy trial duration, and relatively large cohorts needed to test a given treatment. For example, a study designed to test whether the COX-2 inhibitor rofecoxib could delay the progression to Alzheimer's disease in mild cog-

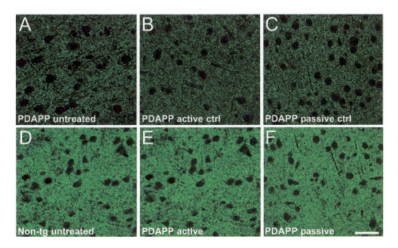

Fig. 2. Synaptophysin immunoreactivity in (A) 18 month old PDAPP mice is decreased compared to (D) non-transgenic mice. Synaptophysin immunoreactivity is preserved in PDAPP mice after (E) active (administration of adjuvanted Aβ 1–42) and (F) passive (administration of anti-Aβ antibodies) treatment paradigms, compared to (B, C) their respective non-treated control groups. Bar = 50 μm.

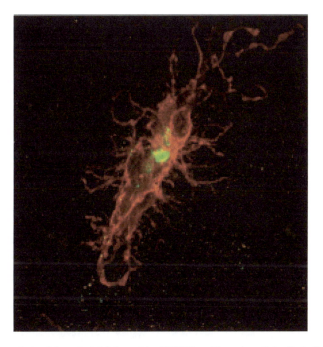

Fig. 3. A confocal image of phagocytosis of deposited Aβ (green) by MHC II-positive microglial cells (red) in a PDAPP mouse brain, after 6 months of immunization with adjuvanted Aβ 1–42.

nitive impairment patients took over 700 patients and 4 years of study to reach a negative conclusion [99]. Clearly animal models that predict clinical outcomes would be invaluable in accelerating the drug discovery process, allowing broad testing of many hypotheses and to potentially simultaneously assess safety and efficacy. Many potential therapies have been described using these models, including some quite unexpected approaches, and certain of these are now in human clinical trials largely due to results from AD-animal model testing. It is not an exaggeration to say that the AD animal models have revolutionized the AD drug discovery process.

4.1. Immunotherapy

The most widely replicated and thoroughly investigated therapeutic approach in these preclinical studies has been the use of anti-Aβ immunotherapies (Reviewed in [34] and [75]). In 1999, our group described the impressive AD-neuropathology preventative effects of immunizing the PDAPP transgenic mouse with Aβ [90]. Subsequent studies in our laboratories and many others demonstrated that anti-Aβ antibodies were capable of reducing amyloid plaques and associated neuropathologies. Also encouraging is the preservation of cortical synaptophysin levels by immunotherapy (Fig. 2), an important correlate of cognitive function in humans.

Further strengthening the case for functional improvement following immunotherapy, a number of studies using transgenic hβAPP and PS1 mice have been published, describing amelioration of established behavioral deficits (Table 2). Long-term Aβ immunization of Tg2576 and βAPP + PS1 mice resulted in improvements in both the radial arm and typical versions of the water maze [51,76]. Passive immunization studies in which Aβ antibodies were given for short-term treatment schedules also resulted in positive cognitive changes in transgenic mice, as PDAPP mice given the monoclonal 266 antibody had improved object recognition performances, while Tg2576 mice given the N-terminus amyloid antibody BAM-10 showed increased spatial memory retention in the water maze relative to controls [23,56].

Precise details of the possible immunotherapeutic mechanisms of action are still an area of spirited scientific discussion. The overall consensus is that antibodies are capable of having several effects including plaque clearance (through both monocyte-mediated [4] (Fig. 3) and direct effects [3] and capture/clearance of soluble Aβ species that are neuroactive/toxic [60]. Recently, antibody-mediated clearance of even intracellular amyloid has been reported [6,81].

Immunization with Aβ1–42 (referred to as AN-1792 in clinical trials) was tested in human AD cases with noteworthy effects. Dosing in the trials was suspended after several cases (eventually 6% of the treated subjects) developed meningoencephalitis [83]. This side effect highlights a limitation of the animal models in that they do not necessarily perfectly predict clinical outcomes, which may be due to limitations in the models' pathology as well as the more genetically varied human population. Interestingly, several cases from these studies have gone to autopsy due to causes other than the immunotherapy, and showed strikingly similar reductions in AD neuropathologies as predicted by the mouse model [28,69,80]. Finally, certain memory related tests, as well as the CSF biomarker tau, seemed improved by therapy [5], [Gilman et al. in press]; these hints of cognitive efficacy and robust pathology reduction are encouraging. A new clinical trial has been initiated using the "passive" administration of an Aβ monoclonal antibody, which differs from the "active" immunization approach used in the original trials. Very recently clinical trials were initiated using a fragment of Aβ as an "active" immunogen that was designed to avoid an inflammatory response.

5. AD-mouse models have identified many novel therapeutic approaches

In the decade since mouse models have emerged, an extensive range of therapies besides immunotherapy have been tested in several different AD-models. Preliminary results from dozens of approaches have been presented in various venues, and a full review of all these studies is beyond the scope of this review. Instead, Table 3 presents a sampling of results involving chronic treatment (> 2 weeks) using transgenic models which have appeared in peer-reviewed journals and which have been selected to illustrate the breadth of potential therapeutic approaches. Small molecules, in many cases orally bioavailable, have shown effectiveness by approaches ranging from natural products that bind Aβ [66], metal chelation [15], lipid metabolism inhibitors [47], to inflammation modulators [50]. As a testament to the creativity of these scientists, the sources of compounds range from curry spice to drugs in clinical trials for other indications. It is hard to imagine that in the pre-transgenic model of AD era that funding and allowance to test even a fraction of these compounds in AD patients would have happened.

As is also evident from Table 3, studies vary widely in the choice of model, duration of therapy, and perhaps most importantly, the age/amyloid burden present when therapy was initiated. This great variability in paradigms exclude head-to head efficacy assessments and predictions. Our experience with immunotherapy suggests that preventing amyloidosis may be easier (when expressed as percent reduction in plaque area) than reducing existing burdens (even though treatment of older plaque bearing animals may result in a larger absolute reduction when expressed as ng of Aβ/gm brain tissue).

One point that is interesting to note in Table 3 is that none of the tested compounds have the same proposed mechanism of action and none are direct inhibitors of the amyloidogenic secretases. Thus the pharmaceu-

Table 2
Behavioral Phenotypes of Transgenic Mouse Models and Cognitive Changes Following Amyloid Immunotherapy

Transgenic Model	Behavioral Phenotypes	Age of Phenotype (mo)	Amyloid-Modifying Treatment	Result	References
PDAPP	Water maze (spatial reference, serial memory)	3, 10, **13, 18**	m266, 1x week for 6 weeks	Treated PDAPP mice displayed improved object recognition performance relative to Untreated PDAPP animals	[23]
	Holeboard maze (**spatial reference memory**)	3–5, **20–26**	4 and 24mo PDAPP mice		
	Radial arm maze	3			
	Object recognition	6, 9–10			
	Operant bar pressing	3, 6			
	Cued fear conditioning	11			
	Eyeblink conditioning	6, 10			
	Hyperactivity	3, 6, 9			
	Perturbed sleep/wake patterns	**3–5, 20–26**			
Tg2576	Water maze (spatial **acquisition**, reference, **retention** memory)	6–11, 12–15, **12–18, 20–25**	Aβ1–42, 1x mo from 7.5mo, Tg2576 mice tested at 11.5, 15.5 mo	Treated Tg2576 mice displayed lesser radial arm water maze error rates, improved spatial acquisition	[76]
	Water maze (visual cued navigation)	**3, 9, 19**			
	Radial arm water maze (spatial acquisition, serial memory)	11.5, **15.5**			
	Holeboard maze (**spatial reference memory**)	3, 7, 9			
	T-maze (alternation forced)	10, 16	BAM-10 antibody, given 1, 4, 6, 12d after initial testing, Tg2576 mice tested at 9-11mo	Treated Tg2576 mice displayed improvements in water maze spatial retention memory	[56]
	Y-maze (alternation)	10, 16–18			
	Contextual fear conditioning (spatial)	16–18			
	Hyperactivity	17			
	Open Field	10, 16			
APP23	Water maze (spatial **acquisition**, retention memory)	3, 6, **18, 25**			
	Passive Avoidance (spatial memory)	25			
	Hyperactivity	1.5–2, 3, 6			
	Open Field	3, 6			
	Rotorod	3, 6			
TgCRND8	Water maze (spatial acquisition, retention memory)	2.75	Aβ1–42, given 1x mo from 6w, TgCRND mice tested at 11, 15, 19, 23w	Treated TgCRND8 mice displayed improvements in water maze spatial reference memory	[51]
	Auditory Startle	1.5, 2.5–3, 3–3.5, **3.5–4.25**			
	Prepulse Inhibition	1.5–2, 3–3.5, **3.5–4.25**			
APP + PS1	Water maze (spatial acquisition learning)	**15–17**	Aβ1–42, 1x mo from 7.5mo, Tg2576 mice tested at 11.5, 15.5 mo	Treated APP + PS1 mice displayed lesser radial arm water maze error rates, improved spatial acquisition	[76]
	Radial arm water maze	4–5, 11.5, 14.5–16.5, 15–17, **15.5**			
	Y-maze (alternation, entries)	3–3.5, 5–7, 6, 9, 15–17			

Boldface type indicates specific behavioral tasks in which hAPP performance progressively worsens with age, and their time of onset in months.

Table 3
A Sampling of the Diverse Approaches Reported to Reduce Alzheimer's Pathology in Transgenic AD Models

Test Article	Proposed Mechanism of Action	Dose and Route	Length	AD Model	Age/Amyloid Burden at Therapy Initiation	Percentage Reduction in Plaque Burden	Other Reported Efficacy	Ref
Curcumim	Amyloid binding anti-oxidant in curry powder	160 and 5000 ppm in chow	6 mo	Tg2576	10 months of age when few plaques present.	@ low dose ~50%; NS at high dose	Reduced levels of oxidized proteins and IL-1B	[66]
iABeta5p	β-sheet disrupting peptide	1 mg, 3x/week I.V.	8 wk	βAPPV717I X PS-1A246E	9 months (3 months after plaques begin to appear).	45% in cortex; 29% in hippocampus	Reduced neuronal death in subiculum	[84]
Lithium	GSK3β Kinase inhibition	2.4 g/kg in chow	7 mo	PDAPP (homozygous)	1 month old, before plaques present.	~75%		[95]
CP-113,818	ACAT inhibitor	7.2 mg/kg/day Subcu-taneous implant	2 mo	Aβ PPSw +Ldn	4.5 months, when plaques are just forming	~90%	Spatial learning improved	[47]
Clioquinol	Copper-Zinc chelation	30 mg/kg/day oral	9 wks	Tg2576	21 months of age, well after plaque initiation	49%		[15]
NCX-2216	NO-releasing NSAID; microglial activation	375 ppm in chow	5 mo	SwAPP X PS-1M146L	7 months, plaque formation evident at that age	45%	Reduced Congo red + deposits	[50]

References were selected from peer-reviewed reports in which therapeutic agents showed efficacy in reducing, at a minimum, amyloid plaque load after chronic (>2 months) treatment. Note that despite very different reported mechanisms of action, all have reported efficacy. The wide variance in animal models, duration and age of treatment, and methods of quantitation preclude direct comparisons between studies.

tical universe of potential amyloid directed therapies is quite diverse and cause for optimism that effective therapies will emerge and be validated clinically in the near future.

6. Summary

While truly effective therapies for AD are still works in progress, the past decade has seen a revolution in potential treatments that may eventually spell the end to one of the most increasingly common and dreaded diseases. The advent of transgenic animal models has exponentially enabled rapid exploration of mechanisms of disease and potential therapies. Testing of hypotheses that could never have been approved or afforded for study in man are now routine because of these animal models. The existence of these mice could not have been imagined 100 years ago, when AD was first described. Hopefully, before the next century is over, living with AD will itself be unimaginable.

Acknowledgement

The authors thank Terry Guido and Dr. Sally Schroeter for assistance with preparation of figures.

References

[1] G.W. Arendash, D.L. King, M.N. Gordon, D. Morgan, J.M. Hatcher, C.E. Hope and D.M. Diamond, Progressive, age-related behavioral impairments in transgenic mice carrying both mutant amyloid precursor protein and presenilin-1 transgenes, Brain Research 891 (2001), 42–53.

[2] J.S. Aucoin, P. Jiang, N. Aznavour, X.K. Tong, M. Buttini, L. Descarries and E. Hamel, Selective cholinergic denervation, independent from oxidative stress, in a mouse model of Alzheimer's disease, Neuroscience 132 (2005), 73–86.

[3] B.J. Bacskai, S.T. Kajdasz, R.H. Christie, C.W. Carter, D. Games, P. Seubert, D. Schenk and B.T. Hyman, Anti-amyloid-beta antibodies promote clearance of amyloid-beta deposits imaged in vivo in PDAPP mice, Society for Neuroscience Abstracts, [print] 26 (2000), Abstract No.

[4] F. Bard, C. Cannon, R. Barbour, R.L. Burke, D. Games, H. Grajeda, T. Guido, K. Hu, J. Huang, K. Johnson-Wood, K. Khan, D. Kholodenko, M. Lee, I. Lieberburg, R. Motter, M. Nguyen, F. Soriano, N. Vasquez, K. Weiss, B. Welch, P. Seubert, D. Schenk and T. Yednock, Peripherally administered antibodies against amyloid beta-peptide enter the central nervous system and reduce pathology in a mouse model of Alzheimer disease, Nature Medicine 6 (2000), 916–919.

[5] A.J. Bayer, R. Bullock, R.W. Jones, D. Wilkinson, K.R. Paterson, L. Jenkins, S.B. Millais and S. Donoghue, Evaluation of the safety and immunogenicity of synthetic Abeta42 (AN1792) in patients with AD, Neurology 64 (2005), 94–101.

[6] L.M. Billings, S. Oddo, K.N. Green, J.L. McGaugh and F.M. Laferla, Intraneuronal Abeta causes the onset of early Alzheimer's disease-related cognitive deficits in transgenic mice, Neuron 45 (2005), 675–688.

[7] L. Bondolfi, M. Calhoun, F. Ermini, H.G. Kuhn, K.H. Wiederhold, L. Walker, M. Staufenbiel and M. Jucker, Amyloid-associated neuron loss and gliogenesis in the neocortex of amyloid precursor protein transgenic mice, *Journal of Neuroscience* **22** (2002), 515–522.

[8] D.R. Borchelt, T. Ratovitski, J. van Lare, M.K. Lee, V. Gonzales, N.A. Jenkins, N.G. Copeland, D.L. Price and S.S. Sisodia, Accelerated amyloid deposition in the brains of transgenic mice coexpressing mutant presenilin 1 and amyloid precursor proteins, *Neuron* **19** (1997), 939–945.

[9] M. Buttini, G.Q. Yu, K. Shockley, Y. Huang, B. Jones, E. Masliah, M. Mallory, T. Yeo, F.M. Longo and L. Mucke, Modulation of Alzheimer-like synaptic and cholinergic deficits in transgenic mice by human apolipoprotein E depends on isoform, aging, and overexpression of amyloid beta peptides but not on plaque formation, *Journal of Neuroscience* **22** (2002), 10539–10548.

[10] C. Casas, N. Sergeant, J.M. Itier, V. Blanchard, O. Wirths, N. van der Kolk, V. Vingtdeux, E. van de Steeg, G. Ret, T. Canton, H. Drobecq, A. Clark, B. Bonici, A. Delacourte, J. Benavides, C. Schmitz, G. Tremp, T.A. Bayer, P. Benoit and L. Pradier, Massive CA1/2 neuronal loss with intraneuronal and N-terminal truncated Abeta42 accumulation in a novel Alzheimer transgenic model, *American Journal of Pathology* **165** (2004), 1289–1300.

[11] P.F. Chapman, G.L. White, M.W. Jones, D. Cooper-Blacketer, V.J. Marshall, M. Irizarry, L. Younkin, M.A. Good, T.V. Bliss, B.T. Hyman, S.G. Younkin and K.K. Hsiao, Impaired synaptic plasticity and learning in aged amyloid precursor protein transgenic mice, *Nature Neuroscience* **2** (1999), 271–276.

[12] M.C. Chartier-Harlin, F. Crawford, H. Houlden, A. Warren, D. Hughes, L. Fidani, A. Goate, M. Rossor, P. Roques, J. Hardy et al., Early-onset Alzheimer's disease caused by mutations at codon 717 of the beta-amyloid precursor protein gene, *Nature* **353** (1991), 844–846.

[13] G. Chen, K.S. Chen, J. Knox, J. Inglis, A. Bernard, S.J. Martin, A. Justice, L. McConlogue, D. Games, S.B. Freedman and R.G. Morris, A learning deficit related to age and beta-amyloid plaques in a mouse model of Alzheimer's disease, *Nature* **408** (2000), 975–979.

[14] I.H. Cheng, J.J. Palop, L.A. Esposito, N. Bien-Ly, F. Yan and L. Mucke, Aggressive amyloidosis in mice expressing human amyloid peptides with the Arctic mutation, *Nat Med* **10** (2004), 1190–1192.

[15] R.A. Cherny, C.S. Atwood, M.E. Xilinas, D.N. Gray, W.D. Jones, C.A. McLean, K.J. Barnham, I. Volitakis, F.W. Fraser, Y. Kim, X. Huang, L.E. Goldstein, R.D. Moir, J.T. Lim, K. Beyreuther, H. Zheng, R.E. Tanzi, C.L. Masters and A.I. Bush, Treatment with a copper-zinc chelator markedly and rapidly inhibits beta-amyloid accumulation in Alzheimer's disease transgenic mice.[see comment], *Neuron* **30** (2001), 665–676.

[16] J. Chin, J.J. Palop, G.Q. Yu, N. Kojima, E. Masliah and L. Mucke, Fyn kinase modulates synaptotoxicity, but not aberrant sprouting, in human amyloid precursor protein transgenic mice, *Journal of Neuroscience* **24** (2004), 4692–4697.

[17] M.A. Chishti, D.S. Yang, C. Janus, A.L. Phinney, P. Horne, J. Pearson, R. Strome, N. Zuker, J. Loukides, J. French, S. Turner, G. Lozza, M. Grilli, S. Kunicki, C. Morissette, J. Paquette, F. Gervais, C. Bergeron, P.E. Fraser, G.A. Carlson, P.S. George-Hyslop and D. Westaway, Early-onset amyloid deposition and cognitive deficits in transgenic mice expressing a double mutant form of amyloid precursor protein 695, *Journal of Biological Chemistry* **276** (2001), 21562–21570.

[18] M. Citron, D. Westaway, W. Xia, G. Carlson, T. Diehl, G. Levesque, K. Johnson-Wood, M. Lee, P. Seubert, A. Davis, D. Kholodenko, R. Motter, R. Sherrington, B. Perry, H. Yao, S. Lieberburg Robert Vv, J. Rommens, S. Kim, D. Schenk, P. Fraser, P. St George Hyslop and J. Selkoe Dennis, Mutant presenilins of Alzheimer's disease increase production of 42-residue amyloid beta-protein in both transfected cells and transgenic mice, *Nature Medicine* **3** (1997), 67–72.

[19] J.P. Cleary, D.M. Walsh, J.J. Hofmeister, G.M. Shankar, M.A. Kuskowski, D.J. Selkoe and K.H. Ashe, Natural oligomers of the amyloid-beta protein specifically disrupt cognitive function, *Nature Neuroscience* **8** (2005), 79–84.

[20] K.A. Corcoran, Y. Lu, R.S. Turner and S. Maren, Overexpression of hAPPswe impairs rewarded alternation and contextual fear conditioning in a transgenic mouse model of Alzheimer's disease, *Learning & Memory* **9** (2002), 243–252.

[21] D.W. Dickson, Building a more perfect beast: APP transgenic mice with neuronal loss.[comment], *American Journal of Pathology* **164** (2004), 1143–1146.

[22] K.T. Dineley, X. Xia, D. Bui, J.D. Sweatt and H. Zheng, Accelerated plaque accumulation, associative learning deficits, and up-regulation of alpha 7 nicotinic receptor protein in transgenic mice co-expressing mutant human presenilin 1 and amyloid precursor proteins, *Journal of Biological Chemistry* **277** (2002), 22768–22780.

[23] J.C. Dodart, K.R. Bales, K.S. Gannon, S.J. Greene, R.B. DeMattos, C. Mathis, C.A. DeLong, S. Wu, X. Wu, D.M. Holtzman and S.M. Paul, Immunization reverses memory deficits without reducing brain Abeta burden in Alzheimer's disease model, *Nature Neuroscience* **5** (2002), 452–457.

[24] J.C. Dodart, H. Meziane, C. Mathis, K.R. Bales, S.M. Paul and A. Ungerer, Behavioral disturbances in transgenic mice overexpressing the V717F beta-amyloid precursor protein, *Behavioral Neuroscience* **113** (1999), 982–990.

[25] K. Duff, C. Eckman, C. Zehr, X. Yu, C.M. Prada, J. Perez-tur, M. Hutton, L. Buee, Y. Harigaya, D. Yager, D. Morgan, M.N. Gordon, L. Holcomb, L. Refolo, B. Zenk, J. Hardy and S. Younkin, Increased amyloid-beta42(43) in brains of mice expressing mutant presenilin 1, *Nature* **383** (1996), 710–713.

[26] A.M. Fagan, M. Watson, M. Parsadanian, K.R. Bales, S.M. Paul and D.M. Holtzman, Human and murine ApoE markedly alters A beta metabolism before and after plaque formation in a mouse model of Alzheimer's disease, *Neurobiology of Disease* **9** (2002), 305–318.

[27] L.A. Farrer, L.A. Cupples, J.L. Haines, B. Hyman, W.A. Kukull, R. Mayeux, R.H. Myers, M.A. Pericak-Vance, N. Risch and C.M. van Duijn, Effects of age, sex, and ethnicity on the association between apolipoprotein E genotype and Alzheimer disease. A meta-analysis. APOE and Alzheimer Disease Meta Analysis Consortium.[see comment], *Jama* **278** (1997), 1349–1356.

[28] I. Ferrer, M. Boada Rovira, M.L. Sanchez Guerra, M.J. Rey and F. Costa-Jussa, Neuropathology and pathogenesis of encephalitis following amyloid-beta immunization in Alzheimer's disease, *Brain Pathology* **14** (2004), 11–20.

[29] S.M. Fitzjohn, R.A. Morton, F. Kuenzi, T.W. Rosahl, M. Shearman, H. Lewis, D. Smith, D.S. Reynolds, C.H. Davies, G.L. Collingridge and G.R. Seabrook, Age-related impairment of synaptic transmission but normal long-term potentiation in transgenic mice that overexpress the human

APP695SWE mutant form of amyloid precursor protein, *Journal of Neuroscience* **21** (2001), 4691–468.

[30] D.G. Flood, A.G. Reaume, K.S. Dorfman, Y.G. Lin, D.M. Lang, S.P. Trusko, M.J. Savage, W.G. Annaert, B. De Strooper, R. Siman and R.W. Scott, FAD mutant PS-1 gene-targeted mice: increased A beta 42 and A beta deposition without APP overproduction, *Neurobiology of Aging* **23** (2002), 335–348.

[31] J.D. Fryer, K. Simmons, M. Parsadanian, K.R. Bales, S.M. Paul, P.M. Sullivan and D.M. Holtzman, Human apolipoprotein E4 alters the amyloid-beta 40:42 ratio and promotes the formation of cerebral amyloid angiopathy in an amyloid precursor protein transgenic model, *Journal of Neuroscience* **25** (2005), 2803–2810.

[32] D. Games, D. Adams, R. Alessandrini, R. Barbour, P. Berthelette, C. Blackwell, T. Carr, J. Clemens, T. Donaldson, F. Gillespie et al., Alzheimer-type neuropathology in transgenic mice overexpressing V717F beta-amyloid precursor protein.[see comment], *Nature* **373** (1995), 523–527.

[33] D. Games, K.M. Khan, F.G. Soriano, P.S. Keim, D.L. Davis, K. Bryant and I. Lieberburg, Lack of Alzheimer pathology after beta-amyloid protein injections in rat brain, *Neurobiology of Aging* **13** (1992), 569–576.

[34] D.S. Gelinas, K. DaSilva, D. Fenili, P. St George-Hyslop and J. McLaurin, Immunotherapy for Alzheimer's disease. [Review] [73 refs], *Proceedings of the National Academy of Sciences of the United States of America* **2** (2004), 14657–14662.

[35] D.C. German, U. Yazdani, S.G. Speciale, P. Pasbakhsh, D. Games and C.L. Liang, Cholinergic neuropathology in a mouse model of Alzheimer's disease, *Journal of Comparative Neurology* **462** (2003), 371–381.

[36] J. Giacchino, J.R. Criado, D. Games and S. Henriksen, In vivo synaptic transmission in young and aged amyloid precursor protein transgenic mice, *Brain Research* **876** (2000), 185–190.

[37] T. Gomez-Isla, J.L. Price, D.W. McKeel, Jr., J.C. Morris, J.H. Growdon and B.T. Hyman, Profound loss of layer II entorhinal cortex neurons occurs in very mild Alzheimer's disease, *Journal of Neuroscience* **16** (1996), 4491–4500.

[38] F. Gonzalez-Lima, J.D. Berndt, J.E. Valla, D. Games and E.M. Reiman, Reduced corpus callosum, fornix and hippocampus in PDAPP transgenic mouse model of Alzheimer's disease, *Neuroreport* **12** (2001), 2375–2379.

[39] G.K. Gouras, J. Tsai, J. Naslund, B. Vincent, M. Edgar, F. Checler, J.P. Greenfield, V. Haroutunian, J.D. Buxbaum, H. Xu, P. Greengard and N.R. Relkin, Intraneuronal Abeta42 accumulation in human brain, *American Journal of Pathology* **156** (2000), 15–20.

[40] K.A. Gyure, R. Durham, W.F. Stewart, J.E. Smialek and J.C. Troncoso, Intraneuronal abeta-amyloid precedes development of amyloid plaques in Down syndrome, *Archives of Pathology & Laboratory Medicine* **125** (2001), 489–492.

[41] M.C. Herzig, D.T. Winkler, P. Burgermeister, M. Pfeifer, E. Kohler, S.D. Schmidt, S. Danner, D. Abramowski, C. Sturchler-Pierrat, K. Burki, S.G. van Duinen, M.L. Maat-Schieman, M. Staufenbiel, P.M. Mathews and M. Jucker, Abeta is targeted to the vasculature in a mouse model of hereditary cerebral hemorrhage with amyloidosis.[see comment], *Nature Neuroscience* **7** (2004), 954–960.

[42] G.A. Higgins and H. Jacobsen, Transgenic mouse models of Alzheimer's disease: phenotype and application, *Behav Pharmacol* **14** (2003), 419–438.

[43] L. Holcomb, M.N. Gordon, E. McGowan, X. Yu, S. Benkovic, P. Jantzen, K. Wright, I. Saad, R. Mueller, D. Morgan, S. Sanders, C. Zehr, K. O'Campo, J. Hardy, C.M. Prada, C. Eckman, S. Younkin, K. Hsiao and K. Duff, Accelerated Alzheimer-type phenotype in transgenic mice carrying both mutant amyloid precursor protein and presenilin 1 transgenes, *Nature Medicine* **4** (1998), 97–100.

[44] K. Hsiao, P. Chapman, S. Nilsen, C. Eckman, Y. Harigaya, S. Younkin, F. Yang and G. Cole, Correlative memory deficits, Abeta elevation, and amyloid plaques in transgenic mice.[see comment], *Science* **274** (1996), 99–102.

[45] L. Hu, T.P. Wong, S.L. Cote, K.F. Bell and A.C. Cuello, The impact of Abeta-plaques on cortical cholinergic and non-cholinergic presynaptic boutons in alzheimer's disease-like transgenic mice, *Neuroscience* **121** (2003), 421–432.

[46] S. Huitron-Resendiz, M. Sanchez-Alavez, R. Gallegos, G. Berg, E. Crawford, J.L. Giacchino, D. Games, S.J. Henriksen and J.R. Criado, Age-independent and age-related deficits in visuospatial learning, sleep-wake states, thermoregulation and motor activity in PDAPP mice, *Brain Research* **928** (2002), 126–137.

[47] B. Hutter-Paier, H.J. Huttunen, L. Puglielli, C.B. Eckman, D.Y. Kim, A. Hofmeister, R.D. Moir, S.B. Domnitz, M.P. Frosch, M. Windisch and D.M. Kovacs, The ACAT inhibitor CP-113,818 markedly reduces amyloid pathology in a mouse model of Alzheimer's disease, *Neuron* **44** (2004), 227–238.

[48] B.T. Hyman, H.L. West, G.W. Rebeck, S.V. Buldyrev, R.N. Mantegna, M. Ukleja, S. Havlin and H.E. Stanley, Quantitative analysis of senile plaques in Alzheimer disease: observation of log-normal size distribution and molecular epidemiology of differences associated with apolipoprotein E genotype and trisomy 21 (Down syndrome), *Proceedings of the National Academy of Sciences of the United States of America* **92** (1995), 3586–3590.

[49] M.C. Irizarry, F. Soriano, M. McNamara, K.J. Page, D. Schenk, D. Games and B.T. Hyman, Abeta deposition is associated with neuropil changes, but not with overt neuronal loss in the human amyloid precursor protein V717F (PDAPP) transgenic mouse, *Journal of Neuroscience* **17** (1997), 7053–7059.

[50] P.T. Jantzen, K.E. Connor, G. DiCarlo, G.L. Wenk, J.L. Wallace, A.M. Rojiani, D. Coppola, D. Morgan and M.N. Gordon, Microglial activation and beta -amyloid deposit reduction caused by a nitric oxide-releasing nonsteroidal anti-inflammatory drug in amyloid precursor protein plus presenilin-1 transgenic mice, *J Neurosci* **22** (2002), 2246–2254.

[51] C. Janus, J. Pearson, J. McLaurin, P.M. Mathews, Y. Jiang, S.D. Schmidt, M.A. Chishti, P. Horne, D. Heslin, J. French, H.T. Mount, R.A. Nixon, M. Mercken, C. Bergeron, P.E. Fraser, P. St George-Hyslop and D. Westaway, A beta peptide immunization reduces behavioural impairment and plaques in a model of Alzheimer's disease.[see comment], *Nature* **408** (2000), 979–982.

[52] K. Johnson-Wood, M. Lee, R. Motter, K. Hu, G. Gordon, R. Barbour, K. Khan, M. Gordon, H. Tan, D. Games, I. Lieberburg, D. Schenk, P. Seubert and L. McConlogue, Amyloid precursor protein processing and A beta42 deposition in a transgenic mouse model of Alzheimer disease, *Proceedings of the National Academy of Sciences of the United States of America* **94** (1997), 1550–1555.

[53] P.H. Kelly, L. Bondolfi, D. Hunziker, H.P. Schlecht, K. Carver, E. Maguire, D. Abramowski, K.H. Wiederhold, C. Sturchler-Pierrat, M. Jucker, R. Bergmann, M. Staufenbiel

and B. Sommer, Progressive age-related impairment of cognitive behavior in APP23 transgenic mice, *Neurobiology of Aging* **24** (2003), 365–378.
[54] M. Kidd, Paired helical filaments in electron microscopy of Alzheimer's disease, *Nature* **197** (1963), 192–193.
[55] D.L. King, G.W. Arendash, F. Crawford, T. Sterk, J. Menendez and M.J. Mullan, Progressive and gender-dependent cognitive impairment in the APP(SW) transgenic mouse model for Alzheimer's disease, *Behavioural Brain Research* **103** (1999), 145–162.
[56] L.A. Kotilinek, B. Bacskai, M. Westerman, T. Kawarabayashi, L. Younkin, B.T. Hyman, S. Younkin and K.H. Ashe, Reversible memory loss in a mouse transgenic model of Alzheimer's disease, *Journal of Neuroscience* **22** (2002), 6331–6335.
[57] L.S. Kulnane and B.T. Lamb, Neuropathological characterization of mutant amyloid precursor protein yeast artificial chromosome transgenic mice, *Neurobiology of Disease* **8** (2001), 982–992.
[58] R. Lalonde, T.L. Lewis, C. Strazielle, H. Kim and K. Fukuchi, Transgenic mice expressing the betaAPP695SWE mutation: effects on exploratory activity, anxiety, and motor coordination, *Brain Research* **977** (2003), 38–45.
[59] B.T. Lamb, K.A. Bardel, L.S. Kulnane, J.J. Anderson, G. Holtz, S.L. Wagner, S.S. Sisodia and E.J. Hoeger, Amyloid production and deposition in mutant amyloid precursor protein and presenilin-1 yeast artificial chromosome transgenic mice, *Nature Neuroscience* **2** (1999), 695–697.
[60] M.P. Lambert, K.L. Viola, B.A. Chromy, L. Chang, T.E. Morgan, J. Yu, D.L. Venton, G.A. Krafft, C.E. Finch and W.L. Klein, Vaccination with soluble Abeta oligomers generates toxicity-neutralizing antibodies, *Journal of Neurochemistry* **79** (2001), 595–605.
[61] T.A. Lanz, D.B. Carter and K.M. Merchant, Dendritic spine loss in the hippocampus of young PDAPP and Tg2576 mice and its prevention by the ApoE2 genotype, *Neurobiol Dis* **13** (2003), 246–253.
[62] J. Larson, G. Lynch, D. Games and P. Seubert, Alterations in synaptic transmission and long-term potentiation in hippocampal slices from young and aged PDAPP mice, *Brain Research* **840** (1999), 23–35.
[63] J.H. Lee, K.F. Lau, M.S. Perkinton, C.L. Standen, B. Rogelj, A. Falinska, D.M. McLoughlin and C.C. Miller, The neuronal adaptor protein X11beta reduces amyloid beta-protein levels and amyloid plaque formation in the brains of transgenic mice, *Journal of Biological Chemistry* **279** (2004), 49099–49104.
[64] J. Lewis, D.W. Dickson, W.L. Lin, L. Chisholm, A. Corral, G. Jones, S.H. Yen, N. Sahara, L. Skipper, D. Yager, C. Eckman, J. Hardy, M. Hutton and E. McGowan, Enhanced neurofibrillary degeneration in transgenic mice expressing mutant tau and APP.[see comment], *Science* **293** (2001), 1487–1491.
[65] J. Lewis, E. McGowan, J. Rockwood, H. Melrose, P. Nacharaju, M. Van Slegtenhorst, K. Gwinn-Hardy, M. Paul Murphy, M. Baker, X. Yu, K. Duff, J. Hardy, A. Corral, W.L. Lin, S.H. Yen, D.W. Dickson, P. Davies and M. Hutton, Neurofibrillary tangles, amyotrophy and progressive motor disturbance in mice expressing mutant (P301L) tau protein.[erratum appears in Nat Genet 2000 Sep;26(1):127], *Nature Genetics* **25** (2000), 402–405.
[66] G.P. Lim, T. Chu, F. Yang, W. Beech, S.A. Frautschy and G.M. Cole, The curry spice curcumin reduces oxidative damage and amyloid pathology in an Alzheimer transgenic mouse, *Journal of Neuroscience* **21** (2001), 8370–8377.
[67] W.L. Lin, J. Lewis, S.H. Yen, M. Hutton and D.W. Dickson, Ultrastructural neuronal pathology in transgenic mice expressing mutant (P301L) human tau, *Journal of Neurocytology* **32** (2003), 1091–1105.
[68] H.J. Luth, J. Apelt, A.O. Ihunwo, T. Arendt and R. Schliebs, Degeneration of beta-amyloid-associated cholinergic structures in transgenic APP SW mice, *Brain Research* **977** (2003), 16–22.
[69] E. Masliah, L. Hansen, A. Adame, L. Crews, F. Bard, C. Lee, P. Seubert, D. Games, L. Kirby and D. Schenk, Abeta vaccination effects on plaque pathology in the absence of encephalitis in Alzheimer disease, *Neurology* **64** (2005), 129–131.
[70] E. Masliah, A. Sisk, M. Mallory and D. Games, Neurofibrillary pathology in transgenic mice overexpressing V717F beta-amyloid precursor protein, *Journal of Neuropathology & Experimental Neurology* **60** (2001), 357–368.
[71] E. Masliah, R.D. Terry, R.M. DeTeresa and L.A. Hansen, Immunohistochemical quantification of the synapse-related protein synaptophysin in Alzheimer disease, *Neurosci Lett* **103** (1989), 234–239.
[72] M.F. McCool, G.B. Varty, R.A. Del Vecchio, T.M. Kazdoba, E.M. Parker, J.C. Hunter and L.A. Hyde, Increased auditory startle response and reduced prepulse inhibition of startle in transgenic mice expressing a double mutant form of amyloid precursor protein, *Brain Research* **994** (2003), 99–106.
[73] E.G. McGeer and P.L. McGeer, Innate immunity in Alzheimer's disease: a model for local inflammatory reactions, *Mol Interv* **1** (2001), 22–29.
[74] M.J. McNamara, T. Gomez-Isla and B.T. Hyman, Apolipoprotein E genotype and deposits of Abeta40 and Abeta42 in Alzheimer disease, *Archives of Neurology* **55** (1998), 1001–1004.
[75] D. Morgan, Antibody therapy for Alzheimer's disease, *Expert Review of Vaccines* **2** (2003), 53–59.
[76] D. Morgan, D.M. Diamond, P.E. Gottschall, K.E. Ugen, C. Dickey, J. Hardy, K. Duff, P. Jantzen, G. DiCarlo, D. Wilcock, K. Connor, J. Hatcher, C. Hope, M. Gordon and G.W. Arendash, A beta peptide vaccination prevents memory loss in an animal model of Alzheimer's disease.[see comment][erratum appears in Nature 2001 Aug 9;412(6847):660], *Nature* **408** (2000), 982–985.
[77] C. Mori, E.T. Spooner, K.E. Wisniewsk, T.M. Wisniewski, H. Yamaguch, T.C. Saido, D.R. Tolan, D.J. Selkoe and C.A. Lemere, Intraneuronal Abeta42 accumulation in Down syndrome brain, *Amyloid* **9** (2002), 88–102.
[78] L. Mucke, E. Masliah, G.Q. Yu, M. Mallory, E.M. Rockenstein, G. Tatsuno, K. Hu, D. Kholodenko, K. Johnson-Wood and L. McConlogue, High-level neuronal expression of abeta 1–42 in wild-type human amyloid protein precursor transgenic mice: synaptotoxicity without plaque formation, *Journal of Neuroscience* **20** (2000), 4050–4058.
[79] J. Murrell, M. Farlow, B. Ghetti and M.D. Benson, A mutation in the amyloid precursor protein associated with hereditary Alzheimer's disease, *Science* **254** (1991), 97–99.
[80] J.A. Nicoll, D. Wilkinson, C. Holmes, P. Steart, H. Markham and R.O. Weller, Neuropathology of human Alzheimer disease after immunization with amyloid-beta peptide: a case report.[see comment], *Nature Medicine* **9** (2003), 448–452.
[81] S. Oddo, L. Billings, J.P. Kesslak, D.H. Cribbs and F.M. LaFerla, Abeta immunotherapy leads to clearance of early, but not late, hyperphosphorylated tau aggregates via the proteasome.[see comment], *Neuron* **43** (2004), 321–332.

[82] S. Oddo, A. Caccamo, J.D. Shepherd, M.P. Murphy, T.E. Golde, R. Kayed, R. Metherate, M.P. Mattson, Y. Akbari and F.M. LaFerla, Triple-transgenic model of Alzheimer's disease with plaques and tangles: intracellular Abeta and synaptic dysfunction, *Neuron* **39** (2003), 409–421.

[83] J.M. Orgogozo, S. Gilman, J.F. Dartigues, B. Laurent, M. Puel, L.C. Kirby, P. Jouanny, B. Dubois, L. Eisner, S. Flitman, B.F. Michel, M. Boada, A. Frank and C. Hock, Subacute meningoencephalitis in a subset of patients with AD after Abeta42 immunization.[see comment], *Neurology* **61** (2003), 46–54.

[84] B. Permanne, C. Adessi, G.P. Saborio, S. Fraga, M.J. Frossard, J. Van Dorpe, I. Dewachter, W.A. Banks, F. Van Leuven and C. Soto, Reduction of amyloid load and cerebral damage in a transgenic mouse model of Alzheimer's disease by treatment with a beta-sheet breaker peptide, *FASEB Journal* **16** (2002), 860–862.

[85] P.N. Pompl, M.J. Mullan, K. Bjugstad and G.W. Arendash, Adaptation of the circular platform spatial memory task for mice: use in detecting cognitive impairment in the APP(SW) transgenic mouse model for Alzheimer's disease, *Journal of Neuroscience Methods* **87** (1999), 87–95.

[86] D. Quon, Y. Wang, R. Catalano, J.M. Scardina, K. Murakami and B. Cordell, Formation of beta-amyloid protein deposits in brains of transgenic mice, *Nature* **352** (1991), 239–241.

[87] J.M. Redwine, B. Kosofsky, R.E. Jacobs, D. Games, J.F. Reilly, J.H. Morrison, W.G. Young and F.E. Bloom, Dentate gyrus volume is reduced before onset of plaque formation in PDAPP mice: a magnetic resonance microscopy and stereologic analysis, *Proceedings of the National Academy of Sciences of the United States of America* **100** (2003), 1381–1386.

[88] M. Sadowski, J. Pankiewicz, H. Scholtzova, Y. Ji, D. Quartermain, C.H. Jensen, K. Duff, R.A. Nixon, R.J. Gruen and T. Wisniewski, Amyloid-beta deposition is associated with decreased hippocampal glucose metabolism and spatial memory impairment in APP/PS1 mice, *Journal of Neuropathology & Experimental Neurology* **63** (2004), 418–428.

[89] A.M. Saunders, W.J. Strittmatter, D. Schmechel, P.H. George-Hyslop, M.A. Pericak-Vance, S.H. Joo, B.L. Rosi, J.F. Gusella, D.R. Crapper-MacLachlan, M.J. Alberts et al., Association of apolipoprotein E allele epsilon 4 with late-onset familial and sporadic Alzheimer's disease.[see comment], *Neurology* **43** (1993), 1467–1472.

[90] D. Schenk, R. Barbour, W. Dunn, G. Gordon, H. Grajeda, T. Guido, K. Hu, J. Huang, K. Johnson-Wood, K. Khan, D. Kholodenko, M. Lee, Z. Liao, I. Lieberburg, R. Motter, L. Mutter, F. Soriano, G. Shopp, N. Vasquez, C. Vandevert, S. Walker, M. Wogulis, T. Yednock, D. Games and P. Seubert, Immunization with amyloid-beta attenuates Alzheimer disease-like pathology in the PDAPP mouse, *Nature* **400** (1999), 173–177.

[91] C. Schmitz, B.P. Rutten, A. Pielen, S. Schafer, O. Wirths, G. Tremp, C. Czech, V. Blanchard, G. Multhaup, P. Rezaie, H. Korr, H.W. Steinbusch, L. Pradier and T.A. Bayer, Hippocampal neuron loss exceeds amyloid plaque load in a transgenic mouse model of Alzheimer's disease.[see comment], *American Journal of Pathology* **164** (2004), 1495–1502.

[92] R. Sherrington, E.I. Rogaev, Y. Liang, E.A. Rogaeva, G. Levesque, M. Ikeda, H. Chi, C. Lin, G. Li, K. Holman et al., Cloning of a gene bearing missense mutations in early-onset familial Alzheimer's disease.[see comment], *Nature* **375** (1995), 754–760.

[93] W.J. Strittmatter, A.M. Saunders, D. Schmechel, M. Pericak-Vance, J. Enghild, G.S. Salvesen and A.D. Roses, Apolipoprotein E: high-avidity binding to beta-amyloid and increased frequency of type 4 allele in late-onset familial Alzheimer disease, *Proceedings of the National Academy of Sciences of the United States of America* **90** (1993), 1977–1981.

[94] C. Sturchler-Pierrat, D. Abramowski, M. Duke, K.H. Wiederhold, C. Mistl, S. Rothacher, B. Ledermann, K. Burki, P. Frey, P.A. Paganetti, C. Waridel, M.E. Calhoun, M. Jucker, A. Probst, M. Staufenbiel and B. Sommer, Two amyloid precursor protein transgenic mouse models with Alzheimer disease-like pathology, *Proceedings of the National Academy of Sciences of the United States of America* **94** (1997), 13287–13292.

[95] Y. Su, J. Ryder, B. Li, X. Wu, N. Fox, P. Solenberg, K. Brune, S. Paul, Y. Zhou, F. Liu and B. Ni, Lithium, a common drug for bipolar disorder treatment, regulates amyloid-beta precursor protein processing, *Biochemistry* **43** (2004), 6899–6908.

[96] N. Suzuki, T.T. Cheung, X.D. Cai, A. Odaka, L. Otvos, Jr., C. Eckman, T.E. Golde and S.G. Younkin, An increased percentage of long amyloid beta protein secreted by familial amyloid beta protein precursor (beta APP717) mutants, *Science* **264** (1994), 1336–1340.

[97] A. Takeuchi, M.C. Irizarry, K. Duff, T.C. Saido, K. Hsiao Ashe, M. Hasegawa, D.M. Mann, B.T. Hyman and T. Iwatsubo, Age-related amyloid beta deposition in transgenic mice overexpressing both Alzheimer mutant presenilin 1 and amyloid beta precursor protein Swedish mutant is not associated with global neuronal loss.[erratum appears in Am J Pathol 2000 Oct;157(4):1413], *American Journal of Pathology* **157** (2000), 331–339.

[98] R.D. Terry, E. Masliah, D.P. Salmon, N. Butters, R. DeTeresa, R. Hill, L.A. Hansen and R. Katzman, Physical basis of cognitive alterations in Alzheimer's disease: synapse loss is the major correlate of cognitive impairment, *Annals of Neurology* **30** (1991), 572–580.

[99] L.J. Thal, Therapeutics and mild cognitive impairment: Current status and future directions, *Alzheimer Disease & Associated Disorders* **17** (2003), S69–S71.

[100] F. Trinchese, S. Liu, F. Battaglia, S. Walter, P.M. Mathews and O. Arancio, Progressive age-related development of Alzheimer-like pathology in APP/PS1 mice, *Annals of Neurology* **55** (2004), 801–814.

[101] J. Tsai, J. Grutzendler, K. Duff and W.B. Gan, Fibrillar amyloid deposition leads to local synaptic abnormalities and breakage of neuronal branches, *Nature Neuroscience* **7** (2004), 1181–1183.

[102] B. Urbanc, L. Cruz, R. Le, J. Sanders, K.H. Ashe, K. Duff, H.E. Stanley, M.C. Irizarry and B.T. Hyman, Neurotoxic effects of thioflavin S-positive amyloid deposits in transgenic mice and Alzheimer's disease, *Proceedings of the National Academy of Sciences of the United States of America* **99** (2002), 13990–13995.

[103] J. Valla, K. Chen, J.D. Berndt, F. Gonzalez-Lima, S.R. Cherry, D. Games and E.M. Reiman, Effects of image resolution on autoradiographic measurements of posterior cingulate activity in PDAPP mice: implications for functional brain imaging studies of transgenic mouse models of Alzheimer's Disease, *Neuroimage* **16** (2002), 1–6.

[104] D. Van Dam, R. D'Hooge, M. Staufenbiel, C. Van Ginneken, F. Van Meir and P.P. De Deyn, Age-dependent cognitive

decline in the APP23 model precedes amyloid deposition, *European Journal of Neuroscience* **17** (2003), 388–396.
[105] M. von Kienlin, B. Kunnecke, F. Metzger, G. Steiner, J.G. Richards, L. Ozmen, H. Jacobsen and H. Loetscher, Altered metabolic profile in the frontal cortex of PS2APP transgenic mice, monitored throughout their life span, *Neurobiology of Disease* **18** (2005), 32–39.
[106] M.A. Westerman, D. Cooper-Blacketer, A. Mariash, L. Kotilinek, T. Kawarabayashi, L.H. Younkin, G.A. Carlson, S.G. Younkin and K.H. Ashe, The relationship between Abeta and memory in the Tg2576 mouse model of Alzheimer's disease, *Journal of Neuroscience* **22** (2002), 1858–1867.
[107] D.T. Winkler, L. Bondolfi, M.C. Herzig, L. Jann, M.E. Calhoun, K.H. Wiederhold, M. Tolnay, M. Staufenbiel and M. Jucker, Spontaneous hemorrhagic stroke in a mouse model of cerebral amyloid angiopathy, *Journal of Neuroscience* **21** (2001), 1619–1627.
[108] O. Wirths, G. Multhaup, C. Czech, N. Feldmann, V. Blanchard, G. Tremp, K. Beyreuther, L. Pradier and T.A. Bayer, Intraneuronal APP/A beta trafficking and plaque formation in beta-amyloid precursor protein and presenilin-1 transgenic mice, *Brain Pathology* **12** (2002), 275–286.
[109] T.P. Wong, T. Debeir, K. Duff and A.C. Cuello, Reorganization of cholinergic terminals in the cerebral cortex and hippocampus in transgenic mice carrying mutated presenilin-1 and amyloid precursor protein transgenes, *Journal of Neuroscience* **19** (1999), 2706–2716.
[110] C.C. Wu, F. Chawla, D. Games, R.E. Rydel, S. Freedman, D. Schenk, W.G. Young, J.H. Morrison and F.E. Bloom, Selective vulnerability of dentate granule cells prior to amyloid deposition in PDAPP mice: digital morphometric analyses, *Proceedings of the National Academy of Sciences of the United States of America* **101** (2004), 7141–7146.
[111] T. Wyss-Coray, L. Feng, E. Masliah, M.D. Ruppe, H.S. Lee, S.M. Toggas, E.M. Rockenstein and L. Mucke, Increased central nervous system production of extracellular matrix components and development of hydrocephalus in transgenic mice overexpressing transforming growth factor-beta 1, *American Journal of Pathology* **147** (1995), 53–67.
[112] T. Wyss-Coray, C. Lin, F. Yan, G.Q. Yu, M. Rohde, L. McConlogue, E. Masliah and L. Mucke, TGF-beta1 promotes microglial amyloid-beta clearance and reduces plaque burden in transgenic mice.[see comment], *Nature Medicine* **7** (2001), 612–618.
[113] T. Wyss-Coray, E. Masliah, M. Mallory, L. McConlogue, K. Johnson-Wood, C. Lin and L. Mucke, Amyloidogenic role of cytokine TGF-beta1 in transgenic mice and in Alzheimer's disease, *Nature* **389** (1997), 603–606.
[114] T. Wyss-Coray, F. Yan, A.H. Lin, J.D. Lambris, J.J. Alexander, R.J. Quigg and E. Masliah, Prominent neurodegeneration and increased plaque formation in complement-inhibited Alzheimer's mice, *Proceedings of the National Academy of Sciences of the United States of America* **99** (2002), 10837–10842.
[115] P.P.B.J.C.S. Zandi, Do NSAIDs prevent Alzheimer's disease? And, if so, why? The epidemiological evidence, *Neurobiology of Aging* **22** (2001), 811–817.

Alzheimer's disease: The amyloid cascade hypothesis: An update and reappraisal

John Hardy
Laboratory of Neurogenetics, National Institute on Aging, Porter Neuroscience Building, 35, Convent Drive, Bethesda, MD20892, USA
Tel.: +1 301 451 6081; E-mail: hardyj@mail.nih.gov

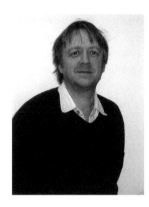

Abstract. Here I recap the scientific and personal background of the delineation of the amyloid cascade hypothesis for Alzheimer's disease that I wrote with Gerry Higgins and the events leading to the writing of that influential review.

My former and wise Head of Department, Bob Williamson, used to quip that the greatest thing about molecular genetics was that knowledge was a handicap and this is certainly why I have enjoyed a career in genetics. By that he meant that all you needed to know about a disease was its mode of inheritance. Positional cloning would lead you to the mutant gene which, unambiguously, caused disease. And after that, there would be no argument: pathogenesis would start from there.

In the 1970's and 1980's there were huge numbers of ideas, mostly rather vague and untestable, about what was the cause of Alzheimer's disease: slow viruses, aluminum exposure, "accelerated aging" (whatever that is, beyond a smokescreen for sloppy thought, has never been clear to me), or an environmental toxin were among the favorite notions. There was also some confusion about the relative importance of, and the relationships between, the different elements of the disease pathology: the plaques, which Glenner [2] and Masters and Beyreuther [12] had shown were made of the amyloid-β peptide in the mid 1980s, the tangles, which Wischik and Goedert [5] had shown was made of tau in the late 1980s, and the neuronal loss.

We geneticists made some missteps: the original linkage report was wrong, and yet had pointed at a chromosomal 21 gene [14]. It took us some time to realize the disease was genetically heterogeneous [15]: however, with this realization and because of the linkage of the amyloid gene to Hereditary Amyloidosis, Dutch Type [11,16], our group suddenly understood that the simplest interpretation of all the genetic data was that AβPP mutations caused a minority of early onset autosomal dominant Alzheimer's disease. We focused our attention on those families that showed evidence for linkage to chromosome 21 markers and immediately began to find mutations in AβPP, close to the amyloid-β part of the molecule [4]. These data were important because they gave us the first defined cause of the disease, and they also gave us the possibility to make transgenic models of the disease. I realized that these findings proved one cause of disease. More importantly, I realized they implied that all causes of disease would share mechanistic relationships with this first cause. Overexpression of AβPP in Down syndrome immediately became an obvious second defined cause, as Glenner had been suggested many years before [3].

Emboldened by these ideas, but aware of my limitations as a discussant of amyloid processing, I contacted David Allsop [1], who had originally worked out the amino acid composition of amyloid, and together we wrote the widely cited review for Trends in Pharmacological Sciences [6]. Dennis Selkoe had also understood the significance of our genetic data and reviewed the field for Cell [13], and these reviews, together with the Science review are widely seen as the start of the dominance of the "Amyloid Cascade Hypothesis" for Alzheimer's disease. I think this attribution is a little unfair: presumably, Glenner [3] and Masters and Beyreuther [12] had isolated amyloid and cloned the amyloid gene because they believed something along the lines of the amyloid cascade hypothesis although they never expressed their ideas clearly.

The story of how the review was written is a little complicated. In late 1991, I had visited the United States to give a talk to Gerry Higgins' group at the National Institute on Aging (coincidentally, my current employer, though no longer Gerry's: in fact, Gerry's former secretary is my Senior Administrator). While I was visiting Gerry's lab, he and I had got on very well, and he showed me a manuscript he had in press in Nature [10], describing the production of transgenic amyloid mice with fulminant Alzheimer pathology, both plaques and tangles. He offered to show me slides from the mice, but he couldn't lay his hands on them at that time. I didn't mind because looking down a microscope is always a waste of time for me. However, the manuscript was stunning, and ostensibly described the full modeling of the disease process. After I was back in London, Gerry and I spoke by 'phone several times, and I suggested we review the genetic and animal data together. He agreed, and contacted a friend of his who was an editor at Science to see if they were interested. To my surprise, they were, and I drafted the paper immediately, with him correcting the draft and supplying the figure: the title was also his choosing. The review took possibly a week to write. At the time, I was organizing a small meeting in London about Alzheimer's disease and I invited him to be the Plenary Lecturer. But as this was all brewing, he began to tell me that people didn't believe him about the pathology in his mice. At last, the day before we were to have the meeting, he 'phoned to say he couldn't come: he was having serious problems at work, and perhaps he should withdraw his name from the paper.

I said of course he should be an author: we had written the paper together, and that is how we left it. Apart from taking him to lunch 5 years later, during a visit of his to Florida to interview to become an administrator at NASCAR, I have never seen or spoken to him since. As the probable fraud of his mouse analysis was uncovered, he resigned, left science and disappeared. So this paper, while it could be seen as the beginning of the amyloid cascade hypothesis, was Gerry's last.

What do I think of it today? First, it is simple, clear and short: too many articles are complicated, muddy and long: even a venture capitalist or a corporate CEO can read to the end of it. Second, while adjudication of final truth depends on successful therapy, I think there can be little doubt that it is largely correct, as we have recently reviewed [8]. Third, as an idea, the amyloid cascade hypothesis has been extremely valuable in focusing research. Fourth, I have found it irritating to be asked time and time again to present and defend it, rather like Procul Harem being asked endlessly to sing "A Whiter Shade of Pale".

Subsequent findings which have supported the basic tenet of the article have included (see ref. [8]):

1) the observation that presenilin mutations have the same effect on amyloid processing as AβPP mutations and presenilin is in fact, part of the enzyme complex which produces Aβ from AβPP,
2) the realization that tau mutations lead to tangles, cell loss and dementia, indicating that tau is indeed downstream from Aβ,
3) the observation that the crossing of an AβPP transgene into a tau transgenic mouse does indeed push tangle formation and this effect is rescued by reducing the amyloid load: (thus, years later, we were indeed able to make mice with pathology similar to those fraudulently described by Gerry).
4) the genetic linkage screens for late onset Alzheimer's disease show up both the AβPP gene and a locus on chromosome 10 which influence AβPP metabolism.

Amyloid-based treatments, the final test of the amyloid cascade hypothesis, are showing some hopeful results, but they are certainly not yet conclusive.

The amyloid cascade hypothesis has been extensively criticized particularly by those who point out that by "amyloid" we originally meant "plaque amyloid" (although I note that at the time, the official name for what we now call Aβ was amyloid-β peptide). While I accept this criticism because most people, including me, now think it is some smaller oligomeric species,

I find it tiresome. Of course, our ideas have changed. If they hadn't, we would have wasted the last 13 years doing research: the article in Science was intended to generate ideas and act as a framework for a research agenda, not to be a definitive statement. I re-read it for the first time in at least 10 years to write this article: when I wrote it, I certainly didn't mean it to be laid down on a tablet of stone and consulted to ascertain ultimate wisdom about Alzheimer's disease. Other criticisms have seemed, to my intolerant ear, to be merely vague murmurings of malcontents who have consistently failed to come up with a viable alternative.

Writing this short memoir enables me to spread the thanks for this work. I wrote the widely cited review, but my thoughts at that time were influenced by the conversations I had with my boss, Bob Williamson, with my postdocs, Alison Goate, Mike Owen, Marie-Christine Chartier-Harlin and Mike Mullan and also with Christine Van Broeckhoven and Peter St George Hyslop. There was a community of ideas and our discussions, both within our group and with Christine and Peter, were free and open: I wish it were always so. Karen Duff, Mike Hutton and Jada Lewis have led subsequent transgenic work, which I think has almost proved the amyloid hypothesis beyond reasonable doubt. Colleagues like these and Dave Morgan have made science both productive and fun for me and most of the collaborations started in those days continue today.

I believe we are close to a therapy for Alzheimer's disease based on the amyloid cascade hypothesis, but time will tell.

"We skipped the light fandango
Turned cartwheels cross the floor.
I was feeling kind of sea sick,
The crowd called out for more.
The room was humming harder
As the ceiling flew away.
When we called out for another drink
The waiter brought a tray
And so it was that later
As the miller told his tale
That her face at first just ghostly
Turned a whiter shade of pale."

References

[1] D. Allsop, M. Landon and M. Kidd, The isolation and amino acid composition of senile plaque core protein, *Brain Res* **259**(2) (24 Jan 1983), 348–352.

[2] G.G. Glenner and M.A. Murphy, Amyloidosis of the nervous system, *J Neurol Sci* **94**(1–3) (Dec 1989), 1–28.

[3] G.G. Glenner and C.W. Wong, Alzheimer's disease and Down's syndrome: sharing of a unique cerebrovascular amyloid fibril protein, *Biochem Biophys Res Commun* **122**(3) (16 Aug 1984), 1131–1135.

[4] A.M. Goate, M.C. Chartier-Harlin, M.C. Mullan, J. Brown, F. Crawford, L. Fidani, L. Giuffra, A. Haynes, N. Irving, L. James, R. Mant, P. Newton, K. Rooke, P. Roques, C. Talbot, M. Pericak-Vance, A. Roses, R. Williamson, M.N. Rossor, M. Owen and J. Hardy, Segregation of a missense mutation in the amyloid precursor protein gene with familial Alzheimer's disease, *Nature* **349** (1991), 704–706.

[5] M. Goedert, C.M. Wischik, R.A. Crowther, J.E. Walker and A. Klug, Cloning and sequencing of the cDNA encoding a core protein of the paired helical filament of Alzheimer disease: identification as the microtubule-associated protein tau, *Proc Natl Acad Sci USA* **85**(11) (June 1988), 4051–4055.

[6] J. Hardy and D. Allsop, Amyloid deposition as the central event in the aetiology of Alzheimer's disease, *Trends Pharm. Sci.* **12** (1991), 383–388.

[7] J. Hardy, K. Duff, K. Gwinn-Hardy, J. Pérez-Tur and M. Hutton, Genetic dissection of Alzheimer's disease and related dementias: amyloid and its relationship to tau, *Nature Neurosci* **1** (1998), 95–99.

[8] J. Hardy and D.J. Selkoe, The amyloid hypothesis of Alzheimer's disease: progress and problems on the road to therapeutics, *Science* **297**(5580) (19 Jul 2002), 353–356.

[9] J.A. Hardy and G.A. Higgins, Alzheimer's disease: the amyloid cascade hypothesis, *Science* **286** (1992), 184–185.

[10] S. Kawabata, G.A. Higgins and J.W. Gordon, Amyloid plaques, neurofibrillary tangles and neuronal loss in brains of transgenic mice overexpressing a C-terminal fragment of human amyloid precursor protein, *Nature* **354**(6353) (12 Dec 1991).

[11] E. Levy, M.D. Carman, I.J. Fernandez-Madrid, M.D. Power, I. Lieberburg, S.G. van Duinen, G.T. Bots, W. Luyendijk and B. Frangione, Mutation of the Alzheimer's disease amyloid gene in hereditary cerebral hemorrhage, Dutch type, *Science* **248**(4959) (1 June 1990), 1124–1126.

[12] C.L. Masters and K. Beyreuther, Neuronal origin of cerebral amyloidogenic proteins: their role in Alzheimer's disease and unconventional virus diseases of the nervous system, *Ciba Found Symp* **126** (1987), 49–64.

[13] D.J. Selkoe, The molecular pathology of Alzheimer's disease, *Neuron* **6**(4) (April 1991), 487–498.

[14] P.H. St George-Hyslop, R.E. Tanzi, R.J. Polinsky, J.L. Haines, L. Nee, P.C. Watkins, R.H. Myers, R.G. Feldman, D. Pollen, D. Drachman et al., The genetic defect causing familial Alzheimer's disease maps on chromosome 21, *Science* **235**(4791) (20 Feb 1987), 885–890.

[15] P. St. George Hyslop et al., Genetic linkage studies suggest that Alzheimer's disease is not a single homogenous disorder, *Nature* **347** (1990), 194–197.

[16] C. Van Broeckhoven, J. Haan, E. Bakker, J.A. Hardy, W. Van Hul, A. Wehnert, M. Vegter-Van der Vlis and R.A.C. Roos, The beta-amyloid precursor protein gene is tightly linked to the locus causing Hereditary Cerebral Hemorrhage with Amyloidosis of Dutch Type, *Science* **248** (1990), 488–490.

Pathways to the discovery of the Aβ amyloid of Alzheimer's disease

Colin L. Masters[a,*] and Konrad Beyreuther[b]
[a]*Department of Pathology, The University of Melbourne, and the Mental Health Research Institute of Victoria, Australia*
[b]*Centre for Molecular Biology, The University of Heidelberg, Germany*

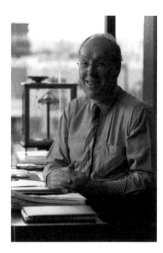

Abstract. Many participants played a role in discovering the composition and sequence of the Aβ amyloid of Alzheimer's disease. This sequence enabled the cloning of the amyloid precursor protein (APP), which elucidated its proteolytic origin from the membrane of neurons. The proteolytic enzymes which process APP and the Aβ fragment itself are now the prime validated drug targets for therapeutic intervention.

Approaching the centennial year of Alzheimer's presentation of a distinct form of neurodegeneration [2], we can look back over the past two decades during which an extraordinary research effort has been underway elucidating the role of Aβ amyloid in the causation of Alzheimer's disease (AD). Our contributions in the 1980's [20,27–33,44] to the purification and N-terminal sequencing of the amyloid plaque cores (APC) of AD and the discovery of its biogenesis from a neuronal precursor (the amyloid protein precursor – APP) by proteolytic cleavages (the β- and α-secretases) needs to be seen on the background of many years of prior research activity from a diverse range of individuals and groups. In this article, we summarize the interconnecting pathways which led to these discoveries and the subsequent torrent of research activity around Aβ amyloid and APP.

1. Prior to the modern era – up to the mid 1960's

For one of us (CLM), the "modern era" commences in the mid-1960s with his initial studies on the nature of spongiform change in the transmissible spongiform encephalopathies. These studies commenced in 1968 as part of a collaborative project between Byron Kakulas, Michael Alpers, Joe Gibbs and Carleton Gajdusek. At that time, Masters was a medical student exploring the morphologic features of the "slow virus" diseases, specifically Creutzfeldt-Jakob disease and kuru, occurring both naturally and after experimental transmission to non-human primates. In addition to the characteristic features of spongiform change, gliosis, and neuronal loss [31], it was well known at that time that a variable feature was the "kuru plaque", an amyloid deposition

*Corresponding author: Colin L. Masters, Department of Pathology, The University of Melbourne, Victoria 3010, Australia. Tel.: +61 3 8344 5868; E-mail: c.masters@unimelb.edu.au.

(as described by Igor Klatzo in 1957). Masters' interest in these kuru plaques began when he observed similar structures in some of the experimentally infected animals being assessed from 1968 to 1975. It was generally recognized at that time that the kuru plaques were morphologically distinct from the Alzheimer's plaque, not only in their intrinsic shapes and in the nature of the surrounding neuritic and glial reaction, but also in their topographic distribution within the brain.

Prior to the mid-1960's, very little progress had been made in understanding the pathological significance and biochemical nature of the amyloid depositions either in the brain (the concept of amyloid dates from Virchow's description of cerebral corpora amylacea) or systemically. Von Braunmühl was among the leaders of the German school of pathologists who attempted to understand the "colloidal" nature of amyloid. The same school had developed the use of the cotton dyes, such as Congo Red, for the differentiation of amyloid from other proteinaceous deposits. The fact that abnormal degenerative and regenerative changes occurred in response to cerebral amyloid deposition was fully appreciated [3,7], but the origin of the cerebral deposits remained enigmatic, particularly since some forms were clearly associated with small blood vessels, the amyloid congophilic angiopathy (ACA) of Pantelakis. The concept of a vascular or hematogenous origin of the cerebral amyloid plaque clearly arose during this period, and as we will see below, was promoted by the general (non-neuropathologically trained) pathologists who were used to evaluating the systemic forms of amyloidosis.

2. Beginning the modern era – mid-1960's to 1970

Three major intellectual streams emerged during the latter half of the 1960's. First, Friede [8] described the histochemical reactivity of the AD "senile" plaque, and observed the enzymatic activity specific for acetylcholinesterase. This eventually developed into the cholinergic theory of AD [43] and the current class of cholinesterase inhibitors useful in the symptomatic treatment of AD. Second, the emergence of the technology behind electron microscopy led to the "great tangle debate" between the schools of Bob Terry and Michael Kidd: was the Alzheimer neurofibrillary tangle (NFT) a paired helical filament or a twisted tubule? Electron microscopy also made major inroads into the filamentous structure of the amyloid plaque core and surrounding neuritic changes. Third, and more productively, the unlocking of the structural basis of the systemic amyloid filament had begun.

3. Early studies on the structural and biochemical nature of the Alzheimer plaque – the 1970's

In the early 1970's, despite the technical advances in histochemistry (including immunocytochemistry), electron microscopy, x-ray crystallography and protein chemistry (including N-terminal sequencing), little progress was made in understanding the amyloid plaques in both AD and the "slow virus" diseases. Remarkably, the first attempts at purifying the APC came from James Austin's group in Denver, Colorado in 1971/72 [35,36], but they had used formalin-fixed tissues. Nevertheless, their studies did reveal the presence of non-proteinaceous elements such as silicon, a forerunner to later interest in aluminum, copper and zinc.

In the first half of the 1970's, George Glenner had made spectacular progress in the biochemical elucidation of the AL types of systemic amyloid [11]. Glenner, who died in 1995 at the age of 67 from the complications of cardiac amyloidosis, was among the first to obtain N-terminal sequences on the amyloid AL light chains derived from plasma cell myelomas (Bence Jones proteins). He had conducted his seminal studies at the NIH in Bethesda, having moved there in 1958. Over the years he had built a reputation as a great biomedical scientist, yet at the same time difficult to deal with at the personal level. He may have had problems with a bi-polar depressive disorder, or he may just have had an ornery personality. One characteristic that colleagues noted was his reluctance to quote the work of other scientists with whom he was directly competing, best illustrated in reference to the late Earl Benditt's work on the systemic amyloids. Other views may yet be forthcoming from the surviving pioneers of these systemic amyloid studies – Merrill Benson, Per Westermark, Martha Skinner, Alan Cohen, Blas Frangione and Mordechai Pras. It was against this background that Masters approached Glenner.

Masters' first post-doctoral position was with EP Richardson in Boston in 1976/77, continuing studies on the AD/CJD amyloid plaques at a morphological level. In late 1977, Masters moved to the NIH laboratories of Carleton Gajdusek and Joe Gibbs, to continue the collaboration which had started in 1968. After some discussion with Joe Gibbs, it was agreed that Masters should start a project on purifying and characterising the amyloid plaques from the human transmissible diseases (kuru, CJD and the Gerstmann-Sträussler Syndrome – see [28,29]). Joe Gibbs, of course, knew of George Glenner's scientific reputation and of his presence on the NIH campus, and suggested that Masters visit Glenner's laboratory. By this time, Glenner had begun to think about the AD-amyloid connection, and had decided that the best approach would be to isolate the AD amyloid from the leptomeningeal vessels, but he had not commenced work on this subject. Masters and Glenner met on two or three occasions, and Glenner then drafted a research proposal which he sent to Joe Gibbs. As a result of this, an intramural NIH conference was convened in 1978, at which Glenner, Masters, Gibbs and others presented ideas on how to approach the general methods involved in purifying the AD/CJD amyloids. From the very start, Glenner assumed that the AD amyloid was derived from the vascular compartment, in the same manner as had been identified for the AA and AL proteins.

Over the ensuing two years (1978–1980), Glenner and Masters met only on one or two occasions in Glenner's laboratory to discuss progress, but at each meeting Glenner remained very secretive and obfuscatory about his own activities. At this stage, samples had not been exchanged between their respective laboratories at the NIH, nor was it clear that Glenner had actually begun dissecting any human AD brain tissues.

Masters' approach at the NIH was to try and adapt the known detergent – high salt extraction methods previously used for the purification of intermediate filaments, relying on the relative insolubility of the APC of both kuru and GSS brains. Because of the scarcity of tissue samples and the low numbers of APC in these conditions, Masters also began using AD brains to establish the methodologies.

While these studies were going on at the NIH from 1978 to mid-1980, other connections and collaborations were being established. In the AD field, several groups were actively engaged in the purification of the NFT, including Denis Selkoe in Boston and Henryk Wisniewski and his team at Staten Island (including Khalid Iqbal and Patricia Merz). On one of their many visits to Salem and Boston, Gajdusek and Masters dropped in unannounced to see Selkoe at his McLean laboratory, to check on progress with his NFT preparations. This would have been in 1979, and it was apparent at that time that Selkoe was not directly working on an APC purification strategy. In contrast, Pat Merz and Steve Bobin at Staten Island were very interested in the amyloid purifications in both scrapie/kuru/GSS and AD. Masters, Bobin and Merz set up a collaboration in which they shared protocols, samples, and techniques. This eventually resulted in a publication in 1983 (submitted in November 1982), which was the first to describe in detail some of the methods that had been jointly developed for the purification of amyloid from AD, GSS and scrapie frozen brains [33]. This paper concentrated on the electron microscopic appearances of the different types of amyloid filaments, which at the time was a very controversial area because of the studies emerging from the Prusiner laboratory in San Francisco. In retrospect, it was evident that we had relatively "pure" preparations of scrapie/GSS amyloid in our laboratories at a time well before Prusiner had "pure" preparations of the prion protein (PrP). If we had been able to solubilize and characterize the scrapie/GSS amyloid protein at that time, it would have led us directly to the PrP protein, pre-empting Prusiner's later discoveries by several years.

4. Dramatic discoveries on many fronts in the 1980's

Masters left the NIH labs in the latter half of 1980 for a year in Heidelberg with Melitta Schachner before returning to Australia in 1981, where he re-commenced studies on the sporadic and genetic cerebral AD/CJD amyloids [28,29]. For uncertain reasons, George Glenner moved to San Diego in 1982, having published a major review on the "β-fibrilloses" in 1980 [10]. His attempts to dominate the amyloid nomenclature debate with his emphasis on their β-pleated sheet structure (emanating from his earlier discoveries) were to be carried forward in his AD studies in California, where he found more ready access to AD brain tissues. During 1982/83, Masters was in communication with Glenner, and samples of pure AD-APC were sent to him on the understanding that it was a collaboration in which he would perform X-ray diffraction studies. It was never clear what became of those samples, as results were never forthcoming from his laboratory. Also, in 1982, Prusiner visited Masters' Australian laboratory while attending the International Congress of Biochemistry in Perth, at which he set up the collaboration with Charles Weissman, which was to lead to the eventual cloning of the PrP gene. During Prusiner's visit, Masters discussed progress in isolating the AD and GSS amyloid. Although Prusiner, at that time and for many years thereafter, maintained that his "prion rods" were distinct from amyloid fibrils and Merz's "scrapie associated fibrils", it came as a great surprise that he subsequently consulted with Glenner, and published observations on the Congo Red negative birefringence of the aggregated prion rods [39].

In 1983, another surprising paper appeared from Michael Kidd, Mike Landon and David Allsop in the Nottingham Medical School [1] disclosing their method of AD-APC purification (discontinuous sucrose gradient with subtilisin pre-digestion) and showing that their total amino acid composition was different from the known AA/AL amyloid proteins. We [33] had not been aware of competitors other than Glenner. Much later, we also learned that Alex Roher had also been working on purified APC [40]. In subsequent discussions with Allsop and Landon, it was clear that they had made plans to determine the N-terminal sequence, but their chosen collaborator failed to deliver. Moreover, they apparently had not discovered a method to solubilize the APC, a pre-condition for determining the N-terminal sequence.

In retrospect, it was clear that Glenner had been very busy and productive during 1983 and 1984, as his two papers on the N-terminal sequence of the AD amyloid protein appeared in May and August 1984 [12,13]. As expected, he had confined himself to the amyloid extractable from the leptomeningeal vasculature, and his method required predigestion with collagenase and (partial) solubilization in 6M guanidine-HCl, followed by Sephadex G100 chromatography. He also found the amyloid was soluble in 88% formic acid for HPLC. In his first paper, he obtained an N-terminal sequence as far as residue 24, with a mistake at residue 11 (identified Gln instead of Glu). He named contents of the two G100 peaks "β_1, β_2 peptide" after the "β-pleated sheet" configuration determined by X-ray crystallography (in contravention to the International Amyloidosis Nomenclature Committee rules which required the A-"x" system). He predicted that the β_1/β_2 peptides would be derived from a unique serum protein precursor, and cited 12 papers (eight of which were his own).

Masters first saw this paper when travelling to an EMBO-sponsored meeting on the Transmissible Spongiform Encephalopathies being organized by Alan Dickinson in Edinburgh. At this meeting, Konrad Beyreuther and Stan Prusiner were present: Beyreuther because of his association with Heino Diringer who had interested him in some of the properties of scrapie fibrils isolated in Diringer's Berlin laboratories, and Prusiner was there with some important unpublished information on the N-terminal sequence of PrP. Masters approached Beyreuther, known for his expertise in amino acid sequencing, to help with his studies on the AD amyloid plaque cores. By that time, Masters had also determined their solubility in strong chaotropes such as guanidine, and had discovered formic acid to be the most effective solvent (a tip derived from the previous generation of Australian wool protein chemists). Beyreuther readily agreed to collaborate, and Masters sent purified AD-APC to him and Gerd Multhaup for sequencing at the Institute for Genetics, Cologne. Our method for the APC purification now consisted of a pepsin digestion, Triton X100/high salt extraction followed by separation on a discontinuous sucrose gradient. Beyreuther and Multhaup were able to solubilize the AD-APC in formic acid and obtain a very ragged N-terminal sequence as far as residue 28 (four more than Glenner!). On SDS gels, dimers and higher order aggregates were readily observed of the 4 kD monomer, which at the time, in conformance with the International Nomenclature rules, we referred to as "A_4" (and the oligomers as A_8, A_{16}, A_{64}, etc., the "A" standing for either *Amyloid* or *Alzheimer*). We noted the pH-dependence of this aggregation process as being typical of protonation of histidines.

Glenner's next paper [13] appeared while we were making rapid progress with our own analyses. He now referred to the "β_1/β_2 peptide" as "the β protein", corrected his sequencing error at residue 11, and predicted that since the amyloid N-terminal sequence from a vascular preparation from a case of Down's syndrome was the same as from AD, that there would be a gene defect on chromosome 21 responsible for AD.

By late 1984, we had assembled enough data from our APC studies to draft a manuscript which was submitted to PNAS, and accepted in January 1985 [32]. In the acknowledgements, we thanked Steve Bobin, Michael Landon and George Glenner for "helpful discussions". This was certainly true for Bobin and Landon, with whom we had developed cordial relationships. Glenner, however, maintained a very "stand-offish" attitude, and even had the presumption to request further supplies of our purified APC (see Fig. 1 – "1 mg would be fine"!). Our PNAS paper [32] was published in June 1985. Subsequent discussions with Glenner showed that he believed that we could never have obtained our results without reference to his 1–24 sequence, and that he was extremely annoyed at our incursion into his domain. For many years thereafter, he maintained that the basic amyloid subunit was 28 residues in length. Initially, we ourselves were uncertain whether the N-terminal raggedness was an artefact of the preparative method, or caused by non-specific degradation of material remaining *in situ* for extended periods. Further studies from our laboratories [16,30] and others [14] suggested that the latter interpretation was more likely. The strong amyloidogenic propensity of synthetic A_4 was easily demonstrable [22,30].

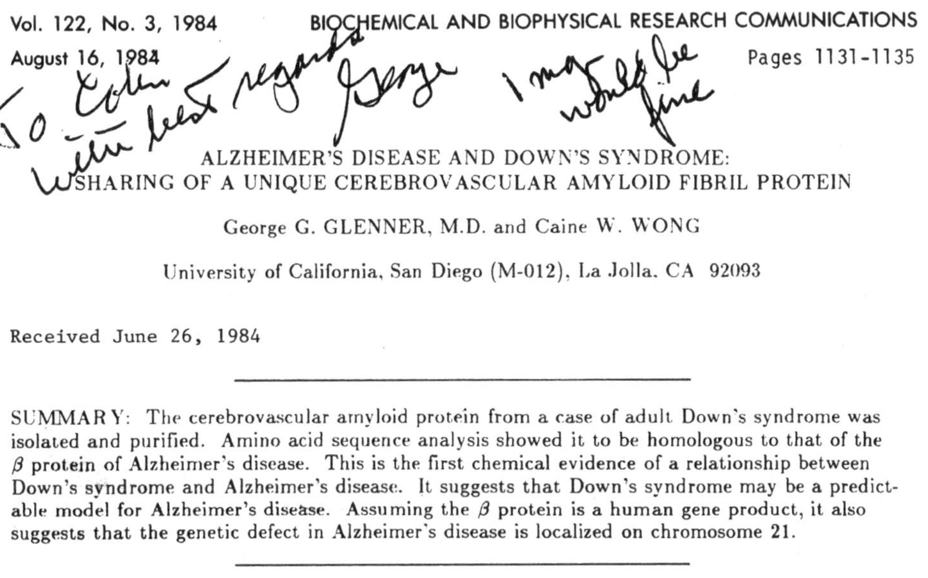

Vol. 122, No. 3, 1984 BIOCHEMICAL AND BIOPHYSICAL RESEARCH COMMUNICATIONS
August 16, 1984 Pages 1131-1135

To Colin with best regards George
1 mg would be fine

ALZHEIMER'S DISEASE AND DOWN'S SYNDROME:
SHARING OF A UNIQUE CEREBROVASCULAR AMYLOID FIBRIL PROTEIN

George G. GLENNER, M.D. and Caine W. WONG

University of California, San Diego (M-012), La Jolla, CA 92093

Received June 26, 1984

SUMMARY: The cerebrovascular amyloid protein from a case of adult Down's syndrome was isolated and purified. Amino acid sequence analysis showed it to be homologous to that of the β protein of Alzheimer's disease. This is the first chemical evidence of a relationship between Down's syndrome and Alzheimer's disease. It suggests that Down's syndrome may be a predictable model for Alzheimer's disease. Assuming the β protein is a human gene product, it also suggests that the genetic defect in Alzheimer's disease is localized on chromosome 21.

Fig. 1. Image of a reprint sent to CLM from George Glenner, at some time in late 1984, with the inscription "1 mg would be fine", referring to the collaboration in which Masters had previously sent him samples of purified AD-APC for X-ray diffraction studies, Glenner was now requesting further supplies. No results ever came from this collaboration.

The most important question which needed to be addressed in early 1985 was the origin of the cerebral amyloid. We immediately set out to raise antisera to the purified and fractionated APC and to a variety of synthetic peptides of A_4 (the Aβ peptide, as it subsequently became known). Using these antisera on AD brain sections, we were privileged to be the first to see the full extent of amyloid deposition in the human AD brain – a major revelation to the eyes of a classically trained neuropathologist! The Nottingham group had drawn attention to the similarity in amino acid composition between APC and NFT preparations [21], and we were very surprised to find similar (but more ragged) N-terminal sequences from our own NFT preparations [16,30]. Even more surprising, some antisera raised to both native and synthetic APC/A_4 reacted with a subpopulation of NFT *in situ* [30]. All of the antisera reacting with APC also strongly reacted with the vascular amyloid (ACA). We [30] also observed that the APC might have a non-proteinaceous component (see also [6]). From these observations we made several bold predictions including that the A_4 (Aβ) subunit would be of neuronal origin, consist of about 40 residues, and would be derived from a precursor protein [30]. The concept of a neuronal origin of an intracerebral amyloidogenic protein (diametrically opposed to the prevailing views of Glenner, Frangione and Wisniewski) received further support with the studies of Ghiso and Frangione who showed that a neuronally-derived protein, cystatin C, was the cause of a rare Icelandic congophilic angiopathy [9,26]. But the more compelling evidence for the neuronal origin of the AD-APC/ACA was to come eventually from the cloning of the Aβ precursor protein (APP) itself [20].

Looking back, what should we say about our conclusions that NFT contain Aβ? Early reports of NFT reacting with antisera to "neurotubules" [15] were followed up with the discoveries of tau [5,18] and ubiquitin [34] in the NFT, which have dominated the field over the past two decades. Initial studies on the biochemical nature of the NFT [17,19,42] did reveal properties in common with the APC, particularly in terms of solubility. At one point, Selkoe's group came very close to believing that the NFT and APC shared a common (vascular) origin [41]. More recent studies have maintained the possibility that Aβ can accumulate in intracellular locations, yet there is still no compelling evidence from either *in vitro* experiments or the transgenic mice AD models for direct Aβ and tau/ubiquitin interactions. We would now conclude that the question of NFT formation in AD is as puzzling today as it was 20 years ago, and leave open the question of whether Aβ has any direct role in the aggregation of tau (phosphorylated or not!).

Further support for the neuronal origin of the AD amyloid came from the parallel studies of the prion protein in CJD/GSS. In our PNAS paper, we made detailed reference to the biochemical similarities between the APC of AD and the chemical profile of inhibiting infectivity of scrapie [32]. At that time (late 1984), the PrP protein had been identified [4], the prion rods/filaments were known to bind Congo Red [39] and the N-terminal sequence of PrP had been published [38]. By the time we had assembled the arguments for the "neuronal origin" paper [30], the full sequence of the PrP cDNA was known [37] and observed to be expressed in the brain (equally in control and in infected animals). Within a short period of time, the PrP-composition of the CJD/GSS/scrapie-amyloid was confirmed by immunological techniques [24] and the neuronal origin of PrP demonstrated [25]. Just as we had observed with AD-APC immunoreactivity for Aβ epitopes, the antigenic enhancement of PrP amyloid with formic acid pre-treatment [27] suggested a common conformation underlay both types of extracellular deposits. Thus, by 1987, we could see that the purified kuru plaques and GSS amyloid that had led us into the AD story were also repositories of the secrets of the inherent infectivity of the PrP protein. It has now taken Prusiner's team and collaborators almost another 20 years to devise the experimental conditions required for the proof of the prion theory. There still remains a major gap in the prion field in that the molecular mechanisms underlying the toxicity (neuronal vacuolation?) leading to neurodegeneration remain unexplained. Our observations in 1985/1986 that the AD brain is under severe oxidative stress [27] were the first to suggest that the accumulation of Aβ in the AD brain might cause damage through some redox-active chemistry. This is currently one of our major strategies directed at therapeutic interventions in AD. It remains probable that similar processes might underlie the damage induced by an abnormal conformer of the PrP protein (and indeed the α-synuclein of Parkinson's disease, the SOD-1 in amyotrophic lateral sclerosis, the polyglutamine expansions of Huntington's disease, the tauopathy of Pick's disease, and complement factor H in age related macular degeneration).

Once we had determined the N-terminal sequence of the AD amyloid, it was clear that the major challenge ahead was to use this information to derive a cDNA clone to uncover the precursor protein. This came to fruition in the second half of 1986 [20,44].

References

[1] D. Allsop, M. Landon and M. Kidd, The isolation and amino acid composition of senile plaque core protein, *Brain Res* **259** (1983), 348–352.

[2] A. Alzheimer, Über eine eigenartige Erkrankung der Hirnrinde, *Allgem. Zeit. Psychiat. und Psych. Gerich. Med.* **64** (1907), 146–148.

[3] M. Bielschowsky, Histopathology of nerve cells, in: *Cytology and Cellular Pathology of the Nervous System*, (Vol. 1), W. Penfield, ed., Hafner Publishing Co., New York (1965 facsimile of 1932 edition), pp. 145–188.

[4] D.C. Bolton, M.P. McKinley and S.B. Prusiner, Identification of a protein that purifies with the scrapie prion, *Science* **218** (1982), 1309–1311.

[5] J.P. Brion, P. van den Bosch de Aguilar and J. Flament-Durand, Senile dementia of the Alzheimer type: morphological and immunocytochemical studies, in: *Senile Dementia of the Alzheimer Type: Early Diagnosis, Neuropathology and Animal Models*, J. Traber and W.H. Gispen, eds, Springer-Verlag, Berlin, 1985, pp. 164–174.

[6] J.M. Candy, J. Klinowski, R.H. Perry, E.K. Perry, A. Fairbairn, A.E. Oakley, T.A. Carpenter. J.R. Atack, G. Blessed and J.A. Edwardson, Aluminosilicates and senile plaque formation in Alzheimer's disease, *Lancet* **1** (1986), 354–357.

[7] O. Fischer, Miliare Nekrosen mit drusigen Wucherungen der Neurofibrillen, eine regelmässige Veränderung der Hirnrinde bei seniler Demenz, *Monat. Psychiatr. Neurol.* **22** (1907), 361–372.

[8] R.L. Friede, Enzyme histochemical studies of senile plaques, *J. Neuropathol. Exp. Neurol.* **24** (1965), 477–491.

[9] J. Ghiso, O. Jensson and B. Frangione, Amyloid fibrils in hereditary cerebral hemorrhage with amyloidosis of Icelandic type is a variant of α-trace basic protein (cystatin C), *Proc. Natl. Acad. Sci. USA* **83** (1986), 2974–2978.

[10] G.G. Glenner, Amyloid deposits and amyloidosis. The beta-fibrilloses, *N. Engl. J. Med.* **302** (1980), 1283–1292 and 1333–1343.

[11] G.G. Glenner, W. Terry, M. Harada, C. Isersky and D. Page, Amyloid fibril proteins: proof of homology with immunoglobulin light chains by sequence analyses, *Science* **172** (1971), 1150–1151.

[12] G.G. Glenner and C.W. Wong, Alzheimer's disease: initial report of the purification and characterization of a novel cerebrovascular amyloid protein, *Biochem. Biophys. Res. Commun.* **120** (1984), 885–890.

[13] G.G. Glenner and C.W. Wong, Alzheimer's disease and Down's syndrome: sharing of a unique cerebrovascular amyloid fibril protein, *Biochem. Biophys. Res. Commun.* **122** (1984), 1131–1135.

[14] P.D. Gorevic, F. Goni, B. Pons-Estel, F. Alvarez, N.S. Peress and B. Frangione, Isolation and partial characterization of neurofibrillary tangles and amyloid plaque core in Alzheimer's disease: immunohistological studies, *J. Neuropathol. Exp. Neurol.* **45** (1986), 647–664.

[15] I. Grundke-Iqbal, A.B. Johnson, H.M. Wisniewski, R.D. Terry and K. Iqbal, Evidence that Alzheimer neurofibrillary tangles originate from neurotubules, *Lancet* **1** (1979), 578–580.

[16] D.C. Guiroy, M. Miyazaki, G. Multhaup, P. Fischer, R.M. Garruto, K. Beyreuther, C.L. Masters, G. Simms, C.J. Gibbs Jr. and D.C. Gajdusek, Amyloid of neurofibrillary tangles of Guamanian parkinsonism-dementia and Alzheimer disease share identical amino acid sequence, *Proc. Natl. Acad. Sci. USA* **84** (1987), 2073–2077.

[17] Y. Ihara, C. Abraham and D.J. Selkoe, Antibodies to paired helical filaments in Alzheimer's disease do not recognize normal brain proteins, *Nature* **304** (1983), 727–730.

[18] Y. Ihara, N. Nukina, R. Miura and M. Ogawara, Phosphorylated tau protein is integrated into paired helical filaments in

[18] ...Alzheimer's disease, *J. Biochem. (Tokyo)* **99** (1986), 1807–1810.
[19] K. Iqbal, T. Zaidi, C.H. Thompson, P.A. Merz and H.M. Wisniewski, Alzheimer paired helical filaments: bulk isolation, solubility and protein composition, *Acta Neuropathol. (Berl)* **62** (1984), 167–177.
[20] J. Kang, H. Lemaire, A. Unterbeck, J.M. Salbaum, C.L. Masters, K. Grzeschik, G. Multhaup, K. Beyreuther and B. Müller-Hill, The precursor of Alzheimer's disease amyloid A4 protein resembles a cell-surface receptor, *Nature* **325** (1987), 733–736.
[21] M. Kidd, D. Allsop and M. Landon, Senile plaque amyloid, paired helical filaments and cerebrovascular amyloid in Alzheimer's disease are all deposits of the same protein, *Lancet* **1** (1985), 278.
[22] D.A. Kirschner, H. Inouye, L.K. Duffy, A. Sinclair, M. Lind and D.J. Selkoe, Synthetic peptide homologous to β protein from Alzheimer disease forms amyloid-like fibrils *in vitro*, *Proc. Natl. Acad. Sci. USA* **84** (1987), 6953–6957.
[23] T. Kitamoto, K. Ogomori, J. Tateishi and S.B. Prusiner, Formic acid pretreatment enhances immunostaining of cerebral and systemic amyloids, *Lab. Invest.* **57** (1987), 230–236.
[24] T. Kitamoto, J. Tateishi, T. Tashima, I. Takeshita, R.A. Barry, S.J. DeArmond and S.B. Prusiner, Amyloid plaques in Creutzfeldt-Jakob disease stain with prion protein antibodies, *Ann. Neurol.* **20** (1986), 204–208.
[25] H.A. Kretzschmar, S.B. Prusiner, L.E. Stowring and S.J. DeArmond, Scrapie prion proteins are synthesized in neurons, *Am. J. Pathol.* **122** (1986), 1–5.
[26] H. Löfberg, A.O. Grubb and A. Brun, Human brain cortical neurons contain α-trace. Rapid isolation, immunohistochemical and physiochemical characterization of human α-trace, *Biomedical Research* **2** (1981), 298–306.
[27] R.N. Martins, C.G. Harper, G.B. Stokes and C.L. Masters, Increased cerebral glucose-6-phosphate dehydrogenase activity in Alzheimer's disease may reflect oxidative stress, *J. Neurochem.* **46** (1986), 1042–1045.
[28] C.L. Masters, D.C. Gajdusek and C.J. Gibbs Jr, The familial occurrence of Creutzfeldt-Jakob disease and Alzheimer's disease, *Brain* **104** (1981), 535–558.
[29] C.L. Masters, D.C. Gajdusek and C.J. Gibbs Jr, Creutzfeldt-Jakob disease virus isolations from the Gerstmann-Sträussler syndrome. With an analysis of the various forms of amyloid plaque deposition in the virus-induced spongiform encephalopathies, *Brain* **104** (1981), 559–587.
[30] C.L. Masters, G. Multhaup, G. Simms, J. Pottgiesser, R.N. Martins and K. Beyreuther, Neuronal origin of a cerebral amyloid: neuro-fibrillary tangles of Alzheimer's disease contain the same protein as the amyloid of plaque cores and blood vessels, *EMBO J* **4** (1985), 2757–2763.
[31] C.L. Masters and E.P. Richardson Jr, Subacute spongiform encephalopathy (Creutzfeldt-Jakob disease). The nature and progression of spongiform change, *Brain* **101** (1978), 333–344.
[32] C.L. Masters, G. Simms, N.A. Weinman, B.L. McDonald, G. Multhaup and K. Beyreuther, Amyloid plaque core protein in Alzheimer disease and Down syndrome, *Proc. Nat. Acad. Sci. USA* **82** (1985), 4245–4249.
[33] P.A. Merz, H.M. Wisniewski, R.A. Somerville, S.A. Bobin, C.L. Masters and K. Iqbal, Ultrastructural morphology of amyloid fibrils from neuritic and amyloid plaques, *Acta Neuropathol. (Berl)* **60** (1983), 113–124.
[34] H. Mori, J. Kondo and Y. Ihara, Ubiquitin is a component of paired helical filaments in Alzheimer's disease, *Science* **235** (1987), 1641–1644.
[35] T. Nikaido, J. Austin, R. Rinehart, L. Trueb, J. Hutchinson, H. Stukenbrok and B. Miles, Studies in aging of the brain I. Isolation and preliminary characterization of Alzheimer plaques and cores, *Arch. Neurol.* **25** (1971), 198–211.
[36] T. Nikaido, J. Austin, L. Trueb and R. Rinehart, Studies in aging of the brain II. Microchemical analyses of the nervous system in Alzheimer patients, *Arch. Neurol.* **27** (1972), 549–554.
[37] B. Oesch, D. Westaway, M. Wälchli, M.P. McKinley, S.B. Kent, R. Aebersold, R.A. Barry, P. Tempst, D.B. Teplow, L.E. Hood et al., A cellular gene encodes scrapie PrP 27–30 protein, *Cell* **40** (1985), 735–746.
[38] S.B. Prusiner, D.F. Groth, D.C. Bolton, S.B. Kent and L.E. Hood, Purification and structural studies of a major scrapie prion protein, *Cell* **38** (1984), 127–134.
[39] S.B. Prusiner, M.P. McKinley, K.A. Bowman, D.C. Bolton, P.E. Bendheim, D.F. Groth and G.G. Glenner, Scrapie prions aggregate to form amyloid-like birefringent rods, *Cell* **35** (1983), 349–358.
[40] A. Roher, D. Wolfe, M. Palutke and D. KuKuruga, Purification, ultrastructure, and chemical analysis of Alzheimer disease amyloid plaque core protein, *Proc. Natl. Acad. Sci. USA* **83** (1986), 2662–2666.
[41] D.J. Selkoe, C.R. Abraham, M.B. Podlisny and L.K. Duffy, Isolation of low-molecular-weight proteins from amyloid plaque fibers in Alzheimer's disease, *J. Neurochem.* **46** (1986), 1820–1834.
[42] D.J. Selkoe, Y. Ihara and F.J. Salazar, Alzheimer's disease: insolubility of partially purified paired helical filaments in sodium dodecyl sulfate and urea, *Science* **215** (1982), 1243–1245.
[43] W.K. Summers, L.V. Majouski, G.M. Marsh, K. Tachiki and A. Kling, Oral tetrahydroaminoacridine in long-term treatment of senile dementia, Alzheimer type, *N. Engl. J. Med.* **315** (1986), 1241–1245.
[44] B.U. Zabel, J.M. Salbaum, G. Multhaup, C.L. Masters, J. Bohl and K. Beyreuther, Sublocalization of the gene for the pre- cursor of Alzheimer's disease amyloid A4 protein on chromosome 21, *Cytogenetics and Cell Genetics* **46** (1987), 725–726.

Amyloid β-peptide is produced by cultured cells during normal metabolism: A reprise

Dennis J. Selkoe

Center for Neurologic Diseases, Harvard Institutes of Medicine, Rm 730, 77 Avenue Louis Pasteur, Boston MA 02115, USA
Tel.: +1 617 525 5200; Fax: +1 617 525 5252; E-mail: dselkoe@rics.bwh.harvard.edu

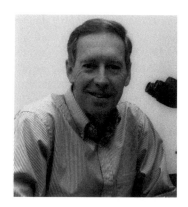

Abstract. In the twenty years since George Glenner identified the amyloid β-protein (Aβ), advances in understanding the biochemical pathology, genetics and cell biology of Alzheimer's disease have led to a detailed molecular hypothesis for the genesis of AD and brought us into human trials of anti-amyloid agents. The ability to study Aβ dynamically in cultured cells and *in vivo* derives from the recognition in 1992 that Aβ is a normal product of cellular metabolism throughout life and circulates as a soluble peptide in biological fluids. Here, I review the background underlying this discovery and then discuss its implications for research on Alzheimer's disease, particularly for the development of disease-modifying therapies.

Keywords: Amyloid β-protein, APP, secretases, Alzheimer's disease, drug discovery

More than two decades have passed since the seminal identification of the amyloid β-protein by George Glenner and Caine Wong [1]. The concept that Alzheimer's disease might share key pathogenic features with other primary amyloidoses motivated Glenner to isolate the subunit protein of cerebrovascular amyloid fibrils and initiated a long and arduous scientific journey that, in my view, is likely to lead to treatments – and even to prevention – of this most common form of mental failure in humans. Glenner's hypothesis about the origin of Alzheimer's disease was based on extensive studies of a range of systemic amyloidotic disorders conducted over the years by many scientists, including him. Although the theory that Alzheimer's disease represents, in essence, a primary cerebral amyloidosis has not been definitively proven at this writing and remains controversial, the wealth of insights about the biology of certain membrane proteins that Glenner's discovery spawned exemplifies the salutary intersection of basic and disease-oriented research.

My own initiation into the complexities of neurodegenerative disease began many years before I met George Glenner and learned about his hypotheses. During the third year of medical school, I developed an enduring fascination with the dysfunction of the human nervous system. Among my initial impressions, I was struck by the fact that some of the most interesting diseases of the brain were assigned to the backs of medical textbooks in short sections that contained little meaningful information. Alzheimer's disease, now recognized as one of the most common disorders of the human brain, was no exception. I began studying neurology the year prior to the report by Blessed, Tomlinson and Roth that the putatively rare "presenile dementia" that Alois Alzheimer had described was similar to, if not virtually indistinguishable from, the major form of common senile dementia [2]. I did not actually come across this fundamental reinterpretation of the nature of Alzheimer's disease until some years later, as I completed my residency in neurology. But I recall that my first encounter as a medical student with a patient with Alzheimer's disease piqued my interest about this obscure disorder that robbed its victims of their most human qualities – insight, judgment, abstraction and memory. Like other authors in this volume and like many investigators worldwide, I have retained my early fascination for understanding the molecular origins of this disorder, which continues to represent an enormous personal and societal tragedy.

By the time my colleagues and I undertook the investigations that led to the subject paper of this review, Glenner's hypothesis and his pursuit of the identity of the amyloid β-protein had been followed by several crucial observations, particularly the recognition that the amyloid fibers comprising the cores of senile plaques were composed of seemingly the same subunit protein that Glenner had described in vascular amyloid [3] and that this subunit was a fragment of a large, single-transmembrane precursor protein (AβPP) [4–7]. The isolation of the first full-length complementary DNA clones of APP by Konrad Beyreuther and co-workers [4] enabled studies on the biology of this previously unrecognized polypeptide to go forward. In my formative laboratory at McLean Hospital, my colleagues and I had already developed a method to purify amyloid plaque cores by fluorescence-activated cell sorting and had recognized the close biochemical relationship of their subunit to Glenner's vascular amyloid protein but its distinction from the protein filaments of neurofibrillary tangles [8]. By 1986, when we published our first study on β-amyloid, I had become convinced that understanding how the small amyloid β-peptide fragment arose in the brain and how it apparently triggered a complex series of neuronal alterations could prove key to deciphering Alzheimer's disease [9].

The work that Christian Haass and Michael Schlossmacher in my laboratory carried out, together with our collaborators, in 1991–1992 [10] constitutes one of the most exciting experiences that I have enjoyed during my time in scientific research. Glenner himself had assumed that there would be a soluble, circulating peptide that served as the subunit of the highly insoluble amyloid fibrils that he first isolated [1]. This idea, coupled with the numerous parallels between the amyloid pathology of Alzheimer's disease and the characteristics of numerous organ-limited and systemic amyloidoses occurring outside of the brain, convinced me that it should be possible to find a soluble form of the amyloid β-protein in biological fluids, including plasma. An intensive search for evidence that the amyloid β-protein circulated in human plasma did not yield a clear signal; in retrospect, this was due to the insensitivity of our initial immunochemical approaches. But closely related work that Michael Schlossmacher and Christian Haass performed on normal cultured cells revealed a small ($\sim$ 4 kDa), entirely soluble peptide in the conditioned medium of the cells that comigrated on electrophoretic gels with synthetic peptides having the sequence of the β-protein obtained from amyloid plaque material (Fig. 1) [10]. We also observed a slightly smaller, 3 kDa peptide in the conditioned medium of the cells, which we subsequently designated "p3". A series of experiments reported in the paper [10] showed that a variety of cell types that express APP naturally secrete Aβ and the smaller 3 kDa fragment into the medium under normal metabolic conditions, including primary neurons cultured from fetal human brain (Fig. 2). Radiosequencing performed by David Teplow and Christian Haass on these two secreted peptides in the medium of human embryonic kidney 293 cells stably transfected with APP_{695} confirmed that the absolute positions and periodicity of the principal radioactive peaks were entirely consistent with those predicted to arise from Aβ and from a truncated Aβ molecule [10]. The main 4 kDa species began at Aspartate-1 and therefore corresponded to the Aβ that had been originally isolated by Glenner and Wong from vascular amyloid and by Masters et al from amyloid plaques. The 3 kDa species began at Leucine 17 or Valine 18 in these cells. Because Leucine 17 was the known amino-terminus of the $\sim$ 10 kDa APP C-terminal fragment produced by α-secretase cleavage of AβPP [11], we speculated that the 3 kDa peptide represented an N-terminal fragment of this species. In this early work, we were unable to detect Aβ peptide in total cell lysates of the APP-expressing 293 cells, whereas it was readily detected in their conditioned medium. This result did not mean that the peptide was not generated intracellularly but rather that our methods were apparently too insensitive at that juncture to detect the small amounts that were generated prior to secretion into the medium.

Our work was performed at the same time as parallel studies by our colleagues, Peter Seubert, Carmen Vigo-Pelfrey, Ivan Lieberburg and Dale Schenk at Athena Neurosciences, who had developed novel, highly sensitive antibodies that allowed the first detection of Aβ by enzyme-linked immunosorbant assays (ELISA) in biological fluids, including cerebrospinal fluid and plasma. This key finding was published in a companion paper

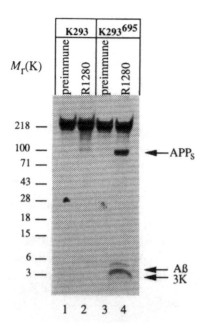

Fig. 1. Peptides of M_r, 4 kDa and 3 kDa are specifically immunoprecipitated from culture medium by various antibodies to Aβ. Comparison of the amounts of 4 kDa and 3 kDa peptides produced by untransfected 293 cells (lane 2) and by 293 cells stably transfected with β-APP$_{695}$ (lane 4). R1280 precipitated substantially more 4 kDa and 3 kDa peptides from the transfected cells. Preimmune serum was negative (lanes 1 and 3). A 218 kDa protein was nonspecifically precipitated in variable amounts by both preimmune and immune sera. From Nature 359, 322–325, 1992. Copyright permission granted by Nature.

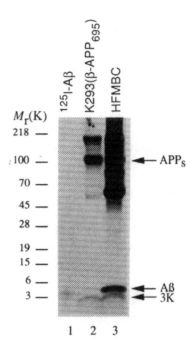

Fig. 2. The 4 kDa and 3 kDa peptides are produced by a variety of different cell types. Conditioned medium from radiolabeled human fetal mixed-brain cultures (HFMBC) (lane 3) and from transfected 293 cells (lane 2) were precipitated with R1280. The 4 kDa and 3 kDa peptides produced by the two cell types comigrate. Lane 1, radioiodinated Aβ. HFMBC consistently produced the highest amounts of Aβ. From Nature 359, 322–325, 1992. Copyright permission granted by Nature.

to ours [12]. Closely similar observations by Mioki Shoji, Steven Younkin and their colleagues [13] were entirely in agreement with our own, and the three studies together established definitively that Aβ was a normal product of cellular metabolism throughout life and circulated in human biological fluids.

My collaborators and I were excited about this discovery and about the opportunities it appeared to open up. In our paper, Haass, Schlossmacher and I pointed out that the cells we studied were morphologically normal and did not admit vital dyes. This observation, coupled with the absence of a detectable signal for intracellular Aβ in the very cells that showed readily detectable extracellular Aβ, made it clear that the generation of Aβ required neither preexisting cellular injury nor aberrant proteolysis of APP (as had been generally assumed) and that the Aβ found in the medium did not represent peptide released from dying cells. This conclusion was strongly supported by the companion observation that Aβ was present in the cerebrospinal fluid and plasma of normal humans [12,13]. At the end of our paper, we commented "The finding that Aβ is generated *in vitro* as a soluble peptide that can readily be quantitated leads us to propose the use of various cultured cells, both neuronal and non-neural, as simple screens to identify synthetic and natural molecules which increase or decrease the production, release or stability of Aβ." Although there were several implications of the discovery of normal Aβ production, I viewed this one as perhaps the most significant. We further hypothesized in our paper that, "chronically enhanced production and/or decreased clearance of soluble, diffusible Aβ could lead to the gradual precipitation of aggregated non-diffusible Aβ in the form of spherical plaques and vascular deposits in Alzheimer's disease and Down's syndrome. Our findings indicate that several cellular sources could contribute to such deposits."

From my perspective, the discovery that soluble Aβ is physiologically secreted by healthy cells in the absence of detectable membrane injury had at least three broad implications for further research on AD and related basic biological questions. *First*, the biochemical and cell biological events underlying Aβ generation could now be studied dynamically and in great detail, both in cell culture and in laboratory animals. Until this time, Aβ had only been obtained painstakingly and in small quantities from the insoluble vascular or plaque amyloid deposits of postmortem human brains via lengthy purification.

Second, the ability to detect and quantify the principal protein constituent of the invariant histological lesion of AD (senile plaques) in CSF and plasma opened up new avenues towards identifying a laboratory marker to support a clinical diagnosis and perhaps monitor progression of the pathology. In this regard, subsequent work indeed demonstrated that decreases in the levels of the 42-residue form of Aβ in CSF correlated with the presence of Alzheimer's disease and could potentially be useful diagnostically [14]. In a review that immediately followed our 1992 papers [15], I speculated: "the possibility that the levels of soluble Aβ in CSF might actually decline during the course of progressive cerebral β-amyloid deposition must also be borne in mind. Such a situation occurs in another familiar cerebrovascular amyloidosis, hereditary cerebral hemorrhage with amyloidosis of the Icelandic type [16]." This was prior to the recognition that Aβ42 levels fell – rather than rose – in patients with Alzheimer's disease. In that review, I noted "it has often been suggested that AD may represent an augmentation of a process that invariably accompanies brain aging, and this concept takes on an important new credibility when it is realized that Aβ is a protein that is produced throughout one's lifespan by each one of us."

The *third* broad implication of the discovery of cellular Aβ production, and arguably the one with the greatest impact, has been its role in the development of amyloid-inhibiting therapeutics. For the first time, investigators had a simple, manipulable cellular screen to identify compounds, whether randomly tested or rationally designed, that alter Aβ production, release or clearance. My colleagues and I assumed that once nontoxic, cell-permeable compounds that decrease Aβ secretion were identified in culture, their effects on soluble Aβ levels in CSF or brain tissue of animals could then be assessed [15]. We hoped that this combined *in vitro* and *in vivo* screening system would offer a practical route toward ultimately validating the hypothesis that Aβ accumulation in regions of the brain serving memory and cognition was responsible for initiating Alzheimer's disease (Fig. 3).

An outcome of the first implication mentioned above developed rather quickly after our report. Martin Citron and others in my laboratory, in collaboration with Tilman Oltersdorf and Ivan Lieberburg, showed that same year that a mutation in APP in familial AD results directly in increased generation of the Aβ peptide by cells [17]. The findings in this paper provided the first direct link between an Alzheimer's disease genotype and the biochemical phenotype of progressive Aβ accumulation in the brain. Closely similar work by Xiao-Dan Cai and Steve Younkin on this particular mutation of APP (the KM $\rightarrow$ NL, or "Swedish", mutation) [18] also supported the concept that mutations causing inherited forms of Alzheimer's disease might produce the disorder by altering the cellular production of Aβ, as has been borne out by many subsequent studies.

Besides its provision of a simple culture system for studying many aspects of Aβ production and clearance, the discovery of Aβ secretion has led to the identification of small molecules that can inhibit the β- and γ-secretase enzymes which generate Aβ. While γ-secretase inhibitors with substantial potency and drug-like properties have only very recently begun to be tested in humans, there remains the hope that chronic modulation of Aβ secretion will slow the progression of Alzheimer's disease or, perhaps more importantly, prevent its initiation. A great deal of further preclinical and clinical research will be needed to bring this hope to full realization.

Finally, among the several criticisms raised about the "Aβ hypothesis" of Alzheimer's disease has been the concern that interfering therapeutically with Aβ generation may prevent its normal function and incur toxicity. In this regard, we had observed in our original report that our "findings raise the possibility that Aβ has a physiological function throughout life" [10]. While its function is not yet clearly established and could well turn out not to be vital, the goal of Aβ-lowering therapy has always been to do so partially, in a way that would return cerebral Aβ levels towards normal but certainly not to sub-physiological levels.

Conclusion

On a personal level, it was enormously exciting and satisfying to be able to participate in the studies reviewed herein. I am deeply indebted to Christian Haass and Michael Schlossmacher and to our innovative and committed collaborators mentioned earlier. Science in the modern era has increasingly flourished on the basis of the sharing of ideas and techniques by colleagues of diverse backgrounds. The particular discovery that I

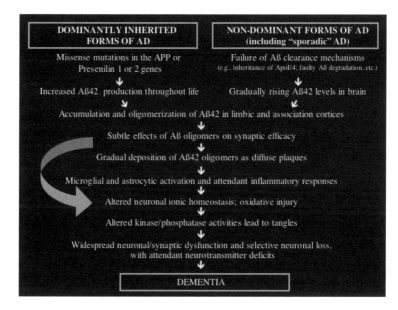

Fig. 3. A hypothetical model of the pathogenesis of Alzheimer's disease based on currently available information.

have reviewed in this article certainly exemplifies that. It is both a privilege and a responsibility to continue this line of research until our field achieves the goal of safe and effective disease-modifying therapy.

References

[1] G.G. Glenner and C.W. Wong, Alzheimer's disease: Initial report of the purification and characterization of a novel cerebrovascular amyloid protein, Biochem. Biophys. Res. Commun. 120 (1984) 885-890.

[2] G. Blessed, B.E. Tomlinson and M. Roth, The association between quantitative measures of dementia and senile change in the cerebral grey matter of elderly subjects, Br. J. Psychiat. 114 (1968) 797-811.

[3] C.L. Masters, G. Simms, N.A. Weinman, G. Multhaup, B.L. McDonald and K. Beyreuther, Amyloid plaque core protein in Alzheimer disease and Down syndrome, Proc. Natl. Acad. Sci. USA 82 (1985) 4245-4249.

[4] J. Kang, H.-G. Lemaire, A. Unterbeck, J.M. Salbaum, C.L. Masters, K.-H. Grzeschik, G. Multhaup, K. Beyreuther and B. Muller-Hill, The precursor of Alzheimer's disease amyloid A4 protein resembles a cell-surface receptor, Nature 325 (1987) 733-736.

[5] D. Goldgaber, M.I. Lerman, O.W. McBridge, V. Saffiotti and D.C. Gajdusek, Characterization and chromosomal localization of a cDNA encoding brain amyloid of Alzheimer's disease, Science 235 (1987) 877-880.

[6] R.E. Tanzi, J.F. Gusella, P.C. Watkins, G.A.B. Bruns, P.H. St. George-Hyslop, M.L. Van Keuren, D. Patterson, S. Pagan, D.M. Kurnit and R.L. Neve, Amyloid β-protein gene: cDNA, mRNA distribution, and genetic linkage near the Alzheimer locus, Science 235 (1987) 880-884.

[7] N.K. Robakis, N. Ramakrishna, G. Wolfe and H.M. Wisniewski, Molecular cloning and characterization of a cDNA encoding the cerebrovascular and the neuritic plaque amyloid peptides, Proc. Natl. Acad. Sci. USA 84 (1987) 4190-4194.

[8] D.J. Selkoe, C.R. Abraham, M.B. Podlisny and L.K. Duffy, Isolation of low-molecular-weight proteins from amyloid plaque fibers in Alzheimer's disease, J. Neurochem. 146 (1986) 1820-1834.

[9] D.J. Selkoe, Molecular pathology of amyloidogenic proteins and the role of vascular amyloidosis in Alzheimer's disease, Neurobiol. Aging 10 (1989) 387-395.

[10] C. Haass, M. Schlossmacher, A.Y. Hung, C. Vigo-Pelfrey, A. Mellon, B. Ostaszewski, I. Lieberburg, E.H. Koo, D. Schenk, D. Teplow and D. Selkoe, Amyloid β-peptide is produced by cultured cells during normal metabolism, Nature 359 (1992) 322-325.

[11] F.S. Esch, P.S. Keim, E.C. Beattie, R.W. Blacher, A.R. Culwell, T. Oltersdorf, D. McClure and P.J. Ward, Cleavage of amyloid β-peptide during constitutive processing of its precursor, Science 248 (1990) 1122-1124.

[12] P. Seubert, C. Vigo-Pelfrey, F. Esch, M. Lee, H. Dovey, D. Davis, S. Sinha, M.G. Schlossmacher, J. Whaley, C. Swindlehurst, R. McCormack, R. Wolfert, D.J. Selkoe, I. Lieberburg and D. Schenk, Isolation and quantitation of soluble Alzheimer's β-peptide from biological fluids, Nature 359 (1992) 325-327.

[13] M. Shoji, T.E. Golde, J. Ghiso, T.T. Cheung, S. Estus, L.M. Shaffer, X. Cai, D.M. McKay, R. Tintner, B. Frangione and S.G. Younkin, Production of the Alzheimer amyloid β protein by normal proteolytic processing, Science 258 (1992) 126-129.

[14] R. Motter, C. Vigo-Pelfrey, D. Kholodenko, R. Barbour, K. Johnson-Wood, D. Galasko, L. Chang, B. Miller, C. Clark, R. Green et al., Reduction of beta-amyloid peptide 42 in the cerebrospinal fluid of patients with Alzheimer's disease, Ann. Neurol. 38 (1995) 643-648.

[15] D.J. Selkoe, Physiological production of the amyloid β-protein and the mechanism of Alzheimer's disease, Trends in Neurosci. 16 (1993) 403-409.

[16] A. Grubb, O. Jensson, G. Gudmundsson, A. Arnason, H. Loefberg and J. Malm, Abnormal metabolism of gamma-trace alkaline microprotein. The basic defect in hereditary cerebral hemorrhage with amyloidosis, N. Engl. J. Med. 311 (1984) 1547-1549.

[17] M. Citron, T. Oltersdorf, C. Haass, L. McConlogue, A.Y. Hung, P. Seubert, C. Vigo-Pelfrey, I. Lieberburg and D.J. Selkoe, Mutation of the β-amyloid precursor protein in familial Alzheimer's disease increases β-protein production, Nature 360 (1992) 672-674.

[18] X.-D. Cai, T.E. Golde and G.S. Younkin, Release of excess amyloid β protein from a mutant amyloid β protein precursor, Science 259 (1993) 514-516.

Tau

Tau protein, the main component of paired helical filaments

Jesús Avila
Centro de Biología Molecular "Severo Ochoa" (CSIC-UAM). Facultad de Ciencias, Campus de Cantoblanco, Universidad Autónoma de Madrid, 28049 – Madrid. Spain
E-mail: javila@cbm.uam.es

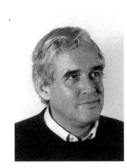

Abstract. In this volume we commemorate the centennial of Alois Alzheimer's discovery of what was later known as Alzheimer's disease, named by Alzheimer's mentor, Emil Kraepelin [1]. In a much more low level, our group remember in this issue a paper published twenty years ago. In that paper it was described that tau can self-polymerize and, at that time, it suggested that tau was not only a component of Alzheimer paired helical filaments, as indicated some months earlier during that year, 1986, but that it was the main component of Alzheimer paired helical filaments.

Keywords: Alzheimer disease, paired helical filament, phosphorylation, tau

1. Introduction

One hundred years ago, Aloïs Alzheimer described in a meeting the disease, a work that was published a year later [2]. In the description, he indicates the presence of two aberrant structures. Today, we know those structures like senile plaques (SP) and neurofibrillary tangles (NFT). Later on, he wrote "... the plaques are not the cause of senile dementia, but only an accompanying feature of senile involution of the central nervous system" [3], suggesting that the other structures were involved in the dementia, as suggested more recently by other authors [4].

The discovery of the main component of senile plaques (always, historically, the plaques were ahead of the tangles) was done in 1984 by Glenner and Wong [5], and at that time almost nothing was known about the component of NFT except that they were composed of paired helical filaments (PHF), as described for the first time by Kidd [6].

Two years later, and after several efforts to characterize and isolate PHF by Iqbal and colleagues [7], the first knowledge about the composition of NFT arises.

1986 was a good year in the identification of NFT components. In a pioneer paper Grundke-Iqbal et al. [8] described that tau was a component of PHF (tau is a microtubule associated protein discovered by Kirschner's group [9]). The observation of Iqbal et al was further supported by two other papers published in the same issue of PNAS [10,11], and by other work published in Japan [12]. Also, another manuscript by Grundke-Iqbal et al. [13], described that tau, in PHF, was in hyperphosphorylated form. Additionally, during that year it was commented a previous publication by Brion et al. [14] that also suggested the presence of tau in PHF. Also in 1986, it has been described that antibodies against PHF reacted with a 68 kD protein [15]. Some years later this protein was identified like hyperphosphorylated tau [16].

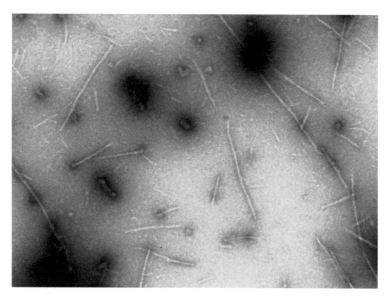

Fig. 1. An example of the assembled tau polymers (see text).

2. The article

Almost at the end of 1986 it was already clear that tau was a component of PHF. However, to prove that it was the main component of PHF, which is involved in making the scaffold of the PHF, it must show that it polymerizes into PHF-like filaments. The objective of the work that is commented in this review was to know if tau was able to polymerize into fibrillar PHF-like polymers. The title of the manuscript was: "Self-assembly of microtubule associated protein tau into filaments ressembling to those found in Alzheimer's disease" by E. Montejo de Garcini, L. Serrano and me, and it was published in Biochem. Biophys. Res. Commun. 141, 790–796, in 1986.

In that report [17], it was suggested that tau was not only a component of PHF but the main component. Also, it was suggested that tau polymerization can be facilitated by deamidation. Some years later, Watanabe et al. [18] described deamidation in tau from paired helical filaments.

3. The self-criticisms of the published paper

At that time our objective, almost our obsession, was to know if tau, a very soluble protein, was able to form (or not) fibrillar polymers. We tested many conditions for that. We knew that tau was able to bind to nucleic acids [19], but when we mixed tau with DNA, no polymers were found. Pierre and Nuñez (1983) [20] described that tau was able to be phosphorylated *in vitro*; we tried that, but polymers were not obtained. Also, we looked for conditions that were able to destroy microtubule polymerization, like the presence of Tris, or the use of urea, since it will denature tubulin but probably not a protein with a structure of random coil like tau [21], but negative results were obtained. Finally, one day we found that tau was able to form filaments *in vitro*, in the presence of urea (see Fig. 1).

Thus, the interest of the work was based in the indication, for the first time, that tau is able to form filamentous polymers *in vitro*. On the other hand, and after 20 years, self-critical reading of the manuscript indicates a fact that occurs *in vitro*, but not *in vivo*. This fact is the deamidation at glutamine residues (urea should deaminate everything, glutamine and asparagines). In the paper it was indicated that deamidation could facilitate tau assembly, mainly at glutamine residues. Several years later, Watanabe et al. [22] described that, indeed deamidation takes place in tau from PHF, but that it occurs mainly at asparagine residues.

Some time later, better conditions to raise *in vitro* tau polymers were obtained, but the observation of its assembly in 1986 was a very strong indication that tau could be the main component of PHF.

4. Other studies on tau polymerization

The fact that tau was the main component of PHF was further clearly supported by the work of C. Wischik in

1988 [23,24], following an approach similar, but more sophisticated, to that done by Glenner and Wong [5] to analyze the component of senile plaques. Additionally, M. Goedert [25], working in the same laboratory, described the whole sequence of this human protein, showing that it was almost identical to that described by Lee et al. (1988) for mouse tau protein, and that it was the main component of PHF.

Also, Wischik et al. [23,24] described that the "core" of PHF was the tau region involved in its binding to MT, previously indicated by Lee et al. 1988. Before that, in 1985, the tubulin binding region bound to tau was described [26].

Also, in 1988, it has been described that a fragment of tau was enough, at high protein concentrations, to assemble into fibrillar polymers resembling PHF [27].

In 1992, tau self-assembly was rediscovered by other groups [28–30], describing that a fragment containing the region involved in the binding of tau to microtubules was sufficient to raise assembled polymers.

A main problem to polymerize tau into fibrillar structures was the huge amount of protein needed for that. Thus, it started a search for compounds to decrease the critical concentration needed for tau assembly. Since G. Perry et al. (1991) described that in NFT there was a non-protein component, heparin; the assembly of tau in the presence of heparin was tested, and positive results were obtained [31]. In a few months, afterwards, Goedert et al. [32] found the same result.

Later on, several groups described other components like polyanions [33], fatty acids [34,35], or some or their oxidized products [36,37], quinones [38], proteins like α-synuclein [39], or 14-3-3 [40], solvents like TFE [41] or others [42] that facilitate tau polymerization. Some of these compounds mainly favour tau assembly when it is in phosphorylated form [38]. In this way, Alonso et al described that phosphorylated tau was the real component of PHF [43]. Then, several studies on tau protein kinases [44] and tau phosphatases [45] have been done. Once we knew those enzymes, tau polymerization in cultured cells was achieved in conditions in which the presence of phosphotau and toxic oxidant products facilitated that polymerization [46]. These experiments will be consistent with the possibility that a previous oxidative damage could be the cause of the onset of some tauopathies [47].

Afterwards, the discovery that one of the causes of a familiar tau frontotemporal dementia linked to chromosome 17 (FTDP-17), was the mutation of tau gene at specific sites [48–50], and the fact that in that disease (tauopathy), aberrant tau filaments were assembled, allowed the raise of several transgenic mice bearing some of those tau mutations. These mice were used as models to study tau polymerization *in vivo* [51]. Also, transgenic mouse models overexpressing tau kinases have been described [52].

Curiously, and previously, Harada et al. [53] described that the presence of tau was not needed for mouse viability, a result that was further confirmed by another group [54].

In summary, our contribution to this volume has allowed us to indicate the past, the present and some of the consequences (there are some other excellent works on tau that have not been commented in this brief review, and I will excuse for that) of the work started in 1986, twenty years ago, that, in my opinion, was a good year to remember, for the people working in tau, like the year when tau presence in PHF was described.

References

[1] E. Kraepelin, Lehrbuch der Psychatrie. Leipzig, *Barth* (1910).

[2] A. Alzheimer, Über eine eigenartige Erkrankung der Hirninde, Z. Psychiatr, *Psych. Gerichtl. Med.* **64** (1907), 146–148.

[3] A. Alzheimer, Ueber eigenartige Krankheitsfaelle des spaeteren Alters, Zeitschrift fuer die gesamte, *Neurologie und Psychiatrie* **4** (1911), 256–286.

[4] P.V. Arriagada, J.H. Growdon, E.T. Hedley-Whyte and B.T. Hyman, Neurofibrillary tangles but not senile plaques parallel duration and severity of Alzheimer's disease, *Neurology* **42** (1992), 631–639.

[5] G.G. Glenner and C.W. Wong, Alzheimer's disease: initial report of the purification and characterization of a novel cerebrovascular amyloid protein, *Biochem. Biophys. Res. Commun.* **120** (1984), 885–890.

[6] M. Kidd, Paired helical filaments in electron microscopy of Alzheimer's disease, *Nature* **197** (1963), 192–193.

[7] K. Iqbal, T. Zaidi, C.H. Thompson, P.A. Merz and H.M. Wisniewski, Alzheimer paired helical filaments: bulk isolation, solubility, and protein composition, *Acta Neuropathol (Berl)* **62** (1984), 167–177.

[8] I. Grundke-Iqbal, K. Iqbal, M. Quinlan, Y.C. Tung, M.S. Zaidi and H.M. Wisniewski, Microtubule-associated protein tau. A component of Alzheimer paired helical filaments, *J Biol Chem* **261** (1986), 6084–6089.

[9] M.D. Weingarten, A.H. Lockwood, S.Y. Hwo and M.W. Kirschner, A protein factor essential for microtubule assembly, *Proc Natl Acad Sci USA* **72** (1975), 1858–1862.

[10] J.G. Wood, S.S. Mirra, N.J. Pollock and L.I. Binder, Neurofibrillary tangles of Alzheimer disease share antigenic determinants with the axonal microtubule-associated protein tau (tau), *Proc Natl Acad Sci USA* **83** (1986), 4040–4043.

[11] K.S. Kosik, C.L. Joachim and D.J. Selkoe, Microtubule-associated protein tau (tau) is a major antigenic component of paired helical filaments in Alzheimer disease, *Proc Natl Acad Sci USA* **83** (1986), 4044–4048.

[12] Y. Ihara, N. Nukina, R. Miura and M. Ogawara, Phosphorylated tau protein is integrated into paired helical filaments in Alzheimer's disease, *J Biochem (Tokyo)* **99** (1986), 1807–1810.

[13] I. Grundke-Iqbal, K. Iqbal, Y.C. Tung, M. Quinlan, H.M. Wisniewski and L.I. Binder, Abnormal phosphorylation of the microtubule-associated protein tau (tau) in Alzheimer cytoskeletal pathology, *Proc Natl Acad Sci USA* **83** (1986), 4913–4917.

[14] J.P. Brion, H. Passareiro, J. Nuñez and J. Flament-Durand, Mise en évidence immunologique de la protéine tau au niveau des lésions dégénérescence neurofibrillaire de la maladie d'Alzheimer, *Arch. Biol. (Brux.)* **95** (1985), 229–235.

[15] B.L. Wolozin, A. Pruchnicki, D.W. Dickson and P. Davies, A neuronal antigen in the brains of Alzheimer patients, *Science* **232** (1986), 648–650.

[16] V.M. Lee, B.J. Balin, L. Otvos, Jr. and J.Q. Trojanowski, A68: a major subunit of paired helical filaments and derivatized forms of normal Tau, *Science* **251** (1991), 675–678.

[17] E. Montejo de Garcini, L. Serrano and J. Avila, Self assembly of microtubule associated protein tau into filaments resembling those found in Alzheimer disease, *Biochem. Biophys. Res. Commun.* **141** (1986), 790–796.

[18] A. Watanabe, K. Takio and Y. Ihara, Deamidation and isoaspartate formation in smeared tau in paired helical filaments – Unusual properties of the microtubule-binding domain of tau, *J Biol Chem* **274** (1999), 7368–7378.

[19] V.G. Corces, J. Salas, M.L. Salas and J. Avila, Binding of microtubule proteins to DNA: specificity of the interaction, *Eur. J. Biochem* **86** (1978), 473–479.

[20] M. Pierre and J. Nunez, Multisite phosphorylation of tau proteins from rat brain, *Biochem Biophys Res Commun* **115** (1983), 212–219.

[21] D.W. Cleveland, S.Y. Hwo and M.W. Kirschner, Physical and chemical properties of purified tau factor and the role of tau in microtubule assembly, *J Mol Biol* **116** (1977), 227–247.

[22] A. Watanabe, M. Hasegawa, M. Suzuki, K. Takio, M. Morishimakawashima, K. Titani, T. Arai, K.S. Kosik and Y. Ihara, Invivo Phosphorylation Sites in Fetal and Adult Rat-Tau, *J Biol Chem* **268** (1993), 25712–25717.

[23] C.M. Wischik, M. Novak, P.C. Edwards, A. Klug, W. Tichelaar and R.A. Crowther, Structural characterization of the core of the paired helical filament of Alzheimer disease, *Proc. Natl. Acad. Sci. USA* **85** (1988), 4884–4888.

[24] C.M. Wischik, M. Novak, H.C. Thogersen, P.C. Edwards, M.J. Runswick, R. Jakes, J.E. Walker, C. Milstein, M. Roth and A. Klug, Isolation of a fragment of tau derived from the core of the paired helical filament of Alzheimer disease, *Proc. Natl. Acad. Sci. USA* **85** (1988), 4506–4510.

[25] M. Goedert, C.M. Wischik, R.A. Crowther, J.E. Walker and A. Klug, Cloning and sequencing of the cDNA encoding a core protein of the paired helical filament of Alzheimer disease: identification as the microtubule-associated protein tau, *Proc Natl Acad Sci USA* **85** (1988), 4051–4055.

[26] L. Serrano, E. Montejo de Garcini, M.A. Hernandez and J. Avila, Localization of the tubulin binding site for tau protein, *Eur J Biochem* **153** (1985), 595–600.

[27] E. Montejo de Garcini, J.L. Carrascosa, I. Correas, A. Nieto and J. Avila, Tau factor polymers are similar to paired helical filaments of Alzheimer's disease, *FEBS Lett* **236** (1988), 150–154.

[28] M. Goedert, E.S. Cohen, R. Jakes and P. Cohen, p42 map kinase phosphorylation sites in microtubule-associated protein tau are dephosphorylated by protein phosphatase 2A1. Implications for Alzheimer's disease, *Febs Lett* **312** (1992), 95–99.

[29] R.A. Crowther, O.F. Olesen, R. Jakes and M. Goedert, The microtubule binding repeats of tau protein assemble into filaments like those found in Alzheimer's disease, *FEBS Lett* **309** (1992), 199–202.

[30] H. Wille, G. Drewes, J. Biernat, E.M. Mandelkow and E. Mandelkow, Alzheimer-like paired helical filaments and antiparallel dimers formed from microtubule-associated protein tau *in vitro*, *J. Cell. Biol.* **118** (1992), 573–584.

[31] M. Perez, J.M. Valpuesta, M. Medina, E. Montejo de Garcini and J. Avila, Polymerization of tau into filaments in the presence of heparin: the minimal sequence required for tau-tau interaction, *J Neurochem* **67** (1996), 1183–1190.

[32] M. Goedert, R. Jakes, M.G. Spillantini, M. Hasegawa, M.J. Smith and R.A. Crowther, Assembly of microtubule-associated protein tau into Alzheimer-like filaments induced by sulphated glycosaminoglycans, *Nature* **383** (1996), 550–553.

[33] T. Kampers, P. Friedhoff, J. Biernat, E.M. Mandelkow and E. Mandelkow, RNA stimulates aggregation of microtubule-associated protein tau into Alzheimer-like paired helical filaments, *FEBS Lett* **399** (1996), 344–349.

[34] T.C. Gamblin, M.E. King, J. Kuret, R.W. Berry and L.I. Binder, Oxidative regulation of fatty acid-induced tau polymerization, *Biochemistry* **39** (2000), 14203–14210.

[35] D.M. Wilson and L.I. Binder, Free fatty acids stimulate the polymerization of tau and amyloid beta peptides. In vitro evidence for a common effector of pathogenesis in Alzheimer's disease, *Am. J. Pathol.* **150** (1997), 2181–2195.

[36] M. Arrasate, M. Perez, R. Armas-Portela and J. Avila, Polymerization of tau peptides into fibrillar structures. The effect of FTDP-17 mutations, *FEBS Lett* **446** (1999), 199–202.

[37] M. Perez, R. Cuadros, M.A. Smith, G. Perry and J. Avila, Phosphorylated, but not native, tau protein assembles following reaction with the lipid peroxidation product, 4-hydroxy-2-nonenal, *FEBS Lett* **486** (2000), 270–274.

[38] I. Santa-Maria, F. Hernandez, C.P. Martin, J. Avila and F.J. Moreno, Quinones facilitate the self-assembly of the phosphorylated tubulin binding region of tau into fibrillar polymers, *Biochemistry* **43** (2004), 2888–2897.

[39] B.I. Giasson, M.S. Forman, M. Higuchi, L.I. Golbe, C.L. Graves, P.T. Kotzbauer, J.Q. Trojanowski and V.M. Lee, Initiation and synergistic fibrillization of tau and alpha-synuclein, *Science* **300** (2003), 636–640.

[40] F. Hernandez, R. Cuadros and J. Avila, Zeta 14-3-3 protein favours the formation of human tau fibrillar polymers, *Neurosci Lett* **357** (2004), 143–146.

[41] R. Kunjithapatham, F.Y. Oliva, U. Doshi, M. Perez, J. Avila and V. Munoz, Role for the alpha-helix in aberrant protein aggregation, *Biochemistry* **44** (2005), 149–156.

[42] J.C. Troncoso, A. Costello, A.L. Watson, Jr. and G.V. Johnson, In vitro polymerization of oxidized tau into filaments, *Brain Res* **613** (1993), 313–316.

[43] A. Alonso, T. Zaidi, M. Novak, I. Grundke-Iqbal and K. Iqbal, Hyperphosphorylation induces self-assembly of tau into tangles of paired helical filaments/straight filaments, *Proc Natl Acad Sci USA* **98** (2001), 6923–6928.

[44] K. Ishiguro Tau protein kinases, in: *Brain Microtubule Associated, Harwood Academic Publ GmbH*, J. Avila, R. Brandt and K.S. Kosik, eds, Poststrasse 22, 7000 Chur, Switzerland, 1997, pp. 73–93.

[45] K. Iqbal, A.D. Alonso, C.X. Gong, S. Khatoon, J.J. Pei, J.Z. Wang and I. GrundkeIqbal Tau phosphatases, in: *Brain Microtubule Associated, Harwood Academic Publ GmbH*, J. Avila, R. Brandt and K.S. Kosik, eds, Poststrasse 22, 7000 Chur, Switzerland, 1997, pp. 95–111.

[46] M. Perez, F. Hernandez, A. Gomez-Ramos, M. Smith, G. Perry and J. Avila, Formation of aberrant phosphotau fibrillar polymers in neural cultured cells, *Eur J Biochem* **269** (2002), 1484–1489.

[47] M.A. Smith, G. Perry, P.L. Richey, L.M. Sayre, V.E. Anderson, M.F. Beal and N. Kowall, Oxidative damage in Alzheimer's, *Nature* **382** (1996), 120–121.

[48] M. Hutton, C.L. Lendon, P. Rizzu, M. Baker, S. Froelich, H. Houlden, S. Pickering-Brown, S. Chakraverty, A. Isaacs, A. Grover, J. Hackett, J. Adamson, S. Lincoln, D. Dickson, P. Davies, R.C. Petersen, M. Stevens, E. de Graaff, E. Wauters, J. van Baren, M. Hillebrand, M. Joosse, J.M. Kwon, P. Nowotny, L.K. Che, J. Norton, J.C. Morris, L.A. Reed, J. Trojanowski, H. Basun, L. Lannfelt, M. Neystat, S. Fahn, F. Dark, T. Tannenberg, P.R. Dodd, N. Hayward, J.B. Kwok, P.R. Schofield, A. Andreadis, J. Snowden, D. Craufurd, D. Neary, F. Owen, B.A. Oostra, J. Hardy, A. Goate, J. van Swieten, D. Mann, T. Lynch and P. Heutink, Association of missense and 5'-splice-site mutations in tau with the inherited dementia FTDP-17, *Nature* **393** (1998), 702–705.

[49] M.G. Spillantini, J.R. Murrell, M. Goedert, M.R. Farlow, A. Klug and B. Ghetti, Mutation in the tau gene in familial multiple system tauopathy with presenile dementia, *Proc Natl Acad Sci USA* **95** (1998), 7737–7741.

[50] L.N. Clark, P. Poorkaj, Z. Wszolek, D.H. Geschwind, Z.S. Nasreddine, B. Miller, D. Li, H. Payami, F. Awert, K. Markopoulou, A. Andreadis, I. DSouza, V.M.Y. Lee, L. Reed, J.Q. Trojanowski, V. Zhukareva, T. Bird, G. Schellenberg and K.C. Wilhelmsen, Pathogenic implications of mutations in the tau gene in pallido-ponto-nigral degeneration and related neurodegenerative disorders linked to chromosome 17, *Proc Natl Acad Sci USA* **95** (1998), 13103–13107.

[51] J. Avila, J.J. Lucas, M. Perez and F. Hernandez, Role of tau protein in both physiological and pathological conditions, *Physiol Rev* **84** (2004), 361–384.

[52] J.J. Lucas, F. Hernandez, P. Gomez-Ramos, M.A. Moran, R. Hen and J. Avila, Decreased nuclear beta-catenin, tau hyperphosphorylation and neurodegeneration in GSK-3beta conditional transgenic mice, *Embo J* **20** (2001), 27–39.

[53] A. Harada, K. Oguchi, S. Okabe, J. Kuno, S. Terada, T. Ohshima, R. Sato-Yoshitake, Y. Takei, T. Noda and N. Hirokawa, Altered microtubule organization in small-calibre axons of mice lacking tau protein, *Nature* **369** (1994), 488–491.

[54] H.N. Dawson, A. Ferreira, M.V. Eyster, N. Ghoshal, L.I. Binder and M.P. Vitek, Inhibition of neuronal maturation in primary hippocampal neurons from tau deficient mice, *J Cell Sci* **114** (2001), 1179–1187.

Immunological demonstration of tau protein in neurofibrillary tangles of Alzheimer's disease

Jean-Pierre Brion*
Laboratory of Histology and Neuropathology, Université Libre de Bruxelles, Campus Erasme, 808 route de Lennik, B-1070 Brussels, Belgium

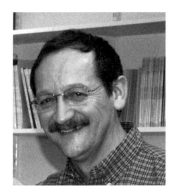

Abstract. Neurofibrillary tangles are one of the neuropathological hallmark of Alzheimer's disease, described early as part of the pathological criteria of the disease. Ultrastructural studies in the sixties showed their unusual features but their molecular composition was not unraveled before the mid-eighties. Initial biochemical studies suggested that they were composed of modified unidentified brain proteins, and several immunocytochemical studies suggested that they contained polypeptides cross-reactive with antibodies to cytoskeletal proteins. In 1985, we demonstrated that neurofibrillary tangles were immunolabelled by antibodies to the microtubule-associated protein tau and that antibodies raised to neurofibrillary tangles cross-reacted with tau proteins. These results were soon confirmed independently in several laboratories. Further studies were devoted to the analysis of tau post-translationnal modifications in the affected tissues and in cellular and animal models.

Keywords: Alzheimer's disease, neurofibrillary tangles, tau proteins, microtubules, phosphorylation

1. Introduction

Neurofibrillary tangles (NFT) were first described by Aloïs Alzheimer in his seminal paper describing the pathological findings in a demented woman aged 51 [2], using Bielschowsky silver staining. Alzheimer's disease (AD) was initially considered as a rare disease, belonging to the group of presenile dementia, until detailed anatomoclinical studies indicated that the characteristics lesions of the disease, senile plaques and NFT, are also common in patients with senile dementia and thus that these conditions constitute a common pathological entity, e.g. [89]. After their initial description, little progress was made for the following decades in the analysis of the molecular composition of NFT, with the exception of the demonstration of their affinity for amyloid dyes, i.e. Congo red, giving a green birefringence when observed under crossed polarization filters [28], suggesting that they were made of orderly arranged subunits.

The early studies of NFT were devoted to the analysis of their unusual ultrastructural characteristics, their pe-

---

*Corresponding author: Dr Jean-Pierre Brion, Laboratory of Histology and Neuropathology, Université Libre de Bruxelles, School of Medicine. 808, route de Lennik, Bldg C-10, 1070 – Brussels, Belgium. Tel.: +32 2 5556505; Fax: +32 2 5556285; E-mail: jpbrion@ulb.ac.be.

culiar biochemical properties and their antigenic composition. Many scientists have contributed to this exciting research avenue. Our own contribution to the initial identification of the molecular components (tau proteins) of NFT is summarized below, tentatively in the frameship of previous works that paved the way towards our own studies and subsequent works by our and other research groups.

2. Ultrastructural studies

A new leap in the description of NFT came with the advent of ultrastructural studies in electron microscopy in the early sixties. These studies showed that NFT were composed of bundles of filaments. These filaments were described as paired helical filaments [60], twisted filaments or tubules [52,87,88]. These filaments were also found in abnormal neurites in senile plaques [41,88]. The term "paired helical filaments" (PHF) is now widely used to describe them [93]. Subsequent studies by negative staining showed that they contained a filamentous substructure [10,92]. Sophisticated ultrastructural studies have however revealed their complex internal structure [21,82,90].

3. Biochemical analysis of PHF

Several groups used the unusual properties of PHF to obtain preparations enriched in PHF for analyzing their molecular composition. Some PHF were observed to be insoluble in denaturing agents such as sodium dodecylsulfate (SDS) and urea [83], properties that impeded the analysis of their molecular components. This property was used to prepare fractions enriched in PHF and use them as immunogenic preparations (see below). Some conflicting results were however reported on the solubility of PHF. In purified preparations of PHF, a least a proportion of them were reported to be soluble in SDS by repeated extraction and these preparations observed to contain major unidentified polypeptides of 57 and 62 kDa [58].

4. Immunocytochemical analysis of PHF

About at the same time, several groups investigated their antigenic composition. The latter approach was taken either by generating antibodies to isolated PHF and studying their cross-reactivity with normal brain proteins, or by generating antibodies to normal proteins and studying their cross-reactivity with PHF. The antibodies raised to PHF preparations were found to react strongly with NFT in light microscopy [54] and in electron microscopy [11]. This labelling was absorbed by brain homogenates from AD patients but not by homogenates from control subjects or only with high concentrations of proteins [19]. Similarly, some anti-PHF serum was observed to react with neither polypeptides of normal brain [47]. These results suggested that PHF contained highly modified proteins exhibiting antigens mainly present in AD brains.

In view of the filamentous appearance of the PHF, several groups studied their immunocytochemical cross-reactivity with antibodies to cytoskeletal proteins. An antiserum to brain microtubules was observed to label NFT in light microscopy [48]; a similar labelling of NFT by some antiserum to microtubules was reported by other groups [79,97] and by our-self [11] and PHF preparations were observed to contain cross-reacting polypeptides detected by an antiserum to microtubules [46], but the cross-reacting polypeptides were not identified in these initial studies. Some antibodies to MAP2 [61,74] and to vimentin [96] also labelled NFT. Early studies also showed an imunolabelling of NFT by some anti-neurofilament antiserum [22,56,59], although the polyspecificity or the ill definition of the antigens was raised as a potential pitfall [37]. However, well-defined monoclonal antibodies to neurofilament polypeptides [4,85] and neurofilament antisera [37] were found to label NFT in situ and even isolated NFT [71,79]. At least some of these neurofilament antibodies were however later found to react also with tau proteins [64,76]. Thus at that time, despite sound efforts to uncover the molecular composition of NFT, although it was suspected that NFT were made of strongly modified normal polypeptides, their clear identity was unknown. The positive reaction of NFT with antibodies raised to complex mixtures of proteins (e.g. microtubules) did not allow the exact identification of the core component of PHF. In addition, several of these antibodies, even well defined monoclonal antibodies, labelled a variable proportion of isolated PHF extracted with SDS, suggesting that some of the normal polypeptides identified in NFT were trapped in NFT rather than authentic component of PHF.

5. The microtubule-associated protein tau is the main antigenic component of PHF

P. Dustin and J. Flament-Durand in the Laboratory of Pathology in Brussels were in the early eighties deeply interested in the study of microtubules and their pathology [29] and I joined their Laboratory at this time. They had previously made several ultrastructural studies of biopsies specimens from AD patients, that convinced them that neurons containing PHF had less normal microtubules and contained accumulations of dense bodies [30,36] and they suggested that disturbances of microtubule assembly might be the cause of an abnormal axoplasmic transport in these cells [30]. Further observation of an accumulation of smooth endoplasmic reticulum also comforted this idea [81]. Although these studies suggested an involvement of microtubules or other filaments in this pathological process, we did not observe a labelling of NFT by anti-tubulin or anti-70 kDa neurofilament antibodies [11]. Other groups [32,97] had also previously reported the absence of tubulin immunoreactivity with well-defined anti-tubulin antibodies in NFT [74]. These observations indicated that PHF did not result from the assembly of tubulin but the labelling of NFT by some antiserums to microtubules [11,48,79,97] suggested the possibility that PHF might result from the pathological assembly of other microtubule proteins. We thus decided to test for the presence of other proteins associated to microtubules in NFT, by generating specific antibodies to some of them. J. Nunez was present in the Free University of Brussels in 1983, in the Laboratory of J. Dumont. He was interested in the developmental study of microtubule-associated proteins and had previously demonstrated that the expression of tau protein isoforms showed a developmental evolution [70]. In collaboration with him, we prepared tau and MAP2 proteins from adult rat brain using the microtubule assembly-disassembly method and the thermostability of tau proteins. We then generated several antisera against tau and MAP2 proteins using polypeptides extracted from polyacrylamide gels after electrophoretic separation by SDS-PAGE. These antisera were characterized by immunoblotting on purified preparations of microtubule-associated proteins and found to react with their cognate antigens. We then tested these antisera by immunocytochemistry on tissue sections from control subjects and AD patients. The anti-MAP2 sera did not label NFT but to our surprise, the anti-tau sera strongly immunolabelled NFT and abnormal neurites around senile plaques, giving an immunolabelling indistinguishable from the labelling with our anti-PHF serum (Fig. 1) [16]. We further characterized this immunoreactivity by immunogold labelling in electron microscopy on tissue sections of AD patients: both the anti-tau and the anti-PHF sera also labelled the PHF on ultrathin sections (Fig. 1) and isolated PHF (Fig. 2). Interestingly, the anti-PHF sera was also observed by western blotting to react with the same set of proteins as the anti-tau sera, confirming that it contained anti-tau antibodies. These results showing that tau was a major component and antigenic determinant of PHF were published [13,16,19] and presented in international meetings [12,19,35].

Several groups [27,44,62,75,95] soon confirmed the identification of tau in PHF independently. The cloning and sequencing of a cDNA encoding the core protein of PHF [40] and the isolation of peptidic fragments from the core of PHF [91] confirmed that tau proteins were an authentic component of PHF. The immunocytochemical analysis of NFT showed that they were composed of the six tau isoforms [39], and in collaboration with B.H. Anderton and his team we also pursued the immunocytochemical and biochemical analysis of NFT, showing that they were composed of the whole tau proteins [14,15], although some NFT (e.g. "ghosts" tangles) were lacking some of the N-and C-termini of tau proteins [14], suggesting that tau proteolysis is part of the pathological process and of the molecular evolution of NFT. The comparison of NFT labeling with anti-PHF/anti-tau antibodies or silver staining showed that it was a robust method correlated to the clinical data [31]. A tau immunoreactivity of fibrillary inclusions observed in other neurodegenerative diseases was soon reported, e.g. in progressive supranuclear palsy [80]. Different neurodegenerative diseases with a peculiar pattern of tau isoforms involvement have now been identified [20]. The spreading of NFT in AD brain follows a relatively stereotyped schema that was established both by neuropathological [9] and biochemical criteria [26].

Several other post-translational modifications of tau proteins in NFT were found in subsequent studies. Tau phosphorylation has been largely documented (see below). The detection of ubiquitin in NFT by immunocytochemistry [78] and after isolation [73] suggested that these fibrillary lesions were hardly handled by the ubiquitn-dependent degradation system. Modification of tau by products of oxidative stress, favouring its aggregation, was also reported later [77].

6. Tau proteins and pathological phosphorylation

Some early results indicated that the tau proteins in PHF were phosphorylated [45,55]. The consequences of tau hyperphosphorylation in AD were then further

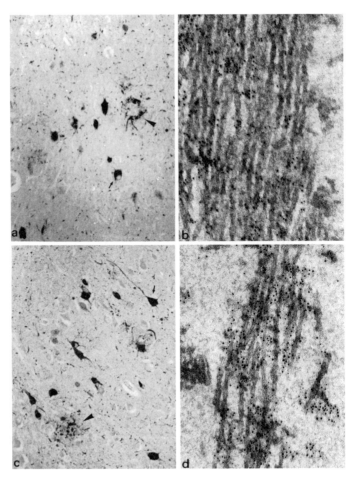

Fig. 1. Immunoabelling on a tissue section of the hippocampus of an AD patient with an antibody to rat tau proteins (A and B) and an antibody to isolated PHF (C and D). The antibodies label only NFT in neurons and in dystrophic neurites in senile plaques, as shown in light microscopy (A and C). The abnormal PHF are also labelled by the antibodies in electron microscopy (immunogold method) (B and D). Reprinted from *Arch. Biol. (Brux)* **95** (1985), 229–235.

shown by studies showing a much-reduced induction of MT assembly in AD brain [57]. We also later observed a reduction of the immunoreactivity for stable microtubules in neurons containing PHF [51]. By comparison with controls, slower migrating tau species were identified in AD tissue homogenates in areas rich in NFT lesions and shown to be highly phosphorylated tau species [34,49]. The "A68" polypeptides [94] identified in Sarkosyl-insoluble preparations of AD brain were found to be modified phosphorylated tau species; they showed an electrophoretic pattern of three main bands [63], contained abundant PHF [65] and reacted with antibodies to different tau isoforms [15]. The mapping of tau phosphorylation sites (serine/threonine residues) by several groups was accomplished using both specific antibodies and mass spectrometry analysis [3]. Tau is a phosphoprotein and even normal adult tau is phosphorylated to some degree. We and others observed that foetal tau is more highly phosphorylated than adult tau [17] but less than PHF-tau; the phosphorylation of tau could be modulated using several experimental treatment of cultured cells, i.e. glutamate, colchicine, Aβ amyloid [24] and oxidative stress [23]. The existence of highly phosphorylated tau species obviously fuelled the search for protein kinases (and phosphatases) responsible for changes in tau phosphorylation. Many kinases are able to generate phosphorylation sites on tau proteins *in vitro*; the glycogen synthase kinase-3β was one of the first neuronal kinase shown to generate typical PHF-tau phosphorylation sites [50, 68,69] that might also play a role in Aβ amyloid toxicity [86]. Other protein kinases might play a role in the abnormal phosphorylation of tau in AD (e.g. cdk5) but GSK-3β remains a prime suspect whose deregulation seems important in AD.

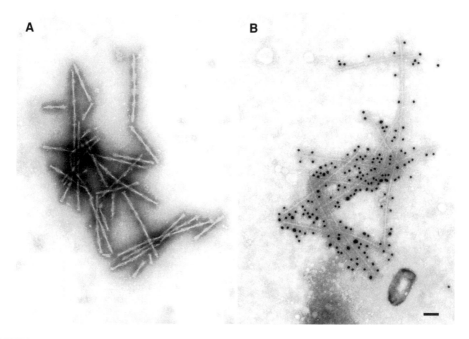

Fig. 2. Isolated PHF from an AD patient, observed in electron microscopy after simple negative staining (A) and after immunolabeling with the original anti-tau antibody to rat tau proteins, used in reference [16]. Scale bar: 100 nm.

The pathogenic role of tau phosphorylation is still a matter of debate; it has been known since early studies that tau phosphorylation modulates its binding to microtubules [67] and its ability to stabilize them. Hyperphosphorylated tau species do not bind well to microtubules and this decreased biological activity would thus be responsible for a "loss of function" in affected neurons. On the other hand, although non-phosphorylated tau proteins can forms filamentous structure in vitro, phosphorylation could favour the aggregation of tau in PHF [1]. The pathological role of PHF themselves is still not well understood: they could mechanically interfere with several cellular processes, e.g. with axoplasmic transport. Soluble or oligomeric forms of phosphorylated tau could also be toxic by themselves [33], leading to a "toxic gain of function". On the other hand, tau phosphorylation/aggregation might well contributes to a protective answer of neurons submitted to various insults; e.g. segregation of harmful proteins in the form of inclusions has been suggested to be protective in Huntington's disease [6].

7. Modelization of NFT

In vitro aggregation of tau in filamentous, PHF-like structures, has been accomplished early [72] and factors affecting this aggregation have been identified [7, 38]. Unexpectedly, several groups including us observed that simple overexpression of wild-type tau in transgenic mice was insufficient to generate NFT [18, 42]. Recent findings however suggest that endogenous murine tau might inhibit NFT formation [5]. The discovery of pathogenic tau mutations in familial forms of frontotemporal dementias [53,84] has fuelled numerous studies aimed at understanding the pathogenic role of these fibrillary lesions and their modelization in cellular and transgenic models. Overexpression of these mutated tau proteins in transgenic animals almost systematically leads to formation of NFT with many of the ultrastructural, biochemical and antigenic properties of human NFT [43]. Others and we observed that expression of some mutants tau affects microtubule assembly [25], a potential "loss of function" property that could play a role in neuronal dysfunction in these diseases.

8. NFT and Aβ amyloid: End of the story?

Independent modelization of both NFT lesions and amyloid deposits has been accomplished in transgenic models (for a review, see [43]. Unexpectedly, others and we observed that animals developing Aβ amyloid deposits did not develop NFT, including animals also expressing a human wild-type tau protein, an unexpected result in the frameship of the amyloid cascade [8]. However, Aβ seems to boost NFT formation if the latter are "forced" to develop at a "basic" level, as observed in double transgenic animals developing Aβ deposits and expressing mutant tau proteins [66]. These tau mutations have however not been identified in AD, and in a perfect model of AD lesions it would be expected that NFT will be generated from wild-type tau proteins in presence of Aβ amyloid.

Alzheimer's disease has, and will still be, a fascinating example of a relatively neglected disease to a major neurobiological research theme. To much extent, it has propelled the interest of the research community for neurodegenerative diseases and the search for the understanding and the treatment of these devastating diseases.

Acknowledgements

The author thanks the belgian F.R.S.M. for its continuous support, the International Alzheimer Research Foundation and Alzheimer Belgique.

References

[1] A.D. Alonso, T. Zaidi, M. Novak, I. Grundke-Iqbal and K. Iqbal, Hyperphosphorylation induces self-assembly of τ into tangles of paired helical filaments/straight filaments, *Proc. Natl. Acad. Sci. USA* **98** (2001), 6923–6928.

[2] A. Alzheimer, Uber eine eigenartige Erkrankung der Hirnrinde, *Allgemeine Zeitschrift fur Psychiatrie* **64** (1907), 146–148.

[3] B.H. Anderton, J. Betts, W. Blackstock, J.P. Brion, S. Chapman, J. Connell, R. Dayanandan, J.J. Gallo, G. Gibb, D.P. Hanger, M. Hutton, E. Kardalinou, K. Leroy, S. Lovestone, T. Mack, H. Reynolds and M. Van Slegtenhorst, Sites of phosphorylation in tau and factors affecting their regulation, *Neuronal Signal Transduction and Alzheimer's disease*, Portland Press, UK, 2001, 73–80.

[4] B.H. Anderton, D. Breinburg, M.J. Downes, P.J. Green, B.E. Tomlinson, J. Ulrich, J.N. Wood and J. Kahn, Monoclonal antibodies show that neurofibrillary tangles and neurofilaments share antigenic determinants, *Nature* **298** (1982), 84–86.

[5] C. Andorfer, Y. Kress, M. Espinoza, R. De Silva, K.L. Tucker, Y.A. Barde, K. Duff and P. Davies, Hyperphosphorylation and aggregation of tau in mice expressing normal human tau isoforms, *J Neurochem* **86** (2003), 582–590.

[6] M. Arrasate, S. Mitra, E.S. Schweitzer, M.R. Segal and S. Finkbeiner, Inclusion body formation reduces levels of mutant huntingtin and the risk of neuronal death, *Nature* **431** (2004), 805–810.

[7] S. Barghorn and E. Mandelkow, Toward a unified scheme for the aggregation of tau into Alzheimer paired helical filaments, *Biochemistry* **41** (2002), 14885–14896.

[8] A. Boutajangout, M. Authelet, V. Blanchard, N. Touchet, G. Tremp, L. Pradier and J.P. Brion, Cytoskeletal abnormalities in mice transgenic for human tau and familial Alzheimer's disease mutants of APP and presenilin-1, *Neurobiology of Disease* **15** (2004), 47–60.

[9] H. Braak and E. Braak, Neuropathological stageing of Alzheimer-related changes, *Acta Neuropathol. (Berl.)* **82** (1991), 239–259.

[10] J.P. Brion, A.M. Couck and J. Flament-Durand, Ultrastructural study of enriched fractions of "tangles" from human patients with senile dementia of the Alzheimer type, *Acta Neuropathol. (Berl.)* **64** (1984), 148–152.

[11] J.P. Brion, A.M. Couck, H. Passareiro and J. Flament-Durand, Neurofibrillary tangles of Alzheimer's disease: an immunohistochemical and immunoelectron study, *J. Submicrosc. Cytol.* **17** (1985), 89–96.

[12] J.P. Brion, J. Flament-Durand and P. Dustin, Microtubules and microtubule-associated proteins (MAPs) in Alzheimer's disease, *3rd International symposium on microtubules and microtubule inhibitors,* Beerse (Belgium), 1985, pp. abst: 33.

[13] J.P. Brion, J. Flament-Durand and P. Dustin, Alzheimer's disease and tau proteins, *Lancet* **ii** (1986), 1098.

[14] J.P. Brion, D.P. Hanger, M.T. Bruce, A.M. Couck, J. Flament-Durand and B.H. Anderton, Tau in Alzheimer neurofibrillary tangles: N- and C-terminal regions are differentially associated with paired helical filaments and the location of a putative abnormal phosphorylation site, *Biochem. J.* **273** (1991), 127–133.

[15] J.P. Brion, D.P. Hanger, A.M. Couck and B.H. Anderton, A68 proteins in Alzheimer's disease are composed of several tau isoforms in a phosphorylated state which affects their electrophoretic mobilities, *Biochem. J.* **279** (1991), 831–836.

[16] J.P. Brion, H. Passareiro, J. Nunez and J. Flament-Durand, Mise en évidence immunologique de la protéine tau au niveau des lésions de dégénérescence neurofibrillaire de la maladie d'Alzheimer, *Arch. Biol. (Brux)* **95** (1985), 229–235.

[17] J.P. Brion, C. Smith, A.M. Couck, J.M. Gallo and B.H. Anderton, Developmental changes in tau phosphorylation: fetal-type tau is transiently phosphorylated in a manner similar to paired helical filament-tau characteristic of Alzheimer's disease, *J. Neurochem.* **61** (1993), 2071–2080.

[18] J.P. Brion, G. Tremp and J.N. Octave, Transgenic expression of the shortest human tau affects its compartmentalization and its phosphorylation as in the pretangle stage of Alzheimer disease, *Am. J. Pathol.* **154** (1999), 255–270.

[19] J.P. Brion, P. van den Bosch de Aguilar and J. Flament-Durand, Senile dementia of the Alzheimer type: morphological and immunocytochemical study, in: *Senile dementia of Alzheimer type. Advances in Applied Neurological Sciences,* (Vol. 2), W.H. Gispen and J. Traber, eds, Springer-Verlag, Berlin, Heidelberg, 1985, pp. 164–174.

[20] L. Buée, T. Bussière, V. Buée-Scherrer, A. Delacourte, and P.R. Hof, Tau protein isoforms, phosphorylation and role in neurodegenerative disorders, *Brain Res. Rev.* **33** (2000), 95–130.

[21] R.A. Crowther and C.M. Wischik, Image reconstruction of the Alzheimer paired helical filament, *EMBO J* **4** (1985), 3661–3665.

[22] D. Dahl, D.J. Selkoe, R.T. Pero and A. Bignami, Immunostaining of neurofibrillary tangles in Alzheimer's senile dementia with a neurofilament antiserum, *J Neurosci* **2** (1982), 113–119.

[23] D.R. Davis, B.H. Anderton, J.P. Brion, H.G. Reynolds and D.P. Hanger, Oxidative stress induces dephosphorylation of

tau in rat brain primary neuronal cultures, *J. Neurochem.* **68** (1997), 1590–1597.

[24] D.R. Davis, J.-P. Brion, A.-M. Couck, J.-M. Gallo, D.P. Hanger, K. Ladhani, C. Lewis, C.C.J. Miller, T. Rupniak, C. Smith and B.H. Anderton, The phosphorylation state of the microtubule-associated protein tau as affected by glutamate, colchicine and β-amyloid in primary rat cortical neuronal cultures, *Biochem. J.* **309** (1995), 941–949.

[25] R. Dayanandan, M. Van Slegtenhorst, T.G.A. Mack, L. Ko, S.H. Yen, K. Leroy, J.P. Brion, B.H. Anderton, M. Hutton and S. Lovestone, Mutations in tau reduce its microtubule binding properties in intact cells and affect its phosphorylation, *FEBS Lett.* **446** (1999), 228–232.

[26] A. Delacourte, J.P. David, N. Sergeant, I. Buée, A. Wattez, P. Vermersch, F. Ghozali, C. Fallet-Bianco, F. Pasquier, F. Lebert, H. Petit and C. Di Menza, The biochemical pathway of neurofibrillary degeneration in aging and Alzheimer's disease, *Neurology* **52** (1999), 1158–1165.

[27] A. Delacourte and A. Defossez, Alzheimer's disease: tau proteins, the promoting factors of microtubule assembly, are major components of paired helical filaments, *J. Neurol. Sci.* **76** (1986), 173–186.

[28] P. Divry, De la nature de l'altération fibrillaire d'Alzheimer, *J. Neurol. Psychiatr.* **34** (1934), 197–201.

[29] P. Dustin, *Microtubules,* (2 ed.), Springer-Verlag, Berlin, 1984.

[30] P. Dustin and J. Flament-Durand, Disturbances of axoplasmic transport in Alzheimer's disease, in: *Axoplasmic Transport in Physiology and Pathology,* D.G. Weiss and A. Gorio, eds, Springer, Berlin, 1982, pp. 131–136.

[31] C. Duyckaerts, J.P. Brion, J.J. Hauw and J. Flament-Durand, Comparison of immunocytochemistry with a specific antibody and Bodian's protargol method. Quantitative assessment of the density of neurofibrillary tangles and senile plaques in senile dementia of the Alzheimer type, *Acta Neuropathol. (Berl.)* **73** (1987), 167–170.

[32] L.F. Eng, L.S. Forno, J.W. Bigbee and K.I. Forno, Immunocytochemcal localization of glial fibrillary acidic protein and tubulin in Alzheimer's disease brain tissue, in: *Aging of the Brain and Dementia,* (Vol. 13), L. Amaducci, A.N. Davison and P. Antuono, eds, Raven Press, New York, 1980, pp. 49–54.

[33] T. Fath, J. Eidenmüller and R. Brandt, Tau-mediated cytotoxicity in a pseudohyperphosphorylation model of Alzheimer's disease, *J. Neurosci.* **22** (2002), 9733–9741.

[34] S. Flament, A. Delacourte, B. Hémon and A. Défossez, Characterization of two pathological tau protein variants in Alzheimer brain cortices, *J. Neurol. Sci.* **92** (1989), 133–141.

[35] J. Flament-Durand and J.P. Brion, Ultrastructural and immunohistochemical study of neurofibrillary tangles in Alzheimer's disease, in: *Xth European Congress of Pathology,* (Vol. 180), E. Grundmann and Münster, eds, Gustav Fisher Pathology Research and Practice, Athens, Greece, 1985, pp. 267.

[36] J. Flament-Durand and A.M. Couck, Spongiform alterations in brain biopsies of presenile dementia, *Acta Neuropathol. (Berl.)* **46** (1979), 159–162.

[37] P. Gambetti, L. Autilio-Gambetti, G. Perry, G. Shecket, and R.G. Crane, Antibodies to neurofibrillary tangles of Alzheimer's disease raised from human and animal neurofilament fractions, *Lab. Invest.* **49** (1983), 430–435.

[38] T.C. Gamblin, R.W. Berry and L.I. Binder, Modeling Tau polymerization *in vitro*: A review and synthesis, *Biochemistry* **42** (2003), 15009–15017.

[39] M. Goedert, M.G. Spillantini, R. Jakes, D. Rutherford and R.A. Crowther, Multiple isoforms of human microtubule-associated protein tau: sequences and localization in neurofibrillary tangles of Alzheimer's disease, *Neuron* **3** (1989), 519–526.

[40] M. Goedert, C.M. Wischik, R.A. Crowther, J.E. Walker and A. Klug, Cloning and sequencing of the cDNA encoding a core protein of the paired helical filament of Alzheimer disease: identification as the microtubule-associated protein tau, *Proc. Natl. Acad. Sci. USA* **85** (1988), 4051–4055.

[41] N.K. Gonatas, W. Anderson and I. Evangelista, The contribution of altered synapses in the senile plaque: an electron microscopic study in Alzheimer's dementia, *J. Neuropathol. Exp. Neurol.* **26** (1967), 25–39.

[42] J. Götz, A. Probst, M.G. Spillantini, T. Schäfer, R. Jakes, K. Bürki and M. Goedert, Somatodendritic localization and hyperphosphorylation of tau protein in transgenic mice expressing the longest human brain tau isoform, *EMBO J.* **14** (1995), 1304–1313.

[43] J. Gotz, J.R. Streffer, D. David, A. Schild, F. Hoerndli, L. Pennanen, P. Kurosinski and F. Chen, Transgenic animal models of Alzheimer's disease and related disorders: Histopathology, behavior and therapy, *Molecular Psychiatry* **9** (2004), 664–683.

[44] I. Grundke-Iqbal, K. Iqbal, M. Quinlan, Y.C. Tung, M.S. Zaidi and H.M. Wisniewski, Microtubule-associated protein tau: a component of Alzheimer paired helical filaments, *J. Biol. Chem.* **261** (1986), 6084–6089.

[45] I. Grundke-Iqbal, K. Iqbal, Y.C. Tung, M. Quinlan, H.M. Wisniewski and L.I. Binder, Abnormal phosphorylation of the microtubule-associated protein tau in Alzheimer cytoskeletal pathology, *Proc. Natl. Acad. Sci. USA* **83** (1986), 4913–4917.

[46] I. Grundke-Iqbal, K. Iqbal, Y.C. Tung, G.P. Wang and H.M. Wisniewski, Alzheimer paired helical filaments: cross-reacting polypeptides normally present in brain, *Acta Neuropathol. (Berl.)* **66** (1985), 52–61.

[47] I. Grundke-Iqbal, K. Iqbal, Y.C. Tung and H.M. Wisniewski, Alzheimer paired helical filaments: immunochemical identification of polypeptides, *Acta Neuropathol (Berl)* **62** (1984), 259–267.

[48] I. Grundke-Iqbal, A.B. Johnson, H.M. Wisniewski, R.D. Terry and K. Iqbal, Evidence that Alzheimer neurofibrillary tangles originate from neurotubules, *Lancet* **1** (1979), 578–580.

[49] D.P. Hanger, J.P. Brion, J.M. Gallo, N.J. Cairns, P.J. Luthert and B.H. Anderton, Tau in Alzheimer's disease and Down's syndrome is insoluble and abnormally phosphorylated, *Biochem. J.* **275** (1991), 99–104.

[50] D.P. Hanger, K. Hughes, J.R. Woodgett, J.P. Brion and B.H. Anderton, Glycogen synthase kinase-3 induces Alzheimer's disease-like phosphorylation of tau: generation of paired helical filaments epitopes and neuronal localization of the kinase, *Neurosci. Lett.* **147** (1992), 58–62.

[51] B.J. Hempen and J.P. Brion, Reduction of acetylated α-tubulin immunoreactivity in neurofibrillary tangle-bearing neurones in Alzheimer's disease, *J. Neuropathol. Exp. Neurol.* **55** (1996), 964–972.

[52] A. Hirano, H.M. Dembitzer, L.T. Kurland and H.M. Zimmerman, The fine structure of some intraganglionic alterations. Neurofibrillary tangles, granulovacuolar bodies and "rod-like" structures as seen in Guam amyotrophic lateral sclerosis and Parkinsonism-dementia complex, *J. Neuropathol. Exp. Neurol.* **27** (1968), 167–182.

[53] M. Hutton, C.L. Lendon, P. Rizzu, M. Baker, S. Froelich, H. Houlden, S. Pickering-Brown, S. Chakraverty, A. Isaacs, A. Grover, J. Hackett, J. Adamson, S. Lincoln, D. Dickson, P. Davies, R.C. Petersen, M. Stevens, E. De Graaff, E. Wauters,

J. Van Baren, M. Hillebrand, M. Joosse, J.M. Kwon and P. Nowotny, Association of missense and 5'-splice-site mutations in tau with the inherited dementia FTDP-17, *Nature* **393** (1998), 702–705.

[54] Y. Ihara, C. Abraham and D. Selkoe, Antibodies to paired helical filaments in Alzheimer's disease do not recognize normal brain proteins, *Nature* **304** (1983), 727–730.

[55] Y. Ihara, N. Nukina, R. Miura and M. Ogawara, Phosphorylated tau protein is integrated into paired helical filaments in Alzheimer's disease, *J. Biochem.* **99** (1986), 1807–1810.

[56] Y. Ihara, N. Nukina, H. Sugita and Y. Toyokura, Staining of Alzheimer's neurofibrillary tangles with antiserum againt 200 K component fo neurofilament, *Proc Jpn Acad* **157** (1981), 152–156.

[57] K. Iqbal, I. Grundke-Iqbal, T. Zaidi, P.A. Merz, G.Y. Wen, S.S. Shaikh and H.M. Wisniewski, Defective brain microtubule assembly in Alzheimer's disease, *Lancet* **i** (1986), 421–426.

[58] K. Iqbal, T. Zaidi, C.H. Thompson, P.A. Merz and H.M. Wisniewski, Alzheimer paired helical filaments: bulk isolation, solubility, and protein composition, *Acta Neuropathol. (Berl.)* **62** (1984), 167–178.

[59] T. Ishii, S. Haga and S. Tokutake, Presence of neurofilament protein in Alzheimer's neurofibrillary tangles (ANT). An immunofluorescent study, *Acta Neuropathol (Berl)* **48** (1979), 105–112.

[60] M. Kidd, Paired helical filaments in electron microscopy of Alzheimer's disease, *Nature* **197** (1963), 192–193.

[61] K.S. Kosik, L.K. Duffy, M.M. Dowling, C. Abraham, A. McCluskey and D.J. Selkoe, Microtubule-associated protein 2: monoclonal antibodies demonstrate the selective incorporation of certain epitopes into Alzheimer neurofibrillary tangles, *Proc. Natl. Acad. Sci. USA* **81** (1984), 7941–7945.

[62] K.S. Kosik, C.L. Joachim and D.J. Selkoe, The microtubule-associated protein, tau, is a major antigenic component of paired helical filaments in Alzheimer's disease, *Proc. Natl. Acad. Sci. USA* **83** (1986), 4044–4048.

[63] H. Ksiezak-Reding, L.I. Binder and S.H. Yen, Alzheimer disease proteins (A68) share epitopes with tau but show distinct biochemical properties, *J. Neurosci. Res.* **25** (1990), 420–430.

[64] H. Ksiezak-Reding, D.W. Dickson, P. Davies and S.H. Yen, Recognition of tau epitopes by anti-neurofilament antibodies that bind to Alzheimer neurofibrillary tangles, *Proc. Natl. Acad. Sci. USA* **84** (1987), 3410–3414.

[65] V.M.Y. Lee, B.J. Balin, L. Otvos and J.Q. Trojanowski, A68 proteins are major subunits of Alzheimer disease paired helical filaments and derivatized forms of normal tau, *Science* **251** (1991), 675–678.

[66] J. Lewis, D.W. Dickson, W.L. Lin, L. Chisholm, A. Corral, G. Jones, S.H. Yen, N. Sahara, L. Skipper, D. Yager, C. Eckman, J. Hardy, M. Hutton and E. McGowan, Enhanced neurofibrillary degeneration in transgenic mice expressing mutant tau and APP, *Science* **293** (2001), 1487–1491.

[67] G. Lindwall and R.D. Cole, Phosphorylation affects the ability of tau protein to promote microtubule assembly, *J. Biol. Chem.* **259** (1984), 5301–5306.

[68] S. Lovestone, C.H. Reynolds, D. Latimer, D.R. Davis, B.H. Anderton, J.-M. Gallo, D. Hanger, S. Mulot, B. Marquardt, S. Stabel, J.R. Woodgett and C.C.J. Miller, Alzheimer's disease-like phosphorylation of the microtubule-associated protein tau by glycogen synthase kinase-3 in transfected mammalian cells, *Curr. Biol.* **4** (1994), 1077–1086.

[69] E.-M. Mandelkow, G. Drewes, J. Biernat, N. Gustke, J. Van Lint, J.R. Vandenheede and E. Mandelkow, Glycogen synthase kinase-3 and the Alzheimer-like state of microtubule-associated protein tau, *FEBS Lett.* **314** (1992), 315–321.

[70] A. Mareck, A. Fellous, J. Francon and J. Nunez, Changes in composition and activity of microtubule-associated proteins during brain development, *Nature* **284** (1980), 353–355.

[71] C.C.J. Miller, J.P. Brion, R. Calvert, T.K. Chin, P.A.M. Eagles, M.J. Downes, M. Haugh, J. Kahn, A. Probst, J. Ulrich and B.H. Anderton, Alzheimer paired helical filaments share epitopes with neurofilaments side arms, *EMBO J.* **5** (1986), 269–276.

[72] E. Montejo de Garcini, L. Serrano and J. Avila, Self assembly of microtubule associated protein tau into filaments resembling those found in Alzheimer disease, *Biochem Biophys Res Commun* **141** (1986), 790–796.

[73] H. Mori, J. Kondo and Y. Ihara, Ubiquitin is a component of paired helical filaments in Alzheimer's disease, *Science* **235** (1987), 1641–1644.

[74] N. Nukina and Y. Ihara, Immunocytochemical study on senile plaques in Alzheimer's disease, *Proc. Jap. Acad.* **59** (1983), 284–292.

[75] N. Nukina and Y. Ihara, One of the antigenic determinants of paired helical filaments is related to tau protein, *J. Biochem.* **99** (1986), 1541–1544.

[76] N. Nukina, K.S. Kosik and D.J. Selkoe, Recognition of Alzheimer paired helical filaments by monoclonal neurofilament antibodies is due to crossreaction with tau protein, *Proc. Natl. Acad. Sci. USA* **84** (1987), 3415–3419.

[77] M. Pérez, R. Cuadros, M.A. Smith, G. Perry and J. Avila, Phosphorylated, but not native, tau protein assembles following reaction with the lipid peroxidation product, 4-hydroxy-2-nonenal, *FEBS Lett.* **486** (2000), 270–274.

[78] G. Perry, R. Friedman, G. Shaw and V. Cahu, Ubiquitin is detected in neurofibrillary tangles and senile plaque neurites of Alzheimer disease brains, *Proc. Natl. Acad. Sci. USA* **84** (1987), 3033–3036.

[79] G. Perry, N. Rizzuto, L. Autilio-Gambetti and P. Gambetti, Paired helical filaments from Alzheimer disease patients contain cytoskeletal components, *Proc. Natl. Acad. Sci. USA* **82** (1985), 3916–3920.

[80] A. Probst, D. Langui, C. Lautenschlager, J. Ulrich, J.P. Brion and B.H. Anderton, Progressive supranuclear palsy: extensive neuropil threads in addition to neurofibrillary tangles, *Acta Neuropathol. (Berl.)* **77** (1988), 61–68.

[81] S. Richard, J.P. Brion, A.M. Couck and J. Flament-Durand, Accumulation of smooth endoplasmic reticulum in Alzheimer's disease: new morphological evidence of axoplasmic flow disturbances, *J. Submicrosc. Cytol.* **21** (1989), 461–467.

[82] G.C. Ruben, K. Iqbal, I. Grundke-Iqbal, H.M. Wisniewski, T.L. Ciardelli and J.E. Johnson, Jr., The microtubule-associated protein tau forms a triple-stranded left-hand helical polymer, *J. Biol. Chem.* **266** (1991), 22019–22027.

[83] D.J. Selkoe, Y. Ihara and F.J. Salazar, Alzheimer's disease: insolubility of partially purified paired helical filaments in sodium dodecyl sulfate and urea, *Science* **215** (1982), 1243–1245.

[84] M.G. Spillantini, J.R. Murrell, M. Goedert, M.R. Farlow, A. Klug and B. Ghetti, Mutation in the tau gene in familial multiple system tauopathy with presenile dementia, *Proc. Natl. Acad. Sci. USA* **95** (1998), 7737–7741.

[85] N.H. Sternberger, L.A. Sternberger and J. Ulrich, Aberrant neurofilament phosphorylation in Alzheimer's disease, *Proc. Natl. Acad. Sci. USA* **82** (1985), 4274–4276.

[86] A. Takashima, K. Noguchi, K. Sato, T. Hoshino and K. Imahori, tau protein kinase I is essential for amyloid β-protein-

induced neurotoxicity, *Proc. Natl. Acad. Sci. USA* **90** (1993), 7789–7793.

[87] R.D. Terry, The fine structure of neurofibrillary tangles in Alzheimer's disease, *J. Neuropathol. Exp. Neurol.* **22** (1963), 629–642.

[88] R.D. Terry, N.K. Gonatas and M. Weiss, Ultrastructural studies in Alzheimer's presenile dementia, *Am. J. Pathol.* **44** (1964), 669–697.

[89] B.E. Tomlinson, G. Blessed and M. Roth, Observations on the brains of demented old people, *J. Neurol. Sci.* **11** (1970), 205–242.

[90] C.M. Wischik, R.A. Crowther, M. Stewart and M. Roth, Subunit structure of paired helical filaments in Alzheimer's disease, *J. Cell Biol.* **100** (1985), 1905–1912.

[91] C.M. Wischik, M. Novak, H.C. Thogersen, P.C. Edwards, M.J. Runswick, R. Jakes, J.E. Walker, C. Milstein, M. Roth and A. Klug, Isolation of a fragment of tau derived from the core of the paired helical filament of Alzheimer disease, *Proc. Natl. Acad. Sci. USA* **85** (1988), 4506–4510.

[92] H.M. Wisniewski, P.A. Merz and K. Iqbal, Ultrastructure of paired helical filaments of Alzheimer's neurofibrillary tangle, *J. Neuropathol. Exp. Neurol.* **43** (1984), 643–657.

[93] H.M. Wisniewski, H.K. Narang and R.D. Terry, Neurofibrillary tangles of paired helical filaments, *J Neurol Sci* **27** (1976), 173–181.

[94] B.L. Wolozin, A. Pruchnicki, D.W. Dickson and P. Davies, A neuronal antigen in the brains of patients with Alzheimer's disease, *Science* **232** (1986), 648–650.

[95] J.G. Wood, S.S. Mirra, N.J. Pollock and L.I. Binder, Neurofibrillary tangles of Alzheimer disease share antigenic determinants with the axonal microtubule-associated protein tau, *Proc. Natl. Acad. Sci. USA* **83** (1986), 4040–4043.

[96] S.H. Yen, F. Gaskin and S.M. Fu, Neurofibrillary tangles in senile dementia of the Alzheimer type share an antigenic determinant with intermediate filaments of the vimentin class, *Am J Pathol* **113** (1983), 373–381.

[97] S.H. Yen, F. Gaskin and R.D. Terry, Immunocytochemical studies of neurofibrillary tangles, *Am J Pathol* **104** (1981), 77–89.

The natural and molecular history of Alzheimer's disease

André Delacourte
Unit Inserm 422, 1, Place de Verdun, 59045 Lille cedex, France
Tel.: +33 3 20 62 20 72; Fax: +33 3 20 62 20 79; E-mail: andre.delacourte@lille.inserm.fr

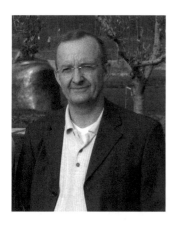

Abstract. Alzheimer's disease (AD) is a very frequent brain pathology of the elderly, with an etiology by far more complicated than thought in the nineties. In particular, the complexity comes from the coexistence of two degenerating processes, tau aggregation and Aβ deposition, that affect polymodal association brain areas, a feature never observed in non-human primates and difficult to model. Genetic studies have shown that AβPP plays a central role in familial and sporadic AD, but the role of tau has been for a long time understated. To apprehend this role, we have developed a spatio-temporal analysis of tauopathy in many brain areas of hundreds of non-demented and demented patients. This prospective and multidisciplinary study showed us that tauopathy always progresses in the brain along a very precise and invariable pathway, from the entorhinal then hippocampal formation to polymodal association areas to end in primary regions and in many subcortical areas. The cognitive impairment follows exactly the progression of the affected brain regions. In strict parallelism, neocortical Aβ deposits increase in quantity and heterogeneity, suggesting a direct link between both neurodegenerative processes. Altogether, our molecular study suggests that AD is a tauopathy fueled by AβPP dysfunction. Restoring AβPP loss of function seems to be the most efficient therapeutic approach.

1. Introduction

First of all, scientists do not forget that Alzheimer's disease (AD) is a devastating disease, not only for the patient, but also for the family. But from a scientific point of view, AD is an exciting field of research. At present, we know that this disease is more complicated than expected, with numerous risk factors. Therefore finding the right lead of research for the scientist working in the Alzheimer field is quite a challenge.

AD is a very complicated disease at the physiopathological level. This was observed by Alois Alzheimer himself who discovered this organic dementing disease with two types of lesions: tangles inside neurons and plaques outside, in the vicinity of degenerating neurons. Alois Alzheimer was probably aware of the importance of intraneuronal lesions, since he also discovered the specific lesions of the fronto-temporal dementia characterized by Arnold Pick, namely Pick bodies of Pick disease.

One century after the princeps paper of Alois Alzheimer, the question of the importance of plaques versus tangles is still a matter of debate. Which lesion is the cause, which one is a consequence, and more importantly, which one will lead to a treatment?

Second, the complexity of the approach comes from the fact that the disease is, on one hand, exclusively present in the brain but, on the other hand, that the brain is inaccessible to molecular investigations, well protected behind the blood brain barrier, then the skull and then by our cultural, social or religious rules.

Third, AD is one of the rare disease that is totally specific to human species. In very old non-human primates such as the baboon or the rhesus monkey, the presence of tangles is strictly limited to the hippocampal formation. The basic neuropathological criteria of AD, namely plaques and tangles in the association cortex, were never found in other non-human species [1, 2].

2. The "amyloid" period

After the discovery of Glenner and Wong in 1984, showing that plaques result from the aggregation of a polypeptide of 39 to 42 amino-acids, successively named A4 then $A\beta$, a number of great discoveries have shown the importance of physiological events linked to plaques [3]. First of all, the discovery by Hardy's team of mutations on the $A\beta$ protein precursor ($A\beta PP$) generated the amyloid cascade hypothesis in 1992 [4]. This theory implies that neuronal dysfunction is generated by amyloid toxicity. Other mutations of FAD located on presenilin 1 and 2 by St Georges Hyslop's team corroborated this cascade hypothesis. Indeed, presenilin cleaves $A\beta PP$ and patients with PS1 mutations release more $A\beta 42$ species [5]. Then transgenic mice with human APP and PS1 mutated genes developing numerous plaques as well as a possible cognitive impairment, corroborated the hypothesis of John Hardy [6]. Nowadays, all scientists agree that $A\beta PP$ dysfunction plays a central role in AD etiopathogenesis.

Legitimately, from the amyloid cascade hypothesis, one can conclude that AD is a simple brain disease, with a unique killer, the neurotoxic $A\beta$ peptide, and a unique and simple therapeutic target: the removal or neutralization of $A\beta$ aggregates. However, the accumulation of data on the natural history of sporadic AD, that represents more than 99% of all cases, has progressively changed our perception of AD physiopathology and revealed that neurofibrillary degeneration is the other inescapable feature that explains AD.

3. The Braak stages

Heiko Braak is a German neuropathologist that has observed both lesions, plaques and tangles, at the spatio-temporal level. Using silver staining on large tissue sections of several thousands of brains of patients at different stages of the pathology, he demonstrated that there is a progressive spreading of neurofibrillary degeneration (NFD), along a precise pathway, from the entorhinal and hippocampal formation towards polymodal association then primary brain regions [7]. Alzheimer dementia is observed when a threshold of neurofibrillary degeneration in the association cortical areas is reached, corresponding to stages IV to VI [8].

The role of tangles to explain Alzheimer dementia was so obvious that the Braak stages were incorporated in the consensus criteria for a definite diagnosis of AD in 1997 [9], in addition to the CERAD criteria based only on the number of amyloid plaques.

4. The natural and molecular history of AD

In the same way, our strategy to study AD was the following: first to study the commonest form of AD, sporadic AD; then to develop a strategy similar to Braak, but using molecular probes rather than histological observations. In our Lille Hospital network, with Prof. Pasquier, Dr Lebert, Prof. Maurage, it has been possible to develop a prospective study combining clinical, neuropathological and molecular data. Of course, this approach on sporadic diseases is a difficult one, and took us two decades to be complete. But we found it was the only way to analyze the basic physiopathological events that generate and fuel the disease.

To be as objective as possible, we studied the development of the two degenerating processes that characterize AD, tangles and plaques, using their basic components as markers, namely tau proteins and $A\beta$ peptides. Then we analyzed if these two degenerating processes were interconnected and their relationship to dementia.

5. Aggregated and hyperphosphorylated tau proteins: A powerful marker of neurofibrillary degeneration

Tau proteins are the basic component of NFD, as observed using histological and biochemical means. Aggregation of tau is easy to observe at the biochemical level, rendering very convenient the quantification of NFD. Indeed, aggregated tau proteins are not dephosphorylated by phosphatases during post-mortem delay, while normal tau proteins are dephosphorylated. Therefore, phosphorylated tau proteins of human brain homogenates detected with phospho-dependant antibodies are those that are aggregated. Using western blots, we have been able to detect and quantify abnormal tau species in AD brains, in that they are aggregated, hyperphosphorylated and abnormally phosphorylated [10], in good agreement with the results of Brion [11] and Iqbal [12]. In addition, we were able to demonstrate that tau proteins in AD are reliable markers of the degenerating process. First we were able to detect two abnormal bands in neocortical areas (Tau 64 and 68) [13], then a third one using more specific antibodies (Tau 60) [14]. These pathological Tau bands were specifically detected by an anti-PHF absorbed with normal tau proteins. The antibody Alz-50 of Peter Davies, that detects so well neurofibrillary degeneration and a group of pathological proteins named A68, was in fact immunostaining those abnormal tau proteins Tau 64 and 68 [15]. This was confirmed later on by Trojanowski's team [16]. At last, using 2D gels and our knowledge that tau proteins contain 6 isoforms [17], we demonstrated the presence of a minor and fourth abnormal tau protein at 72 kDa [18] (MW are those given in the literature these days).

Interestingly enough, using the same approach, we demonstrated that these tau aggregates were different in other neurodegenerative dementing disorders, and that there is a code-bar of tauopathies. In PSP and CBD, we observed a specific characteristic upper doublet (Tau 64 and 69), due to the aggregation of tau isoforms with 4 repeats (4R tauopathy) [19,20], while in Pick's disease, there is a lower doublet (Tau 60 and 64), resulting from the aggregation of 3R isoforms [21,22]. Other diseases have other tau profiles such as the singulet in myotonic dystrophy (DM1) [23,24], and soluble tauopathy in dementia lacking distinctive histology (DLDH) [25]. For DLDH, an heterogeneous group, it has been clearly shown by Zhukareva et al. that a subgroup has a defect in the synthesis of tau proteins [26].

All these specific biochemical signatures and different sets of tau isoforms aggregated in specific subsets of neuronal populations began to demonstrate that tangles are not this unique and late answer to different types of neuronal insults. Indeed, many demented disorders result from a defect of tau proteins [27]. Therefore, the question was to determine the natural history of tau pathology in the aging human brain that develops or not Alzheimer's disease.

6. The spatio-temporal biochemical pathway of tau pathology in aging and sporadic AD

6.1. Tau pathology spreading in cortical areas is invariable and hierarchical

A prospective and multidisciplinary study of more than 200 cases, including 70 non-demented patients was undertaken. We gathered clinical and neuropathological data, and in parallel studied the presence of neurofibrillary degeneration at the biochemical level, using the triplet of abnormal tau proteins as a marker. In Alzheimer brains, we observed that tau pathology always extends along ten stages, corresponding to ten brain areas that are successively affected. Paired helical filaments (PHF)-tau pathology was systematically found to be present in variable amounts in the entorhinal and hippocampal regions of non-demented patients aged over 75 years. When tau pathology was found in other brain areas, it was always along a stereotyped, sequential, hierarchical pathway. The progression was categorized into ten stages according to the brain regions affected: transentorhinal cortex (S1), entorhinal cortex (S2), hippocampus (S3), anterior temporal cortex (S4), inferior temporal cortex (S5), mid temporal cortex (S6), polymodal association areas (prefrontal, parietal inferior, temporal superior) (S7), unimodal areas (S8), primary motor (S9a) or sensory (S9b, S9c) areas, and all neocortical areas (S10) [28].

6.2. Lessons given by tau staging

6.2.1. Relationship with Braak staging
Together, there is a perfect agreement on the pathway of progression of the degenerating process described by Braak, ranked from stage I to VI at the histochemical level, and our staging at the biochemical level. Surprisingly, our biochemical approach was more precise than the neuropathological one, in that we observed precisely that the temporal pole was affected just after the hippocampus and prior to the inferior temporal cortex. This step is included in our staging. Also we were able to distinguish a transentorhinal stage prior to the entorhinal stage and then to the hippocampal stage, showing that the scalpel can also makes the approach very precise.

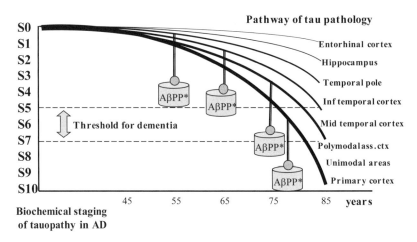

Fig. 1. Pathway of tau pathology in aging and in Alzheimer's disease.
First, neurofibrillary tangles (i.e. tau pathology) are age-related but not age-dependent brain lesions. They appear in the entorhinal cortex of 20% of people with an average age of 25 years. The ratio increases at 50% at the age of 50 years to affect all people at the age of 70 years or older, as shown by Braak et al and in our study. This vulnerability varies dramatically among individuals. A few nonagenarians of our study were very mildly affected. Therefore, the entorhinal formation is a vulnerable area always affected by tau pathology at old age (stages 1 and 2 of tau pathology).
Second, tauopathy in aging tends to spread from the affected vulnerable area to other connected neuronal population, along a neuron-to-neuron propagation that resembles a chain reaction or a domino effect. This spreading can be observed up to the temporal pole (stage 4 of tau pathology) without Aβ deposition.
Third, the extension of tauopathy toward polymodal association areas is systematically observed in the presence of Aβ x-42 deposits (amyloid stage of 1 to 4), as if these aggregates, directly (neurotoxicity) or indirectly (markers of AβPP dysfunction) were fueling tau spreading. This step represents the beginning of incipient AD.
Fourth, when neuroplasticity will be no more able to compensate the progressing neurodegenerative process, clinical impairment and dementia will appear. The cognitive impairment observed in Alzheimer's disease is well explained by the brain areas that are successively affected by tau pathology, from mild cognitive impairment (stages 3 to 6) to the different AD stages, from stage 6 to stage 10 of tau pathology. The amyloid burden will also increase, in parallel to tau staging, with an amyloid staging between 5 and 10.
Fifth, tau pathology will continue its conquest of the brain toward primary regions and subcortical areas.

6.2.2. Relationship with aging

At the present time, we have probably studied more than 500 patients comprising non-demented patients and demented patients with different neurodegenerative brain diseases, at the exception of prion diseases. First we observed that all patients aged over 75 years, controls or affected by a brain pathology, had at least a tau pathology in the entorhinal formation, and very frequently in the hippocampal formation. Since 100% of patients have a tau pathology at the age of 75 years, this means that tau pathology is an inevitable degenerating process that occurs in the human brain (Fig. 1). This vulnerability to tau pathology in the entorhinal and hippocampal formations is also present in a few non-human species such as the baboon or the rhesus monkey [1,2]. Immunohistochemistry is more sensitive than biochemistry to analyze the formation of tau pathology in some specific subsets of neuronal populations. Braak demonstrated that neurofibrillary degeneration can begin very early in the human brain. Using the same histological approach and antibodies against specific tau phosphorylated sites such as ser 199P, we observed similar findings. Together, these studies show that tauopathy is observed in 2 patients out of 10 at the second to third decade of age. At the age of 50 years, probably 1 patient out of 2 has a small but significant entorhinal tau pathology. The frequency increases with age to be constant at the age of 75 years using either histochemical of biochemical means (Fig. 1).

From these results one could speculate that entorhinal tau pathology is an age-associated process, but in fact it is more a vulnerability that is revealed during aging. Indeed, we have been able to study the brain of non-demented centenarians. A few of these patients had a very mild entorhinal tauopathy, demonstrating the absence of a direct link with aging.

6.2.3. Brain lesion burden in mild cognitive impairment (MCI)

There is no clinical method to determine if a patient with MCI has incipient AD. Some will progress to AD with dementia, or have a benign form of MCI without progression. Our prospective study led us to collect all data on the cognitive status as well as the extent of tau and Aβ pathology of patients with MCI [28,29]. We observed that all 13 MCI patients from our brain bank had a tau pathology, but not necessarily Aβ pathology. Furthermore, all patients of our prospective study with a mild tau pathology did not have MCI, probably because tau burden for these patients was compensated by neuronal plasticity. These results are in perfect agreement with those of the Mesulam group [30] showing that tau pathology is more closely related to cognitive impairment than is Aβ. However, from our knowledge of Aβ aggregation in AD (following chapters), we know that the presence of Aβ deposits in the brain of MCI patients, as well as a decrease of Aβ x-42 in the CSF [31], is the marker of incipient AD.

6.2.4. The threshold for dementia

Another interesting point of our staging of tau pathology is the clinical status of patients at stage 7, with a mild to moderate tau pathology in polymodal association areas. All of them are cognitively impaired, but at very different levels. Altogether, we observed that the patients that are fully demented at stage 7 have generally in addition a significant vascular pathology. The logical explanation is that vascular pathology has an additional deleterious effect on neuronal plasticity, that decreases the compensation effect of the not-yet affected neuronal populations, and therefore increases the cognitive deficit. These observations strengthen the idea that clinical impairment results from an imbalance between a progressing degenerating process and decreasing compensatory effects from not-yet affected neurons (Fig. 1). The best illustration comes from Parkinson disease, with extra-pyramidal signs expressed only if more than 50 to 90% of dopaminergic neurons are affected.

6.2.5. The mechanism of progression of tau pathology

The mechanism of tauopathy spreading is likely to open relevant therapeutic avenues in the neuroprotection domain. From the study of AD, we observe that this spreading is not diffuse, but on the contrary along precise neuron-to-neuron connections, from the limbic structures toward the neocortical association areas. Interestingly enough, we observe a similar mechanism of spreading in other sporadic tauopathies, such as progressive supranuclear palsy (PSP). Neurodegeneration in PSP is observed first in the brain stem, then in the striatum, to conquer after the primary motor frontal neocortical area (Broadmann area 4), then the unimodal frontal areas and at last a spreading in all neocortical and limbic areas [20]. In other words, the basic mechanism of tau spreading in sporadic tauopathies is likely starting in a specific vulnerable neuronal population (layer II of the entorhinal formation in AD; occulomotor nuclei for PSP). Then, this local tauopathy will destabilize the connected neuronal populations that had a cross-talk with the vulnerable area, and this degenerating process will extend, with a domino effect, to other neuronal populations along a neuron-to-neuron propagation phenomenon [32]. Knowing better this mechanism of propagation will certainly open therapeutic strategies for AD as well as for other sporadic tauopathies and synucleopathies.

6.3. The relationship between tauopathy and amyloidosis in aging and sporadic AD

It is not surprising that tau pathology is well correlated with cognitive impairment, since it shows the neurodegeneration process and its extent. However, we do not know the factors that generate tauopathy and its extension in brain areas. AβPP dysfunction is the best candidate, as revealed by genetic studies. Therefore, we quantified all AβPP metabolic products to see a possible relationship with the different stages of tau pathology. AβPP holoproteins, AβPP-CTFs and Aβ species were analyzed in the different brain areas of all our non-demented and demented patients. First, Aβ species were studied. Insoluble Aβ-42 and -40 species were fully solubilized and quantified after their extraction in formic acid. In order to simplify the interpretation of the results, we propose the following biochemical staging for the quantification of either Aβ 40 or Aβ x-42 aggregates [29]:

Aβ quantification (μg/g of tissue)	Stage
From trace to 2.5	1
2.5 to 5	2
5 to 10	3
10 to 25	4
25 to 50	5
50 to 100	6
100 to 200	7
200 to 400	8
400 to 800	9
Over 800	10

The quantities of both Aβ species were compared to the extent of tau pathology, as well as to cognitive impairment. Aβ x-42 aggregates were observed at the early stages of tau pathology in non-demented patients and all along AD pathology (Aβ stages 1 to 4), while Aβ x-40 aggregates are markers of the last stages of AD. During the progression of the disease, Aβ x-42 aggregates increase in quantity and heterogeneity (Aβ stages 4 to 10), in close parallelism to the extension of tau pathology. But unexpectedly, there was no spatial overlap between Aβ aggregation that is widespread and heterogeneously distributed in cortical areas and tau pathology that is progressing sequentially, stereotypically, and hierarchically. Hence, there is a synergetic effect of AβPP dysfunction on the neuron-to-neuron propagation of tau pathology. Indeed, tau pathology can be found in the hippocampal area without Aβ deposits, as mentioned by Braak [33]. In contrast, the extension of tau pathology in polymodal association areas was systematically found in the presence of Aβ deposits (Aβ stages 4 to 10), as if these Aβ species, directly or indirectly, were necessary to stimulate the progression of tau pathology (Fig. 1). Altogether, our study clearly demonstrated that amyloid deposits do not precede tau pathology in sporadic AD, as mentioned in the amyloid cascade hypothesis. Interestingly enough, our proteomic analysis of the first Aβ 42 deposits that appear in the aging human brain and in incipient AD are not full length Aβ 1–42, but N-truncated species. In other words, the first Aβ species that initiate amyloidosis are not physiological species, but pathological species. This was observed at the biochemical and immunohistochemical levels. This discovery could improve dramatically the vaccination approach [34].

7. Relationship between tau pathology and amyloid β protein precursor dysmetabolism

The parallelism and synergy between tau and Aβ aggregation led us to search an AβPP molecular event linking the two degenerating processes. AβPP is an ubiquitous protein found in all cell types of all species, suggesting a basic and important role that remains to be identified. A neurotrophic activity for AβPP and secreted sAβPP is often mentioned [35]. Therefore a loss of function of AβPP rather than a gain of toxic function of Aβ could be also a reasonable hypothesis to explain the stimulation of tau pathology and neurodegeneration (Fig. 1).

Complementary to this study of Aβ species, we found no obvious modification of AβPP holoprotein and its secreted sAβPP in correlation with the pathology. However, AβPP -CTFs were found to be significantly diminished during the course of AD and well correlated with the progression of tau pathology [36]. Beta, alpha and gamma stubs were also significantly decreased in the brain tissue of individuals having an inherited form of AD linked to mutations of presenilin 1, showing a general defect common to familial and sporadic forms of AD. An important role of gamma stub, also named AICD (AβPP intracellular domain), as a gene regulator could explain its involvement in the disease if these fragments are lacking [37].

In fact these observations directly lead to other therapeutic strategies concentrated around the concept of a loss of function of AβPP stimulating tau pathology, in good agreement with other teams mentioning that Aβ may be a planet, but AβPP is central [38–40]. From our study on tau and Aβ in the human brain, we propose the following criteria for a good anti-Alzheimer drug: the drug should 1) reduce the production of Aβ x-42 species and in parallel 2) should stimulate the production of the "good" AβPP-CTFs, namely the alpha and gamma stubs. Theoretically, this drug should be able to reduce or to stop the deleterious effect of AβPP dysfunction, and therefore to stop the burden that fuels tau pathology and provoke dementia in AD.

8. Conclusion

Altogether, many converging studies show that AD is not a pure pathology of Aβ, nor it is a pure tauopathy. We propose the following definition: AD is a tauopathy fueled by AβPP dysfunction. The natural and molecular history of sporadic AD shows that both AβPP and tau are equally involved in the etiopathogenesis (Fig. 1). Both are also therapeutic targets and the good news is that βAPists and tauoists must work together. From observations of the human brain, relevant animal models are most likely those that demonstrate a synergy between AβPP and tau lesions. Some interesting models have already been described [41,42]. Another one with a severe neuronal loss is also interesting to understand the loss of function of AβPP as well as the role of intracellular Aβ deposition [43].

At last, one can see that most dementing neurodegenerative disorders are tauopathies, that most demented patients have a tau pathology in neocortical areas and that many different types of tau dysfunction lead to dementia: mutations on tau gene in FTDP-17 (fronto temporal dementia with Parkinsonism linked to chromosome 17) [44], the haplotype H1H1 which is a risk factor for PSP and CBD [45], the abnormal tau splicing in DM1 [24], tau-less DLDH [26], and the vulnerability of specific brain areas to tauopathy as observed in the entorhinal cortex and hippocampus for AD [46], or in the brain stem nuclei for PSP and CBD.

References

[1] W. Hartig, C. Klein, K. Brauer, K.F. Schuppel, T. Arendt, G. Bruckner et al., Abnormally phosphorylated protein tau in the cortex of aged individuals of various mammalian orders, *Acta Neuropathol (Berl)* **100**(3) (2000), 305–312.

[2] C. Schultz, G.B. Hubbard, U. Rub, E. Braak and H. Braak, Age-related progression of tau pathology in brains of baboons, *Neurobiology of Aging* **21**(6) (2000), 905–912.

[3] G.G. Glenner and C.W. Wong, Alzheimer's disease and Down's syndrome: sharing of a unique cerebrovascular amyloid fibril protein, *Biochem Biophys Res Commun* **122**(3) (1984), 1131–1135.

[4] J.A. Hardy and G.A. Higgins, Alzheimer's disease: the amyloid cascade hypothesis, *Science* **256**(5054) (1992), 184–185.

[5] R. Sherrington, E.I. Rogaev, Y. Liang, E.A. Rogaeva, G. Levesque, M. Ikeda et al., Cloning of a gene bearing missense mutations in early-onset familial Alzheimer's disease, *Nature* **375**(6534) (1995), 754–760.

[6] K. Duff, C. Eckman, C. Zehr, X. Yu, C.M. Prada, J. Perez-tur et al., Increased amyloid-beta42(43) in brains of mice expressing mutant presenilin 1, *Nature* **383**(6602) (1996), 710–713.

[7] H. Braak and E. Braak, Development of Alzheimer-related neurofibrillary changes in the neocortex inversely recapitulates cortical myelogenesis, *Acta Neuropathol (Berl)* **92**(2) (1996), 197–201.

[8] H. Braak and E. Braak, Neuropathological stageing of Alzheimer-related changes, *Acta Neuropathol* **82**(4) (1991), 239–259.

[9] B.T. Hyman and J.Q. Trojanowski, Consensus recommendations for the postmortem diagnosis of Alzheimer disease from the National Institute on Aging and the Reagan Institute Working Group on diagnostic criteria for the neuropathological assessment of Alzheimer disease, *J Neuropathol Exp Neurol* **56**(10) (1997), 1095–1097.

[10] A. Delacourte and A. Defossez, Alzheimer's disease: Tau proteins, the promoting factors of microtubule assembly, are major components of paired helical filaments, *J Neurol Sci* **76**(2–3) (1986), 173–186.

[11] J.P. Brion, A.M. Couck, E. Passareiro and J. Flament-Durand, Neurofibrillary tangles of Alzheimer's disease: an immunohistochemical study, *J Submicrosc Cytol* **17**(1) (1985), 89–96.

[12] I. Grundke-Iqbal, K. Iqbal, Y.C. Tung, M. Quinlan, H.M. Wisniewski and L.I. Binder, Abnormal phosphorylation of the microtubule-associated protein tau (tau) in Alzheimer cytoskeletal pathology, *Proc Natl Acad Sci USA* **83**(13) (1986), 4913–4917.

[13] S. Flament, A. Delacourte, B. Hemon and A. Defossez, Characterization of two pathological tau protein variants in Alzheimer brain cortices, *J Neurol Sci* **92**(2–3) (1989), 133–141.

[14] A. Delacourte, S. Flament, E.M. Dibe, P. Hublau, B. Sablonniere, B. Hemon et al., Pathological proteins Tau 64 and 69 are specifically expressed in the somatodendritic domain of the degenerating cortical neurons during Alzheimer's disease. Demonstration with a panel of antibodies against Tau proteins, *Acta Neuropathol* **80**(2) (1990), 111–117.

[15] S. Flament and A. Delacourte, Tau marker? *Nature* **346**(6279) (1990), 22.

[16] J.H. Lee, B.J. Balin, L. Otvos and J.Q. Trojanowski, A68: a major subunit of paired helical filaments and derivatized forms of normal Tau, *Science* (1991).

[17] M. Goedert, M.G. Spillantini, N.J. Cairns and R.A. Crowther, Tau proteins of Alzheimer paired helical filaments: abnormal phosphorylation of all six brain isoforms, *Neuron* **8**(1) (1992), 159–168.

[18] N. Sergeant, J.P. David, M. Goedert, R. Jakes, P. Vermersch, L. Buee et al., Two-dimensional characterization of paired helical filament-tau from Alzheimer's disease: demonstration of an additional 74-kDa component and age-related biochemical modifications, *J Neurochem* **69**(2) (1997), 834–844.

[19] S. Flament, A. Delacourte, M. Verny, J.J. Hauw and F. Javoy-Agid, Abnormal Tau proteins in progressive supranuclear palsy. Similarities and differences with the neurofibrillary degeneration of the Alzheimer type, *Acta Neuropathol* **81**(6) (1991), 591–596.

[20] N. Sergeant, A. Wattez and A. Delacourte, Neurofibrillary degeneration in progressive supranuclear palsy and corticobasal degeneration: tau pathologies with exclusively "exon 10" isoforms, *J Neurochem* **72**(3) (1999), 1243–1249.

[21] A. Delacourte, Y. Robitaille, N. Sergeant, L. Buee, P.R. Hof, A. Wattez et al., Specific pathological Tau protein variants characterize Pick's disease, *J Neuropathol Exp Neurol* **55**(2) (1996), 159–168.

[22] A. Delacourte, N. Sergeant, A. Wattez, D. Gauvreau and Y. Robitaille, Vulnerable neuronal subsets in Alzheimer's and Pick's disease are distinguished by their tau isoform distribution and phosphorylation, *Ann Neurol* **43**(2) (1998), 193–204.

[23] P. Vermersch, N. Sergeant, M.M. Ruchoux, H. Hofmann-Radvanyi, A. Wattez, H. Petit et al., Specific tau variants in the brains of patients with myotonic dystrophy, *Neurology* **47**(3) (1996), 711–717.

[24] N. Sergeant, B. Sablonniere, S. Schraen-Maschke, A. Ghestem, C.A. Maurage, A. Wattez et al., Dysregulation of human brain microtubule-associated tau mRNA maturation in myotonic dystrophy type 1, *Hum Mol Genet* **10**(19) (2001), 2143–2155.

[25] P. Vermersch, R. Bordet, F. Ledoze, M.M. Ruchoux, F. Chapon, P. Thomas et al., Demonstration of a specific profile of pathological Tau proteins in frontotemporal dementia cases, *C R Acad Sci III* **318**(4) (1995), 439–445.

[26] V. Zhukareva, V. Vogelsberg-Ragaglia, V.M. Van Deerlin, J. Bruce, T. Shuck, M. Grossman et al., Loss of brain tau defines novel sporadic and familial tauopathies with frontotemporal dementia, *Ann Neurol* **49**(2) (2001), 165–175.

[27] M. Goedert and M.G. Spillantini, Tau mutations in frontotemporal dementia FTDP-17 and their relevance for Alzheimer's disease, *Biochim Biophys Acta* **1502**(1) (2000), 110–121.

[28] A. Delacourte, J.P. David, N. Sergeant, L. Buee, A. Wattez, P. Vermersch et al., The biochemical pathway of neurofibrillary degeneration in aging and Alzheimer's disease, *Neurology* **52** (1999), 1158–1165.

[29] A. Delacourte, N. Sergeant, D. Champain, A. Wattez, C.A. Maurage, F. Lebert et al., Nonoverlapping but synergetic tau and APP pathologies in sporadic Alzheimer's disease, *Neurology* **59**(3) (2002), 398–407.

[30] A.L. Guillozet, S. Weintraub, D.C. Mash and M.M. Mesulam, Neurofibrillary tangles, amyloid, and memory in aging and mild cognitive impairment, *Arch Neurol* **60**(5) (2003), 729–736.

[31] K. Blennow, CSF biomarkers for mild cognitive impairment, *J Intern Med* **256**(3) (2004), 224–234.

[32] A. Delacourte, The biochemical pathway of neurofibrillary degeneration in aging and Alzheimer's disease, *Neurology* **54** (2000), 538.

[33] H. Braak and E. Braak, Frequency of stages of Alzheimer-related lesions in different age categories, *Neurobiol Aging* **18**(4) (1997), 351–357.

[34] N. Sergeant, S. Bombois, A. Ghestem, H. Drobecq, V. Kostanjevecki, C. Missiaen et al., Truncated beta-amyloid peptide species in pre-clinical Alzheimer's disease as new targets for the vaccination approach, *J Neurochem* **85** (2003), 1581–1591.

[35] P.R. Turner, K. O'Connor, W.P. Tate and W.C. Abraham, Roles of amyloid precursor protein and its fragments in regulating neural activity, plasticity and memory, *Prog Neurobiol* **70**(1) (2003), 1–32.

[36] N. Sergeant, J.P. David, D. Champain, A. Ghestem, A. Wattez and A. Delacourte, Progressive decrease of amyloid precursor protein carboxy terminal fragments (APP-CTFs), associated with tau pathology stages, in Alzheimer's disease, *J Neurochem* **81**(4) (2002), 663–672.

[37] X. Cao and T.C. Sudhof, Dissection of amyloid-beta precursor protein-dependent transcriptional transactivation, *J Biol Chem* **279**(23) (2004), 24601–24611.

[38] R.L. Neve and N.K. Robakis, Alzheimer's disease: a re-examination of the amyloid hypothesis, *Trends Neurosci* **21**(1) (1998), 15–19.

[39] R.L. Neve, A beta may be a planet, but APP is central, *Neurobiology of Aging* **22**(1) (2001), 151–154.

[40] H.G. Lee, G. Casadesus, X. Zhu, A. Takeda, G. Perry and M.A. Smith, Challenging the amyloid cascade hypothesis: senile plaques and amyloid-beta as protective adaptations to Alzheimer disease, *Ann N Y Acad Sci* **1019** (2004), 1–4.

[41] J. Gotz, F. Chen, J. van Dorpe and R.M. Nitsch, Formation of neurofibrillary tangles in P301l tau transgenic mice induced by Abeta 42 fibrils, *Science* **293**(5534) (2001), 1491–1495.

[42] J. Lewis, D.W. Dickson, W.L. Lin, L. Chisholm, A. Corral, G. Jones et al., Enhanced neurofibrillary degeneration in transgenic mice expressing mutant tau and APP, *Science* **293**(5534) (2001), 1487–1491.

[43] C. Casas, N. Sergeant, J.M. Itier, V. Blanchard, O. Wirths, N. van der Kolk et al., Massive CA1/2 neuronal loss with intraneuronal and N-terminal truncated Abeta42 accumulation in a novel Alzheimer transgenic model, *Am J Pathol* **165**(4) (2004), 1289–1300.

[44] M.G. Spillantini, J.R. Murrell, M. Goedert, M.R. Farlow, A. Klug and B. Ghetti, Mutation in the tau gene in familial multiple system tauopathy with presenile dementia, *Proc Natl Acad Sci USA* **95**(13) (1998), 7737–7741.

[45] M. Baker, I. Litvan, H. Houlden, J. Adamson, D. Dickson, J. Perez-Tur et al., Association of an extended haplotype in the tau gene with progressive supranuclear palsy, *Hum Mol Genet* **8**(4) (1999), 711–715.

[46] A. Delacourte, N. Sergeant, A. Wattez, C.A. Maurage, F. Lebert, F. Pasquier et al., Tau aggregation in the hippocampal formation: an ageing or a pathological process? *Exp Gerontol* **37**(10–11) (2002), 1291–1296.

Tau protein, the paired helical filament and Alzheimer's disease

Michel Goedert*, Aaron Klug and R. Anthony Crowther
MRC Laboratory of Molecular Biology, Hills Road, Cambridge CB2 2QH, UK

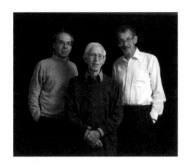

Abstract. In 1906, Alzheimer described the clinical and neuropathological characteristics of the disease that was subsequently named after him. Although the paired helical filament was identified as the major component of the neurofibrillary pathology of Alzheimer's disease in 1963, its molecular composition was only uncovered in the 1980s. In 1988, work at the MRC Laboratory of Molecular Biology in Cambridge (UK) provided direct proof that tau protein is an integral component of the paired helical filament. The paper highlighted here [Goedert M., Wischik C.M., Crowther R.A., Walker J.E. and Klug A. (1988) Cloning and sequencing of a core protein of the paired helical filament of Alzheimer disease: Identification as the microtubule-associated protein tau. Proc. Natl. Acad. Sci. USA 85, 4051–4055] also reported the first sequence of a human tau isoform and paved the way for the identification of the six brain tau isoforms that are expressed by alternative mRNA splicing from a single gene. By the early 1990s, it was clear that tau protein is the major component of the paired helical filament and that the latter is made of all six tau isoforms, each full-length and hyperphosphorylated.

Keywords: Alzheimer disease, neurofibrillary tangles, paired helical filament, tau

1. The tangle discovery

On 3 November 1906, Alois Alzheimer, then head of the Anatomical Laboratory at the Royal Psychiatric Clinic of the Ludwig-Maximilians University in Munich, presented a paper at the 37th meeting of the Society of Southwest German Psychiatrists in Tübingen. In it he described for the first time the clinical and neuropathological characteristics of the form of dementia that was later named after him, following a suggestion by Emil Kraepelin, Director of the Royal Psychiatric Clinic. The work in question was published in the short paper of 1907 and in the more extensive article of 1911.

The paper of 1907 [1] gave the clinicopathological description of the case of Auguste D., who presented with clinical symptoms at age 51 and died aged 56. In her cerebral cortex, Alzheimer saw abundant neurofibrillary tangles and neuritic plaques by Bielschowsky silver staining (the original clinical file and histological preparations were recently recovered [45,75] (Fig. 1). Alzheimer described neurofibrillary tangles (he called them "sehr merkwürdige Veränderungen der Neurofibrillen", or "very odd changes of the neurofibrils") for the first time [1]. He later referred to the tangle as "eigentümliche Fibrillenveränderung der Ganglienzellen", or "peculiar fibrillary change of nerve cells" [2]. Plaques were first described in 1892 by Blocq and Marinesco in the brain of an elderly patient affected by epilepsy [7]. In 1898, Redlich described them as "*miliare Sklerose*", or "miliary sclerosis", in two cases of senile dementia [92]. This was followed by Fischer's 1907 description of plaques in 12 out of 16 cases of senile dementia and their absence in controls and in cases

*Corresponding author. Tel.: +1 44 1223 402036; Fax: +1 44 1223 402197; E-mail: mg@mrc-lmb.cam.ac.uk.

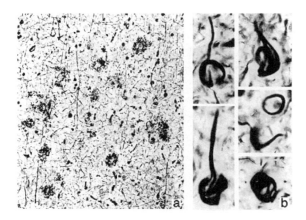

Fig. 1. Sections from the cerebral cortex of Auguste D. stained using Bielschowsky silver (from Alzheimer's original collection). (a), Numerous neurofibrillary tangles and neuritic plaques are in evidence. (b), Examples of neurofibrillary tangles. Reprinted from Graeber et al., Neurogenetics 1, 223–228 (1998), with permission from Springer.

of progressive paralysis and functional psychosis [28]. He concluded that they are a specific feature of senile dementia. Like plaques, the clinical characteristics of dementia had been described before Alzheimer, most notably by Esquirol in 1838 [27].

However, the combination of clinical dementia with its histological counterpart of plaques and tangles and extensive nerve cell loss in cerebral cortex had not been described before and was suggestive of a new clinical syndrome. By the time the 1911 article was published, several additional cases of what appeared to be the same disease had been identified by Alzheimer, Benvoglio and Perusini. Kraepelin described the condition as presenile dementia in the 8th edition of his textbook of Psychiatry, which was published in 1910, and proposed that it be called "Alzheimer's disease" [63]. He created the distinction between presenile and senile dementia as distinct diseases, which was overturned only much later, when it became clear that the two types of dementia were similar, both clinically and neuropathologically [6].

The article of 1911 [2] was devoted mostly to the nosology of Alzheimer's disease. It contains a prescient discussion of the possible relationships between plaques and tangles and their relevance for the disease process. Towards the end, Alzheimer compares cases with plaques and tangles with two cases of circumscribed lobar atrophy that he had recently examined. Similar cases of what is now called "frontotemporal dementia" had been described clinically by Arnold Pick in 1892 [89]. Alzheimer reported on the absence of plaques and the presence of the "eigentümliche Fibrillenveränderung der Ganglienzellen" in the cases with lobar atrophy. The fibrillary changes had a characteristic round shape (he called them "Kugeln", or "balls"), which distinguished them from the tangles of Alzheimer's disease. They are now called Pick bodies and the clinicopathological entity Pick's disease. Over the past twenty years, it has become clear that the fibrillary deposits of Alzheimer's disease and Pick's disease are made of the same protein. In many respects, Alzheimer's 1911 article set the scene for much of what was to come, some of which is described below.

2. The paired helical filament

In the 1960s electron microscopy of tissue sections was used to investigate the fine structure of neurofibrillary tangles in Alzheimer's disease brain. Bundles of abnormal cytoplasmic filaments were observed for the first time in nerve cell bodies and their processes [57, 58,102,103]. In 1963, Michael Kidd described the characteristic paired helical nature of the vast majority of filaments [57] (Fig. 2A). He named the "paired helical filament (PHF)", because it appears to consist of two filaments wound helically around one another, with a longitudinal spacing between crossovers of about 80 nm and a width of 30 nm at the widest point and 15 nm at the narrowest. There was discussion about the molecular nature of the PHF, with some arguing that it is made of neurofilaments [102,103], and Kidd himself favouring the view that it is unrelated to the normal cytoskeleton [57,58]. Also found in the neurofibrillary tangles of Alzheimer's disease, as a minority species, is the so-called straight filament (SF), a filament about 15 nm wide that does not exhibit the modulation in width shown by the PHF (Fig. 2A). It was first described by Hirano and collaborators in 1968 [52]. It took another 20 years before the biochemical identity of the Alzheimer filaments became known.

3. Molecular composition of the paired helical filament

The molecular composition of the PHF was elucidated in the 1980s. Immunological studies identified several candidate proteins, such as neurofilaments [76], vimentin [114], microtubule-associated protein 2 [61, 83], microtubule-associated protein tau [12,20,47,62, 85,113], amyloid-β [74] and ubiquitin [77,87]. Such studies suggested that these molecules may share epi-

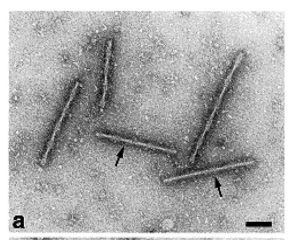

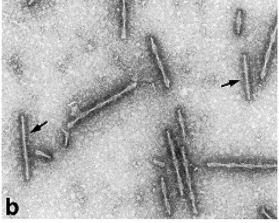

Fig. 2. Electron micrographs of dispersed filament preparations from brains of (a) a sporadic Alzheimer's disease case and (b) a case of frontotemporal dementia and parkinsonism linked to chromosome 17 (FTDP-17) with the V337M mutation in the tau gene. The PHFs in each disease appear to have an identical morphology and in each there is a minority of straight filaments (indicated by arrows). Scale bar, 100 nm. Reprinted from Spillantini et al., Acta Neuropathologica 92, 42–48 (1996), with permission from Springer.

topes with the PHF. However, they suffered from the inherent inability to distinguish between molecules that form an integral part of the PHF and material that is merely associated with or adheres to the filamentous structures. This difficulty was compounded by the fact that different proteins (e.g., neurofilaments and microtubule-associated proteins) possess epitopes in common [64,84]. Furthermore, the insolubility of the filamentous material precluded quantitative biochemical purification.

Martin Roth, the Professor of Psychiatry at the University of Cambridge, had brought the tangle problem to Aaron Klug, then the Joint Head of the Structural Studies Division at the MRC Laboratory of Molecular Biology (LMB), who involved Tony Crowther, a member of the Scientific Staff of that Division. Claude Wischik moved from the Department of Psychiatry to the Division of Structural Studies, in order to isolate tangles from Alzheimer brains. Crowther and Wischik studied the morphology and structural organization of the PHF by electron microscopy and image processing [16,109].

Subsequently, the following approach was developed by the Cambridge group in order to determine unambiguously the molecular composition of the PHF. The PHF is inert and defined only by its ultrastructural appearance, but electron microscopy alone is unsuitable for identification of an intrinsic chemical constituent of the PHF. What was required was a label that identifies both intact individual filaments in microscopy and at the same time the protein bands obtained by gel electrophoresis from successively purified tangle preparations. The protein bands could then be sequenced and this information used for the isolation of cDNA clones encoding the protein sequence. This approach established that tau protein is an integral component of the PHF [34,110,111].

Wischik used proteases to break down the insoluble tangles. In order to obtain a label for following the purification of PHF constituents, Cesar Milstein, the Joint Head of the Division of Protein and Nucleic Acid Chemistry at the LMB, Michal Novak from that Division and Wischik produced monoclonal antibodies, one of which (called 6–423) decorated individual proteolysed PHFs isolated from tangle fragments in electron microscopy and labeled a 12 kDa protein band extracted from purified PHF preparations. A chemical label was also used in the early stages to help identifying tangles in the brain extracts. John Walker and Michael Runswick, then in the Division of Protein and Nucleic Acid Chemistry, determined the partial amino acid sequence of the 12 kDa band, which made it possible to isolate cDNA clones encoding the PHF protein.

Michel Goedert, then in the Director's Section of the LMB, was enlisted into the project. He designed two mixed synthetic oligonucleotides corresponding to the amino acid sequence QIVYKP found in the 12 kDa band and used them to screen a cDNA library that he had made from the frontal cortex of an Alzheimer's disease patient. Screening of 650,000 clones yielded one positive. A hybridization-positive 160 bp fragment from the insert of this clone was found to encode the sequence QIVYKP, when it was subjected to DNA sequencing by Goedert and Crowther. This fragment was then used to screen a second cDNA library (made from the brain of a 15 week-old human fetus).

Screening of 50,000 clones gave 34 positives. Two of these (with inserts of 2.8 and 2.9 kb) were sequenced and found to encode a predicted protein of 352 amino acids, which was unrelated to any sequence known at the time. The most striking feature of this sequence was a stretch of three repeats, 31 or 32 amino acids each, in the carboxy-terminal half, with each repeat displaying a distinctive PGGG motif. The QIVYKP sequence was found in the first of these repeats. By RNA blotting using the 160 bp fragment as the probe, a major 6 kb and a minor 2 kb band were observed in a number of brain regions, but not in heart, kidney or adrenal gland. This pattern of bands was recognized by Goedert as being similar to that described by David Drubin and Marc Kirschner for mouse tau [25]. The same blot was therefore rehybridized with the insert from mouse tau clone pTA2, which Goedert had obtained from Kirschner. The patterns of hybridization and tissue distribution were identical to those obtained with the 160 bp fragment, strongly suggesting that we had cloned the cDNA for human tau. The identification was confirmed with the publication in early 1988 of the predicted amino acid sequence of a mouse tau isoform with three repeats by Lee, Cowan and Kirschner [66], part of which Kirschner had kindly communicated to Klug in late 1987. Although there had been several studies reporting the presence of tau-like immunoreactivity in neurofibrillary tangles or PHFs, the first by Jean-Pierre Brion and colleagues [12], our work provided direct proof that tau protein is present in the PHF.

Klug, Goedert and Wischik presented these findings at the Banbury conference organized by Caleb Finch and Peter Davies at Cold Spring Harbor in April 1988. The paper highlighted here [34], which was published in June 1988, was the first in a series of three by the Cambridge group. The second paper [110] described the purification of protein fragments monitored by antibody 6–423. The third paper [111] justified the use of antibody 6–423 in the biochemical work by immunoelectron microscopy of filament cores that had been stripped of some of the surface material but remained morphologically intact. In November 1988, Yasuo Ihara and collaborators also reported on the presence of the carboxy-terminal third of tau protein in the PHF [60].

4. Six isoforms of tau in adult human brain

In the 1988 paper [34], we mentioned that we had identified a second form of tau, with sequence variation in the first repeat, and suggested that tau mRNA was undergoing alternative splicing. Southern blotting had shown that there was only one tau gene in the human genome [82]. The second form of tau was identified upon the sequencing of clones isolated from a cDNA library prepared from frontal cortex of an adult control individual [35]. It was identical in sequence to the first form of tau, with the exception of an additional inserted stretch of 31 amino acids. This extra sequence encoded an additional repeat of the type present in the previously reported human tau sequence [34]. It was inserted within the first repeat in a way that preserved the periodic pattern. Upon sequencing of genomic clones, the extra repeat was found to be encoded by a separate exon (now known as exon 10), flanked by consensus splice acceptor and donor sequences. Probes derived from cDNA clones encoding the three repeat (type I) and four repeat (type II) tau protein isoforms detected mRNAs for both forms in all adult human brain areas examined. However, in foetal brain, only type I mRNA was found. Type I and type II mRNAs were present in pyramidal cells in hippocampus and cerebral cortex, with hippocampal granule cells expressing only type I mRNA. This work, which was published in early 1989 [35], uncovered the existence of at least two types of tau isoforms in human brain, those with three repeats and those with four repeats. The protein sequencing [110] had indicated the presence of two distinct sequences in the core of the PHF and the present work established that they corresponded to three and four repeats of tau.

Sequencing of a large number of cDNA clones revealed the existence of additional tau isoforms with inserts of 29 and 58 amino acids, in combination with both three and four tandem repeats [36]. With the isoforms described previously, this gave a total of six human brain tau isoforms ranging from 352 to 441 amino acids in length (Fig. 3). Transcripts encoding the 29 and 58 amino acid inserts were found in adult, but not foetal brain, as we had found previously for transcripts encoding tau isoforms with three repeats. We raised anti-peptide antibodies spanning the tau sequence and found that they all stained the neurofibrillary pathology of Alzheimer's disease in a similar way, demonstrating the presence of multiple isoforms. These findings, which were published towards the end of 1989 [36], established the existence of at least six tau isoforms in human brain. They provided a molecular underpinning to the long-known heterogeneity of tau protein [13].

This work left open the question as to whether we had identified the full complement of tau isoforms ex-

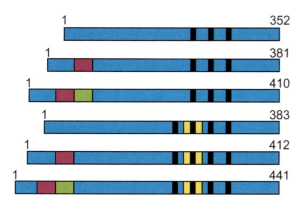

Fig. 3. Schematic representation of the six tau isoforms expressed in adult human brain. The regions common to all isoforms are shown in blue, with the N-terminal inserts in red and green, respectively. The alternatively spliced exon 10 in the repeat region is shown in yellow and the microtubule-binding repeats are indicated by black bars.

pressed in human brain. To investigate this directly, we expressed all six isoforms individually in *E. coli* from full-length cDNA clones and compared the running pattern of the purified proteins on SDS-PAGE with that of dephosphorylated tau from foetal and adult human brain. Native tau was dephosphorylated with alkaline phosphatase, because phosphorylation was a known post-translational modification of tau that could lead to a change in its mobility [71].

By SDS-PAGE, the recombinant tau isoforms gave a set of six characteristically spaced bands, ranging from 48–67 kDa in apparent molecular mass (Fig. 4). The pattern consisted of a triplet of bands corresponding to isoforms with three repeats and an equivalent but displaced triplet of bands corresponding to isoforms with four repeats. The recombinant isoforms were biologically active, as assessed by their ability to promote microtubule assembly. The rates of assembly were 2.5–3.0 times faster for isoforms containing four repeats when compared with three repeat-containing isoforms, with no significant contribution by the amino-terminal inserts. These findings were in keeping with experiments using tau fragments synthesized *in vitro* and synthetic peptides, which had shown that the tau repeats constitute microtubule binding units [26,67].

In adult cerebral cortex, following alkaline phosphatase treatment, four major tau bands and two minor bands were observed, which aligned with the six recombinant isoforms. This showed that we had identified all the brain tau isoforms by cDNA cloning. The four major bands aligned with the three- and four-repeat containing isoforms without amino-terminal inserts and the three- and four-repeat containing isoforms with the 29 amino acid amino-terminal insert. The two minor

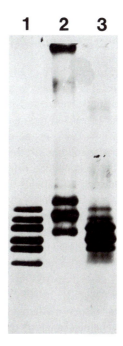

Fig. 4. Immunoblot of PHF tau before and after dephosphorylation compared with recombinant tau isoforms. Lane 1 represents the six recombinant human brain tau isoforms, lane 2 represents PHF tau before dephosphorylation and lane 3 represents PHF tau after dephosphorylation with E. coli alkaline phosphatase at high temperature. Antiserum 133, which recognizes the N-terminus of tau, was used for immunoblotting. Note the presence of three strong (of 60, 64 and 68 kDa) and one weak (of 72 kDa) PHF tau bands (lane 2). Note also the alignment of PHF tau bands after dephosphorylation (lane 3) with the recombinant isoforms (lane 1). Reprinted from Goedert et al., Neuron 8, 159–168 (1992), with permission from Elsevier.

bands aligned with three- and four-repeat containing isoforms with the 58 amino acid amino-terminal insert. In foetal brain, following alkaline phosphatase treatment, a 48 kDa band was present that aligned with the shortest recombinant tau isoform. A second, broader band of 50 kDa was also observed, probably because of incomplete dephosphorylation. These findings, which were published at the end of 1990 [37], showed that the three repeat-containing isoform with no inserts is the major foetal form of human tau and that isoforms with three and four repeats, with and without amino-terminal inserts, are expressed in adult brain. They also showed that similar levels of three-repeat and four-repeat containing tau isoforms are expressed in normal adult human brain. Two years later, we and others reported the amino acid sequence of "big tau", an isoform with a large alternatively spliced insert in the amino-terminal region of the longest isoform from brain [15,39]. Big tau is expressed in the peripheral nervous system, but not in brain or spinal cord.

5. Dispersed filaments are made of full-length, hyperphosphorylated tau protein

The insolubility of the bulk of PHFs and SFs from tangle fractions had been a major impediment towards their biochemical purification and molecular characterization. It also precluded the quantitative analysis of tau pathology. In 1990, in the development of a preparation method involving sarkosyl extraction [94], Greenberg and Davies obtained a fraction consisting of dispersed filaments, the tangles themselves having been removed in the first step of centrifugation [46]. By immunoblotting, three major tau bands of 60, 64 and 68 kDa apparent molecular mass were observed (a minor fourth band of 72 kDa was described later [80]). It was realized that these bands were probably the same as the previously described A68 and SDS-soluble abnormal tau bands [29,112]. In 1991, Virginia Lee and colleagues purified dispersed filaments to homogeneity and used protein chemical analysis to demonstrate that they were made of tau protein [68]. Crowther showed that PHFs and SFs represent different assemblies of an identical or closely related structural subunit [17]. This work established that tau is the major component of the PHF and SF and removed any lingering doubt about potential additional components that remained to be discovered.

Lee and colleagues also showed that tau protein from their purified filament preparations was hyperphosphorylated. Earlier studies by Inge Grundke-Iqbal and colleagues and by Ihara and collaborators had already suggested that tau protein is hyperphosphorylated in Alzheimer's disease brain [48,54]. In 1992, we showed that after extensive dephosphorylation the PHF tau bands aligned with the six recombinant brain tau isoforms, indicating that PHF tau consists of all six tau isoforms in an abnormally hyperphosphorylated state [38] (Fig. 4). The relative amounts of the different isoforms recovered were similar to those observed in normal human brain.

Dispersed filaments were strongly decorated by antibodies directed against the N- and C-terminal regions of tau, but not by an antibody specific for the repeat region (the latter antibody labelled PHF tau bands by immunoblotting, indicating that its epitope was not accessible in the core of the filament) (Fig. 5). Together with the earlier work [34,110,111] these findings demonstrated that full-length tau assembles through its microtubule-binding repeats, with the N- and C-terminal regions extending from the filament surface, forming the fuzzy coat (first described in [111]) around the filament. Treatment of filaments with pronase was found to remove the fuzzy coat, leaving a pronase-resistant core, which retains the characteristic appearance of the starting filament (Fig. 5). Filaments in extracellular tangles, the remnants of neurofibrillary deposits left after a tangle-containing cell has died, show a similar partial proteolysis of the constituent tau protein [8]. Similar to truncation, the ubiquitination of tau was also found to be a secondary event that occurs after filament assembly [78]. More recently, we showed that PHFs and SFs have a cross-β structure, which is the defining feature of amyloid fibres [5]. There had been some controversy in the literature with regard to the internal molecular fine structure of the filaments.

From the above work, hyperphosphorylation of tau emerged as a potential trigger of filament formation. PHF tau was found to have a greatly reduced ability to bind to microtubules and this functional impairment was shown to result from hyperphosphorylation [11, 115]. This finding was in line with earlier work, which had reported that phosphorylation negatively affects the ability of tau to interact with microtubules [70]. During the 1990s, many phosphorylation sites in tau were identified through mass spectrometry and the use of phosphorylation-dependent antibodies [42,50,79]. The latter provided sensitive and specific markers of tau pathology [96] (Fig. 6a,c,e). The vast majority of phosphorylation sites was located outside the repeat region and many sites were found to be Ser/Thr-Pro sequences. Most phosphorylation-dependent antibodies did not label normal adult brain tau, or recognized it only weakly. By contrast, the same antibodies strongly labelled fetal tau, the PHF-tau bands and isolated tau filaments [41,56]. This indicated that in Alzheimer's disease brain the six adult brain tau isoforms are abnormally phosphorylated in a way similar to the normal phosphorylation of the single fetal tau isoform. Candidate protein kinases for the hyperphosphorylation of tau were identified. They included mitogen-activated protein (MAP) kinase [23], glycogen synthase kinase-3 (GSK3) [49,73], cyclin-dependent kinase 5 (CDK5) [59], microtubule affinity regulating kinase (MARK) [24] and stress-activated protein (SAP) kinases [44]. Protein phosphatase 2A was identified as the major brain tau phosphatase [40].

6. Synthetic tau filaments

Hyperphosphorylation is believed to be an early event in the pathway that leads from soluble to insol-

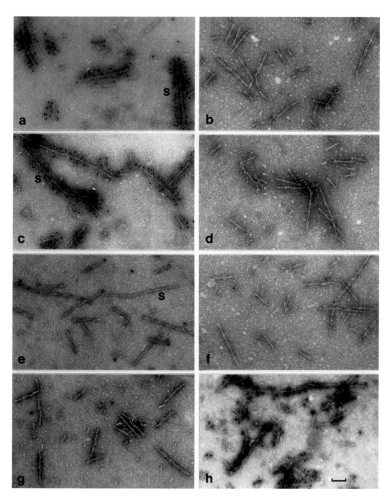

Fig. 5. Immunoelectron microscopy of dispersed paired helical filament preparations, showing the presence of full-length tau and that the N- and C-termini are cleaved by mild pronase treatment. (a), (c), (e) and (g) represent native material; in (b), (d), (f) and (h) the grids were treated with pronase prior to immunodecoration. The antibodies used were as follows: 133, which recognizes the N-terminus of tau (a and b); 134, which recognizes the C-terminus of tau; 135, which recognizes the microtubule-binding repeat region of tau (e and f); 6–423, which recognizes tau truncated at residue 391 (g and h). Some straight filaments are indicated (S). Note immunodecoration of some but not all filaments with antiserum 133 in (a), of almost all filaments with antiserum 134 in (c), and of almost all filaments with antibody 6–423 in (h). Antiserum 135 failed to decorate filaments (e and f). Scale bar, 100 nm. Reprinted from Goedert et al., Neuron 8, 159–168 (1992), with permission from Elsevier.

uble and filamentous tau protein. However, it remains unclear whether it is sufficient for assembly into filaments. The availability of large quantities of recombinant human tau isoforms and the ease with which tau fragments can be expressed facilitated studies aimed at producing synthetic tau filaments. Early experiments had shown that PHF-like filaments can be assembled *in vitro* from bacterially expressed, non-phosphorylated three repeat fragments of tau [18,107]. The formation of these filaments lent strong support to the view that the repeat region of tau is the only component necessary for the morphological appearance of the PHF. However, these studies failed to provide any insight into filament formation *in vivo*, because the tau filaments were obtained only with truncated tau under non-physiological conditions.

Subsequently, experiments using sulphated glycosaminoglycans (GAGs) to stimulate phosphorylation of tau by a number of protein kinases led to the observation that sulphated GAGs induce the assembly of full-length tau into filaments [43,86]. By immunoelectron microscopy, these filaments were decorated by antibodies directed against the N- and C-terminal regions of tau, but not by an antibody against the microtubule-binding repeat region, exactly like the tau filaments from Alzheimer's disease [43] (Fig. 7). The assembly of tau is a nucleation-dependent phenomenon [31] and a short amino acid sequence (VQIVYK) in the third

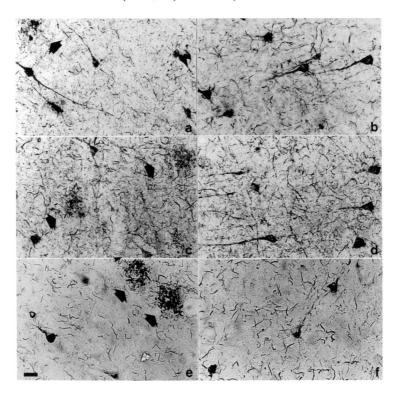

Fig. 6. Immunohistochemical localisation of neurofibrillary pathology using phosphorylation-dependent anti-tau antibodies. (a,c,e), Cerebral cortex from a sporadic Alzheimer's disease case. (b,d,f), Cerebral cortex from a case of frontotemporal dementia and parkinsonism linked to chromosome 17 (FTDP-17) with the V337M mutation in the tau gene. The phosphorylation-dependent anti-tau antibodies were: (a,b), AT8 (pS202 and pT205), (c,d), AT100 (pT212 and pS214) and (e,f), AT180 (pT231). The arrows in (a), (c) and (e) point to neuritic plaques, which are characteristic of Alzheimer's disease. Cases of FTDP-17 lack significant plaque pathology. Scale bar, 50 μm. Reprinted from Spillantini et al., Acta Neuropathologica 92, 42–48 (1996), with permission from Springer.

microtubule-binding repeat was found to be essential for heparin-induced filament assembly [105]. Subsequently, RNA and arachidonic acid were also found to induce the bulk assembly of full-length recombinant tau into filaments [51,55,108]. This work provided robust methods for the assembly of full-length tau into filaments. Two recent studies have used heparin-induced assembly of tau to identify small molecule inhibitors of filament formation [90,101]. Pathological co-localization of sulphated GAGs and RNA with hyperphosphorylated tau protein has suggested that these findings may also be relevant for the assembly of tau in Alzheimer's disease brain [32,88,104].

7. Tauopathies and neurodegeneration

By the early 1990s, the presence of tau protein had also been described in the filamentous deposits of Pick's disease, progressive supranuclear palsy and corticobasal degeneration [69]. Unlike Alzheimer's disease, these diseases lack significant $A\beta$ pathology. Subsequently, filamentous tau deposits were described in many other neurodegenerative diseases, now often referred to as tauopathies (Table 1).

Hyperphosphorylation of tau is a feature common to all diseases with tau filaments. The phosphorylated sites are similar, with only minor differences between diseases. However, the pattern of abnormal tau bands was found to vary. Thus, Alzheimer's disease and other conditions (such as the Parkinsonism-dementia complex of Guam) are characterized by three major bands of 60, 64 and 68 kDa and a minor band of 72 kDa. By contrast, filamentous tau from brains of patients with progressive supranuclear palsy and corticobasal degeneration lacks the 60 kDa band [30,65], whereas pathological tau from Pick's disease brain shows major 60 and 64 kDa bands [21]. Differences in the tau isoform composition of the pathological filaments explain these patterns of bands. This work revealed that the biochemical composition of tau filaments is not uniform.

The molecular dissection of the PHF and SF of Alzheimer's disease gave quite a complete description of the composition of the filaments. It also pro-

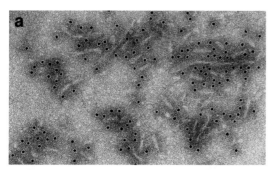
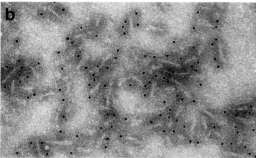
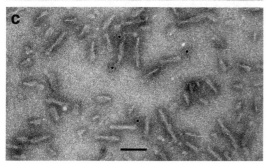

Fig. 7. Immunoelectron microscopy of synthetic paired helical-like filaments formed following incubation of recombinant tau protein with heparin. The antibodies used were as follows: 133, which recognizes the N-terminus of tau (a); 134, which recognizes the C-terminus of tau (b); 135, which recognizes the microtubule-binding repeat region of tau (c). Note immunodecoration with 133 and 134, but not with 135, as for Alzheimer filaments (see Fig. 5). Scale bar, 100 nm. Reprinted from Goedert et al., Nature 383, 550–553 (1996), with permission from Macmillan.

Table 1
Diseases in which tau deposits have been described

Alzheimer's disease
Amyotrophic lateral sclerosis/parkinsonism-dementia complex
Argyrophilic grain disease
Autosomal-dominant Parkinson's disease
Autosomal-dominant parkinsonism
Autosomal-recessive juvenile parkinsonism
Corticobasal degeneration
Dementia pugilistica
Diffuse neurofibrillary tangles with calcification
Down's syndrome
Familial British dementia
Frontotemporal dementia and parkinsonism linked to chromosome 17
Gerstmann-Sträussler-Scheinker disease
Guadeloupean parkinsonism
Hallervorden-Spatz disease
Myotonic dystrophy
Niemann-Pick disease, type C
Non-Guamanian motor neuron disease with neurofibrillary tangles
Pick's disease
Postencephalitic parkinsonism
Prion protein cerebral amyloid angiopathy
Progressive subcortical gliosis
Progressive supranuclear palsy
Subacute sclerosing panencephalitis
Tangle only dementia

vided clues regarding the mechanisms of filament formation. However, it did not provide any direct information about the relevance of tau dysfunction and filament formation for the disease process. This had been suspected to be the case, largely because of the good correlation between neurofibrillary pathology and nerve cell degeneration [3,8,10]. However, the identification in 1991 and 1995, respectively, of causative mutations in the amyloid β-protein precursor gene and the presenilin genes in familial cases of Alzheimer's disease [33,72,81,93,95], led many to believe that tau-positive inclusions were epiphenomena of little or no consequence. For some, this was further compounded by the presence of filamentous tau deposits in a number of apparently unrelated conditions. What was missing was genetic evidence linking dysfunction of tau protein to neurodegeneration and dementia.

In 1994, an autosomal-dominantly inherited form of frontotemporal dementia with parkinsonism was linked to chromosome 17q21.2, a region that contains the tau gene [106]. This was followed by the identification of other forms of frontotemporal dementia that were linked to this region, resulting in the denomination "frontotemporal dementia and parkinsonism linked to chromosome 17" (FTDP-17) for this class of disease. Cases of FTDP-17 were found to exhibit filamentous tau-positive inclusions, including Pick bodies and Alzheimer-type tangles with PHFs and SFs, in the absence of Aβ deposits [19,96,98,100] (Figs 2B, 6b,d,f). The now widely used term "tauopathy" was introduced, because of the sheer abundance of tau inclusions in a family with frontotemporal dementia [97]. In June 1998, exactly ten years after the publication of our paper describing the presence of tau protein in the core of the PHF, the first mutations in the tau gene in FTDP-17 were identified [31,91,99]. At the time of writing, 37 different mutations, mostly affecting the sequence or splicing of the repeat region, have been reported. The study of FTDP-17 has established that primary lesions in tau can lead to neurodegeneration and dementia, with the formation of tau filaments being the likely gain of toxic function. It follows that dysfunction of tau is most probably also of central importance for the pathogenesis of sporadic diseases with a filamentous tau pathology. This is strongly supported by the extensive evidence implicating the tau gene as a susceptibility locus for progressive supranuclear palsy and corticobasal degeneration [4,14,22].

References

[1] A. Alzheimer, Über eine eigenartige Erkrankung der Hirnrinde, *Allg Z Psychiat Psych Gerichtl Med* **64** (1907), 146–148.

[2] A. Alzheimer, Über eigenartige Krankheitsfälle des späteren Alters, *Z Ges Neurol Psychiat* **4** (1911), 356–385.

[3] P.V. Arriagada, J.H. Growdon, E.T. Hedley-White and B.T. Hyman, Neurofibrillary tangles but not senile plaques parallel duration and severity of Alzheimer's disease, *Neurology* **42** (1992), 631–639.

[4] M. Baker, I. Litvan, H. Houlden, J. Adamson, D. Dickson, J. Perez-Tur, J. Hardy, T. Lynch, E. Bigio and M. Hutton, Association of an extended haplotype in the tau gene with progressive supranuclear palsy, *Hum Mol Genet* **8** (1999), 711–715.

[5] J. Berriman, L.C. Serpell, K.A. Oberg, A.L. Fink, M. Goedert and R.A. Crowther, Tau filaments from human brain and from *in vitro* assembly of recombinant protein show cross-β structure, *Proc Natl Acad Sci USA* **100** (2003), 9034–9038.

[6] G. Blessed, B.E. Tomlinson and M. Roth, The association between quantitative measures of dementia and of senile change in the cerebral grey matter of elderly subjects, *Brit J Psychiat* **114** (1968), 797–811.

[7] P. Blocq and G. Marinesco, Sur les lésions et la pathogénie de l'épilepsie dite essentielle, *Sem Méd* **12** (1892), 445–446.

[8] W. Bondareff, C.M. Wischik, M. Novak, W.B. Amos, A. Klug and M. Roth, Molecular analysis of neurofibrillary degeneration in Alzheimer's disease, *Am J Pathol* **137** (1990), 711–723.

[9] W. Bondareff, C.Q. Mountjoy, C.M. Wischik, D.L. Hauser, L.D. LaBree and M. Roth, Evidence of subtypes of Alzheimer's disease and implications for etiology, *Arch Gen Psychiat* **50** (1993), 350–356.

[10] H. Braak and E. Braak, Neuropathological staging of Alzheimer-related changes, *Acta Neuropathol* **82** (1991), 239–259.

[11] G.T. Bramblett, M. Goedert, R. Jakes, S.E. Merrick, J.Q. Trojanowski and V.M.-Y. Lee, Abnormal tau phosphorylation at Ser396 in Alzheimer's disease recapitulates development and contributes to reduced microtubule binding, *Neuron* **10** (1993), 1089–1099.

[12] J.P. Brion, H. Passareiro, J. Nunez and J. Flament-Durand, Mise en évidence immunologique de la protéine tau au niveau des lésions de dégénérescence neurofibrillaire de la maladie d'Alzheimer, *Arch Biol* **95** (1985), 229–235.

[13] D.W. Cleveland, S.-Y. Hwo and M.W. Kirschner, Physical and chemical properties of purified tau factor and the role of tau in microtubule assembly, *J Mol Biol* **116** (1977), 227–247.

[14] C. Conrad, A. Andreadis, J.Q. Trojanowski, D.W. Dickson, D. Kang, X. Chen, W. Wiederholt, L. Hansen, E. Masliah, L.J. Thal, R. Katzman, Y. Xia and T. Saitoh, Genetic evidence for the involvement of tau in progressive supranuclear palsy, *Ann Neurol* **41** (1997), 277–281.

[15] D. Couchie, C. Mavilia, I.S. Georgieff, R.K. Liem, M.L. Shelanski and J. Nunez, Primary structure of high molecular weight tau present in the peripheral nervous system, *Proc Natl Acad Sci USA* **89** (1992), 4378–4381.

[16] R.A. Crowther and C.M. Wischik, Image reconstruction of the Alzheimer paired helical filament, *EMBO J* **4** (1985), 3661–3665.

[17] R.A. Crowther, Straight and paired helical filaments in Alzheimer disease have a common structural unit, *Proc Natl Acad Sci USA* **88** (1991), 2288–2292.

[18] R.A. Crowther, O.F. Olesen, R. Jakes and M. Goedert, The microtubule binding repeats of tau protein assemble into filaments like those found in Alzheimer's disease, *FEBS Lett* **309** (1992), 199–202.

[19] R.A. Crowther and M. Goedert, Abnormal tau-containing filaments in neurodegenerative diseases, *J Struct Biol* **130** (2000), 271–279.

[20] A. Delacourte and A. Défossez, Alzheimer's disease: tau proteins, the promoting factors of microtubule assembly, are major antigenic components of paired helical filaments, *J Neurol Sci* **76** (1986), 173–186.

[21] A. Delacourte, Y. Robitaille, N. Sergeant, L. Buée, P.R. Hof, A. Wattez, A. Laroche-Cholette, J. Mathieu, P. Chagnon and D. Gauvreau, Specific pathological tau protein variants characterize Pick's disease, *J Neuropathol Exp Neurol* **55** (1996), 159–168.

[22] E. di Maria, M. Tabaton, T. Vigo, G. Abruzzese, E. Bellone, C. Donati, E. Frasson, R. Marchese, P. Montagna, D.G. Munoz, P.P. Pramstaller, G. Zanusso, F. Ajmar and P. Mandich, Corticobasal degeneration shares a common genetic background with progressive supranuclear palsy, *Ann Neurol* **47** (2000), 374–377.

[23] G. Drewes, B. Lichtenberg-Kraag, F. Döring, E.M. Mandelkow, J. Biernat, M. Dorée and E. Mandelkow, Mitogen-activated protein (MAP) kinase transforms tau protein into an Alzheimer-like state, *EMBO J* **11** (1992), 2131–2138.

[24] G. Drewes, A. Ebneth, U. Preuss, E.M. Mandelkow and E. Mandelkow, MARK, a novel family of protein kinases that phosphorylate microtubule-associated proteins and trigger microtubule disruption, *Cell* **89** (1997), 297–308.

[25] D.G. Drubin, D. Caput and M.W. Kirschner, Studies on the expression of the microtubule-associated protein, tau, during mouse brain development, with newly isolated complementary DNA probes, *J Cell Biol* **98** (1984), 1090–1097.

[26] D.J. Ennulat, R.K.H. Liem, G.A. Hashim and M.L. Shelanski, Two separate 18-amino acid domains of tau promote the polymerization of tubulin, *J Biol Chem* **264** (1989), 5327–5330.

[27] J. Esquirol, *Des maladies mentales*, Baillière, Paris 1838.

[28] O. Fischer, Miliare Nekrosen mit drusigen Wucherungen der Neurofibrillen, eine regelmässige Veränderung der Hirnrinde bei seniler Demenz, *Monatsschr Psychiat Neurol* (1907), 361–372.

[29] S. Flament and A. Delacourte, Abnormal tau species are produced during Alzheimer's disease neurodegenerating process, *FEBS Lett* **247** (1989), 213–216.

[30] S. Flament, A. Delacourte, M. Verny, J.J. Hauw and F. Javoy-Agid, Abnormal tau proteins in progressive supranuclear palsy. Similarities and differences with the neurofibrillary

degeneration of the Alzheimer type, *Acta Neuropathol* **81** (1991), 591–596.

[31] P. Friedhoff, M. von Bergen, E.M. Mandelkow, P. Davies and E. Mandelkow, A nucleated assembly mechanism of Alzheimer paired helical filaments, *Proc Natl Acad Sci USA* **95** (1998), 15712–15717.

[32] S.D. Ginsberg, J.E. Galvin, T.S. Chiu, V.M.-Y. Lee, E. Masliah and J.Q. Trojanowski, RNA sequestration to pathological lesions of neurodegenerative diseases, *Acta Neuropathol* **96** (1998), 487–494.

[33] A. Goate, M.C. Chartier-Harlin, M. Mullan, J. Brown, F. Crawford, L. Fidani, L. Giuffra, A. Haynes, N. Irving, L. James, R. Mant, P. Newton, K. Rook, P. Roques, C. Talbot, M. Pericak-Vance, A. Roses, R. Williamson, M. Rossor, M. Owen and J. Hardy, Segregation of a missense mutation in the amyloid precursor protein gene with familial Alzheimer's disease, *Nature* **349** (1991), 704–706.

[34] M. Goedert, C.M. Wischik, R.A. Crowther, J.E. Walker and A. Klug, Cloning and sequencing of the cDNA encoding a core protein of the paired helical filament of Alzheimer disease, *Proc Natl Acad Sci USA* **85** (1988), 4051–4055.

[35] M. Goedert, M.G. Spillantini, M.C. Potier, J. Ulrich and R.A. Crowther, Cloning and sequencing of the cDNA encoding an isoform of microtubule-associated protein tau containing four tandem repeats: differential expression of tau protein mRNAs in human brain, *EMBO J* **8** (1989), 393–399.

[36] M. Goedert, M.G. Spillantini, R. Jakes, D. Rutherford and R.A. Crowther, Multiple isoforms of human microtubule-associated protein tau: Sequences and localization in neurofibrillary tangles of Alzheimer's disease, *Neuron* **3** (1989), 519–526.

[37] M. Goedert and R. Jakes, Expression of separate isoforms of human tau protein: Correlation with the tau pattern in brain and effects on tubulin polymerization, *EMBO J* **9** (1990), 4225–4230.

[38] M. Goedert, M.G. Spillantini, N.J. Cairns and R.A. Crowther, Tau proteins of Alzheimer paired helical filaments: Abnormal phosphorylation of all six brain isoforms, *Neuron* **8** (1992), 159–168.

[39] M. Goedert, M.G. Spillantini and R.A. Crowther, Cloning of a big tau microtubule-associated protein charcteristic of the peripheral nervous system, *Proc Natl Acad Sci USA* **89** (1992), 1983–1987.

[40] M. Goedert, E.S. Cohen, R. Jakes and P. Cohen, MAP kinase phosphorylation sites in microtubule-associated protein tau are dephosphorylated by protein phosphatase 2A1, *FEBS Lett* **312** (1992), 95–99.

[41] M. Goedert, R. Jakes, R.A. Crowther, J. Six, U. Lübke, M. Vandermeeren, P. Cras, J.Q. Trojanowski and V.M.-Y. Lee, The abnormal phosphorylation of tau protein at Ser-202 in Alzheimer disease recapitulates phosphorylation during development, *Proc Natl Acad Sci USA* **90** (1993), 5066–5070.

[42] M. Goedert, R. Jakes, R.A. Crowther, P. Cohen, E. Vanmechelen, M. Vandermeeren and P. Cras, Epitope mapping of monoclonal antibodies to the paired helical filaments of Alzheimer's disease: identification of phosphorylation sites in tau protein, *Biochem J* **301** (1994), 871–877.

[43] M. Goedert, R. Jakes, M.G. Spillantini, M. Hasegawa, M.J. Smith and R.A. Crowther, Assembly of microtubule-associated protein tau into Alzheimer-like filaments induced by sulphated glycosaminoglycans, *Nature* **383** (1996), 550–553.

[44] M. Goedert, M. Hasegawa, R. Jakes, S. Lawler, A. Cuenda and P. Cohen, Phosphorylation of microtubule-associated protein tau by stress-activated protein kinases, *FEBS Lett* **409** (1997), 57–62.

[45] M.B. Graeber, S. Kösel, E. Grasbon-Frodl, H.J. Möller and P. Mehraein, Histopathology and APOE genotype of the first Alzheimer disease patient, Auguste D., *Neurogenetics* **1** (1998), 223–228.

[46] S. Greenberg and P. Davies, A preparation of Alzheimer paired helical filaments that displays distinct tau proteins by polyacrylamide gel electrophoresis, *Proc Natl Acad Sci USA* **87** (1990), 5827–5831.

[47] I. Grundke-Iqbal, K. Iqbal, M. Quinlan, Y.-C. Tung, M.S. Zaidi and H.M. Wisniewski, Microtubule-associated protein tau, a component of Alzheimer paired helical filaments, *J Biol Chem* **261** (1986), 6084–6089.

[48] I. Grundke-Iqbal, K. Iqbal, Y.-C. Tung, M. Quinlan, H.M. Wisniewski and L.I. Binder, Abnormal phosphorylation of the microtubule-associated protein tau in Alzheimer cytoskeletal pathology, *Proc Natl Acad Sci USA* **83** (1986), 4913–4917.

[49] D.P. Hanger, K. Hughes, J.R. Woodgett, J.P. Brion and B.H. Anderton, Glycogen synthase kinase-3 induces Alzheimer's disease-like phosphorylation of tau: generation of paired helical filament epitopes and neuronal localization of the kinase, *Neurosci Lett* **147** (1992), 58–62.

[50] M. Hasegawa, M. Morishima-Kawashima, K. Takio, M. Suzuki, K. Titani and Y. Ihara, Protein sequence and mass spectrometric analyses of tau in the Alzheimer's disease brain, *J Biol Chem* **267** (1992), 17047–17054.

[51] M. Hasegawa, R.A. Crowther, R. Jakes and M. Goedert, Alzheimer-like changes in microtubule-associated protein tau induced by sulfated glycosaminoglycans. Inhibition of microtubule binding, stimulation of phosphorylation, and filament assembly depend on the degree of sulfation, *J Biol Chem* **272** (1997), 33118–33124.

[52] A. Hirano, H.M. Dembitzer, L.T. Kurland and H.M. Zimmerman, The fine structure of some intraganglionic alterations, *J Neuropathol Exp Neurol* **27** (1968), 167–182.

[53] M. Hutton, C.L. Lendon, P. Rizzu, M. Baker, S. Froelich, H. Houlden, S. Pickering-Brown, S. Chakraverty, A. Isaacs, A. Grover, J. Hackett, J. Adamson, S. Lincoln, D. Dickson, P. Davies, R.C. Petersen, M. Stevens, E. de Graaff, E. Wauters, J. van Baren, M. Hillebrand, M. Joosse, J.M. Kwon, P. Nowotny, L.K. Che, J. Norton, J.C. Morris, L.A. Reed, J. Trojanowski, H. Basun, L. Lannfelt, M. Neystat, S. Fahn, F. Dark, T. Tannenberg, P.R. Dodd, N. Hayward, J.B.J. Kwok, P.R. Schofield, A. Andreadis, J. Snowden, D. Craufurd, D. Neary, F. Owen, B.A. Oostra, J. Hardy, A. Goate, J. van Swieten, D. Mann, T. Lynch and P. Heutink, Association of missense and 5'-splice-site mutations in tau with the inherited dementia FTDP-17, *Nature* **393** (1998), 702–705.

[54] Y. Ihara, N. Nukina, R. Miura and M. Ogawara, Phosphorylated tau protein is integrated into paired helical filaments in Alzheimer's disease, *J Biochem (Tokyo)* **99** (1986), 1807–1810.

[55] T. Kampers, P. Friedhoff, J. Biernat, E.M. Mandelkow and E. Mandelkow, RNA stimulates aggregation of microtubule-associated protein tau into Alzheimer-like paired helical filaments, *FEBS Lett* **399** (1996), 344–349.

[56] K. Kanemura, K. Takio, R. Miura, K. Titani and Y. Ihara, Fetal-type phosphorylation of the tau in paired helical filaments, *J Neurochem* **58** (1992), 1667–1675.

[57] M. Kidd, Paired helical filaments in electron microscopy of Alzheimer's disease, *Nature* **197** (1963), 192–193.

[58] M. Kidd, Alzheimer's disease – an electron microscopical study, *Brain* **87** (1964), 307–320.
[59] S. Kobayashi, K. Ishiguro, A. Omori, M. Takamatsu, M. Atioka, K. Imahori and T. Uchida, A cdc-related kinase PSSALRE/cdk5 is homologous with the 30 kDa subunit of tau protein kinase II, a proline-directed protein kinase associated with microtubules, *FEBS Lett* **335** (1993), 171–175.
[60] J. Kondo, T. Honda, H. Mori, Y. Hamada, R. Miura, M. Ogawara and Y. Ihara, The carboxyl third of tau is tightly bound to paired helical filaments, *Neuron* **1** (1988), 827–834.
[61] K.S. Kosik, L.K. Duffy, M.M. Dowling, C.R. Abraham, A. McCluskey and D.J. Selkoe, Microtubule-associated protein 2: monoclonal antibodies demonstrate the selective incorporation of certain epitopes into Alzheimer neurofibrillary tangles, *Proc Natl Acad Sci USA* **81** (1984), 7941–7945.
[62] K.S. Kosik, C.L. Joachim and D.J. Selkoe, Microtubule-associated protein tau is a major antigenic component of paired helical filaments in Alzheimer's disease, *Proc Natl Acad Sci USA* **83** (1986), 4044–4048.
[63] E. Kraepelin, *Psychiatrie. Ein Lehrbuch für Studierende und Ärzte*, II. Band, Klinische Psychiatrie. Verlag Johann Ambrosius Barth, Leipzig 1910.
[64] H. Ksiezak-Reding, D.W. Dickson, P. Davies and S.-H. Yen, Recognition of tau epitopes by anti-neurofilament antibodies that bind to Alzheimer neurofibrillary tangles, *Proc Natl Acad Sci USA* **84** (1987), 3410–3414.
[65] H. Ksiezak-Reding, K. Morgan, L.A. Mattiace, P. Davies, W.K. Liu, S.-H. Yen, K. Weidenheim and D.W. Dickson, Ultrastructure and biochemical composition of paired helical filaments in corticobasal degeneration, *Am J Pathol* **145** (1994), 1496–1508.
[66] G. Lee, N. Cowan and M.W. Kirschner, The primary structure and heterogeneity of tau protein from mouse brain, *Science* **239** (1988), 285–288.
[67] G. Lee, R.L. Neve and K.S. Kosik, The microtubule binding domain of tau protein, *Neuron* **2** (1989), 1615–1624.
[68] V.M.-Y. Lee, B.J. Balin, L. Otvos and J.Q. Trojanowski, A68 – a major subunit of paired helical filaments and derivatized forms of normal tau, *Science* **251** (1991), 675–678.
[69] V.M.-Y. Lee, M. Goedert and J.Q. Trojanowski, Neurodegenerative Tauopathies, *Annu Rev Neurosci* **24** (2001), 1121–1159.
[70] G. Lindwall and R.D. Cole, Phosphorylation affects the ability of tau protein to promote microtubule assembly, *J Biol Chem* **259** (1984), 5301–5305.
[71] G. Lindwall and R.D. Cole, The purification of tau protein and the occurrence of two phosphorylation states of tau in brain, *J Biol Chem* **259** (1984), 12241–12245.
[72] E. Levy-Lahad, W. Wasco, P. Poorkaj, D.M. Romano, J. Oshima, W.H. Pettingell, C.E. Yu, P.D. Jondro, S.D. Schmift, K. Wang, A.C. Crowley, Y.H. Fu, S.Y. Guenette, D. Galas, E. Nemens, E.M. Wijsman, T.D. Bird, G.D. Schellenberg and R.E. Tanzi, Candidate gene for the chromosome 1 familial Alzheimer's disease locus, *Science* **269** (1995), 973–977.
[73] E.M. Mandelkow, G. Drewes, J. Biernat, N. Gustke, J. van Lint, J.R. Vandenheede and E. Mandelkow, Glycogen synthase kinase-3 and the Alzheimer-like state of microtubule-associated protein tau, *FEBS Lett* **314** (1992), 315–321.
[74] C.L. Masters, G. Multhaup, G. Simms, J. Pottgiesser, R.N. Martins and K. Beyreuther, Neuronal origin of cerebral amyloid: Neurofibrillary tangles of Alzheimer's disease contain the same protein as the amyloid of plaque cores and blood vessels, *EMBO J* **4** (1985), 2757–2763.

[75] K. Maurer, S. Volk and H. Gerbaldo, Auguste D. and Alzheimer's disease, *Lancet* **349** (1997), 1546–1549.
[76] C.C.J. Miller, J.P. Brion, R. Calvert, T.K. Chin, P.A.M. Eagles, M.J. Downes, J. Flament-Durand, M. Haugh, J. Kahn, A. Probst, J. Ulrich and B.H. Anderton, Alzheimer's paired helical filaments share epitopes with neurofilament side arms, *EMBO J* **5** (1986), 269–276.
[77] H. Mori, J. Kondo and Y. Ihara, Ubiquitin is a component of paired helical filaments in Alzheimer's disease, *Science* **235** (1987), 1641–1644.
[78] M. Morishima-Kawashima, M. Hasegawa, K. Takio, M. Suzuki, K. Titani and Y. Ihara, Ubiquitin is conjugated with N-terminally processed tau in paired helical filaments, *Neuron* **10** (1993), 1151–1160.
[79] M. Morishima-Kawashima, M. Hasegawa, K. Takio, M. Suzuki, H. Yoshida, K. Titani, and Y. Ihara, Proline-directed and non-proline-directed phosphorylation of PHF-tau, *J Biol Chem* **270** (1995), 823–829.
[80] S.F.C. Mulot, K. Hughes, J.R. Woodgett, B.H. Anderton and D.P. Hanger, PHF-tau from Alzheimer's brain comprises four species on SDS-PAGE which can be mimicked by *in vitro* phosphorylation of human tau by glycogen synthase kinase-3β, *FEBS Lett* **349** (1994), 359–364.
[81] J.R. Murrell, M. Farlow, B. Ghetti and M.D. Benson, A mutation in the amyloid precursor protein associated with hereditary Alzheimer's disease, *Science* **254** (1991), 97–99.
[82] R.L. Neve, P. Harris, K.S. Kosik, D.M. Kurnit and T.A. Donlon, Identification of cDNA clones for the human microtubule-associated protein tau and chromosomal localization of the genes for tau and microtubule-associated protein 2, *Brain Res* **387** (1986), 271–280.
[83] N. Nukina and Y. Ihara, Immunocytochemical study on senile plaques in Alzheimer's disease. II. Abnormal dendrites in senile plaques as revealed by anti-microtubule-associated proteins (MAPs) immunostaining, *Proc Jpn Acad* **59** (1983), 284–292.
[84] N. Nukina, K.S. Kosik and D.J. Selkoe, Recognition of Alzheimer paired helical filaments by monoclonal neurofilament antibodies is due to crossreaction with tau protein, *Proc Natl Acad Sci USA* **84** (1987), 3415–3419.
[85] N. Nukina and Y. Ihara, One of the antigenic determinants of paired helical filaments is related to tau protein, *J Biochem (Tokyo)* **99** (1986), 1541–1544.
[86] M. Pérez, J.M. Valpuesta, M. Medina, E. Montejo de Garcini and J. Avila, Polymerization of tau into filaments in the presence of heparin: the minimal sequence requirement for tau-tau interaction, *J Neurochem* **67** (1996), 1183–1190.
[87] G. Perry, R. Friedman, G. Shaw and V. Chau, Ubiquitin is detected in neurofibrillary tangles and senile plaque neurites of Alzheimer disease brains, *Proc Natl Acad Sci USA* **84** (1987), 3033–3036.
[88] G. Perry, S.L. Siedlak, P. Richey, M. Kawai, P. Cras, R.N. Kalaria, P.G. Galloway, J.M. Scardina, B. Cordell, B.D. Greenberg, S.R. Ledbetter and P. Gambetti, Association of heparan sulphate proteoglycan with the neurofibrillary tangles of Alzheimer's disease, *J Neurosci* **11** (1991), 3679–3683.
[89] A. Pick, Über die Beziehungen der senilen Hirnatrophie zur Aphasie, *Prager Med Wochenschr* **17** (1892), 165–167.
[90] M. Pickhardt, Z. Gazova, M. von Bergen, I. Khlistunova, Y. Wang, A. Hascher, E.M. Mandelkow, J. Biernat and E. Mandelkow, Anthraquinones inhibit tau aggregation and dissolve Alzheimer's paired helical filaments *in vitro* and in cells, *J Biol Chem* **280** (2005), 3628–3635.

[91] P. Poorkaj, T.D. Bird, E. Wijsman, E. Nemens, R.M. Garruto, L. Anderson, A. Andreadis, W.C. Wiederholt, M. Raskind and G.D. Schellenberg, Tau is a candidate gene for chromosome 17 frontotemporal dementia, *Ann Neurol* **43** (1998), 815–825.

[92] E. Redlich, Über miliare Sklerose der Hirnrinde bei seniler Atrophie, *Jahrb Psychiat Neurol* **17** (1898), 208–216.

[93] E.I. Rogaev, R. Sherrington, E.A. Rogaeva, G. Levesque, M. Ikeda, Y. Liang, H. Chi, C. Lin, K. Holman, T. Tsuda, L. Mar, S. Sorbi, B. Nacmias, S. Piacentini, L. Amaducci, I. Chumakov, D. Cohen, L. Lannfelt, P.E. Fraser, J.M. Rommens and P.H. St George-Hyslop, Familial Alzheimer's disease in kindreds with missense mutations in a gene on chromosome 1 related to the Alzheimer's disease type 3 gene, *Nature* **376** (1995), 775–778.

[94] R. Rubenstein, R.J. Kascsak, P.A. Merz, H.M. Wisniewski, R.I. Carp and K. Iqbal, Paired helical filaments associated with Alzheimer disease are readily soluble structures, *Brain Res* **372** (1986), 80–88.

[95] R. Sherrington, E.I. Rogaev, Y. Liang, E.A. Rogaeva, G. Levesque, M. Ikeda, H. Chi, C. Lin, G. Li, K. Holman, T. Tsuda, L. Mar, J.F. Foncin, A.C. Bruni, M.P. Montesi, S. Sorbi, I. Rainero, L. Pinessi, L. Nee, I. Chumakov, D. Pollen, A. Brookes, P. Sanseau, R.J. Polinsky, W. Wasco, H.A.R. da Silva, J.L. Haines, M.A. Pericak-Vance, R.E. Tanzi, A.D. Roses, P.E. Fraser, J.M. Rommens and P.H. St George-Hyslop, Cloning of a gene bearing missense mutations in early-onset familial Alzheimer's disease, *Nature* **375** (1995), 754–760.

[96] M.G. Spillantini, R.A. Crowther and M. Goedert, Comparison of the neurofibrillary pathology in Alzheimer's disease and familial presenile dementia with tangles, *Acta Neuropathol* **92** (1996), 42–48.

[97] M.G. Spillantini, M. Goedert, R.A. Crowther, J.R. Murrell, M.J. Farlow and B. Ghetti, Familial multiple system tauopathy with presenile dementia: a disease with abundant neuronal and glial tau filaments, *Proc Natl Acad Sci USA* **94** (1997), 4113–4118.

[98] M.G. Spillantini, T.D. Bird and B. Ghetti, Frontotemporal dementia and parkinsonism linked to chromosome 17: a new group of tauopathies, *Brain Pathol* **8** (1998), 387–402.

[99] M.G. Spillantini, J.R. Murrell, M. Goedert, M.R. Farlow, A. Klug and B. Ghetti, Mutation in the tau gene in familial multiple system tauopathy with presenile dementia, *Proc Natl Acad Sci USA* **95** (1998), 7737–7741.

[100] M.G. Spillantini, R.A. Crowther, W. Kamphorst, P. Heutink and J.C. van Swieten, Tau pathology in two Dutch families with mutations in the microtubule-binding region of tau, *Am J Pathol* **153** (1998), 1359–1363.

[101] S. Taniguchi, N. Suzuki, M. Masuda, S. Hisanaga, T. Iwatsubo, M. Goedert and M. Hasegawa, Inhibition of heparin-induced tau filament formation by phenothiazines, polyphenols and porphyrins, *J Biol Chem* **290** (2005), 7614–7623.

[102] R.D. Terry, The fine structure of neurofibrillary tangles in Alzheimer's disease, *J Neuropathol Exp Neurol* **22** (1963), 629–642.

[103] R.D. Terry, N.K. Gonatas and M. Weiss, Ultrastructural studies in Alzheimer's presenile dementia, *Am J Pathol* **44** (1964), 269–297.

[104] M.M. Verbeek, I. Otte-Höller, J. van den Born, L.P.W.J. van den Heuvel, G. David, P. Wesseling and R.M.W. de Waal, Agrin is a major heparan sulfate proteoglycan accumulating in Alzheimer's disease brain, *Am J Pathol* **155** (1999), 2115–2125.

[105] M. von Bergen, P. Friedhoff, J. Biernat, J. Heberle, E.M. Mandelkow and E. Mandelkow, Assembly of tau protein into Alzheimer paired helical filaments depends on a local sequence motif ((306)VQIVYK(311)) forming beta structure, *Proc Natl Acad Sci USA* **97** (2000), 5129–5134.

[106] K.C. Wilhelmsen, T. Lynch, E. Pavlou, M. Higgins and T.G. Nygaard, Localization of disinhibition-dementia-parkinsonism-amyotrophy complex to 17q21–22, *Am J Hum Genet* **55** (1994), 1159–1165.

[107] H. Wille, G. Drewes, J. Biernat, E.M. Mandelkow and E. Mandelkow, Alzheimer-like paired helical filaments and antiparallel dimers formed from microtubule-associated protein tau *in vitro*, *J Cell Biol* **118** (1992), 573–584.

[108] D.M. Wilson and L.I. Binder, Free fatty acids stimulate the polymerization of tau and amyloid beta peptides. In vitro evidence for a common effector of pathogenesis in Alzheimer's disease, *Am J Pathol* **150** (1997), 2181–2195.

[109] C.M. Wischik, R.A. Crowther, M. Stewart and M. Roth, Subunit structure of paired helical filaments in Alzheimer's disease, *J Cell Biol* **100** (1985), 1905–1912.

[110] C.M. Wischik, M. Novak, H.C. Thogersen, P.C. Edwards, M.J. Runswick, R. Jakes, J.E. Walker, C. Milstein, M. Roth and A. Klug, Isolation of a fragment of tau derived from the core of the paired helical filament of Alzheimer disease, *Proc Natl Acad Sci* **85** (1988), 4506–4510.

[111] C.M. Wischik, M. Novak, P.C. Edwards, A. Klug, W. Tichelaar and R.A. Crowther, Structural characterization of the core of the paired helical filament of Alzheimer disease, *Proc Natl Acad Sci USA* **85** (1988), 4884–4888.

[112] B.L. Wolozin, A. Pruchnicki, D.W. Dickson and P. Davies, A neuronal antigen in the brains of Alzheimer patients, *Science* **232** (1986), 648–650.

[113] J.G. Wood, S.S. Mirra, N.J. Pollock and L.I. Binder, Neurofibrillary tangles of Alzheimer disease share antigenic determinants with the microtubule-associated protein tau, *Proc Natl Acad Sci USA* **83** (1986), 4040–4043.

[114] S.-H. Yen, F. Gaskin and S.M. Fu, Neurofibrillary tangles in senile dementia of the Alzheimer type share an antigenic determinant with intermediate filaments of the vimentin class, *Am J Pathol* **113** (1983), 373–381.

[115] H. Yoshida and Y. Ihara, Tau in paired helical filaments is functionally distinct from fetal tau: assembly incompetence of paired helical filament tau, *J Neurochem* **61** (1993), 1183–1186.

Neurofibrillary tangles/paired helical filaments (1981–83)

Yasuo Ihara
Department of Neuropathology, Faculty of Medicine, University of Tokyo, 7-3-1 Hongo, Bunkyo-ku, Tokyo 113, Japan
Tel.: +81 3 5841 3541; Fax: +81 3 5800 6854; E-mail: yihara@m.u-tokyo.ac.jp

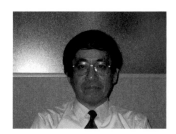

Abstract. Neurofibrillary tangles, one of the hallmarks of Alzheimer's disease, had been a target of modern neuropathology based on electron microscopy. In 1960s their unit fibrils were found to be paired helical filaments (PHF), the unique appearance of which attracted many researchers to their nature. In the late 1970s, a keen interest in their constituents at the molecular levels had increasingly grown, but electron microscopic approach failed to address the issue. I describe here what was going on at the turning point when electron microscopic study yielded immunocytochemical approach and direct characterization by isolation, with some emphasis on the situation in Japan. Personal memories are provided about Dr Selkoe's lab (1981–1982) in Mailman Research Center, Belmont, Boston, where we encountered a series of remarkable properties of PHF. How insolubility of PHF, and smearing on the blot was found is described.

1. Introduction

When I was a resident of neurology (1973–75), I happened to take from the desk in a resident room a small brochure that was distributed by a pharmaceutical company in Japan. The cover photo showed neurofibrillary tangles (NFT) in Alzheimer's disease (AD), the unusual morphology of which so impressed me at a stage when there was insufficient knowledge about its neuropathology. Soon I learned that their nature had been the target of modern neuropathology. I also came to learn about an attempt by Dr Khalid Iqbal to isolate NFT and determine their major components by SDS-PAGE. The paper written by Dr Iqbal, though only a short communication [6], had a great impact upon many young neurologists/psychiatrists. It was probably this paper that made young Khalid Iqbal world-famous. This is why in 1976 I joined the lab of Dr Yoshito Kaziro, Institute of Medical Sciences, University of Tokyo, for the study of microtubules (MT), simply because they have fibrous structures somehow resembling NFT. I never imagined at that time that the NFT I had started to struggle with three years later were closely related to MT.

2. NFT before 1980

The introduction of electron microscopy to neuropathology in the 1960s revolutionized morphological studies; fine structures of many inclusion bodies were uncovered for the first time. NFT were a representative example. They were shown to be composed of unusual filaments, paired helical filaments (PHF), which consist of two 10 nm filaments wound around each other, giving regular constrictions every 80 nm [20]. Because of their unique morphology, PHF allow us to easily distinguish them from neurofilaments (NF) and MT, which are two major cytoskeletal elements in neurons. In addition, they are found only in humans, not in other species, including nonhuman primates. Something specific to humans – this was also why I was highly attracted to NFT.

It was postulated in the late 1970s that PHF are derived from normal cytoskeletons, and this possibility has been extensively examined by electron microscopy. Although there were few observations showing transition of NF into PHF [12,21], they were not confirmed by other researchers. Nevertheless, many researchers seemed to assume that PHF are altered NF, because (i) NF are neuron-specific 10 nm filaments, and PHF were believed to exist only in neuronal processes, and (ii) NF can be transformed into a twisted configuration *in vitro* [13].

Immunocytochemical studies of NFT began around the late 1970s, an approach where various antibodies are examined for their ability to stain NFT in the section [7]. In particular, NF were highlighted. Many researchers competed to generate antibodies to NF, and test them for reactivity to NFT. On the other hand, in the 1970s, Dr Nishimura and his colleagues at Osaka University had initiated a series of pioneering works [11]. They attempted to isolate NFT from brain homogenates from unfixed AD and control brains by sucrose density gradient centrifugation. Each interface was subjected to fluorescence microscopy using thioflavin T and polyacrylamide gel electrophoresis. Although their attempts were not successful, their challenge inspired many young researchers and medical students in Japan.

3. Earlier immunocytochemical works on NFT

Electron microscopic observations had never added important information about the components of NFT, despite intensive efforts. Thus, it was natural that many researchers were going to focus on different approaches to identify PHF components. By 1980, there were a couple of research groups seeking to identify the PHF components, mainly using an immunocytochemical approach. Drs P. Gambetti and D. Dahl described how the antibodies to chick NF can intensely stain NFT in formalin-fixed, paraffin-embedded sections [3]. Their preliminary immunocytochemical data had already been published in a certain proceeding. I also learned that Dr B Anderton was going to apply monoclonal techniques to identify the components of NFT [1].

On the other hand, I became aware that a major problem was that there was no brain bank in Japan. Pathologists hated the idea of providing someone else with unfixed brains for biochemical studies. This kind of atmosphere was most prevalent in Japan, and it was almost impossible for us to obtain unfixed brains from pathologists, before 1990. Thus, I was forced to take an immunocytochemical approach by using a panel of well-characterized antibodies. At about the same time, "Immunocytochemistry", a famous monograph written by Ludwig A. Sternberger, was published. According to the monograph, conventional formalin-fixed, paraffin-embedded sections and light microscope were sufficient for the newly emerging immunoperoxidase method.

I thought that the specificities of the antibodies used for this purpose were a vital issue and they were not paid sufficient attention or not fully characterized: it was possible that the polyclonal antibodies used were contaminated with antibodies to unknown antigens, leading to an incorrect identification of the component. I decided to generate well-characterized antibodies to NF using gel-purified NF-H, NF-M, and NF-L. Partially purified NF from rat spinal cords were subjected to SDS-PAGE everyday, and the gel band corresponding to each component was excised and extracted. Each pooled antigen was used to immunize a rabbit. At the end of March 1981, just before joining Selkoe's laboratory, I found that the first lot of NF-H antisera stained a substantial fraction of NFT in the section [5]. This was very exciting. For the first time monospecific antibodies to NF-H were confirmed to label at least some NFT and senile plaque neurites in the AD hippocampus. This immunocytochemical result seemed to me to be quite reasonable, and strongly suggested that PHF were altered NF.

4. Dr Selkoe's lab in the Mailman Research Center (1981–82)

In 1979–80, I reached the age when I was allowed to spend two or three years conducting research in foreign countries, most commonly the US. Of course, I applied to Dr Terry and to Dr Iqbal, the most active researchers in this field, but my application was politely declined. In 1980, when I was a manager of the department, Dr Edward D. Bird visited us, who was well known for his work on the GABA depletion in Huntington's disease brain. I learned that he was running a brain bank in McLean Hospital in Boston. He kindly asked me what I wanted to study in the US. Answering my wish, he said "I know of only one person in the center who is interested in Alzheimer's. I can pass your letter onto him". This was the start of my correspondence with

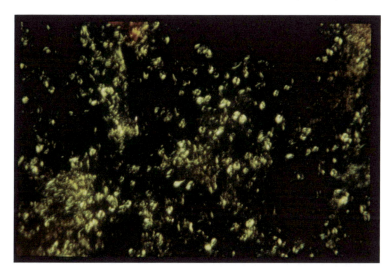

Fig. 1. SDS-NFT under polarized light microscope. Pieces from AD cortices were homogenized in 2% SDS buffer containing 1% β-mercaptoethanol and heated to 90°C for 10 min. SDS-insoluble stuff was collected by low-speed centrifugation, and smeared on glass slides, followed by staining with 0.1% Congo red, and viewed under polarized light. A great number of ring-shaped, globose-typed NFT maintain their configurations and show Congo-red birefringence. Original magnification, x200. Taken from *Jikken Igaku* (cover; Vol 4, No 11, 1986) with permission.

Dennis J. Selkoe. At that time, Dennis was only a newcomer, and known to only a limited number of people for his work on aluminum-induced fibrous pathology at Dr Shelanski's laboratory [14].

In the middle of April 1981, I arrived at Logan airport. It was a gloomy day, typical of Boston in early spring. I picked up my luggage and stepped down the staircase to the exit. A handsome young man was at the end of the staircase, and whispered to me just as I passed him, "Dr Ihara". It was Dennis J Selkoe, who was working at the Mailman Research Center, McLean Hospital, Belmont. The next morning, Dennis and I discussed in his very small office what I should do for the next two years in his laboratory. Dennis showed me a memo pad on which about twenty project titles were listed. I replied, "I have no interest in any but this". It read "purification of NFT from AD brain". "It will be difficult," said Dennis. "Is that all right with you?" "No problem!" I replied.

It was quite a small lab. Besides Dennis, there were only three people working there: Kenneth S. Kosik as a post doc, Carmela Abraham as a technician, and one more technician, who soon left the lab. A secretary told me that it had been more than 20 years since she had met Japanese researchers at the Folch-Pi lab. The best thing for me was that there were many nonfixed AD brain slices in the deep freezer that should have contained abundant NFT: this was what had brought me to the US. But I was a little discouraged by the poor equipment in the research center. In particular, there was only an old-fashioned ultracentrifuge (for example, a Beckman type L centrifuge, which I had never seen in Japan) and no SW50.1 rotor (Beckman), which was the most convenient for subcellular fractionation. We borrowed a rotor from a lab at the Eunice Kennedy Shriver Center (Waltham, MA) not far from our laboratory, but on which only two buckets could hook. I was also surprised to see that many old machines were carefully maintained and still working. A huge Zeiss fluorescence microscope in the core facility was made in the 1950s! One thing I brought to the US with me was a mini gel system, which I had rightly thought was not available in the US.

5. Insolubility of NFT/PHF

I started to work in the lab in the middle of May 1981. Of course, my goal was the purification of PHF and identification of their components. At that time, Dennis confirmed that PHF are insoluble in 2% Triton X-100, as judged by electron microscopy and, using the detergent, he obtained a PHF-enriched fraction, but found no difference in the bands on 1D gel or in the spots on 2D gel between AD and control brains. In particular, he could not find the so-called PHF-P (PHF protein) at $\sim$ 50 kD, persistently claimed to be a PHF component [6]. Dennis was absolutely puzzled by the conflicting observations, and I believed that the purifi-

Fig. 2. Purified SDS-NFT under polarized light microscope. An aliquot from 1.4/2.0 M sucrose interface was smeared on a glass slide, followed by addition of 0.1% Congo red. Globose NFT were overwhelmed by needle-like tangles, which resemble velvet. Original magnification, x200.

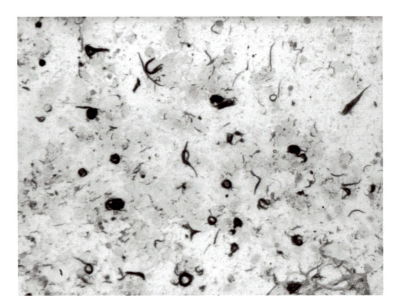

Fig. 3. NFT stained specifically with an antiserum to SDS-NFT. Pieces of AD cortex were Dounce-homogenized in Tris saline (TS) buffer, followed by differential centrifugation. Nuclear fraction was saved and aliquots were smeared on glass slides, which was processed for immunostaining with anti-PHF. Original magnification, x200.

cation was not adequate for detecting PHF components.

What I tried first was to establish an easy method of quantifying NFT under a light microscope. If one had to depend on EM for identification and quantification of PHF every time, it would be highly time-consuming. I remember it took me more than one week for electron microscopic observation, and only when the technician agreed to Dennis's urgent request. Regarding the assay method, I had already performed some preliminary experiments in Japan, and had found that thioflavin T was never good for raw materials: it gave so much nonspecific fluorescence as to interfere with NFT identification. I tested Congo-red birefringence of NFT. The dye was not so sensitive for NFT in the formalin-fixed, paraffin-embedded section (for example, neuropil threads were not visualized), but as far as unfixed materials are used, it was highly sensitive and specific under polarized microscopy (Fig. 1). Dipping in 0.1% Congo red solution for < 1 min was enough for their

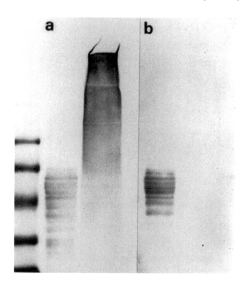

Fig. 4. Western blot with anti-PHF of TS-soluble (left lanes in a and b) and Sarkosyl-insoluble fractions (right lanes in a and b) from AD (a) and control brain homogenates (20%) (b). Specimens from 10% brain homogenates did not give such strong signals in the TS-soluble fraction. Several bands clustered at mid molecular range represent tau. A strongly stained smear (a, right) is seen in AD but not control brain.

observation!

Now that I had a semiquantitative assay method for NFT, I was in a position to examine each purification step for its effectiveness quite easily. From Dennis' data, NFT were insoluble in the nonionic detergent. I selected urea, the most frequently used denaturant, to try differential solubilization: an old and somewhat tricky technique. One day in June 1981, I tested the solubility of NFT by increasing the concentrations of urea in the NFT suspension: 2 M, 4 M, to 6 M, step by step. Most surprisingly, 6 M urea did not solubilize NFTs in the suspension at all as judged by polarized microscopy. This was true even with 8 M urea. I immediately moved to 6 M guanidine-HCl and 2% SDS, and finally heated 2% SDS with or without 1% β-mercaptoethanol [15]. NFT were present with no noticeable morphological alterations! (Fig. 1) NFT are indeed insoluble in such harsh denaturants and detergents, which were the most commonly used reagents to solubilize any protein. This was when I learned that even a strong detergent that is believed to solubilize any protein cannot bring NFT into solution. Immediately I realized that this insolubility could explain Dennis's enigmatic observations that even PHF-enriched fraction never showed a protein that was not also found in control brains. We had simply confirmed that in the SDS/urea-solubilized fraction there was no significant difference between AD and control brains. If that were the case, so-called PHF-P should not be the component of PHF, but presumably represent GFA (glial fibrillary acidic protein). This was also suggested by the observation on the protein composition of Huntington's disease brain [17]. It was as if I had got a beautiful whole picture at the summit when the clouds had suddenly cleared.

SDS–NFT became excellent specimens for determining whether the antibodies bind to integral components making up the PHF framework, rather than their associated proteins. As electron microscopic pictures showed, after SDS treatment, individual PHF became thinner and cleaner on their surface [15]. Thus SDS–NFT were believed to be composed exclusively of the integral component(s). If a certain antiserum can label SDS–NFT, it would be a particular antibody that reacted with the real component but not loosely associated proteins. Using SDS-NFT specimens and several NF antibodies, by the fall of 1982 I had a strong feeling that PHF were not altered NF. I heard from Dennis that major researchers who were interested in NFT/PHF agreed at a semiclosed meeting in the summer that PHF are derived from NF.

Then why are NFT or PHF insoluble in harsh denaturants or detergents? A possible explanation for me was that the component was cross-linked to make up PHF. I had never come across the idea that a certain noncovalent bond could be quite resistant to the detergent, exhibiting apparent insolubility. Through reading a certain volume of Methods in Enzymology, I came to know transglutaminase that can catalyze the formation of a covalent bond between free amine groups (e.g., protein- or peptide-bound lysine) and the gamma-carboxyamide group of protein- or peptide-bound glutamine. It is known that transglutaminase forms extensively crosslinked generally insoluble protein polymers. Carmela mixed transglutaminase and isolated NF *in vitro*, but could not generate PHF, although insoluble NF polymers were produced [16]. Besides ε–γ cross-linking, dityrosine was another well-characterized one. One day I noted a white-blue fluorescence at the 1.4/2.0 M interface where purified PHF are located (see below), but its emission spectrum was found later to be different from that of dityrosine, which emits a real blue fluorescence.

6. Preparation of PHF antibodies and PHF-smear

This insolubility characteristic makes NFT purification quite easy: homogenizing AD cortical pieces in

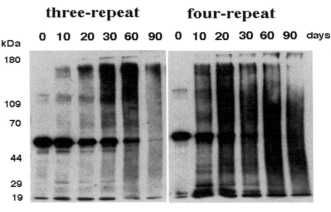

Fig. 5. Smearing of recombinant three- and four-repeat tau by prolonged incubation. Purified recombinant three- and four-repeat tau (0.1 mg/mL) were incubated in 0.1 M sodium phosphate buffer, pH 7.4, at 37°C, under sterile conditions for 10 to 90 days. The SDS sample buffer was added to each tube at the indicated day, followed by western blotting with TM2, a monoclonal antibody to carboxyl terminal portion of tau. Extensive smears emerged after 20-day incubation. Four-repeat tau disappeared significantly faster than did three-repeat tau.

hot SDS buffer containing 1% β-mercaptoethanol, followed by centrifugation to collect the insoluble product in which NFT should become enriched. Thus, the insoluble stuff was further fractionated by sucrose density gradient centrifugation. PHF were mainly collected at the interface of 1.4/2.0 M. As you can see in Fig. 2, fine or thinner bundles as well as typical perikaryal NFT were also enriched in the interface and showed Congo-red birefringence. When sucrose layers were made of 1.0/1.2/1.4/1.8/2.0 M, large NFT were recovered at the interface of 1.8/2.0 M, while needle-like NFT were exclusively seen at the 1.4/1.8 M interface. At first, I did not realize that the stuff showing velvet-like birefringence (see Fig. 2) also represented PHF. Only time-consuming electron microscopy confirmed my assumption. Senile plaque cores were also insoluble in SDS, and only partial separation from PHF was possible: cores were heavier than NFT and recovered in the 2.0 M sucrose layer below the 1.4/2.0 M interface. Thanks to insolubility, I finally succeeded in substantially purifying PHF, but had one problem: protein determination. Because of the high insolubility of PHF, conventional methods cannot be applied, and I had to undertake an alkaline hydrolysis method that I had never attempted before. The method took me more than half a day for protein determination of several samples! At most, 2–4 mg of PHF from 1 g of wet weight AD cortex (corresponding to ∼1/20–1/40 of the total protein) was recovered at the 1.4/2.0 M interface.

I then moved to the next step: identification of the PHF component. I thought that I could soon identify the component by releasing peptides from PHF using specific proteases, but it turned out not to be the case until 1987 [9]. This is because purified SDS-NFT was resistant to any protease. Even proteinase K, an unusually nonspecific protease, cannot eliminate the Congo-red birefringence of NFT. I applied many proteases without success. At the end of 1981, I gave up this direction.

I came to the conclusion that if it is very difficult to handle the insoluble product, then one should deal with its precursor, which must be soluble in the cytoplasm. Thus, to identify the precursor, one must generate specific antibodies to PHF, and purified PHF were in my hands. I was rather skeptical about my chances of obtaining specific antibodies because of its resistance to proteases, but had no other good ideas. SDS-purified PHF were immunized to two rabbits. Most unexpectedly, both rabbits raised specific antibodies: the antisera stained isolated NFT very strongly (see Fig. 3), and those in the formalin-fixed, paraffin-embedded section intensely. Moreover, besides NFT, we observed for the first time extensive networks of thread-like structures (later called neuropil threads or curly fibers) throughout the AD neocortex [4]. The presence of curly fibers is consistent with an observation that innumerable needle-like small tangles, besides large NFT, are recovered from AD brains (see Fig. 2).

Now that I had confirmed specific labeling of NFT by the antibody, I was ready to identify a particular (SDS-) soluble precursor(s) for PHF in the AD brain homogenate. In May 1982, I prepared several brain homogenates from AD and control brains, and subjected them to western blotting using one of the antisera. At

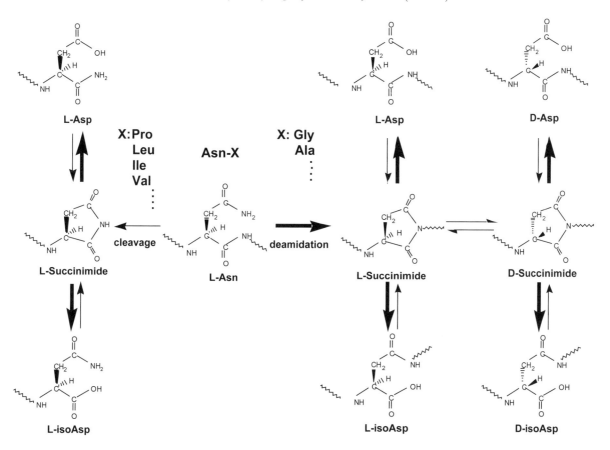

Fig. 6. Pathways for deamidation/isoaspartate formation and peptide bond cleavage through a succinimide intermediate. L-Asparaginyl residues can be converted spontaneously via a succinimidyl intermediate to form L-isoaspartyl and L-aspartyl residues (right). This reaction tends to occur when asparaginyl residues are followed by a small residue such as glycine. In contrast, when bulky residues, especially leucyl or prolyl residue, follow an asparaginyl residue, the peptide bond cleavage can occur through a succinimide intermediate (left).

the final stage of DAB (3, 3'-diaminobenzidine) development, Dennis and Carmela joined me just in time to observe the result. We had no doubt we would see in the next moment a distinct band(s) on the blot that can be labeled by the antiserum. "Something's coming out," shouted Carmela. Only in lanes for AD brain homogenates, but not for control homogenates, emerged smears [4] (later we called this PHF-smear) from high-molecular weight regions to low-molecular weight regions but no discrete bands. We had no words, and it was the first time we had seen such a peculiar western blot pattern. "This tells us something", said Dennis after a pause. I repeated the same experiments using total homogenates (10%) and soluble fractions. The results were the same: AD, but not control, samples always gave strong smears and no discrete bands. Of course, homogenates from AD cerebella did not show any reaction. In other words, smearing was a phenomenon specific to AD cortices and for NFT abundance. I sometimes came across several bands clustered around

~ 50 kD in the supernatant in AD and control brain homogenates, but never thought that these were significant because such bands were seen as well in the supernatants from control brains. I was very disappointed with these peculiar results and, at the same time, the smears of unknown origins were deeply etched on my memory. I never imagined that their elucidation would wait for another 20 years [18,19].

One day in June 1982, Dr Toyokura, professor of neurology, University of Tokyo Hospital, gave me a call and asked me to return to Japan by the fall. I knew that many senior staff had left the department, which was in a difficult situation regarding maintaining the levels of clinical practice. I continued experiments until the end of July 1982, and Carmela took over the experiments. The following year, we were able to submit a short paper to Nature [4], although the nature of the smears was not known.

7. Smears, twenty years later

In 1987–88, the two molecules, tau [8] and ubiquitin [9], were definitively identified as the major components of PHF, but the cause or significance of the smear on the blot have remained an enigma. The smear on the blot ranged from the gel top to ~10 kD, with the high molecular mass region showing the most intense immunoreactivity (Fig. 4). This smear is not an artifact during electrophoresis, but appears to represent a real molecular form, because (i) it was fractionated according to molecular sizes on gel filtration [10]; (ii) a close inspection of the blot reveals that the smear in the low molecular mass range consists of very fine, closely spaced, discrete bands; the minimal unit of reactive bands may migrate at 10–20 kD; and (iii) the smear reacts strongly with tau antibodies to the carboxyl-terminal portion, but not at all or only faintly with those to the amino-terminal portion [19]. Thus, I speculated that the smear was composed of carboxyl-terminal fragments that should have a strong tendency to aggregate into oligomers.

Ubiquitin was found to be bound to smeared tau, which raised the possibility that ubiquitin is responsible for the smearing, but this was not the case. There are two kinds of smears: ubiquitin-positive and ubiquitin-negative smears [10]. Thus, the ubiquitin-negative smeared tau was subjected to extensive protein chemical analysis. This was in late 1990s. The major difference between the soluble and smeared forms of tau was the presence of structurally altered asparaginyl and aspartyl residues in the microtubule-binding domain (Fig. 5). There was site-specific deamidation and isoaspartate formation (Asn-381 and Asp-387) in the domain from smeared tau *in vivo*, which had a stronger tendency to aggregate independently of disulfide bond formation [10].

Deamidation and isomerization are phenomena frequently seen in peptides and proteins that have been stored for a long time *in vitro* or have a long life *in vivo*, and have been interpreted as representing protein aging [2]. In view of this, we investigated the effect on carboxymethylated (SH-blocked) tau of prolonged incubation under near physiological conditions (at the concentrations of ~ 0.1 mg/mL). We finally found that prolonged incubation of recombinant tau *in vitro* leads to: (i) a smear on the blot very close to that originally described [4] (Fig. 6); (ii) site-specific deamidation and isomerization; and (iii) nonenzymatic cleavage at the carboxyl side of asparaginyl residues that are followed by a bulky residue (most of the asparaginyl residues are clustered within the microtubule-binding domain of tau). Furthermore, the sequencing of smeared tau *in vivo* obtained from AD brain identified similar degradation products starting from bulky residues next to asparaginyl residues. Thus, deamidation/isomerization and nonenzymatic cleavage at asparaginyl residues through a succinimide intermediate is the basis for smear formation on the blot, a unique characteristic of AD brain [18]. Elucidation of the nature of the smears has taken me more than twenty years! What is learned in the cradle is carried to the grave.

References

[1] B.H. Anderton, D. Breinburg, M.J. Downes, P.J. Green, B.E. Tomlinson, J. Ulrich, J.N. Wood and J. Kahn, Monoclonal antibodies show that neurofibrillary tangles and neurofilaments share antigenic determinants, *Nature* **298** (1982), 84–86.

[2] D.W. Aswad, in: *Deamidation and isoaspartate formation in peptides and proteins*, D.W. Aswad, ed., CRC Press, Boca Raton, FL, 1995, pp. 1–6.

[3] P. Gambetti, G. Shecket, B. Ghetti, A. Hirano and D. Dahl, Neurofibrillary changes in human brain. An immunocytochemical study with a neurofilament antiserum, *J. Neuropathol. Exp. Neurol.* **42** (1983), 69–79.

[4] Y. Ihara, C. Abraham and D.J. Selkoe, Antibodies to paired helical filaments in Alzheimer's disease do not recognize normal brain proteins, *Nature* **304** (1983), 727–729.

[5] Y. Ihara, N. Nukina, H. Sugita and Y. Toyokura, Staining of Alzheimer's neurofibrillary tangles with antiserum against 200 K component of neurofilament, *Proc. Japan Acad.* **58B** (1981), 152–156.

[6] K. Iqbal, H.M. Wisniewski, M.L. Shelanski, S. Brostoff, B.H. Liwnicz and R.D. Terry, Protein changes in senile dementia, *Brain Res.* **77** (1974), 337–343.

[7] T. Ishii, S. Haga and S. Tokutake, Presence of neurofilament protein in Alzheimer's neurofibrillary tangles (ANT). An immunofluorescent study, *Acta Neuropathol.* **48** (1979), 105–112.

[8] J. Kondo, T. Honda, H. Mori, Y. Hamada, R. Miura, M. Ogawara and Y. Ihara, The carboxyl third of tau is tightly bound to paired helical filaments, *Neuron* **1** (1988), 827–834.

[9] H. Mori, J. Kondo and Y. Ihara, Ubiquitin is a component of paired helical filaments in Alzheimer's disease, *Science* **235** (1987), 1641–1644.

[10] M. Morishima-Kawashima, M. Hasegawa, K. Takio, M. Suzuki, K. Titani and Y. Ihara, Ubiquitin is conjugated with amino-terminally processed tau in paired helical filaments, *Neuron* **10** (1993), 1151–1160.

[11] T. Nishimura, S. Hariguchi and Z. Kaneko, *Changes in brain water-soluble proteins in presenile and senile dementia*, VIIth International Congress of Neuropathology, Excerpta Medica, Amsterdam, 1975, 139–142.

[12] S. Oyanagi, An electron microscopic observation on senile dementia, with special references to transformation of neurofilaments to twisted tubules and a structural connection of Pick bodies to Alzheimer's neurofibrillary changes, *Shinkei Kenkyuu No Shimpo* **18** (1974), 77–88.

[13] W.W. Schlaepfer, Deformation of isolated neurofilaments and the pathogenesis of neurofibrillary pathology, *J. Neuropathol. Exp. Neurol.* **38** (1978), 244–254.

[14] D.J. Selkoe, R.K. Liem, S.H. Yen and M.L. Shelanski, Biochemical and immunological characterization of neurofilaments in experimental neurofibrillary degeneration induced by aluminum, *Brain Res.* **16** (1979), 235–252.

[15] D.J. Selkoe, Y. Ihara and F.J. Salazar, Alzheimer's disease: insolubility of partially purified paired helical filaments in sodium dodecyl sulfate and urea, *Science* **215** (1982), 1243–1245.

[16] D.J. Selkoe, C. Abraham and Y. Ihara, Brain transglutaminase; In vitro crosslinking of human neurofilament proteins into insoluble polymers, *Proc. Natl. Acad. Sci. USA* **79** (1982), 6070–6074.

[17] D.J. Selkoe, F.J. Salazar, C. Abraham and K.S. Kosik, Huntington's disease: changes in striatal proteins reflect astrocytic gliosis, *Brain Res.* **245** (1982), 117–125.

[18] A. Watanabe, W.-K. Hong, N. Dohmae, K. Takio, M. Morishima-Kawashima and Y. Ihara, Molecular aging of tau: disulfide-independent aggregation and nonenzymatic degradation *in vitro* and *in vivo*, *J. Neurochem.* **90** (2004), 1302–1311.

[19] A. Watanabe, K. Takio and Y. Ihara, Deamidation and isoaspartate formation in smeared tau in paired helical filaments-unusual properties of the microtubule-binding domain of tau, *J. Biol. Chem.* **274** (1999), 7368–7378.

[20] H.M. Wisniewski, H.K. Narang and R.D. Terry, Neurofibrillary tangles of paired helical filaments, *J. Neurol. Sci.* **27** (1976), 173–181.

[21] N. Yoshimura, Evidence that paired helical filaments originate from neurofilaments-electron microscope observations of neurites in senile plaques in the brain in Alzheimer's disease, *Clin Neuropathol.* **3** (1984), 22–27.

Discoveries of Tau, abnormally hyperphosphorylated tau and others of neurofibrillary degeneration: A personal historical perspective

Khalid Iqbal* and Inge Grundke-Iqbal
New York State Institute for Basic Research, in Developmental Disabilities, Department of Neurochemistry, 1050 Forest Hill Road, Staten Island, New York 10314-6399, USA
E-mail: iqbalk@worldnet.att.net, i_g_iqbal@yahoo.com

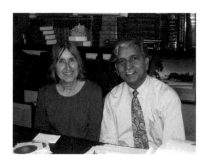

Abstract. Alzheimer disease was described by Alois Alzheimer in 1907, but it was not until ∼ 60–70 years later that any new significant developments were reported on the pathology of this disease. The discoveries that laid down the foundation for the exciting research that has been carried out during the last ∼ 20 years and that have significantly enhanced our understanding of the disease are the ultrastructure of neurofibrillary tangles and neuritic (senile) plaques, the clinical-pathological correlation of these lesions to the presence of dementia, and the bulk isolation and protein composition of paired helical filaments and plaque amyloid. We discovered tau as the major protein subunit of paired helical filaments/neurofibrillary tangles, the abnormal hyperphosphorylation of this protein in this lesion and in Alzheimer brain cytosol and the gain of toxic function by the cytosolic abnormally hyperphosphorylated tau in Alzheimer brain. Here we present a personal historical account of the work in our laboratories that led, in 1986, to the discoveries of tau and its abnormal hyperphosphorylation in paired helical filaments and Alzheimer brain cytosol. This article also describes several major findings which subsequently resulted from the abnormal hyperphosphorylation of tau and in a large part account for the current understanding of the role of this lesion in Alzheimer disease and other tauopathies.

Keywords: Tau, abnormally hyperphosphorylated tau, neurofibrillary tangles, paired helical filaments, self-assembly of tau, protein phosphatase-2A, protein phosphatase-1, microtubule assembly, MAP1, MAP2, glycogen synthase kinase-3β, cyclin-dependent protein kinase-5, protein kinase A

Neurofibrillary degeneration and neuritic (senile) plaques are the two histopathological hallmarks of Alzheimer disease (AD) which were described by Alois Alzheimer in 1907. The number of laboratories involved and the pace of research on AD remained quite slow till the 1980s. Since then our understanding of the various mechanisms of the disease involved has been progressing at a very encouraging rate. The discoveries that laid the foundation for the exciting research that has been carried out during the last ∼ 20 years and that have resulted in very significant findings are (1) the ultrastructure of neurofibrillary tangles and neuritic (senile) plaques by Kidd [73,74] and by Terry [127, 128], and the quantitation of tangles and plaques and the clinical-pathological correlation of these lesions to

*Corresponding author.

the presence and the degree of dementia by Roth et al. [130]; and (2) the biochemical isolation of neurofibrillary tangles and plaque amyloid and the discoveries of the abnormally hyperphosphorylated tau as the major protein subunit of paired helical filaments (PHF) by our team [47,48,59,60], and of Aβ peptide as the major constituent of cerebral vascular and plaque amyloid by Glenner [31,147].

In 1973, Robert D. Terry and Robert Katzman organized a one-day symposium on aging and dementia at the Albert Einstein College of Medicine where we presented a preliminary report of bulk isolation and enrichment of PHF from AD brain. George Glenner, a senior investigator and expert on amyloids, gave a detailed talk on amyloids and their tinctorial properties. Later that afternoon, Henry Wisniewski hosted George Glenner, and K. Iqbal was also invited. George was very friendly and inquisitive about our work on the isolation of PHF. Several years later, he described the first successful isolation of amyloid-β (Aβ) and its β-peptide [31,147], and we showed the isolation of PHF and identification of tau and its abnormal hyperphosphorylation [47,48, 60].

This chapter describes the work that led to the bulk isolation of neurofibrillary tangles from AD brain, the discoveries of tau as the major protein subunit of PHF and of the abnormal hyperphosphorylation of tau in AD, and some of the advances made in the field in our laboratories since these discoveries.

1. Bulk isolation of neurofibrillary tangles, their polypeptide composition, and the identification of tau as the major protein subunit of PHF

Bulk isolation of PHF/neurofibrillary tangles from AD brain: In 1972, we developed a method for the bulk isolation of neuronal and glial cells from fresh and frozen human autopsied brains [57]. Because neurofibrillary tangles are seen in the perikarya of affected neurons, and the number of neurofibrillary tangles was known to correlate with the degree of dementia, the bulk isolation of the neuronal perikarya from the affected areas of AD brain could serve as an important initial step for the isolation of tangles/PHF.

Robert D. Terry, at that time the Head of Research on AD and the Chairman of the Department of Pathology at the Albert Einstein College of Medicine, Bronx, New York, recognized the importance of the newly developed technique and approached us to investigate the molecular composition of tangles/PHF.

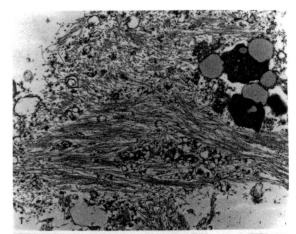
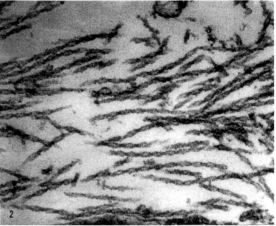

Fig. 1. An electron micrograph of a TT-enriched fraction obtained from the hippocampus of a patient with senile dementia. A: X 9,000 and b: X 60,000.
Reproduced with permission from Iqbal et al., Brain Res. 77:337–343, 1974.

Employing the protocol that we had developed for subcellular fractionation of neuronal perikarya isolated from Huntington disease brains [58], we succeeded in obtaining a tangles/PHF-enriched fraction by subcellular fractionation of neurons isolated from AD brain [59]. For these studies, the presence of tangles/PHF at all stages of tissue fractionation, from isolation of neuronal perikarya to the tangles/PHF-enriched fraction, was carried out by transmission electron microscopy (Fig. 1). All this laborious electron microscopic evaluation of the preparations was carried out by Henry M. Wisniewski.

After our 1974 report [59] was published, different protocols for the isolation of PHF were developed by different laboratories (Table 1). All of these subsequent methods, including those we developed [42,60,109],

Table 1
Methods for Bulk Isolation of PHF

Authors	Method
Iqbal et al., 1974 [59]	Nondenaturing conditions; isolation of neuronal perikarya, followed by conventional subcellular fractionation.
Grundke-Iqbal et al., 1981* [42] Iqbal et al., 1984 [60]	Isolation of neuronal perikarya, followed by treatment with 2% SDS at room temperature for 3–5 min. and sucrose density gradient centrifugations; Yield: 10–100 μg protein/g tissue
Selkoe et al., 1982 [113]	Differential centrifugation of tissue homogenate, followed by extraction in 2% Triton X-100; Yield: 1–2 mg protein/g tissue.
Ihara et al., 1983 [55]	Boiling of tissue homogenate in 2% SDS and 0.1 M β-mercaptoethanol buffered with 0.05 M Tris, pH 7.6; Yield: 50–80 μg/g tissue.
Masters et al., 1985 [91]	Extraction of tissue homogenate with salts and Triton X-100, followed by digestion with pepsin, sucrose discontinuous density gradient centrifugations, and extraction with 2% SDS.
Rubenstein et al., 1986 [109]	Differential and rate zonal centrifugation of tissue homogenate digested with proteinase-K and micrococcal nuclease and extracted by sonication with sarcosyl and sulfobetain 3–14; Yield: 0.2 μg/g tissue.
Greenberg and Davies, 1990 [39]	Treatment of 27,200 x g brain extract with 1% sarkosyl, followed by sedimentation at $\sim$ 80,000 x g and sucrose density gradient centrifugation; Yield: 7 μg/g tissue.

*Isolation of PHF employing treatment with SDS, polypeptide composition of isolated PHF and aggregation of PHF polypeptides at the top of the gel was presented for the first time at the Annual Meeting of the American Association of Neuropathologists in 1981.

involved the use of detergents for the purification of PHF.

1.1. Protein composition of PHF/neurofibrillary tangles

In the early 1970s, SDS-PAGE was a relatively new technique that became available to study the protein compositions of complex mixtures and to isolate microamounts of proteins purified by this technique. SDS-PAGE of the tangles/PHF-enriched preparations revealed the presence of five prominent protein bands, two of the upper three of which co-migrated with tubulin (Fig. 2). We named one of these protein bands neuronal protein (NP) and another, the $\sim$ 50 kDa band, enriched fraction band (EFP). We did so one year before microtubule-associated protein tau was described [143] and before any biochemical studies on AD were available in the literature. During those days, slab gel PAGE was a relatively new technique and the slab gel electrophoresis equipment and as well glass plates were handmade in the machine workshop of Albert Einstein College of Medicine.

1.2. Generation of the first antibody to PHF/neurofibrillary tangles and identification of PHF protein as a non-high molecular weight microtubule-associated protein

To confirm that EFP, which we renamed PHF protein (PHFP) was a protein subunit of PHF, we raised rabbit antibodies to this protein, purified by cutting out the protein band from Coomassie blue-stained slab gels of SDS-PAGE of the PHF-enriched fraction. The antiserum to PHFP stained neurofibrillary tangles and dystrophic neuritis of neuritic (senile) plaques in AD brain and produced a reaction line of identity with brain microtubule-associated protein (MAP) by Ouchterlony double diffusion test [40,41]. Employing the Ouchterlony double diffusion test, we demonstrated that PHFP reacted with a brain microtubule-associated protein (MAP) other than tubulin and higher-molecular weight (HMW) MAP [41]. We also raised an antiserum to human brain microtubules that reacted with PHFP and labeled neurofibrillary tangles in AD brain [40]. On the basis of these findings, we were confident that we had the PHFP and that it was a MAP other than the HMW MAPs. At this stage, we took a two-pronged approach: (1) to further purify the PHF-enriched fraction and study its protein composition, and (2) to purify the MAP with which the Alzheimer neurofibrillary tangles (ANT) crossreacted, the ANT-crossreacting antigen (ANTCA).

During our studies on the purification of tangles/PHF from AD brains, we observed that the isolated tangles looked like very clean preparations after staining with Congo red, producing beautiful apple-green birefringence. However, when viewed by phase contrast microscopy, the same preparations showed heavy contamination with what appeared to be mostly membranes. To achieve higher purity of tangles/PHF, we first tried treatment with TritonX-100 and then replaced it with the inclusion of 2% SDS in the sucrose gradient solutions [60]. With this detergent treatment, we were able to isolate highly purified PHF/tangles (Fig. 3).

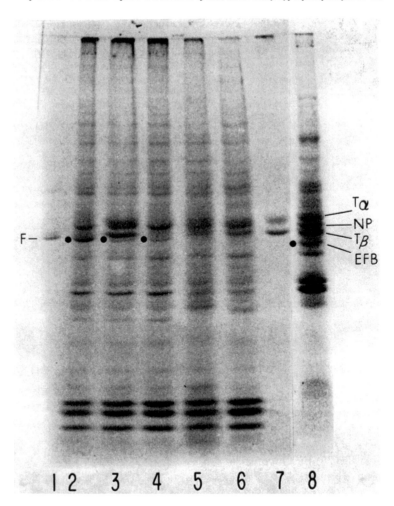

Fig. 2. Sodium dodecyl sulfate (SDS)-polyacrylamide slab gels showing protein patterns of: 1: purified bovine neurofilament protein (F). Mol. Wt. of major band is 51,000; 2: total neuronal proteins from a case of senile dementia mixed with the filament protein; 3: total neuronal proteins as in 2 but mixed with purified human brain tubulin; 4, 5, 6: total neuronal proteins respectively from a case of senile dementia, a normal adult control, and a normal young (5-year-old) control; 7: purified human brain tubulin, β-monomer, mol. Wt. 56,000, β-monomer, mol. Wt. 53,000; 8: a separate but similar gel with TT-enriched fraction from another senile dementia patient. F is the major neurofilament protein subunit; T_α and T_β are the α- and β-monomers of tubulin respectively; NP is a neuronal protein which migrates between the two tubulin monomers; and EFB is the new band corresponding to the enrichment of twisted tubules. Dots on the left side of samples 2, 3, 4 and 8 indicate the position of the band (EFB). Other differences seen in the electrophoretic patterns between diseased and control brain fractions were not consistent. Reproduced with permission from Iqbal, et al., Brain Res. 77:337–343, 1974.

1.3. Controversy on the solubility of PHF

A serious setback in the field: At the 1981 Annual Meeting of the American Association of Neuropathologists, we presented our technique for the bulk isolation of PHF/tangles using detergent and showed that PHF were made of proteins with molecular weights of around 50–70 kDa. Dennis Selkoe contradicted our findings, stating that the tangles were insoluble structures and that their protein composition could not be studied. The paper by Selkoe et al. [113] that appeared in Science, the first paper on AD ever published in that journal, claimed that tangles/PHF, like β-crystallines in senile cataracts [90], probably were made up of polypeptides crosslinked by γ-glutamyl-ε-lysine, and their protein composition could not be studied by SDS-PAGE.

The significant impact that Selkoe's Science paper had on the field was astonishing and concerning. Nobody critically evaluated that we had, over several years demonstrated the biochemical isolation of tangles/PHF, identified a protein in these preparations, and shown that antibodies to this protein labeled tangles in AD brain and that antibodies to a MAP with which this pro-

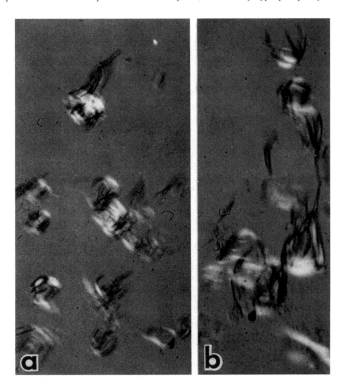

Fig. 3. Congo red birefringence of isolated ANT. A light micrograph of ANT isolated from an Alzheinmer brain and stained with congo red showing birefringence in polarized light; a, ANT isolated by long procedure and b, by short procedure as described in Materials and Methods. X 490.
Reproduced with permission from Iqbal et al., Acta Neuropathol. (Berl) 62:167–177, 1984.

tein crossreacted had also labeled AD tangles [40,41, 59]. Most of the prominent AD researchers accepted the thesis proposed in the *Science* paper, which did not provide any data on γ-glutamyl-ε-lysine crosslinks in tangles/PHF. Several reviews, including a major one in *Scientific American*, were published, accepting the insolubility of PHF and its γ-glutamyl-ε-lysine hypothesis. Even scientists in our own Institute accepted the γ-glutamyl-ε-lysine crosslinking hypothesis and raised questions about our several years of work on PHF protein composition. Henry M. Wisniewski, the Director of our Institute at that time, even assigned some scientists at our Institute to test the solubility of PHF. All this led us to carry out further extensive studies to purify PHF from AD brain and to quantitatively demonstrate their solubility and protein composition by SDS-PAGE. These studies took almost three years and showed that the solubility of PHF was wide-ranging, from being easily soluble in detergent to requiring repeated extractions with SDS-β-mercaptoethanol and that PHF were made up mostly of proteins from 45–70 kDa and their oligomers of proteins of a whole range of molecular sizes [64].

1.4. Generation of monoclonal and polyclonal antibodies to PHF isolated from AD brains and immunolabeling of tangles/PHF in tissue sections and 45 kDa–62 kDa polypeptides in isolated PHF preparations

We generated both monoclonal [60] and polyclonal [43–45] antibodies against PHF purified from AD brains [60]. These antibodies labeled neurofibrillary tangles and plaque neurites in AD brain sections, and six protein bands in the 50-kDa–70-kDa area, a typical tau pattern on Western blots of isolated PHF. By immunoabsorption of the polyclonal antibodies to PHF and antisera to microtubules which labeled tangles on tissue sections, with tubulin, HMW MAP, neurofilament triplet, keratin, and fibroblast lysates as a source of tubulin and vimentin, we concluded that PHF polypeptides were MAP of $\sim$ 50 kDA–70 kDa [44].

2. Discovery of tau as the major protein subunit of PHF

While on one hand our work on purification of tangles/PHF from AD brains, their protein composition and development of their Western blots with antibodies to PHF had led us to patterns of molecular sizes of MAP-tau, we had also in parallel studies pursued the identification of the tangle-crossreacting antigen in brain microtubules, based on our 1979 observations [40]. We observed that the tangle staining of anti-PHF serum and of anti-microtubule sera could be absorbed only with tau and not with HMW MAP. However, having endured almost four years of intense controversy and arguments on the solubility of PHF, we had become very careful not to publish any new findings without being certain of them by several forms of evidence.

Since we had established that PHF protein was a normal brain microtubule protein other than tubulin and HMW MAP, we purified tau from bovine brain by five different methods. All of these tau preparations reacted specifically with antibodies to PHF [47]. Employing these purified tau preparations, we affinity-purified antibodies to each of the six brain tau isoforms from the anti-PHF serum and showed that antibodies to each tau isoform reacted with most neurofibrillary tangles on AD brain sections and with all six tau isoforms in normal brain tau as well as in isolated PHF on Western blots (Fig. 4). Employing PHF purified from AD brains, we also demonstrated colocalization of the PHF polypeptides with the six brain tau isoforms by SDS-PAGE [47]. We were most excited that our systematic approach of the previous ∼12 years had finally resulted in the identification of tau as a major protein subunit of PHF.

The immunohistochemical staining of PHF/neurofibrillary tangles with antibodies to neurofilaments [8,25,30,67,103], vimentin [150], HMW-MAP [77], somatostatin [108], and tau [16,27,56,78,148] was observed by several laboratories. However, immunohistochemical crossreactivity between two proteins does not necessarily allow one to assume any precursor-product relationship. The size of an antigenic site detected by an antibody is relatively small, and identical or closely related antigenic sites comprising a few amino acid residues have been found on molecules that are otherwise unrelated, e.g., between the transforming proteins of Rous sarcoma virus and tubulin, myosin, and vimentin [95]; between thymus and neuronal cell surface proteins [34]; and between rabbit IgG and PHF/tangles [46]. Furthermore, it is not possible to determine with immunohistochemical techniques alone whether crossreactivities may be due to similarities in primary amino acid sequence or to antigenic sites created from folding of different regions of a polypeptide chain, i.e., conformation site(s) [13].

We completed our manuscript on tau by early summer of 1985. We took this manuscript and one on abnormal hyperphosphorylation of tau (see below) with us on our vacation to Germany for final editing. We knew we had an important discovery at hand and decided to submit our paper to Lancet. On September 20, 1985, we received acknowledgement of the receipt of this paper from Lancet. After several days, the editor of Lancet returned our manuscript without reviews, stating that he had a large backlog of papers and did not want to increase this backlog with our paper. We then submitted it to the Journal of Cell Biology, whose reviewers suggested that we try a specialty journal. We then submitted the paper for publication in the Journal of Biological Chemistry (J. Biol. Chem.), where a reviewer stated that our previous paper published in Acta Neuropathologica [45] had unmistakably shown tau bands in Western blots of PHF. To our surprise, this reviewer also pointed out that John Brion, in the Journal of Submicroscopic Cytology [17], had already shown immunohistochemical labeling of neurofibrillary tangles in AD brain with an antibody to tau. We were shocked that we did not know of this finding, especially because John Brion and his collaborator, Flamment Durrand, had inquired of us a lot about our data on the identification of the protein composition of PHF at the International Neuropathology Meeting but never mentioned that they were carrying out similar studies. We asked our Institute librarian to get a copy of J. Brion's publication through interlibrary service. We were greatly relieved to see this publication, because it reported that antisera to PHF could not be absorbed with normal brain proteins including the microtubule preparations.

We had revised our J. Biol. Chem. manuscript and put together a cover letter to the editor, enclosing J. Brion's paper and showing that prior to us, nobody had shown the presence of tau in PHF. It was December 23, 1985, and we had a second manuscript on abnormal hyperphosphorylation of tau ready for submission for publication in the Proceedings of the National Academy of Sciences, USA (Proc. Natl. Acad. Sci. USA) (see below). Because of unreliable mail during the Christmas season, we had decided to drive to Rockefeller University, New York, NY, which is about a 45-minute drive from our Institute, to personally submit the Proc. Natl. Acad. Sci. USA manuscript to Philip Siekevitz, who had agreed earlier to handle our manuscript as a member editor of the National Academy of Sciences. We parked our car on the street in front of Rockefeller University and put our briefcases

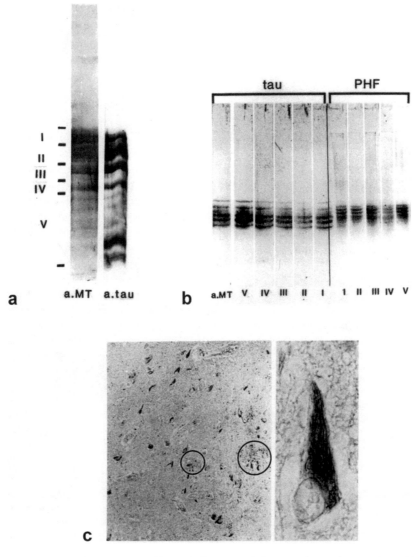

Fig. 4. Labeling of tau and PHF polypeptides on Western blots and of tangles and plaque neurites on tissue sections with antibodies purified by immunoaffinity from five different molecular species of tau. For a, tau (Method 3) was electrophoresed on SDS-polyacrylamide gels (12.5% acrylamide, 16 X 11 cm) and transferred to nitrocellulose paper. Strips were cut from the sides and developed with anti-MT (PHF) serum (*a. MT*) and monoclonal antibody to tau (*a, tau*). The remaining blot was sued for affinity isolation of anti-tau antibodies from the anti-MT(PHF) serum. Roman numerals (*I–V*) indicate the areas of tau species from which the antibodies wre purified. For details see "Materials and Methods". In *b*, immunoblots of tau and PHF polypeptides with affinity-purified antibodies from tau polypeptides of areas I–V are shown. Electro-transfer from SDS gel, 7–10% acrylamide (8 X 6 cm). Differences in the staining intensities of the different antibodies are due to small individual viations in the amounts of the samples applied to the gel. C shows immunocytochemical staining of tangles (some of the tangles marked with *arrows*) and neurites of plaques (marked with *circles*) in paraffin sections of Alzheimer hippocampus with antibodies eluted from tau area I (*left panel*); the background staining might correspond to the normal distribution of tau. The *right panel* shows at high magnification a neuron with the fibrils of its tangle darkly stained by the antibody. Original magnifications: *left panel*, X 130; *right panel*, X 1500. Identical staining was obtained with antibodies eluted from the other four tau areas; plaque amyloid was not stained with any of these five antibodies.
Reproduced with permission from Grundke-Iqbal et al., J. Biol. Chem. 261:6084–6089, 1986.

in the car trunk. When we reached home after seeing Philip Siekevitz, we found that our two briefcases and the Christmas shopping we had done were all gone, because somebody had broken into our car trunk and stolen everything. The biggest loss was our revised J. Biol. Chem. manuscript, the reviewers' comments, and all the relevant papers and calculations. We called the editor (Edward D. Korn) the next day and left a message on requesting that he resend us the reviewer comments. It took a grueling two weeks of work to

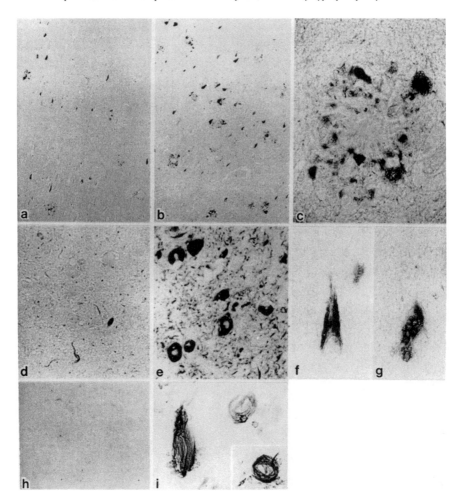

Fig. 5. Immunocytochemical staining with mAb to τ and the effect of dephosphorylation. (*a–c, f, g*) Sections of Alzheimer hippocampus and (*d, e*) temporal cortex; (*h*) section of hippocampus of a 80-year-old non-Alzheimer dementia individual; (*i*) tangle-enriched preparation that had been washed twice with 2% (wt/vol) NaDodSO$_4$ in a boiling water bath. (*b, c, e–h*) Sections were dephosphorylated with alkaline phosphatase prior to immunolabeling; (*a and d*) nondephosphorylated controls; adjacent sections and corresponding areas to *b* and *e* treated identically except that the alkaline phosphatase was substituted with buffer. Numbers of immunostained tangles, plaques, and neuropil threads are very much increased in the dephosphorylated tissue sections in *b* and *e* as compared to the control treated sections in *a* and *d*. (*c*) Staining of plaque neurites but not of central core amyloid; (*f*) a neuron with immunolabeled tangle extending into the apical dendrite; (*g*) a neuron with granulovacuolar inclusions; (*h*) no staining is seen in the non0Alzheimer hippocampus even after dephosphorylation. (*a, b*) X 75; (*c, f, g*, and *I*) X 750; (*d, e*) X 300; (*h*) X 150.
Reproduced with permission from Grundke-Iqbal et al., Proc. Natl. Acad. Sci. USA 83:4913–4917, 1986.

find and recalculate some data and to revise and resubmit the manuscript, which was accepted and then was published in the May 5th, 1986, issue of J. Biol. Chem. [47].

3. Discovery of the abnormal hyperphosphorylation of tau

In December 1984, we attended a conference of the New York Academy of Sciences on Dynamic Aspects of Microtubule Biology, where Lester (Skip) I. Binder presented on the immunohistochemical localization of tau using monoclonal antibody (mAb) Tau-1 to tau, which he and his colleagues had generated [14]. We met him for the first time at this meeting and asked him if we could have some Tau-1, which he very graciously provided us. When we tested Tau-1, although it reacted very nicely and specifically with all six isoforms of normal brain tau on Western blots, we found that it immunostained only a small number of neurofibrillary tangles in AD brain sections compared to our anti-PHF serum and immunoaffinity-purified tau antibodies. We wanted to know the reason for this discrepancy. We called Skip Binder and inquired if Tau-1 was phosphodependent and found that he had not studied this aspect and could not help us with this information. We undertook this study and found that Tau-1 labeled practically all tangles and plaque neurites when tissue was first pretreated with alkaline phosphatase (Fig. 5). This finding suggested that Tau-1 was phosphodependent and recognized only dephosphorylated tau at the epitope recognized by this antibody, and that tau in tangles/PHF was in an abnormally phosphorylated state [48]. Furthermore, we found that Tau-1 could label PHF polypeptides on Western blots only when they were first dephosphorylated either in a test tube prior to SDS-PAGE, or on the nitrocellulose membrane used for the Western blots (Fig. 6). Because tau, a phosphoprotein, was phosphorylated in PHF/AD brain differently than that from normal brain tau, we coined the term "the abnormally phosphorylated tau" [48].

We were thrilled with the discovery that tau in tangles/PHF was abnormally phosphorylated. When the manuscript was completed for submission for publication in Proc. Natl. Acad. Sci. USA, we felt that although Skip Binder had supplied us the mAb Tau-1 as a gift, we should offer him co-authorship of the article. We called Skip and described to him the discovery we had made employing his tau antibody. He was totally surprised, both by the fact that his mAb Tau-1 was phosphodependent and that tau in PHF was abnormally hyperphosphorylated. He was very happy that we offered him co-authorship, which he readily accepted. We sent Skip a copy of the manuscript for his input. He called back after going through the manuscript, disclosing that he had been working with John Wood (Emory University) on immunohistochemical staining of AD brain using his mAb Tau-1, and after reading our manuscript, he (Skip Binder) understood why they could not immunostain more than a few tangles with Tau-1. Furthermore, Skip informed us that they had no idea about the possibility of abnormal phosphorylation of tau in tangles/PHF and that John (Wood) "fell from his chair" when he (Skip) informed him of our findings. Skip also told us that they had a paper on their work on immunohistochemical staining of tangles with Tau-1 in review for Proc. Natl. Acad. Sci. USA. The paper by Wood et al. appeared in the June 1986, issue of Proc. Natl. Acad. Sci. USA [148] and, to our horror, it included dephosphorylation studies and claimed that tau was abnormally phosphorylated – without citing or acknowledging that they had carried out those studies on the basis of information from us via Skip Binder. After our strong protest, they agreed to publish a correction (Proc. Natl. Acad. Sci. USA, 83:9773, 1986) citing our paper [48] which was in press at that time.

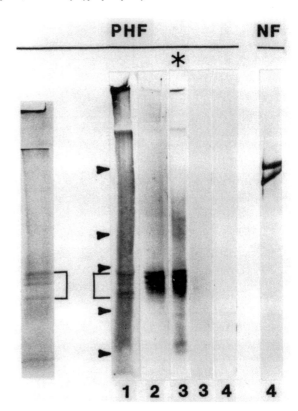

Fig. 6. Immunoblots of PHF polypeptides with (lane 1) antiserum to isolated PHF, 1:1,000 dilution; (lane 2) PHF-reactive anti-microtubule serum, 1:3,000 dilution; (lane 3) mAb to τ at 0.1 μg/ml on dephosphorylated (*) and nondephosphorylated blots and (lane 4) blots of PHF and neurofilament (NF) polypeptides with mAb to NF, SMI 34, 1:10,000 dilution. (#) The dephosphorylation of PHF polypeptides on the paper blots was carried out with alkaline phosphatase (43 μg/ml) before incubation with antibody. Preoteins were electrotransferred from NaDodSO$_4$/polyacrylamide gel, 5–15% acrylamide gradient. Arrowheads indicate positions of M_t markers from tot to bottom: myosin (200,000), phosphorylase b (92,500), bovine serum albumin (68,000), ovalbumin (43,000), α-chymotrypsinogen (25,700). Not shown in this figure, even at a 10-fold increase in the antibody concentration mAb SMI 34 did not label PHF polypeptides. The background smear and the low M_t bands in lane 1 most probably represent oligomers and breakdown products, respectively, of the PHF polypeptides (3–5); similar immunostaining pattern is obtained with mAb to PHF (5). The far left lane shows the Coomassie blue-stained polypeptide pattern of isolated PHF (5-030T acrylamide gradient).
Reproduced with permission fro Grundke-Iqbal et al., Proc. Natl. Acad. Sci. USA, 83:4913–4917, 1986.

4. Discovery of the microtubule assembly defect and the cytosolic abnormal hyperphosphorylation of tau in AD brain

Since our observation reported in 1979 [40] that a microtubule-associated protein crossreacted with PHF protein, we had initiated studies to prepare microtubules by *in vitro* assembly from short-term post-

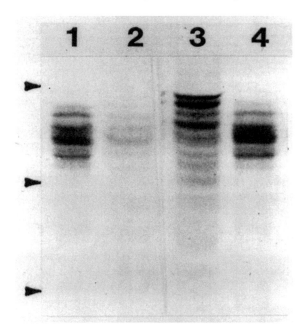

Fig. 7. Western blots of microtubules assembled *in vitro* from a normal human brain (lanes 1 and 4) and an identically treated Alzheimer brain (lanes 2 and 3) developed with monoclonal antibody to tau. *Reproduced with permission from Iqbal et al., Lancet 2:421–426, 1986.*

mortem AD and control brains. After considerable effort, we had finally worked out a program whereby we, a local hospital, and our neuropathologist coordinated to collect brains by six hours postmortem. Over a period of six years, we collected several AD and control brains, mostly during off hours, and processed them for up to two cycles of *in vitro* assembly of microtubules. We observed that we could assemble microtubules from control aged brains but not from AD brains [61]. We could, however, assemble microtubules from both AD and control brains by DEAE-Dextran, a polycation that mimics tau in promoting microtubule assembly. We traced the *in vitro* microtubule assembly defect in AD brain to the presence of abnormally hyperphosphorylated tau in the cytosol (Fig. 7). This was the first study demonstrating a functional impairment of the abnormal hyperphosphorylation of tau in AD brain.

5. Discovery of neuropil threads

Heiko Braak and Eva Braak visited our Institute in 1985. We showed them micrographs of immunostaining of AD brain sections with our antiserum to PHF, which, along with neurofibrillary tangles and plaque neurites, also labeled numerous thread-like structures. They told us that they had observed similar structures in Gallaya's silver-stained AD brain sections. Our collaboration, employing both immunohistochemical staining and Gallaya's silver staining of AD brain sections, resulted in the identification of neuropil threads as a third location of PHF outside of neurofibrillary tangles and neuritic plaques [15].

6. Generation of the first monoclonal antibodies to PHF and the first demonstration of increased PHF immunoreactivity in CSF of patients with AD

Employing the technique we had developed earlier for bulk isolation of highly purified PHF as the immunogen [60], we generated three clones that secreted mAb to PHF [139]. Employing mAb secreted by the clone 5–25, we demonstrated an increase in the PHF immunoreactivity in lumbar CSF of patients with AD [92,139]. This was the first demonstration of the presence and elevation of a brain-lesion associated protein in CSF of AD patients.

7. Discovery of glycosylation of tau in PHF

We discovered that, unlike normal tau, the abnormally hyperphosphorylated tau in AD brain is glycosylated and that glycan(s) maintains the helicity of PHF, but does not have any apparent effect on the ability of tau to promote the assembly of tubulin into microtubules [141]. Removal of glycans by enzymatic deglycosylation converted PHF into bundles of straight filaments 2.5 ± 0.5 mm in diameter, suggesting the involvement of glycosylation in the maintenance of the PHF structure. Subsequent studies from our laboratory showed that the glycosylation of tau precedes its abnormal hyperphosphorylation and aggregation into PHF, and that the glycosylation makes tau a more favorable substrate for abnormal hyperphosphorylation [86,87, 111].

8. Generation of the first cell culture model of neurofibrillary degeneration and demonstration of the role of PP-2A/PP-1 activities in the regulation of the phosphorylation of tau

We demonstrated that tau in SY5Y neuroblastoma cells cultured in low serum was hyperphosphorylated at several of the same sites in AD brain. As in AD, the hyperphosphorylated tau accumulated in the cultured cells, and it did not bind to microtubules [124]. Employing the cell culture model, we subsequently showed that the inhibition of PP-2A/PP-1 activities by okadaic acid upregulated the activities of MAPK and cdk5 and resulted in abnormal hyperphosphorylation of tau, a decrease in stable microtubules, and an increase in cell death; taxol inhibited this okadaic acid-induced cell death [125]. We subsequently confirmed the regulation of the phosphorylation of tau by PP-2A in mammalian brain [11,12,38].

9. Generation and role of abnormally hyperphosphorylated tau in neurodegeneration

After the discoveries of tau as the major protein subunit of PHF, its abnormal phosphorylation, and the *in vitro* microtubule assembly defect in AD, the next two most important questions have been (1) if and how the abnormal phosphorylation of tau might cause neurodegeneration and cognitive deficit, and (2) what causes the abnormal phosphorylation of tau.

9.1. How abnormal hyperphosphorylation of tau might lead to neurodegeneration and cognitive deficit

Our discovery of the abnormal phosphorylation of tau in AD brain cytosol and inhibition of microtubule assembly from the AD brain cytosol [61] provided the critical lead. In collaboration with the group of Chris Bancher, Hans Lassmann, and Kurt Jellinger, we demonstrated immunohistochemically the presence of pretangle accumulation of abnormally hyperphosphorylated tau [10]. These lesions, which we termed "pretangles", showed as mostly amorphous protein aggregates and, unlike mature tangles, had no ubiquitin associated with them. This study suggested that the abnormal hyperphosphorylation of tau most probably preceded its polymerization into PHF/tangles.

The primary structure of tau was not known. We generated the CNBr peptides of tau purified from bovine brain and determined their amino terminal sequences. While the manuscript was in preparation, Lee et al. [80] published the cloning and the cDNA-derived amino acid sequence of murine tau. We found that while the amino acid sequences of two of the three bovine CNBr peptides could be seen in the murine tau sequence, one sequence did not match [62,63]. We raised rabbit antibodies to a synthetic peptide corresponding to the bovine specific tau sequence and confirmed it to belong to tau. While our paper was in press, Himmler [52] and Goedert et al. [32] published the cDNA-derived sequences of bovine and human taus to which our sequence matched. Antibodies to the bovine tau peptide we had raised were phosphodependent and revealed that tau was abnormally phosphorylated at Ser46 [63]. These studies provided the first evidence of a difference between the primary structures of murine and bovine taus and of abnormal hyperphosphorylation at other than the mAb Tau-1 site.

We quantitated the level of tau in AD and age-matched control brains and found that the AD brains contained as much normal tau as the control brains, plus up to $\sim$ 8-fold abnormally hyperphosphorylated tau [70,71]. These findings became a basis for investigation of CSF levels of tau as a biomarker and of a potential diagnostic test for AD by a number of laboratories (e.g. [53,133]). Furthermore, up to 40% of the abnormally phosphorylated tau was found in the cytosol [76]. Separation of the cytosolic abnormally phosphorylated tau from non-hyperphosphorylated tau (normal-like tau) was carried out from AD brain by phosphocellulose chromatography, and the former was found to contain 5–9 moles of phosphates as compared with 2–3 moles of phosphate per mole of the protein in the latter [76]. These findings demonstrated that, like PHF [79], AD P-tau was also hyperphosphorylated. We found that tau polymerized into PHF was unable to promote *in vitro* assembly of tubulin into microtubules, but enzymatic dephosphorylation restored the ability of PHF-tau to promote the assembly [64].

Studies on the cytosolic abnormally hyperphosphorylated tau (AD P-tau) and normal-like tau separated from AD brain revealed that the normal-like AD tau could readily promote microtubule assembly, but the AD P-tau, instead of promoting microtubule assembly, inhibited it and, when added to pre-assembled microtubules, disassembled them [1]. Furthermore, we discovered that the AD P-tau caused the inhibition and disruption of microtubules by sequestering normal tau [1]. Subsequent studies from our laboratory showed that the binding of normal tau to AD P-tau was a polymer reaction that could not be saturated by increasing concentrations of normal tau and formed bundles of straight tau filaments [2]. Essentially, the same phenomenon was observed several years later in transgenic mice, when tangles of straight tau filaments were found continuing to grow even when the expression of P301L mutated tau was inhibited at four months of age in these animals [110]. The AD P-tau sequestered not only normal tau but also MAP1 and MAP2 *in vitro* and in situ [1,3].

We found that tau promoted microtubule assembly by stimulating the binding of GTP to the exchangeable site of tubulin, and that the abnormally hyperphosphorylated tau from AD depressed the GTP binding [72]. Thus, it appears that the abnormal hyperphosphorylation of tau in AD not only results in the loss of normal tau functions but in a gain of toxic function in which the abnormal tau sequesters normal tau, MAP1, and MAP2 and compromises the microtubule network. The loss of microtubules probably results in inhibition of axoplasmic flow, leading to a retrograde neurodegeneration and loss of synapses and cognition in AD patients. Most recently, we have demonstrated that the abnormal hyperphosphorylation of tau produced experimentally in normal adult rats by activation of brain cAMP-dependent protein kinase (PKA) by forskolin or isoproterenol results in impairment of spatial memory [89,123]. Abnormal hyperphosphorylation of tau-induced memory deficit has also been confirmed in a number of transgenic mouse models (see e.g. [96]). Thus, it appears that the abnormally hyperphosphorylated tau, instead of promoting assembly and stabilizing microtubules, sequesters normal tau, MAP1 and MAP2, causing inhibition and disassembly of microtubules, which results in a retrograde neurodegeneration due to compromised axoplasmic flow, and results in dementia. Such a scenario of neurodegeneration, the tau hypothesis, was proposed by us several years earlier [61].

9.1.1. Self-assembly of tau into PHF

Our previous studies had shown (1) that the *in vitro* dephosphorylation of Alzheimer neurofibrillary tangles/PHF by protein phosphatase (PP)-2A and PP-2B disaggregated PHF, and the dephosphorylated tau thereby released readily stimulated the *in vitro* assembly of tubulin into microtubules [140]; and (2) that the normal tau bound to the AD abnormally hyperphosphorylated tau (AD P-tau) in a non-saturation manner and the product of the association of these taus were bundles of straight tau filaments [2]. Since the major protein subunit of PHF is the abnormally hyperphosphorylated tau [48], we investigated whether the abnormal hyperphosphorylation of tau alone was sufficient to induce self-assembly of tau in PHF. We found that AD P-tau readily self-assembled into tangles of PHF *in vitro*, and its prior dephosphorylation, but not deglycosylation, inhibited the self-assembly [4]. Furthermore, we demonstrated that *in vitro* hyperphosphorylation of all six recombinant human brain isoforms promoted their self-assembly into tangles of PHF. This was the first demonstration of self-assembly of tau into PHF under physiological conditions (Fig. 8). Previous studies were able to achieve assembly of tau into straight filaments (SF) and PHF-like structures using urea treatment for 60 hours; incubations with unsaturated fatty acids, tRNA, heparin or polyglutamic acid; and employing a tau fragment, tau concentrations of up to 12 mg/ml, and incubation times up to several days [24,29,33,68,93,102,112,135,144,145,149].

9.2. How and what causes the abnormal hyperphosphorylation of tau

AD is multifactorial. In less than 1% of all cases, AD cosegregates with certain mutations in amyloid β protein precursor (AβPP), presenilin-1 (PS-1), and presenilin-2 (PS-2) [18]. In over 99% of AD cases, to date, no mutation has been associated with the disease. Independent of the etiology, neurofibrillary degeneration of the abnormally hyperphosphorylated tau and β-amyloidosis are the two hallmark lesions of AD. These two lesions occur in disproportionate numbers in AD, and neither of these lesions are unique to AD. Some of the normal human aged brains contain as much Aβ burden, in the form of compact senile plaques, as in typical cases of AD [27,28,69]. In hereditary cerebral hemorrhage with amyloidosis of the Dutch type and sporadic cerebral amyloid angiopathy, the Aβ burden is considerably greater than in AD but without any neurofibrillary degeneration [23,81,134]. On the other hand, a family of dementia disorders, called tauopathies, such as frontotemporal dementia with Parkinsonism linked to chromosome 17 (FTDP-17), progressive supranuclear palsy, cortico basal degeneration, Pick disease, Guam Parkinsonism-dementia complex, dementia pugilistica, and argyrophillic grain disease, are characterized by neurofibrillary degeneration of the abnormally hyperphosphorylated tau, but in the absence of β-amyloidosis (see for review [129]). The inherited FTDP-17 is caused by certain mutations in the tau gene that involve either alternate splicing of its mRNA, resulting in an increase in four-repeat to three-repeat tau ratio, or missense mutations, in which a single amino acid residue in tau protein is changed to a different amino acid [54,104,122]. Thus, tau pathology alone, in the absence of β-amyloidosis, is sufficient to produce the disease. β-amyloidosis and neurofibrillary degeneration of abnormally hyperphosphorylated tau are probably produced by some common event such as alteration in some signal transduction pathway(s)

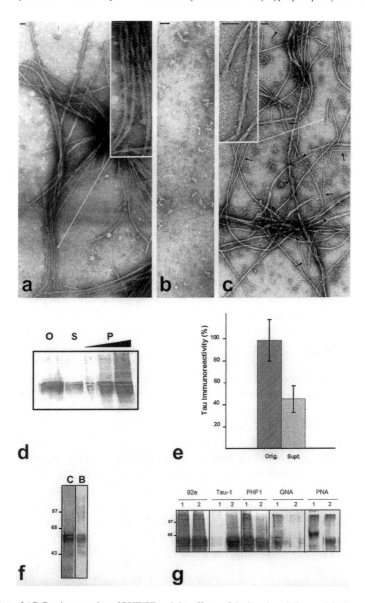

Fig. 8. *In vitro* polymerization of AD P-τ into tangles of PHF/SF and the effects of dephosphorylation and deglycosylation. AD P-τ, 0.4 mg/ml, without treatment (*a*), dephosphorylated by AP (*b*), or deglycosylated by endoglycosidase F/N-glycosidase F (*c*), was incubated for 90 min, and the products of the assembly were examined by NSEM. Dephosphorylation, but not deglycosylation, completely abolished AD P-τ polymerization. Bar represents 50 nm. (*Insets*) PHF at higher magnifications. Arrows label examples of 10–15 nm (straight) and 4 nm (arrowhead) filaments. (*d*) AD P-τ, 0.4 mg/ml, was incubated as above to induce assembly, and the aggregated protein was separated from the non-aggregated protein by centrifugation at 35°C and 100,000 X g for 15 min. The pellet (P) was resuspended to its original volume, and equivalent samples of the original mixture (O), the supernatant (S), and the pellet (1, 2, and 4X) were analyzed by Western blots by using Tau0-1 antibody and dephosphorylation of the proteins on the blot with AP. (*e*) The amount (mean × SD of 4 values) of AD P-τ present in the original and the supernatant fractions was quantitated by scanning the immunoblots. (*f*) SDS/PAGE (10% gel) of AD P-τ and blot of a lane from the same gel developed with Tau-1 antibody after dephosphorylation. One strip (8 μg of protein/lane) was stained with Coomassie blue (*c*), and another strip (2 μg of protein/lane) was stained with Tau-1 antibody after dephosphorylation of the proteins on the membrane (B). (*g*) For *in vitro* dephosphorylation and deglycosylation of AD P-τ aliquots of AD P-τ were treated with (2) or without (1) the addition of AP to dephosphorylate (panels labeled 92e, Tau-1 and PHF1) or endoglycosidase F/N-glycosidase F to deglycosylate (panels labeled GNA and PNA) the proteins as described. The immunoblots were developed with 92e (dilution 1/5,000) to detect the total amount of, Tau-1 (1/50,000) to detect dephosphorylated τ, and PHF1 (1/250) to detect phosphorylated τ. The increase in Tau-1 staining and decrease in PHF1 staining show dephosphorylation of AD P-τ. The immunoblots were developed with lectin GNA or PNA to detect glycosylation. Decrease in the staining with the lectins shows deglycosylation of AD P-τ by the glycosidase.

Reproduced with permission of Alonso et al., Proc. Natl. Acad. Sci. USA 98:6923–6928, 2001.

(see [65]), rather than as a result of the direct neurotoxicity of one lesion to the other, which was suggested by the amyloid cascade hypothesis.

The state of phosphorylation of a phosphoprotein is a function of the balance between the activities of protein kinases and protein phosphatases that regulate its phosphorylation. Tau, which is phosphorylated at more than 30 serine/threonine residues in AD [50, 94], is a substrate for several protein kinases [66, 116,118,120,121]. Among these kinases, glycogen synthase kinase-3 (GSK-3), cyclin-dependent protein kinase 5 (cdk5), protein kinase A (PKA), calcium, calmodulin-dependent protein kinase-II (CaMKII), mitogen-activated protein kinase ERK1/2, and stress-activated protein kinases have been implicated the most in the abnormal hyperphosphorylation of tau (see [66]). Our laboratory led the studies on the role of site-site interaction in the abnormal hyperphosphorylation of tau [89,114,117,119,123,142]. We were the first to demonstrate that phosphorylation of tau by non-proline dependent protein kinases PKA, PKC, CaMKII and casein kinase-1 (CK1) primed it for subsequent phosphorylation by proline directed protein kinases (PDPK) cdk5 and GSK-3, showed quantitative inhibition of the binding of tau to microtubules at various sites, and identified Ser262 and Thr231 to be the two major sites, phosphorylation of which inhibits the binding of tau to microtubules [115,117,119]. In collaboration with Jin-Jing Pei (Karolinska Institute, Stockholm, Sweden), we demonstrated the association of GSK-3β and cdk5 with neurofibrillary degeneration at all Braak stages of this pathology [98–100].

9.2.1. Discovery of decrease in activities of protein phosphatase (PP)-2A and PP-1 in AD brain and the role of these enzymes in the regulation of the phosphorylation of tau

We investigated both the phosphoseryl/phosphothreonyl protein phosphatases involved in regulation of the phosphorylation of tau and the activities of those enzymes in AD and age-matched control brains. We were the first to discover that the activities of protein phosphatase-2A (PP-2A) and PP-1 were compromised by $\sim$ 20% in AD brain [35] and that this decrease in AD brain phosphatase activity was also towards the abnormally hyperphosphorylated tau isolated from AD brain [37]. Subsequently, we demonstrated that the phosphorylation of tau that suppresses its microtubule binding and assembly activities in adult mammalian brain is regulated by PP-2A [11,12,36,38]. PP-2A also regulates the activities of several tau kinases in brain.

We showed that inhibition of PP-2A activity by okadaic acid in cultured cells and in metabolically active rat brain slices results in abnormal hyperphosphorylation of tau at several of the same sites as in AD, not only by a decrease in dephosphorylation, but also indirectly by promoting the activities of CaM Kinase II [12], PKA [85,125], MAP kinase kinase (MEK1/2), extracellular regulated kinase (ERK1/2), and P70S6 kinase [7,101]. Thus, barring the fact that tau is not the only neuronal substrate of these protein kinases and phosphatases, it should be possible to inhibit the abnormal hyperphosphorylation of tau by inhibiting the activity of one or more tau kinases and/or restoring or upregulating the activity of PP-2A.

Although the brain has several tau phosphatase activities [19,20,105,106], PP-2A and PP-1 make more than 90% of the serine/threonine protein phosphatase activity in mammalian cells [97]. The intracellular activities of these enzymes are regulated by endogenous inhibitors. PP-1 activity is regulated mainly by a 18.7-kDa heat-stable protein called inhibitor-1 (I-1) [21,22]. In addition, a structurally related protein, DARPP-32 (dopamine and cAMP-regulated phosphoprotein of apparent molecular weight 32,000), is expressed predominantly in the brain [137]. I-1 and DARPP-32 are activated on phosphorylation by protein kinase A and inactivated at basal calcium level by PP-2A. Thus, inhibition of PP-2A activity would keep I-1 and DARPP-32 in active form and thereby result in a decrease in PP-1 activity. In AD, a reduction in PP-2A activity might have decreased PP-1 activity by allowing upregulation of I-1/DARPP-32 activity.

9.2.2. Discovery of cleavages and translocation of a PP-2A inhibitor from neuronal nucleus to cytoplasm

PP-2A is inhibited in the mammalian tissue by two heat-stable proteins: (1) the I_1^{PP2A}, a 30-kDa cytosolic protein [82] that inhibits PP-2A with a Ki of 30 nM and (2) I_2^{PP2A}, a 39-kDa nuclear protein that inhibits PP-2A with a Ki of 23 nM [83]. Both I_1^{PP2A} and I_2^{PP2A} have been cloned from human kidney [84,132] and, in our laboratory, from human brain [131]. I_1^{PP2A} has been found to be the same protein as the putative histocompatibility leukocyte antigen class II-associated protein (PHAP-1). This protein, which has also been described as mapmodulin, pp32, and LANP [136], is 249 amino acids long and has an apparent molecular weight of 30 kDa on SDS-PAGE. I_2^{PP2A}, which is the same as TAF-1β or PHAPII, is a nuclear protein that is a homologue of the human SETα protein. We discovered that in AD brain the I2 PP2A is cleaved into amino terminal and carboxy terminal halves and is translocated from neuronal nucleus to cytoplasm [126]. Both I_1^{PP2A} and I_2^{PP2A} interact with the catalytic subunit of PP2A (Chen et al., in preparation). We discovered that the level of I_1^{PP2A} is $\sim$ 20% greater in AD brains than in age-matched control brains, which probably is a cause of the decrease in PP-2A activity in AD brain.

9.3. Substrate regulation of the phosphorylation of tau

In addition to the activities of the tau kinases and phosphatases, the phosphorylation of tau is also regulated by its conformational state. Free tau is more readily hyperphosphorylated than is microtubule-bound tau. The rate and extent of tau phosphorylation by PKA, CaM Kinase II, C-kinase, casein kinase (CK)-I, cdk5, and GSK-3 are dependent on its initial phosphorylation state. For instance, we demonstrated that when recombinant human brain tau is prephosphorylated by one of several non-PDPKs, i.e., PKA, CaM Kinase II or C-kinase, its subsequent phosphorylations catalyzed by the PDPK cdk5 or GSK-3 are stimulated severalfold [117,119]. In addition, the rate and extent to which various tau isoforms are phosphorylated also depend on whether tau contains three or four repeats and zero, one, or two N-terminal inserts [121].

We discovered that in addition to abnormal hyperphosphorylation, tau is also abnormally glycosylated, and that in AD brain, the latter appears to precede the former [86,87,141]. Furthermore, we found by *in vitro* studies that the abnormal glycosylation promotes tau phosphorylation with PKA, GSK-3β, and ckd5 and inhibits dephosphorylation of tau with PP2A and PP5 [9, 87]. In addition, like some other neuronal phosphoproteins, tau is also O-GlcNAcylated [51]. In contrast to classical N- or O-glycosylation, O-GlcNAcylation which involves the addition of a single sugar at serine/threonine residues of a protein, dynamically post-translationally modifies cytoplasmic and nuclear proteins in a manner analogous to protein phosphorylation (see [88]). In collaboration with Cheng-Xin Gong, we discovered that O-GlcNAcylation and phosphorylation of tau reciprocally regulate each other, and that decreased glucose metabolism in cultured cells and in mice, which decreases the O-GlcNAcylation of tau, produces abnormal hyperphosphorylation of this protein. Furthermore, we found that in AD, probably as a result of impaired glucose uptake/metabolism, there is a global decrease in O-GlcNAcylation.

In inherited frontotemporal dementia linked to chromosome-17 (FTDP-17), certain mutations in the tau gene co-segregate with the disease. The most studied of these mutations are the missense mutations G272V, P301L, V337M, and R406W. We found that tau with these mutations is a more favorable substrate for hyperphosphorylation than the wild-type tau; the mutated taus are hyperphosphorylated much faster and polymerize into filaments at lower stoichiometry than the identically treated wild-type tau [6]. Thus, all these studies taken together suggest that, in addition to the levels of the activities of tau kinases and phosphatases, the phosphorylation of tau is regulated at the substrate (tau) level. Impaired glucose metabolism via downregulation of O-GlcNAcylation in AD and mutations in tau gene in FTDP-17 probably contribute to neurofibrillary degeneration.

9.4. Discovery of intraneuronal Aβ and its coexistence with neurofibrillary tangles

Since the first description of plaque amyloid by Alois Alzheimer in 1907, all subsequent histopathological studies by many laboratories had shown Aβ to be only extracellular. George Glenner had demonstrated the isolation and sequence of Aβ from the extracellular amyloid from the meninges [31,147]. We were the first to demonstrate the intraneuronal localization of Aβ and its presence both in tangle bearing and non-tangle-bearing neurons in AD brain [49]. This discovery (Fig. 9) was made possible by using several mAbs to Aβ that we had generated earlier [75]. Although at present, it is increasingly believed that intraneuronal Aβ is the major neurotoxic source and might lead to neurofibrillary degeneration, this view is not universally supported, especially by studies of the brains of normal aged and AD (see, for review [65]).

10. Phosphorylation sites involved in converting normal functional tau into a toxic molecule

Tau is abnormally hyperphosphorylated at more than 30 sites in AD. However, not all of these sites may be involved in converting normal tau into a toxic molecule. Identification of these critical sites has been most difficult. We demonstrated that phosphorylation of tau at Ser-262, Thr-231, and Ser-235 inhibits its binding to microtubules by $\sim$ 35, $\sim$ 25, and 10%, respectively [115]. We observed that hyperphosphorylation of tau at the level of 4–6 moles phosphate/mole of the

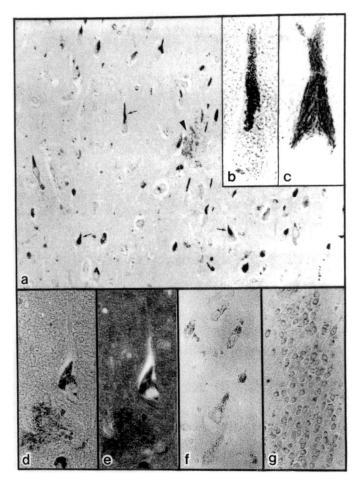

Fig. 9. Immunostaining of Alzheimer (*a–e*) and 38-year-old control (*f and g*) hippocampus with mAb to amyloid (*a, b and d–g*) or anti-PHF serum (*c*). (*a*) mAb to amyloid stains plaques (arrowhead) and intraneuronal material (arrows), which at low power looks like neurofibrillary tangles. However, at high magnification (*b*), it presents a tightly packed granular material and can be easily distinguished from the tangles, which are fibrillar when stained with anti-PHF serum (*c*) or thioflavine S (*e*). (*d and e*) Amyloid-immunoreactive material and thioflavine S-positive fluorescent tangles frequently occur in the same neuron. (*a*, X 200; *b* and *c*, X 1000; *d* and *e*, X 420; *f* and *g*, x 280).
Reproduced with permission from Grundke-Iqbal et al., Proc. Natl. Acad. Sci. USA 86:2853–2857, 1989.

protein induces the toxic property whereby it sequesters normal tau [6]. Additional phosphorylation to a level of ~ 10 phosphates per mole of the protein is required to induce its self-assembly into filaments. We showed that taus with the FTDP-17 mutations G272V, P301L, V337M, and R406W are phosphorylated much faster than the wild-type tau and self-assemble at lower levels of phosphorylation than the wild-type protein. Time kinetics of phosphorylation of these mutated and wild-type taus at various abnormally phosphorylated sites and the ability of these proteins to bind normal tau suggest Ser-199/202/205, Thr-212, Thr-231/Ser-235, Ser-262/356, and Ser-404 to be among the critical sites that convert tau to a toxic-like protein. Further phosphorylation at Thr-231, Ser-396, and Ser-422 promotes self-assembly of tau into filaments [6]. These sites are known to be substrates of PKA, CaMKII, GSK-3β and cdk5, among other protein kinases.

11. Inhibition of neurofibrillary degeneration and outcome measures

AD is multifactorial and heterogeneous. Aβ and neurofibrillary tangles are more likely products than causes of AD. Our last three decades of studies have led us to hypothesize the involvement of different signal transduction pathways as primary pathogenetic events in AD (Fig. 10). These signaling abnormalities could be results of different metabolic abnormalities such

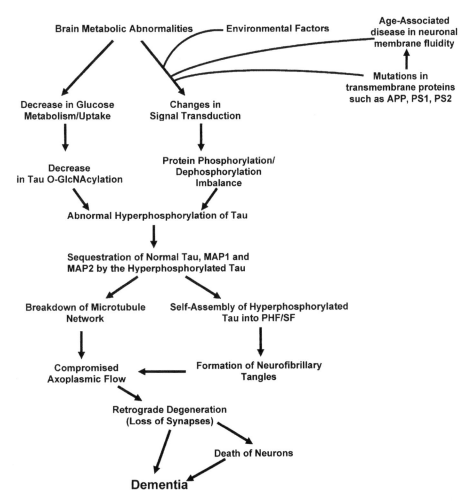

Fig. 10. A schematic showing different major steps of the "Metabolic/signal transduction hypothesis". AD and other tauopathies require a genetic predisposition. They are triggered by a variety of environmental factors affecting one or more specific signal transduction pathways, which result in a protein phosphorylation/dephosphorylation imbalance and the abnormal hyperphosphorylation of tau. This leads to neurofibrillary degeneration and dementia. In Ad, the protein phosphorylation/dephosphorylation imbalance in the affected neurons is generated at least in part by a decrease in the activities of tau phosphatases, i.e., PP2A and PP1; the activities of tau kinases such as cdk5, GSK-3, CaM kinase II and PKA might also be increased in the affected neurons. This protein phosphorylation/dephosphorylation imbalance probably involves an alteration of a specific signal transduction pathway(s) produced by an increase in the levels of an extracellular signal, e.g., FGF2 or an alteration in the molecular topology of the neuronal cell membrane or both. With age, the molecular topology of the ell membranes is altered due to a decrease in membrane fluidity. The mutations in transmembrane proteins, such as β-APP, PS1 and PS2, increase the vulnerability of the cell membrane to alteration in pathological signal transduction. The increased risk for AD in the carriers of $APOE_4$ allele as opposed to $APOE_2$ or $APOE_3$ alleles might also involve alteration of signal transduction through the interaction of $APOE_4$ with the neuronal cell membrane. Any mutation or post-translational modification of tau that will make it a better substrate for abnormal hyperphosphorylation will also increase the risk for the disease. High cholesterol might be involved in decreasing membrane fluidity. Decreased glucose metabolism/uptake might lead to the abnormal hyperphosphorylation of tau through a decrease in its O-GlcN-acylation.
Reproduced with permission from Iqbal and Grundke-Iqbal, Acta Neuropathol. (berl) 109:25–31, 2005.

as impaired brain glucose metabolism and as well as certain mutations in transmembrane proteins such as AβPP, PS-1 and PS-2. These alterations in different signal transduction pathways probably lead to a common downstream deleterious functional effect – the hyperphosphorylation of tau. Thus, therapeutic interventions that can overcome the deleterious effect/s of the pathological tau appear promising.

The most promising therapeutic approaches to inhibit neurofibrillary degeneration and consequently AD are (1) to inhibit sequestration of normal MAPs by the AD P-tau and (2) to inhibit the abnormal hyperphosphorylation of tau. The latter can be carried out either by restoring the PP-2A activity in the affected areas of the brain to normal levels or by inhibiting the activity of one or more tau kinases that are critically involved in converting normal tau into an abnormal state whereby it sequesters normal MAP. In collaboration with Jian-Zhi Wang, we demonstrated that the activation of PKA with forskolin or isoproterenol primes tau for abnormal hyperphosphorylation by the constitutive GSK-3β activity in adult rats, and the spatial memory of these animals is impaired [89,123]. Co-treatment of these animals with forskolin and RP-cAMPS, a PKA inhibitor, inhibited the abnormal hyperphosphorylation of tau and the impairment of spatial memory. We discovered that memantine, a low- to moderate-affinity NMDA receptor antagonist, which improves mental function and the quality of daily living of patients with moderate to severe AD [107,146], restores the okadaic acid-induced inhibition of PP-2A activity, the abnormal hyperphosphorylation of tau at Ser-262, and the associated neurodegeneration in hippocampal slice cultures from adult rats [85]. Furthermore, the restoration of the PP-2A activity to normal levels by memantine also results in the restoration of the expression of MAP2 in the neuropil and a reversal of the hyperphosphorylation and the accumulation of neurofilament H and M subunits.

Inhibition of the abnormal hyperphosphorylation of tau and sequestration of normal MAPs by the hyperphosphorylated tau are among the most promising therapeutic targets for AD and other tauopathies. Approaches to inhibit the abnormal hyperphosphorylation of tau include the inhibition of the one or more tau kinase activities, activation of one or more tau phosphatases, and the enhancement of brain glucose metabolism, which directly affects the O-GlcNAcylation of tau.

12. Concluding remarks

We have been most fortunate to study the biology of AD and related conditions and to have been able to make several key discoveries in the field. We were among the first to study the molecular pathology of AD. When we started studying AD in 1973, only morphological descriptions of the histopathology of AD and the correlation of those brain lesions to clinical expression of the disease, i.e., the dementia, were available. Our persistence in carrying out systematic studies on neurodegeneration in AD led us to several key discoveries, which include (1) the isolation and protein composition of PHF [59,60]; (2) identification of tau and its abnormally hyperphosphorylated state as the major protein subunit of PHF [47,48]; (3) the presence of the abnormally hyperphosphorylated tau in AD brain cytosol and the inhibition of microtubule assembly by the pathological tau [61]; (4) the decrease in the activities of PP-2A and PP-1 in AD brain as a cause of the abnormal hyperphosphorylation of tau [35,37]; (5) the sequestration of normal tau, MAP1, and MAP2 by the abnormally hyperphosphorylated tau as a molecular mechanism of neurofibrillary degeneration [1–3]; (6) the promotion of the self-assembly of tau into tangles of PHF by its hyperphosphorylation [4]; and (7) the intraneuronal localization of Aβ [49].

During our more than 30 years of research work on AD, we have had the fortune of collaborating with a large number of senior scientists, and in our own research group with graduate students, postdoctoral fellows, and young scientists. We would like to acknowledge Robert D. Terry, at whose initiative and with whose support we entered the AD field. Henry M. Wisniewski carried out the morphological evaluation of the PHF preparations for our first study and fought for us during the PHF solubility controversy in the early 1980s. Sabiha Khatoon's discovery of normal levels of normal-like tau and of the several-fold increase in abnormally hyperphosphorylated tau in AD not only laid the foundation of subsequent studies on the molecular mechanisms of neurofibrillary degeneration, but also stimulated research on studies on the CSF levels of tau and phosphor-tau as a potential diagnostic biomarker. Gian Ping Wang was the first to generate monoclonal antibodies to PHF, and he and Takashi Kudo demonstrated the elevated level of conjugated ubiquitin in AD CSF. Cheng-Xin Gong's discovery of the decrease in PP-2A/PP-1 activities in AD brain identified a cause of abnormal hyperphosphorylation of tau and demonstrated the involvement of these phosphatases in neurofibrillary degeneration. Alejandra del C. Alonso discovered the sequestration of normal tau, MAP1, and MAP2 by the abnormally hyperphosphorylated tau as a key likely step in the molecular mechanism of neurofibrillary degeneration and demonstrated that abnormal hyperphosphorylation alone is sufficient to cause self-assembly of tau into tangles of PHF. Jian-Zhi Wang found that neurofibrillary tangles/PHF could be dissociated by PP-2A or PP-2B, releasing dephosphorylated tau, which was biologically active in promoting microtubule assembly. She also discovered that, unlike normal brain tau, tau in PHF was glycosylated and that the generation of AD-like abnormally hyperphosphorylated tau, which results in its self-assembly into PHF, requires catalysis by cdk5 and GSK-3β, or one of these kinases along with PKA and CaMKII. Jin-Jing Pei demonstrated the association of GSK-3β and cdk5 with neurofibrillary pathology from early Braak stages. Toshihisa Tanaka generated the first cell culture model of neurofibrillary pathology. Fei Liu discovered that O-GlcNAcylation and phosphorylation of tau reciprocally regulate each other and that, due to decreased brain glucose metabolism, there is most likely a global decrease in O-GlcNAcylation in AD brain. Hitoshi Tanimukai and Ichiro Tsujio discovered a decrease in the mRNAs of PP-2A inhibitors and translocation of the N-terminal half of the I2 of PP-2A from neuronal nucleus to the cytoplasm in AD brains. Last but not least, our two research assistants, Tanweer Zaidi and Yunn Chyn Tung, helped develop the technique for the bulk isolation and solubilization of PHF, and the generation of antibodies and the identification of tau as the major component of PHF, respectively.

Acknowledgements

We thank Janet Biegelson and Sonia Warren for providing secretarial assistance, including the preparation of this manuscript, and Maureen Marlow for copy editing. Currently, our studies on neurofibrillary degeneration are supported in part by the New York State Office of Mental Retardation and Developmental Disabilities and a National Institutes of Health/National Institute on Aging grant AG19158.

References

[1] del C. Alonso, T. Zaidi, I. Grundke-Iqbal and K. Iqbal, Role of abnormally phosphorylated tau in the breakdown of microtubules in Alzheimer disease Proc, *Natl. Acad. Sci. USA* **91** (1994), 5562–5566.

[2] del C. Alonso, I. Grundke-Iqbal and K. Iqbal, Alzheimer's disease hyperphosphorylated tau sequesters normal tau into tangles of filaments and disassembles microtubules, *Nature Med* **2** (1996), 783–787.

[3] del C. Alonso, I. Grundke-Iqbal, H.S. Barra and K. Iqbal, Abnormal phosphorylation of tau and the mechanism of Alzheimer neurofibrillary degeneration: Sequestration of MAP1 and MAP2 and the disassembly of microtubules by the abnormal tau, *Proc. Natl. Acad. Sci. USA* **94** (1997), 298–303.

[4] del C. Alonso, T. Zaidi, M. Novak, I, Grundke-Iqbal and K. Iqbal, Hyperphosphorylation induces self – assembly of tau into tangles of paired helical filaments/straight filaments, *Proc. Natl. Acad. Sci. USA* **98** (2001), 6923–6928.

[5] del C. Alonso, T. Zaidi, Q. Wu, M. Novak, H.S. Barra, I. Grundke-Iqbal and K. Iqbal, Interaction of tau isoforms with Alzheimer's disease abnormally hyperphosphorylated tau and *in vitro* phosphorylation into the disease-like protein, *J. Biol. Chem.* **276** (2001), 37967–37973.

[6] del C. Alonso, A. Mederlyova, M. Novak, I. Grundke-Iqbal and K. Iqbal, Promotion of hyperphosphorylation by frontotemporal dementia tau mutations, *J. of Biol. Chem.* **279** (2004), 34878–34881.

[7] W.L. An, R.F. Cowburn, L. Li, H. Braak, I. Alafuzoff, K. Iqbal, I. Grundke-Iqbal, B. Winblad and J.J. Pei, Upregulation of phosphorylated/activated p70 S6 kinase and its relationship to neurofibrillary pathology in Alzheimer's disease, *Am. J. Pathol.* **163** (2003), 591–607.

[8] B.H. Anderton, D. Breinburg, M.J. Downes, P.J. Green, B.E. Tomlinson, J. Ulrich, J.N. Wood and J. Kahn, Monoclonal antibodies show that neurofibrillary tangles and neurofilaments share antigenic determinants, *Nature (Lond.)* **298** (1982), 84–86.

[9] C.S. Arnold, G.V. Johnson, R.N. Cole, D.L. Dong, M. Lee and G.W. Hart, The microtubule-associated protein tau is extensively modified with O-linked N0-acetylglucosamine, *J. Biol. Chem.* **271** (1996), 28741–28744.

[10] C. Bancher, C. Brunner, H. Lassmann, H. Budka, K. Jellinger, G. Wiche, F. Seitelberger, I. Grundke-Iqbal, K. Iqbal and H.M. Wisniewski, Accumulation of abnormally phosphorylated tau precedes the formation of neurofibrillary tangles in Alzheimer's disease, *Brain Res* **477** (1989), 90–99.

[11] M. Bennecib, C.X. Gong, J. Wegiel, M.H. Lee, I. Grundke-Iqbal and K. Iqbal, Inhibition of protein phosphatases and regulation of tau phosphorylation in rat brain, *Alzheimer's Reports* **3** (2000), 295–304.

[12] M. Bennecib, C.X. Gong, I. Grundke-Iqbal and K. Iqbal, Inhibition of PP-2A upregulates CaMKII in rat forebrain and induces hyperphosphorylation of tau at Ser 262/356, *FEBS Lett* **490** (2001), 15–22.

[13] J.A. Berzofsky, G.K. Buckenmeyer, G. Hicks, F.R. Gurd, R.J. Feldmann and J. Minna, Topographic antigenic determinants recognized by monoclonal antibodies to sperm whale myoglobin, *J. Biol. Chem.* **257** (1982), 3189–3198.

[14] L.I. Binder, A. Frankfurter and L.I. Rebhun, The distribution of tau in the mammalian central nervous system, *J. Cell Biol.* **101** (1985), 1371–1378.

[15] H. Braak, E. Braak, I. Grundke-Iqbal and K. Iqbal, Occurrence of neuropil threads in the senile human brain and in Alzheimer's disease: A third location of paired helical filaments outside of neurofibrillary tangles and neuritic plaques, *Neurosci. Lett.* **65** (1986), 351–355.

[16] J.P. Brion, H. Passareiro, J. Nunez and J. Flament-Durand, Mise en évidence immunologique de la protéine tau au niveau des lésions dégénérescence neurofibrillaire de la maladie d'Alzheimer, *Arch. Biol. (Brux)* **95** (1985), 229–235.

[17] J.P. Brion, A.M. Couck, E. Passareiro and J. Flament-Durand, Neurofibrillary tangles of Alzheimer's disease an immunohistochemical study, *J. Submicrosc. Cytol.* **17** (1985), 89–96.

[18] D. Campion, C. Dumanchin, D. Hannequin, D. Dubois, S. Belliard, M. Puel, C. Thomas-Anterion, A. Michon, C. Martin, F. Charbonnier, G. Raux, A. Camuzat, C. Penet, V. Mesnage, M. Martinez, F. Clerget-Darpoux, A. Brice and T. Frebourg, Early-onset autosomal dominant Alzheimer disease

[19] L.Y. Cheng, J.Z. Wang, C.X. Gong, J.J Pie, T. Zaidi, I. Grundke-Iqbal and K. Iqbal, Multiple forms of phosphates from human brain isolation and partial characterization of affi-gel blue binding phosphatases, *Neurochem. Res.* **25** (2000), 107–120.

[20] L.Y. Cheng, J.-Z. Wang, C.-X. Gong, J.-J. Pei, T. Zaidi, I. Grundke-Iqbal and K. Iqbal, Multiple forms of phosphatase from human brain isolation and partial characterization of affi-gel blue nonbinding phosphatase activities, *Neurochem. Res.* **26** (2001), 425–438.

[21] P. Cohen, S. Alemany, B.A. Hemmings, T.J. Resink, P. Stralfors and H.Y.L. Tung, Protein phosphatase-1 and protein phosphatase-2A from rabbit skeletal muscle, *Meth. Enzymol.* **159** (1988), 390–408.

[22] P. Cohen, The structure and regulation of protein phosphatases, *Annu. Rev. Biochem.* **58** (1989), 453–508.

[23] F. Corio, E.M. Castano and B. Frangione, Brain amyloid in normal aging and cerebral amyloid angiopathy is antigenically related to Alzheimer's disease beta-protein, *Am. J. Pathol.* **129** (1987), 422–428.

[24] R.A. Crowther, O.F. Olesen, R. Jakes and M. Goedert, The microtubule binding repeats of tau protein assemble into filaments like those found in Alzheimer's disease, *FEBS Lett* **309** (1992), 199–202.

[25] D. Dahl, D.J. Selkoe, R.T. Pero and A. Bignami, Immunostaining of neurofibrillary tangles in Alzheimer's senile dementia with a neurofilament antiserum, *J. Neurosci.* **2** (1982), 113–119.

[26] A. Delacourte and A. Defossez, Alzheimer's disease tau proteins, the promoting factors of microtubule assembly, are major components of paired helical filaments, *J. Neurol. Sci.* **76** (1986), 173–186.

[27] D.W. Dickson, J. Farlo, P. Davies, H. Crystal, P. Fuld and S.H. Yen, Alzheimer's disease, A double-labeling immunohistochemical study of senile plaques, *Am. J. Pathol.* **132** (1988), 86–101.

[28] D.W. Dickson, H.A. Crystal, L.A. Matttiace, D.M. Masur, A.D. Blau, P. Davies, S.H. Yen and M. Aronson, Identification of normal and pathological aging in prospectively studied nondemented elderly humans, *Neurobiol. Aging* **13** (1991), 179–189.

[29] P. Friedhoff, M. von Bergen, E.M. Mandelkow and E. Mandelkow, Structure of tau protein and assembly into paired helical filaments, *Biochim. Biophys. Acta.* **1502** (2000), 122–132.

[30] P. Gambetti, G. Scheket, B. Ghetti, A. Hirano and D. Dahl, Neurofibrillary changes in human brain. An immunocytochemical study with a neurofilament antiserum, *J. Neuropathol. Exper. Neurol.* **42** (1983), 69–79.

[31] G.G. Glenner and C.W. Wong, Alzheimer's disease and Down's syndrome sharing of a unique cerebrovascular amyloid fibril protein, *Biochem. Biophys. Res. Commun.* **122** (1984), 1131–1135.

[32] M. Goedert, M.G. Spillantini, M.C. Potier, J. Ulrich and R.A. Crowther, Cloning and sequencing of the cDNA encoding an isoform of microtubule-associated protein tau containing four tandem repeats: differential expression of tau protein mRNAs in human brainm EMBO, *J.* **8** (1989), 393–399.

[33] M. Goedert, R. Jakes, M.G. Spillantini, M. Hasegawa, M.J. Smith and R.A. Crowther, Assembly of microtubule-associated protein tau into Alzheimer-like filaments induced by sulphated glycosaminoglycans, *Nature* **383** (1996), 550–553.

[34] E.S. Golub and E.D. Day, Localization of brain-associated hematopoietic antigens in the neuronal fraction of brain, *Cell Immunol* **16** (1975), 427–431.

[35] C.X. Gong, T.J. Singh, I. Grundke-Iqbal and K. Iqbal, Phosphoprotein phosphatase activities in Alzheimer disease brain, *J. Neurochem.* **61** (1993), 921–927.

[36] C.X. Gong, I. Grundke-Iqbal and K. Iqbal, Dephosphorylation of Alzheimer disease abnormally phosphorylated tau by protein phosphatase-2A, *Neurosci* **61** (1994), 765–772.

[37] C.X. Gong, S. Shaikh, J.Z. Wang, T. Zaidi, I. Grundke-Iqbal and K. Iqbal, Phosphatase activity towards abnormally phosphorylated τ decrease in Alzheimer disease brain, *J. Neurochem.* **65** (1995), 732–738.

[38] C.X. Gong, T. Lidsky, J. Wegiel, L. Zuck, I. Grundke-Iqbal and K. Iqbal, The phosphorylation state of microtubule-associated protein tau is regulated by protein phosphatase 2A in mammalian brain, *J. Biol. Chem.* **275** (2000), 5534–5544.

[39] S.G. Greenberg and P. Davies, A preparation of Alzheimer paired helical filaments that displays distinct tau proteins by polyacrylamide gel electrophoresis, *Proc. Natl. Acad. Sci. USA* **87** (1990), 5827–5831.

[40] I. Grundke-Iqbal, A.B. Johnson, H.M. Wisniewski, R.D. Terry and K. Iqbal, Evidence that Alzheimer neurofibrillary tangles originate from neurotubules, *Lancet* **I** (1979), 578–580.

[41] I. Grundke-Iqbal, A.B. Johnson, R.D. Terry, H.M. Wisniewski and K. Iqbal, Alzheimer neurofibrillary tangles Antiserum and immunohistological staining, *Ann. Neurol.* **6** (1979), 532–537.

[42] I. Grundke-Iqbal, K. Iqbal, P. Merz and H.M. Wisniewski. Isolation and properties of Alzheimer neurofibrillary tangles, *J. Neuropathol. Exp. Neuro.* **40** (1981), 312.

[43] I. Grundke-Iqbal, K. Iqbal, Y.C. Tung and H.M. Wisniewski, Alzheimer paired helical filaments: Immunochemical identification of polypeptides, *Acta Neuropathol* **62** (1984), 259–267.

[44] I. Grundke-Iqbal, K. Iqbal, Y.C. Tung, G.P. Wang and H.M. Wisniewski, Alzheimer paired helical filaments: Cross-reacting polypeptide/s normally present in brain, *Acta Neuropathol* **68** (1985), 52–61.

[45] I .Grundke-Iqbal, G.P. Wang, K. Iqbal, Y.C. Tung and H.M.Wisniewski, Alzheimer paired helical filaments: Identification of polypeptides with monoclonal antibodies, *Acta Neuropathol* **68** (1985), 279–283.

[46] I. Grundke-Iqbal, K. Iqbal and H.M. Wisniewski, Alzheimer neurofibrillary tangles and plaque neurites crossreact with IgG, *J. Neuropathol. Exp. Neurol.* **44** (1985), 368.

[47] I. Grundke-Iqbal, K. Iqbal, M. Quinlan, Y.C. Tung, M.S. Zaidi and H.M. Wisniewski, Microtubule-associated protein tau: A component of Alzheimer paired helical filaments, *J. Biol. Chem.* **261** (1986), 6084–6089.

[48] I. Grundke-Iqbal, K. Iqbal, Y.C. Tung, M. Quinlan, H.M. Wisniewski and L.I. Binder, Abnormal phosphorylation of the microtubule-associated protein τ (tau) in Alzheimer cytoskeletal pathology, *Proc. Natl. Acad. Sci. USA* **93** (1986), 4913–4917.

[49] I. Grundke-Iqbal, K. Iqbal, L. George, Y.C. Tung, K.S. Kim and H.M. Wisniewski, Amyloid protein and neurofibrillary tangles coexist in the same neuron in Alzheimer disease, *Proc. Natl. Acad. Sci. USA* **86** (1989), 2853–2857.

[50] D.P. Hanger, J.B. Betts, T.L. Loviny, W.P. Blackstock, B.H. Anderton, New phosphorylation sites identified in hy-

perphosphorylated tau (paired helical filament-tau) from Alzheimer's disease brain using nanoelectrospray mass spectrometry, *J. Neurochem.* **71** (1998), 2465–2476.
[51] G.W. Hart, Dynamic O-linked glycosylation of nuclear and cytoskeletal proteins, *Annu. Rev. Biochem.* **66** (1997), 315–335.
[52] A. Himmler, Structure of the bovine tau gene alternatively spliced transcripts generate a protein family, *Mol. Cell. Biol.* **9** (1989), 1389–1396.
[53] F. Hulstaert, K. Blennow, A. Ivanoiu, H.C. Schoonderwaldt, M. Riemenschneider, P.P. De Devn, C. Bancher, P. Cras, J. Wiltfang, P.D. Mehta, K. Iqbal, H. Pottel, E. Vanmechelen and H. Vanderstichele, Improved discrimination of AD patients using beta-amyloid(1–42) and tau levels in CSF, *Neurology* **52** (1999), 1555–1562.
[54] M. Hutton, C.L. Lendon, P. Rizzu, M. Baker, S. Froelich, H. Houlden, S. Pickering-Brown, S. Chakraverty, A. Isaacs, A. Grover, J. Hackett, J. Adamson, S. Lincoln, D. Dickson, P. Daview, R.C. Petersen, M. Stevens, E. de Grafff, E. Wauters, J. van Baren, M. Hillebrand, M. Joosse, J.M. Kwon, P. Nowotny, L.K. Che, J. Norton, J.C. Morris, L.A. Reed, J. Trojanowski, H. Basun, L. Lannfelt, M. Nevstat, S. Fahn, F. Dark, T. Tannenberg, P.R. Dodd, N. Hayward, J.B. Kowk, P.R. Schofield, A. Andreadis, J. Snowden, D. Craufurd, D. Neary, F. Owen, B.A. Oostra, J. Hardy, A. Goate, J. van Swieten, D. Mann, T. Lynch and P. Heutink, Association of missense and 5′-splice-site mutations in tau with the inherited demential FTDP-17, *Nature* **393** (1998), 702–705.
[55] Y. Ihara, C. Abraham and D.J. Selkoe, Antibodies to paired helical filaments in Alzheimer's disease do not recognize normal brain proteins, *Nature* **3034** (1983), 727–730.
[56] Y. Ihara, N. Nukina, R. Miura and M. Ogawara, Phosphorylated tau protein is integrated into paired helical filaments in Alzheimer's disease, *J. Biochem. (Tokyo)* **99** (1986), 1807–1810.
[57] K. Iqbal and I. Tellez-Nagel, Isolation of neurons and glial cells from normal and pathological human brains, *Brain Research* **45** (1972), 296–301.
[58] K. Iqbal, I. Tellez-Nagel and I. Grundke-Iqbal, Protein abnormalities in Huntington's Chorea, *Brain Research* **76** (1974), 178–184.
[59] K. Iqbal, H.M. Wisniewski, M.L. Shelanski, S. Brostoff, B.L. Liwnicz and R.D. Terry, Protein changes in senile dementia, *Brain Research* **77** (1974), 337–343.
[60] K. Iqbal, T. Zaidi, C.H. Thompson, P.A. Merz and H.M. Wisniewski, Alzheimer paired helical filaments bulk isolation, solubility and protein composition, *Acta Neuropathol. (Berl)* **62** (1984), 167–177.
[61] K. Iqbal, I. Grundke-Iqbal, T. Zaidi, P.A. Merz, G.Y. Wen, S.S. Shaikh, H.M. Wisniewski, I. Alafuzoff and B. Winblad, Defective brain microtubule assembly in Alzheimer's disease, *Lancet* **2** (1986), 421–426.
[62] K. Iqbal, A.J. Smith, T. Zaidi and I. Grundke-Iqbal, Microtubule-associated protein tau Identification of a novel peptide from bovine brain, *FEBS Lett* **248** (1989), 87–91.
[63] K. Iqbal, I. Grundke-Iqbal, A.J. Smith, L. George, Y.C. Tung and T. Zaidi, Identification and localization of a tau peptide to paired helical filaments of Alzheimer disease, *Proc. Natl. Acad. Sci. USA* **86** (1989), 5646–5650.
[64] K. Iqbal, T. Zaidi, C. Bancher and I. Grundke-Iqbal, Alzheimer paired helical filaments Restoration of the biological activity by dephosphorylation, *FEBS Lett* **349** (1994), 104–108.

[65] K. Iqbal and I. Grundke-Iqbal, Metabolic/signal transduction hypothesis of Alzheimer's disease and other tauopathies, *Acta Neuropathol. (Berl)* **109** (2005), 25–31.
[66] K. Iqbal, A. del C. Alonso, M.O. Chohan, E. El-Akkad, C.X. Gong, S. Khatoon, B. Li, F. Liu, A. Rahman, H. Tanimukai and I. Grundke-Iqbal, Tau pathology in Alzheimer disease and other tauopathies, *Biochim. Biophys. Acta.* **1739** (2005), 198–210.
[67] T. Ishii, S. Haga and S. Tobutake, Presence of neurofilament protein in Alzheimer's neurofibrillary tangles (ANF); an immunofluorescent study, *Acta. Neuropathol. (Berl.)* **48** (1979), 105–112.
[68] T. Kampers, P. Friedhoff, J. Biernat, E.M. Mandelkow and E. Mandelkow, RNA stimulates aggregation of microtubule-associated protein tau into Alzheimer-like paired helical filaments, *FEBS Lett* **399** (1996), 344–349.
[69] R. Katzman, R.D. Terry, R. DeTeresa, R. Brown, P. Davies, P. Fuld, X. Renling and A. Peck, Clinical, pathological and neurochemical changes in dementia a subgroup with preserved mental status and numerous neocortical plaques, *Ann. Neurol.* **23** (1988), 138–144.
[70] S. Khatoon, I. Grundke-Iqbal and K. Iqbal, Brain levels of microtubule-associated protein tau are elevated in Alzheimer's disease brain: a radioimmunoslot-blot assay for nanograms of the protein, *J. Neurochem.* **59** (1992), 750–753.
[71] S. Khatoon, I. Grundke-Iqbal and K. Iqbal, Levels of normal and abnormally phosphorylated tau in different cellular and regional compartments of Alzheimer disease and control brains, *FEBS Lett* **351** (1994), 80–84.
[72] S. Khatoon, I. Grundke-Iqbal and K. Iqbal, Guanosine triphosphate binding to -subunit of tubulin in Alzheimer's disease brain Role of microtubule-associated protein τ, *J. Neurochem.* **64** (1995), 777–787.
[73] M. Kidd, Paired helical filaments in electron microscopy of Alzheimer's disease, *Nature* **197** (1963), 192–193.
[74] M. Kidd, Alzheimer's disease an electron microscopical study, *Brain* **87** (1964), 307–320.
[75] K.S. Kim, D.L. Miller, C.M.J. Chen, V.J. Sapienza, C. Bai, I. Grundke-Iqbal, J.R. Currie and H.M. Wisniewski, Production and characterization of monoclonal antibodies reactive to synthetic cerebrovascular amyloid peptide, *Neurosci. Res. Commun.* **2** (1988), 121–130.
[76] E. K?pke, Y.C. Tung, S. Shaikh, A. del C. Alonso, K. Iqbal and I. Grundke-Iqbal, Microbutule associated protein tau abnormal phosphorylation of a non-paired helical filament pool in Alzheimer disease, *J. Biol. Chem.* **268** (1993), 24374–24384.
[77] K. Kosik, L.K. Duffy, M.M. Dowling, C. Abraham, A. McCluskey and D. Selkoe, Microtubule-associated protein 2 monoclonal antibodies demonstrate the selective incorporation of certain epitopes into Alzheimer neurofibrillary tangles, *Proc. Natl. Acad. Sci. USA* **81** (1984), 7941–7945.
[78] K.S. Kosik, C.L. Joachim and D.J. Selkoe, The microtubule-associated protein, tau, is a major antigenic component of paired helical filaments in Alzheimer's disease, *Proc. Natl. Acad. Sci USA* **83** (1986), 4044–4048.
[79] H. Ksiezak-Reding, W.K. Liu and S.H. Yen, Phosphate analysis and dephosphorylation of modified tau associated with paired helical filaments, *Brain Res* **597** (1992), 209–219.
[80] G. Lee, N. Cowan and M. Kirschner, The primary structure and heterogeneity of tau protein from mouse brain, *Science* **239** (1988), 285–288.
[81] E. Levy, M.D. Carman, I.J. Fernandez-Madrid, M.D. Power, I. Lieberburg, S.G. van Duinen, G.T. Bots, W. Luyendijk and

B. Frangione, Mutation of the Alzheimer's disease amyloid gene in hereditary cerebral hemorrhage, Dutch type, *Science* **248** (1990), 24–26.

[82] M. Li, H. Guo and Z. Damuni, Purification and characterization of two potent heat-stable protein inhibitors of protein phosphatase 2A from bovine kidney, *Biochemistry* **34** (1995), 1988–1996.

[83] M. Li, A. Makkinje and Z. Damuni, Molecular identification of I_1^{PP2A}, a novel potent heat-stable inhibitor protein of protein phosphatase 2A, *Biochemistry* **35** (1996), 6998–7002.

[84] M. Li, A. Makkinje and Z. Damuni, The myeloid leukemia-associated protein SET is a potent inhibitor of protein phosphatase 2A, *J. Biol. Chem.* **271** (1996), 11059–11062.

[85] L. Li, A. Sengupta, N. Haque, I. Grundke-Iqbal and K. Iqbal, Memantine inhibits and reverses the Alzheimer type abnormal hyperphosphorylation of tau and associated neurodegeneration, *FEBS Lett* **566** (2004), 261–269.

[86] F. Liu, T. Zaidi, K. Iqbal, I. Grundke-Iqbal, R.K. Merkle, and C.X. Gong, Role of glycosylation in hyperphosphorylation of tau in Alzheimer's disease, *FEBS Lett* **512** (2002), 101–106.

[87] F. Liu, T. Zaidi, I. Grundke-Iqbal, K. Iqbal and C.X. Gong, Aberrant glycosylation modulates phosphorylation of tau by protein kinase A and dephosphorylation of tau by protein phosphatase 2A and 5, *Neuroscience* **115** (2002), 829–837.

[88] F. Liu, K. Iqbal, I. Grundke-Iqbal, G.W. Hart and C.-X. Gong, O-GlcNAcylation regulates phosphorylation of tau a novel mechanism involved in Alzheimer's disease, *Proc. Natl. Acad. Sci. USA* **101** (2004), 10804–10809.

[89] S.J. Liu, J.Y. Zhang, H.L. Li, Z.Y. Fang, Q. Wang, H.M. Deng, C.X. Gong, I. Grundke-Iqbal, K. Iqbal and J.Z. Wang, Tau becomes a more favorable substrate for GSK-3 when it is prephosphorylated by PKA in rat brain, *J. Biol. Chem.* **279** (2004), 50078–50088.

[90] L. Lorand, L.K. Hsu, G.E. Siefring Jr. and N.S. Rafferty, Lens transglutaminase and cataract formation, *Proc. Natl. Acad. Sci. USA* **78** (1981), 1356–1360.

[91] C.L. Masters, G. Multhaup, G. Sims, J. Pottigiesser, R.N. Martins and K. Beyreuther, neuronal origin of cerebral amyloid: neurofibrillary tangles of Alzheimer's disease contain the same protein as the amyloid of plaque cores and blood vessels, *EMBO J* **4** (1985), 2757–2763.

[92] P.D. Mehta, L. Thal, H.M. Wisniewski, I. Grundke-Iqbal and K Iqbal, Paired helical filament antigen in CSF, *Lancet* **2** (1985), 35.

[93] E. Montejo de Garcini, L. Serrano and J. Avila, Self-assembly of microtubule-associated protein tau into filaments resembling those found in Alzheimer disease, *Biochem. Biophys. Res. Commun.* **141** (1986), 790–796.

[94] M. Morishima-Kawashima, M. Hasegawa, K. Takio, M. Suzuki, H. Yoshida, K. Titani and Y. Ihara, Proline-directed and non-proline-directed phosphorylation of PHF-tau, *J. Biol. Chem.* **270** (1995), 823–829.

[95] E.A. Nigg, G. Walter and S.J. Singer, On the nature of cross-reactions observed with antibodies directed to defined epitopes, *Proc. Natl. Acad. Sci. USA* **79** (1982), 5939–5943.

[96] S. Oddo, L. Billings, J.P. Kesslak, D.H. Cribbs and F.M. LaFerla, Abeta immunotherapy leads to clearance of early, but not late, hyperphosphorylated tau aggregates via the proteasome, *Neuron* **43** (2004), 321–332.

[97] C.J. Oliver and S. Shenolikar, Physiologic importance of protein phosphatase inhibitors, *Frontiers Biosci* **3** (1998), 961–972.

[98] J.J. Pei, T. Tanaka, Y.C. Tung, E. Braak, K. Iqbal and I. Grundke-Iqbal, Distribution, levels and activity of glycogen synthase kinase-3 in the Alzheimer Disease brain, *J. Neuropathol. Exp. Neurol.* **56** (1997), 70–78.

[99] J.J. Pei, I. Grundke-Iqbal, K. Iqbal, N. Bogdanovic, B. Winblad and R. Cowburn, Accumulation of cyclin-dependent kinase-5 (cdk5) in neurons with early stages of Alzheimer's disease neurofibrillary degeneration, *Brain Res* **797** (1998), 267–277.

[100] J.J. Pei, E. Braak, H. Braak, I. Grundke-Iqbal, K. Iqbal, B. Winblad and R.F. Cowburn, Distribution of active Glycogen Synthase Kinase 3β (GSK-3β) in brains staged for Alzheimer's disease neurofibrillary changes, *J. Neuropathol. Exper. Neurol.* **58** (1999), 1010–1019.

[101] J.J. Pei, C.X. Gong, W.L. An, B. Winblad, R.F. Cowburn, I. Grundke-Iqbal and K. Iqbal, Okadaic-Acid-Induced inhibition of protein phosphatase 2A produces activation of mitogen-activated protein kinases ERK1/2, MEK1/2, and p70 S6, similar to that in Alzheimer's disease, *Am. J. Pathol.* **163** (2003), 845–858.

[102] M. Perez, J.M. Valpuesta, M. Medina, E. Montejo de Garcini and J. Avila, Polymerization of tau into filaments in the presence of heparin the minimal sequence required for tau-tau interaction, *J. Neurochem.* **67** (1996), 1183–1190.

[103] G. Perry, N. Rizzuto, L. Autilio-Gambetti and P. Gambetti, Alzheimer's paired helical filaments contain cytoskeletal components, *Proc. Natl. Acad. Sci. USA* **82** (1985), 3916–3920.

[104] P. Poorkaj, T.D. Bird, E. Wijsman, E. Nemens, R.M. Garruto, L. Anderson, A. Andreadis, W.C. Wiederholt, M. Raskind and G.D. Schellenberg, Tau is a candidate gene for chromosome 17 frontotemporal dementia, *Ann. Neurol.* **43** (1998), 815–825.

[105] A. Rahman, I. Grundke-Iqbal and K. Iqbal, Phosphothreonine-212 of Alzheimer abnormally hyperphosphorylated tau is a preferred substrate of protein phosphatase-1, *J. Neurochem. Res.* **30** (2005), 277–287.

[106] A. Rahman, I. Grundke-Iqbal and K. Iqbal, PP2B isolated from human brain preferentially dephosphorylates Ser-262 and Ser-396 of the Alzheimer Disease abnormally hyperphosphorylated tau, *J. Neural. Transm.* (2005), (Epub ahead of print).

[107] B. Reisberg, R. Doody, A. SToffler, F. Schmitt, S. Ferris and H.J. Mobius, Memantine in moderate-to-severe Alzheimer's disease, *N. Engl. J. Med.* **348** (2003), 1333–1341.

[108] G.W. Roberts, T.J. Crow and J.M. Polak, Location of neuronal tangles in somatostatin neurones in Alzheimer's disease, *Nature* **314** (1985), 92–94.

[109] R. Rubenstein, R. J. Kascsak, P.A. Merz, H.M. Wisniewski, R.I. Carp and K. Iqbal, Paired helical filaments associated with Alzheimer disease are readily soluble structures, *Brain Res* **372** (1986), 80–88.

[110] K. SantaCruz, J. Lewis, T. Spires, J. Paulson, L. Kotilinek, M. Ingelsson, A. Guimaraes, M. DeTure, M. Ramsden, E. McGowan, C. Forster, M. Yue, J. Orne, C. Janus, A. Mariash, M. Kuskowski, B. Hyman, M. Hutton and K.H. Ashe, Tau suppression in a neurodegenerative mouse model improves memory function, *Science* **308** (2005), 476–481.

[111] Y. Sato, Y. Naito, I. Grundke-Iqbal, K. Iqbal and T. Endo, Analysis of N-glycans of pathological tau possible occurrence of aberrant processing of tau in Alzheimer's disease, *FEBS Lett* **496** (2001), 152–160.

[112] O. Schweers, E.M. Mandelkow, J. Biernat and E. Mandelkow, Oxidation of cysteine-322 in the repeat domain of microtubule-associated protein τ controls the *in vitro* assem-

[113] bly of paired helical filaments, *Proc. Natl. Acad. Sci. USA* **92** (1995), 8463–8467.

[113] D.J. Selkoe, Y. Ihara and F.J. Salazar, Alzheimer's disease insolubility of partially purified paired helical filaments in sodium dodecyl sulfate and urea, *Science* **215** (1982), 1243–1245.

[114] A. Sengupta, Q. Wu, I. Grundke-Iqbal, K. Iqbal and T.J. Singh, Potentiation of GSK-3-catalyzed Alzheimer-like phosphorylation of human tau by cdk5, *J. Mol. Cell Biochem.* **167** (1997), 99–105.

[115] A. Sengupta, J. Kabat, M. Novak, Q. Wu, I. Grundke-Iqbal and K. Iqbal, Phosphorylation of tau at both Thr 231 and Ser 262 is required for maximal inhibition of its binding to microtubules, *Arch. Biochem. Biophys.* **357** (1998), 299–309.

[116] T.J. Singh, I. Grundke-Iqbal, B. McDonald and K. Iqbal, Comparison of the phosphorylation of microtubule-associated protein tau by non-proline dependent protein kinases, *Mol. Cell. Biochem.* **131** (1994), 181–189.

[117] T.J. Singh, T. Zaidi, I. Grundke-Iqbal and K. Iqbal, Modulation of GSK-3-catalyzed phosphorylation of microtubule-associated protein tau by non-proline dependent protein kinases, *FEBS Lett.* **358** (1995), 4–8.

[118] T.J. Singh, I. Grundke-Iqbal and K. Iqbal, Phosphorylation of tau protein by casein kinase-1 converts it to an abnormal Alzheimer-like state, *J. Neurochem.* **64** (1995), 1420–1423.

[119] T.J. Singh, N. Haque, I. Grundke-Iqbal and K. Iqbal, Rapid Alzheimer-like phosphorylation of tau by the synergistic actions of non-proline-dependent protein kinases and GSK-3, *FEBS Lett* **358** (1995), 267–272.

[120] T.J. Singh, T. Zaidi, I. Grundke-Iqbal and K. Iqbal, Non-proline-dependent protein kinases phosphorylate several sites found in tau from Alzheimer disease brain, *Mol. and Cell. Biochem.* **154** (1996), 143–151.

[121] T.J. Singh, I. Grundke-Iqbal, Q. Wu, V. Chauhan, M. Novak, E. Kontzekova and K. Iqbal, Protein kinase C and calcium/calmodulin-dependent protein kinase II phosphorylate three-repeat and four-repeat tau isoforms at different rates, *Mol. Cell. Biochem.* **168** (1997), 141–148.

[122] M.G. Spillantini, J.R. Murrell, M. Goedert, M.R. Farlow, A. Klug and B. Ghetti, Mutation in the tau gene in familial multiple system tauopathy with presenile dementia, *Proc. Natl. Acad. Sci. USA* **95** (1998), 7737–7741.

[123] L. Sun, X. Wang, S. Liu, Q. Wang, J.Z. Wang, M. Bennecib, C.X. Gong, A. Sengupta, I. Grundke-Iqbal and K. Iqbal, Bilateral injection of isoproterenol into hippocampus induces Alzheimer-like hyperphosphorylation of tau and spatial memory deficit in rat, *FEBS Lett* **579** (2005), 251–258.

[124] T. Tanaka, K. Iqbal, E. Trenkner, D.J. Liu and I. Grundke-Iqbal, Abnormally phosphorylated tau in SY5Y human neuroblastoma cells, *FEBS Lett* **360** (1995), 5–9.

[125] T. Tanaka, J. Zhong, K. Iqbal, E. Trenkner and I. Grundke-Iqbal, The Regulation of Phosphorylation of τ in SY5Y Neuroblastoma Cells The Role of Protein Phosphatases, *FEBS Lett* **426** (1998), 248–254.

[126] H. Tanimukai, I. Grundke-Iqbal and K. Iqbal, Upregulation of Inhibitors of Protein Phosphatase-2A in Alzheimer Disease, *Am. J. Pathol.* **166** (2005), 1761–1771.

[127] R.D. Terry, The fine structure of neurofibrillary tangles in Alzheimer's disease, *J. Neuropathol. Exp. Neurol.* **22** (1963), 629–642.

[128] R.D. Terry, N.K. Gonatas and M. Weiss, Ultrastructural studies in Alzheimer's presenile dementia, *Am. J. Pathol.* **44** (1964), 269–297.

[129] M. Tolnay and A. Probst, Tau protein pathology in Alzheimer's disease and related disorders, *Neuropathol. Appl. Neurobiol.* **25** (1999), 171–187.

[130] B.E. Tomlinson, G. Blessed and M. Roth, Observations on the brains of demented old people, *J. Neurol. Sci.* **11** (1970), 205–242.

[131] I. Tsujio, T. Zaidi, J. Xu, L. Kotula, I. Grundke-Iqbal and K. Iqbal, Inhibitors of protein phosphatase-2A from human brain structures, immunocytological localization and activities towards dephosphorylation of the Alzheimer type hyperphosphorylated tau, *FEBS Lett.* **579** (2005), 363–372.

[132] N. Ulitzur, C. Rancano and S.R. Pfeffer, Biochemical characterization of mapmodulin, a protein that binds microtubule-associated proteins, *J. Biol. Chem.* **272** (1997), 30577–30582.

[133] M. Vandermeeren, M. Mercken, E .Vanmechelen, J. Six, A. van de Voorde, J.J. Martin and P, Cras, Detection of tau proteins in normal and Alzheimer's disease cerebrospinal fluid with a sensitive sandwich enzyme-linked immunosorbent assay, *J. Neurochem.* **61** (1993), 1828–1834.

[134] S.G. van Duinen, E.M. Castano, F. Prelli, G.T. Bots, W. Luyendijk and B. Frangione, Hereditary cerebral hemorrhage with amyloidosis in patients of Dutch origin is related to Alzheimer disease, *Proc. Natl. Acad. Sci. USA* **84** (1987), 5991–5994.

[135] M. von Bergen, P. Friedhoff, J. Biernat, J. Heberle, E.M. Mandelkow and E. Mandelkow, Assembly of tau protein into Alzheimer paired helical filaments depends on a local sequence motif ((306)VQIVYK(311)) forming beta structure, *Proc. Natl. Acad. Sci. USA* **97** (2000), 5129–5134.

[136] M. von Lindern, S. van Baal, J. Wiegant, A. Raap, A. Hagemeijer and G. Grosveld, can, a putative ongogene associated with Myeloid Leukomogenesis, may be activated by fusion of its 3' half to different genes characterization of the set gene, *Mol. Cell. Biol.* **12** (1992), 3346–3355.

[137] S.I. Walaas and P. Greengard, Protein phosphorylation and neuronal function, *Pharmacol. Rev.* **43** (1991), 299–349.

[138] G.P. Wang, I. Grundke-Iqbal, R.J. Kascsak, K. Iqbal and H.M. Wisniewski, Alzheimer neurofibrillary tangles monoclonal antibodies to inherent antigen/s, *Acta. Neuropathol. (Berl.)* **62** (1984), 268–275.

[139] G.P. Wang, S. Khatoon, K. Iqbal, and I. Grundke-Iqbal, Brain ubiquitin is markedly elevated in Alzheimer disease, *Brain Res* **566** (1991), 146–151.

[140] J.Z. Wang, C.X. Gong, T. Zaidi, I. Grundke-Iqbal and K. Iqbal, Dephosphorylation of Alzheimer paired helical filaments by protein phosphatase-2A and -2B, *J. Biol. Chem.* **270** (1995), 4854–4860.

[141] J.Z. Wang, I. Grundke-Iqbal and K. Iqbal, Glycosylation of microtubule-associated protein tau An abnormal posttranslational modification in Alzheimer's disease, *Nature Med* **2** (1996), 871–875.

[142] J.Z. Wang, Q. Wu, A. Smith, I. Grundke-Iqbal and K. Iqbal, τ is phosphorylated by GSK-3 at several sites found in Alzheimer disease and its biological activity markedly inhibited only after it is prephosphorylated by A-kinase, *FEBS Lett* **436** (1998), 28–34.

[143] M.D. Weingarten, A.H. Lockwood, S.Y. Hwo and M.W. Kirschner, A protein factor essential for microtubule assembly, *Proc. Natl. Acad. Sci. USA* **72** (1975), 1858–1862.

[144] H. Wille, G. Drewes, J. Biernat, E.M. Mandelkow and E. Mandelkow, Alzheimer-like paired helical filaments and antiparallel dimers formed from microtubule-associated protein tau *in vitro*, *J. Cell Biol.* **118** (1992), 573–584.

[145] D.M. Wilson and L.I. Binder, Polymerization of microtubule-associated protein tau under near-physiological conditions, *J. Biol. Chem.* **270** (1995), 24306–24314.

[146] B. Winblad and N. Poritis, Memantine in severe dementia: results of the 9M-Best Study (Benefit and efficacy in severely demented patients during treatment with memantine), *Int. J. Geriatr. Psychiatry* **14** (1999), 135–146.

[147] C.W. Wong, V. Ouaranta and G.G. Glenner, Neuritic plaques and cerebrovascular amyloid in Alzheimer disease are antigenically related, *Proc. Natl. Acad. Sci. USA* **82** (1985), 8729—8732.

[148] J.G. Wood, S.S. Mirra, N.J. Pollock and L.I. Binder, Neurofibrillary tangles of Alzheimer disease share antigenic determinants with the axonal microtubule-associated protein tau (tau), *Proc. Natl. Acad. Sci. USA* **83** (1986), 4040–4043. Erratum in *Proc. Natl. Acad. Sci. USA* **83** (1986), 9773.

[149] H. Yanagawa, S.H. Chung, Y. Ogawa, K. Sato, T. Shibata-Seki, J. Masai and K. Ishiguro, Protein anatomy C-tail region of human tau protein as a crucial structural element in Alzheimer's paired helical filament formation *in vitro*, *Biochemistry* **37** (1998), 1979–1988.

[150] S.H. Yen, F. Gaskin and S.M. Fu, Neurofibrillary tangles in senile dementia of the Alzheimer type share an antigenic determinant with intermediate filaments of the vimentin class, *Am. J. Pathol.* **113** (1983), 373–381.

Tau phosphorylation and proteolysis: Insights and perspectives

Gail V.W. Johnson*
Department of Psychiatry, University of Alabama at Birmingham, Birmingham, AL 35294, USA

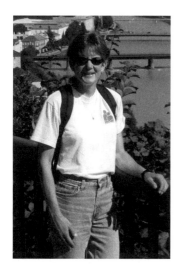

Abstract. In 1992 little was known about the specific protein kinases that phosphorylate tau and the proteases that regulate tau turnover. Although we had already demonstrated that tau was a substrate of the calcium-activated protease calpain (Johnson et al. (1989), Biochem Biophys Res Commun 163, 1505–1511), our publication entitled, "Phosphorylation by cAMP-dependent protein kinase inhibits the degradation of tau by calpain" (Litersky and Johnson (1992), J Biol Chem 267, 1563–1568) was the first demonstration that phosphorylation by a specific kinase could inhibit the proteolysis of tau by calpain. At the time these findings suggested that the abnormal phosphorylation of tau in Alzheimer's disease brain could result in impaired tau turnover and thus result in an abnormal accumulation of the protein that could contribute to the formation of pathological lesions. Since this initial finding, much has been learned about the proteolysis of tau, not only by calpain, but by other proteases as well. However, much remains unknown about how phosphorylation regulates tau turnover *in vivo* and the specific proteases involved. In this article we give a brief history of our initial findings and then discuss subsequent studies from our laboratory, as well as others, on tau proteolysis and modulation by phosphorylation and how these findings contribute to our understanding of the posttranslational processing of tau in Alzheimer's disease.

1. Tau proteolysis by calpain: a retrospect

The decisive year for the field of tau research was 1986, as this was the year that it was first demonstrated that the major antigenic component of the paired helical filaments (PHFs) and the neurofibrillary tangles (NFTs) in Alzheimer's disease brain was hyperphosphorylated tau [13,14,21,41]. Even though tau had been discovered as a protein factor that facilitated microtubule assembly in 1975 [40], very little was known about tau in 1986 other than it was a microtubule-associated phosphoprotein [5] and that phosphorylation negatively impacted its ability to promote microtubule assembly [24]. Nonetheless, soon after the initial discovery, it was speculated that the hyperphosphorylation of tau might make it more resistant to proteolysis and thus more likely to accumulate in neurons contributing to the formation of the PHFs and NFTs. However no one at the time knew which proteolytic systems were responsible for the turnover of tau.

---

*Corresponding author: Gail V.W. Johnson, Ph.D., Professor, Department of Psychiatry, 1720 7th Avenue South, SC1061, University of Alabama at Birmingham, School of Medicine, Birmingham, AL 35294-0017, USA. Tel.: +1 205 934 2465; Fax: +1 205 934 2500; E-mail: gvwj@uab.edu.

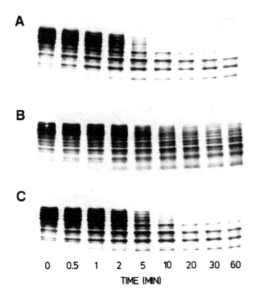

Fig. 1. Immunoblots of the calpain-induced proteolysis of control tau (A), tau phosphorylated by the catalytic subunit of PKA (B), and tau dephosphorylated by alkaline phosphatase (C). Tau was proteolyzed by calpain at an enzyme-to-substrate ratio of 1:20. Samples were subjected to SDS-PAGE and immunoblotted (Tau 2, 1:15,000). Reactions were stopped at times indicated below each lane. Reprinted from [25] with permission from the publisher.

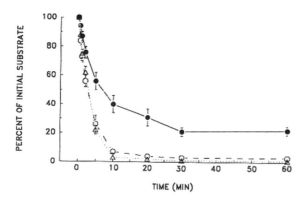

Fig. 2. Quantitative analysis of the calpain-induced (1:20, enzyme-to-substrate ratio) proteolysis of control tau (open circle), tau phosphorylated by PKA (closed circle), or tau dephosphorylated by alkaline phosphatase (open triangle). Reprinted from [25] with permission from the publisher.

Although little was known about the proteases that degraded tau, in the early 1980's Nixon and colleagues provided evidence that neurofilaments, which are also cytoskeletal proteins, were degraded by a calcium-activated proteinase [30] and in 1986 Wisniewski's group verified that neurofilaments were substrates of the calcium-activated neutral proteases [27], which are also known as calpains. Given that calpains are present in brain at high concentrations with neuronal localization [32,39], and it had been demonstrated that they could degrade cytoskeleton proteins such as neurofilaments [27], we decided to test the hypothesis that tau is a substrate for calpain. For these initial studies we used two different preparations of tau, both isolated from bovine brain. We made twice-cycled microtubules and subsequently purified tau from this preparation, and also isolated tau from total brain without microtubule cycling. Using these two preparations we found that tau was a substrate of calpain, but that the two preparations of tau showed differential sensitivity to the protease. Tau isolated from twice-cycled microtubules was degraded extremely rapidly by calpain, while the total brain tau was degraded at a significantly slower rate [19]. This was the first demonstration that tau was a substrate of calpain and that there were at least two populations of tau in the brain based on calpain sensitivity. At the time we did not know what contributed to this differential sensitivity of tau to calpain proteolysis. However, given that Pant had shown the year before that dephosphorylating neurofilaments increased their sensitivity to calpain [31] and the fact that tau in Alzheimer's disease brain is hyperphosphorylated [14], we speculated that it was likely that the phosphorylation state of tau was regulating its sensitivity to degradation by calpain. This speculation was also supported by the fact that tau that was dephosphorylated bound microtubules more efficiently, and thus would be expected to be enriched in the twice-cycled microtubule tau preparation [24]. This initial finding and subsequent speculations are what lead us to carry out the studies that were published in our classic study [25] that is highlighted in this special issue of the *Journal of Alzheimer's Disease*. In the next paragraph we give a retrospective of the studies in this paper.

To examine how phosphorylation affects the proteolysis of tau by calpain, we needed to find a protein kinase that efficiently phosphorylated tau. Fifteen years ago very little was known about the protein kinases that phosphorylate tau. An earlier study by Pierre and Nunez [34] had shown that cAMP-dependent protein kinase (PKA) could phosphorylate tau. This finding along with the report by Chen and Stracher that phosphorylation of actin-binding protein by PKA stabilizes it against degradation by calpain [3] encouraged us to examine how phosphorylation of tau by PKA modulated its susceptibility to calpain-mediated degradation. In this study we used bovine brain tau isolated from twice-cycled microtubules and first showed that tau was efficiently phosphorylated by PKA *in vitro* and that this phosphorylation decreased its electrophoretic

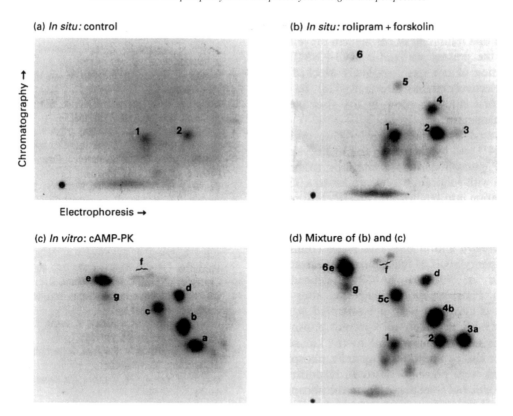

Fig. 3. Autoradiographs of two-dimensional phosphopeptide mapping of tau resulting from basal phosphorylation *in situ* (a), rolipram (a phosphodiesterase inhibitor) and forskolin (an activator of adenylyl cyclase) stimulated phosphorylation (b), tau phosphorylated *in vitro* by PKA (c), or a combination of (b) and (c) (d). Slices were treated as indicated, and tau was excised from polyacrylamide gels, digested with proteases and subjected to electrophoresis on cellulose TLC plates, followed by ascending chromatography. Peptides phosphorylated *in situ* are indicated by numbers (a, b and d) and peptides phosphorylated *in vitro* by letters (c and d). Reproduced with permission from Fleming and Johnson (1995), *Biochemical Journal* **309**, 41–47. ©The Biochemical Society.

mobility. This was intriguing given the fact that the migration of PHF-tau on SDS polyacrylamide gels was also reduced, albeit to a greater extent than tau that had been phosphorylated by PKA [23]. We then went on to clearly demonstrate that phosphorylation of tau by PKA increased its resistance to calpain-mediated degradation (Figs 1 and 2). This was the first demonstration that phosphorylation of tau by a specific kinase results in increased resistance to proteolysis by calpain [25]. Interestingly, although calcium/calmodulin-dependent protein kinase II also phosphorylated tau, phosphorylation of tau by this kinase did not alter its sensitivity to proteolysis by calpain [18]. These data suggest that the inhibition of calpain-mediated tau proteolysis after phosphorylation by PKA was a selective rather than general effect. At the time we hypothesized that abnormal phosphorylation by PKA, or other protein kinases, could result in a protease resistant population of tau, thus increasing tau levels and contributing to PHF formation in Alzheimer's disease.

2. Tau phosphorylation by PKA in situ and the effects of phosphorylation on calcium-dependent proteolysis

After the discovery that phosphorylation of tau *in vitro* by PKA increased its resistance to calpain-mediated proteolysis [25], we wanted to determine whether tau was an *in situ* substrate of PKA. To do this we labeled rat brain slices with ^{32}Pi, activated PKA by stimulating adenylyl cyclase and inhibiting phosphodiesterase activity, and subsequently isolated tau and determined if this treatment increased tau ^{32}P-phosphorylation. The results of these studies clearly demonstrated that increasing cAMP levels in the cell resulted in an increase in tau phosphorylation, and further by two dimensional phosphopeptide mapping we demonstrated that many of the sites on tau that are phosphorylated *in situ* in response to activation of PKA were the same as those phosphorylated by PKA *in vitro* (Fig. 3) [9]. We also observed an increase in tau phos-

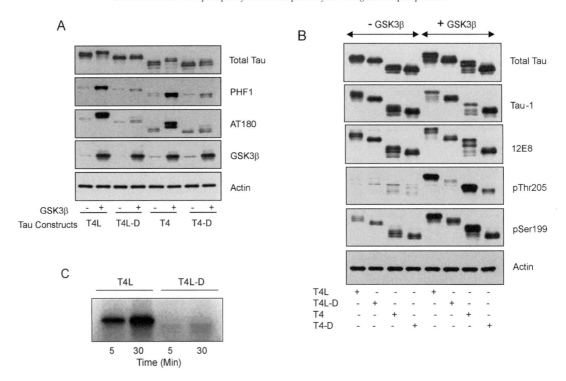

Fig. 4. Asp421 truncated tau constructs are not phosphorylated by GSK3β as efficiently as full-length tau constructs. **A.** and **B.** Cells were transiently transfected with T4L (Tau + exons 2,3 and 10), T4L-D421 (T4-D), T4 (Tau − exons 2 and 3, + exon 10), or T4-D421 (T4-D) alone, or in combination with glycogen synthase kinase 3β (GSK3β) (The D421 constructs were truncated at Asp421 to mimic caspase-cleaved tau). The expression level of all tau constructs was similar and GSK3β expression levels were also the same in all the transiently transfected cells. Representative immunoblots with Tau5/5A6 (Total tau) showed that overexpression of GSK3β reduced the electrophoretic mobility of T4L and T4 compared with the mobility observed in the absence of GSK3β. **A.** Phosphorylation of full-length tau (T4L or T4) by GSK3β resulted in a robust increase in PHF-1 (Ser396/404) and AT180 (Thr231) immunoreactivity compared to that when tau was expressed alone. In contrast, co-expression of GSK3β with the Asp421 truncated tau constructs (T4L-D4 or T4-D) resulted in minimal increases in PHF1 and AT180 immunoreactivity. The actin blots demonstrate that equal amounts of protein were loaded in each lane. **B.** Expression of GSK3β also resulted in a robust increase in the phosphorylation of full-length tau (T4L or T4), but not the Asp421 truncated tau constructs (T4L-D4 or T4-D), at the Tau-1 epitope (Tau-1 recognizes a dephosphorylated epitope so decreased immunoreactivity indicates increased phosphorylation), Thr205 and Ser199. 12E8 immunoreactivity was the same for all constructs in the absence (−) or presence (+) of GSK3β. The actin blots shows that same amount of protein was loaded in each lane. **C.** Representative autoradiograph (of 4 separate experiments) showing the phosphorylation of recombinant T4L and T4L-D421 by recombinant GSK3β in an *in vitro* kinase assay. The tau constructs were incubated with GSK3β for the times indicated. The data show that T4L is phosphorylated by GSK3β much more efficiently than T4L-D421. Reprinted from [4] with permission from the publisher.

phorylation in response to increasing cAMP levels in a cell culture model system [26]. Overall these studies strongly indicate that tau is an *in vivo* substrate of PKA.

In 1993 Scott et al. [37] identified the sites on tau that are phosphorylated *in vitro* by PKA, and Davies and colleagues [17] used this information to make antibodies that specifically recognize two of these phosphoepitopes on tau, Ser214 and Ser409. Davies and colleagues then went on to demonstrate that these antibodies stained tau pathology in Alzheimer's disease brain, but did not stain normal brain. In addition, they provided evidence that PKA, as well as a PKA anchoring protein (AKAP79), are tightly associated with NFT pathology thus suggesting that PKA may contribute to the abnormal phosphorylation of tau in Alzheimer's disease [17]. There is also data to suggest that PKA may be involved in creating the Alzheimer's disease-selective epitope on tau that is recognized by the AT100 antibody [45]. Further, α-synuclein stimulates PKA-catalyzed phosphorylation of tau [16], which is intriguing given the recent findings that α-synuclein induces fibrillization of tau, and α-synuclein and tau co-localize to filamentous inclusions in the brain [11]. Overall, these and other studies strongly suggest that PKA phosphorylates tau in physiological as well as in pathological conditions *in vivo*.

Although we had clearly demonstrated that tau is an *in vitro* substrate of calpain, it was also important to demonstrate that tau is an *in situ* substrate of calpain and that the phosphorylation state of tau regulates its sus-

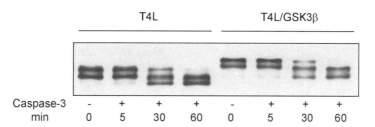

Fig. 5. Tau and Tau phosphorylated by glycogen synthase kinase 3β (GSK3β) are cleaved by active caspase-3 at the same rate and to the same extent. Lysates from cells transfected with either T4L (Tau + exons 2,3 and 10) alone or T4L and GSK3((T4L/GSK3β) were incubated with active caspase-3 for the times indicated and subsequently immunoblotted for total tau levels with Tau5/5A6. These data demonstrate that T4L and phosphorylated T4L are equivalent substrates of caspase-3. Reprinted from [4] with permission from the publisher.

ceptibility to proteolysis. Therefore in our next study we demonstrated that tau undergoes calcium-dependent proteolysis *in situ*, and that increasing the phosphorylation state of tau significantly inhibits calcium-mediated proteolysis [26]. Further, we also showed that the calcium-mediated degradation of tau was blocked by calpain inhibitors [42]. It is also interesting to note that in a recent study it was demonstrated that proteasomal inhibition paradoxically results in tau proteolysis and that this is likely due to calpain activation as a calpain inhibitor effectively blocked the degradation of tau in response to proteasome inhibitors [7]. Taken together, these studies strongly indicate that tau is an *in vivo* substrate of calpain. Induction of apoptosis in granule cells results in the formation of a dephosphorylated tau breakdown product, and the formation of this proteolytic fragment is inhibited by both calpain and caspase inhibitors indicating that tau is a substrate of both proteases *in vivo* [1]. Indeed, in stress-induced cell death models, tau dephosphorylation appears to precede proteolysis.

Even though there is good evidence that tau is a bona fide *in vivo* substrate of calpain, how site-specific phosphorylation modulates calpain-mediated proteolysis *in vivo* remains unclear. Differentially phosphorylated fetal tau isoforms are degraded at the same rate by calpain, indicating that these phosphorylation events do not regulate calpain-mediated proteolysis [29]. However, it needs to be considered that tau is rapidly dephosphorylated postmortem and therefore tau purified from human brain is not truly representative of the *in vivo* phosphorylation state of tau [28]. PHF-tau, which is extensively phosphorylated, is extremely resistant to calpain-mediated hydrolysis [29], but whether the resistance of PHF-tau to calpain-mediated degradation is due to phosphorylation state, conformation state [43, 44] or a combination of both remains to be clearly established.

3. Tau proteolysis by caspases

In recent years there have been a growing number of studies on the proteolysis of tau by proteases other than calpain, and how phosphorylation affects these cleavage events. It is now well-documented that in certain cell models tau is proteolyzed by caspases in response to apoptotic-inducing stressors [1,22]. Caspases are a family of cysteine aspartyl proteases that play critical roles in apoptosis. The predominant site on tau that is cleaved by many caspases is Asp421/Ser422 [10]. Using antibodies that specifically recognize tau truncated at Asp421 (and hence caspase-cleaved), it has been demonstrated that tau that has been proteolyzed by caspases is present in Alzheimer's disease brain but not in control brain [10,35,36], and that most of the tau pathologies contain caspase-cleaved tau. It is also intriguing that tau truncated at Asp421 is more fibrillogenic than full-length tau in *in vitro* polymerization assays [10]. Interestingly, tau truncated at Asp421 is inefficiently phosphorylated both *in situ* and *in vitro* when compared to full-length tau, however phosphorylation of tau does not alter its sensitivity to caspase-mediate proteolysis (Figs 4 and 5). These data suggest that in Alzheimer's disease brain, tau phosphorylation may precede caspase cleavage [4]. It is also intriguing to note that a combination of phosphorylation and cleavage was required to induce the formation of sarkosyl insoluble tau inclusions in a cell culture model (Fig. 6) [4], suggesting that caspase cleavage events and abnormal phosphorylation may synergize to facilitate tau fibrillization and aggregation in Alzheimer's disease.

4. Tau degradation by the proteasome

There is also evidence that the proteasome may play a role in regulating tau turnover. In an *in vitro* assay tau

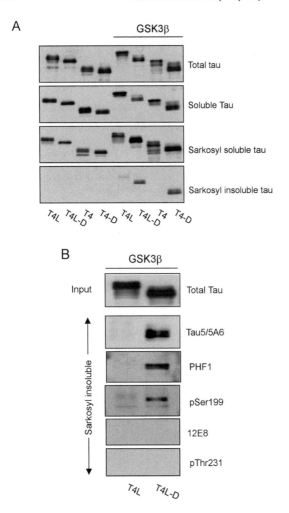

Fig. 6. The Asp421 truncated tau constructs become sarkosyl insoluble in the presence of glycogen synthase kinase 3β (GSK3β). **A**. Cells were transiently transfected with tau constructs alone or with GSK3β. Cell lysates were then fractionated into soluble, sarkosyl soluble and sarkosyl insoluble fractions. The expression of the tau constructs was equivalent for all conditions (Total tau). Co-expression of GSK3β resulted in both T4L-D421 (T4L-D) and T4-D421 (T4-D) partitioning into the sarkosyl insoluble fraction. Even in the presence of GSK3β, the full-length tau constructs were never observed in the sarkosyl insoluble fraction. **B**. The sarkosyl-insoluble fractions from cells transfected with GSK3β and either T4L or T4L-D421 were probed with the phospho-tau independent tau antibodies Tau5/5A6 or the phospho-dependent antibodies, PHF1, phospho-Ser199, 12E8 or phospho-Thr231. These results show that the T4L-D421 in the sarkosyl insoluble fractions is phosphorylated at the PHF1 and Ser199 epitopes. The top panel (input) shows that the amount of tau in the samples was equivalent prior to the preparation of the sarkosyl insoluble fractions. Reprinted from [4] with permission from the publisher.

is efficiently degraded by isolated proteasomes [2], the degradation occurs at both ends of the tau molecule and relatively stable intermediates are produced because of the less efficient proteolysis of the microtubule binding domains [6]. Treatment of human neuroblastoma cells with the irreversible proteasome inhibitor lactacystin attenuates the turnover of tau [6]. Likewise, when an oligodendroglia cell line engineered to overexpress tau was treated with the proteasome inhibitor MG-132 a decrease in tau proteolysis was observed [12]. These studies suggest that tau may be degraded by the proteasome through an ubiquitin-independent pathway. However, more recent studies now suggest that tau may also be degraded by the proteasome through ubiquitin-dependent pathways. The heat shock proteins hsp/hsc70 and hsp90 bind tau [8,33,38], and this recruits in the E3 ligase CHIP, which results in the ubiquitylation of tau [33, 38]. Overexpression of CHIP has been shown to result in an increase in tau degradation and a reduction in the formation of detergent insoluble tau, suggesting that tau degradation by the proteasome can be ubiquitin dependent [15]. In one study data was presented suggesting that phosphorylated tau is selectively ubiquitylated by the CHIP-hsc/hsp70 complex [38], however in another study non-phosphorylated tau was readily ubiquitylated by CHIP-hsc/hsp70 [33]. Therefore it is unclear at this point whether or not the phosphorylation state of tau modulates the process of ubiquitylation and subsequent degradation. Intriguingly, PHF-tau co-precipitates with the proteasome and proteasomal activity was inversely correlated with the amount of PHF-tau that co-precipitated. These data suggest that PHF-tau may inhibit proteasome activity, perhaps due to the fact that it cannot be efficiently degraded, and thus contribute to neuronal dysfunction and death in Alzheimer's disease brain [20].

5. Summary

There is now significant evidence that tau is an *in vivo* substrate of calpain, as well as caspases and the proteasome. Further, site-specific phosphorylation of tau regulates its susceptibility to calpain-mediated proteolysis, however whether or not hyperphosphorylation of specific sites on tau in Alzheimer's disease brain make it more resistant to calpain hydrolysis and thus contribute to the tau pathogenic cascade remains to be determined. It is also presently unclear how phosphorylation impacts tau proteolysis by the caspases or the proteasome, and how dysregulation of these proteolytic systems in Alzheimer's disease may facilitate the formation of tau pathology. Nonetheless, in the years since our initial discovery that tau is a substrate of calpain and that phosphorylation by PKA inhibits tau proteolysis by calpain [19,25] important advances have been made in understanding the processes that regulate tau turnover and the role dysregulation of these events may play in the pathogenesis of Alzheimer's disease.

Acknowledgements

The work from the author's laboratory cited in this review was supported by NIH grants and grants from the Alzheimer's Association. Tori A. Matthews is gratefully acknowledged for critically reading the manuscript and providing helpful comments and suggestions.

References

[1] N. Canu, L. Dus, C. Barbato, M.T. Ciotti, C. Brancolini, A.M. Rinaldi, M. Novak, A. Cattaneo, A. Bradbury and P. Calissano, Tau cleavage and dephosphorylation in cerebellar granule neurons undergoing apoptosis, *J Neurosci* 18 (1998), 7061–7074.

[2] C. Cardozo and C. Michaud, Proteasome-mediated degradation of tau proteins occurs independently of the chymotrypsin-like activity by a nonprocessive pathway, *Arch Biochem Biophys* 408 (2002), 103–110.

[3] M. Chen and A. Stracher, In situ phosphorylation of platelet actin-binding protein by cAMP-dependent protein kinase stabilizes it against proteolysis by calpain, *J Biol Chem* 264 (1989), 14282–14289.

[4] J.H. Cho and G.V. Johnson, Primed phosphorylation of tau at Thr231 by glycogen synthase kinase 3beta (GSK3beta) plays a critical role in regulating tau's ability to bind and stabilize microtubules, *J Neurochem* 88 (2004), 349–358.

[5] D.W. Cleveland, S.Y. Hwo and M.W. Kirschner, Physical and chemical properties of purified tau factor and the role of tau in microtubule assembly, *J Mol Biol* 116 (1977), 227–247.

[6] D.C. David, R. Layfield, L. Serpell, Y. Narain, M. Goedert and M.G. Spillantini, Proteasomal degradation of tau protein, *J Neurochem* 83 (2002), 176–185.

[7] P. Delobel, O. Leroy, M. Hamdane, A.V. Sambo, A. Delacourte and L. Buee, Proteasome inhibition and Tau proteolysis: an unexpected regulation, *FEBS Lett* 579 (2005), 1–5.

[8] F. Dou, W.J. Netzer, K. Tanemura, F. Li, F.U. Hartl, A. Takashima, G.K. Gouras, P. Greengard and H. Xu, Chaperones increase association of tau protein with microtubules, *Proc Natl Acad Sci USA* 100 (2003), 721–726.

[9] L.M. Fleming and G.V. Johnson, Modulation of the phosphorylation state of tau in situ: the roles of calcium and cyclic AMP, *Biochem J* 309(Pt 1) (1995), 41–47.

[10] T.C. Gamblin, F. Chen, A. Zambrano, A. Abraha, S. Lagalwar, A.L. Guillozet, M. Lu, Y. Fu, F. Garcia-Sierra, N. LaPointe, R. Miller, R.W. Berry, L.I. Binder and V.L. Cryns, Caspase cleavage of tau: linking amyloid and neurofibrillary tangles in Alzheimer's disease, *Proc Natl Acad Sci USA* 100 (2003), 10032–10037.

[11] B.I. Giasson, M.S. Forman, M. Higuchi, L.I. Golbe, C.L. Graves, P.T. Kotzbauer, J.Q. Trojanowski and V.M. Lee, Initiation and synergistic fibrillization of tau and alpha-synuclein, *Science* 300 (2003), 636–640.

[12] O. Goldbaum, M. Oppermann, M. Handschuh, D. Dabir, B. Zhang, M.S. Forman, J.Q. Trojanowski, V.M. Lee and C. Richter-Landsberg, Proteasome inhibition stabilizes tau inclusions in oligodendroglial cells that occur after treatment with okadaic acid, *J Neurosci* 23 (2003), 8872–8880.

[13] I. Grundke-Iqbal, K. Iqbal, M. Quinlan, Y.C. Tung, M.S. Zaidi and H.M. Wisniewski, Microtubule-associated protein tau. A component of Alzheimer paired helical filaments, *J Biol Chem* 261 (1986), 6084–6089.

[14] I. Grundke-Iqbal, K. Iqbal, Y.C. Tung, M. Quinlan, H.M. Wisniewski and L.I. Binder, Abnormal phosphorylation of the microtubule-associated protein tau (tau) in Alzheimer cytoskeletal pathology, *Proc Natl Acad Sci USA* 83 (1986), 4913–4917.

[15] S. Hatakeyama, M. Matsumoto, T. Kamura, M. Murayama, D.H. Chui, E. Planel, R. Takahashi, K.I. Nakayama and A. Takashima, U-box protein carboxyl terminus of Hsc70-interacting protein (CHIP) mediates poly-ubiquitylation preferentially on four-repeat Tau and is involved in neurodegeneration of tauopathy, *J Neurochem* 91 (2004), 299–307.

[16] P.H. Jensen, H. Hager, M.S. Nielsen, P. Hojrup, J. Gliemann and R. Jakes, alpha-synuclein binds to Tau and stimulates the protein kinase A-catalyzed tau phosphorylation of serine residues 262 and 356, *J Biol Chem* 274 (1999), 25481–25489.

[17] G.A. Jicha, C. Weaver, E. Lane, C. Vianna, Y. Kress, J. Rockwood and P. Davies, cAMP-dependent protein kinase phosphorylations on tau in Alzheimer's disease, *J Neurosci* 19 (1999), 7486–7494.

[18] G.V. Johnson, Differential phosphorylation of tau by cyclic AMP-dependent protein kinase and Ca^{2+}/calmodulin-dependent protein kinase II: metabolic and functional consequences, *J Neurochem* 59 (1992), 2056–2062.

[19] G.V. Johnson, R.S. Jope and L.I. Binder, Proteolysis of tau by calpain, *Biochem Biophys Res Commun* 163 (1989), 1505–1511.

[20] S. Keck, R. Nitsch, T. Grune and O. Ullrich, Proteasome inhibition by paired helical filament-tau in brains of patients with Alzheimer's disease, *J Neurochem* 85 (2003), 115–122.

[21] K.S. Kosik, C.L. Joachim and D.J. Selkoe, Microtubule-associated protein tau (tau) is a major antigenic component of paired helical filaments in Alzheimer disease, *Proc Natl Acad Sci USA* 83 (1986), 4044–4048.

[22] P.K. Krishnamurthy, J.L. Mays, G.N. Bijur and G.V. Johnson, Transient oxidative stress in SH-SY5Y human neuroblastoma cells results in caspase dependent and independent cell death and tau proteolysis, *J Neurosci Res* 61 (2000), 515–523.

[23] V.M. Lee, B.J. Balin, L. Otvos, Jr. and J.Q. Trojanowski, A68: a major subunit of paired helical filaments and derivatized forms of normal Tau, *Science* 251 (1991), 675–678.

[24] G. Lindwall and R.D. Cole, Phosphorylation affects the ability of tau protein to promote microtubule assembly, *J Biol Chem* 259 (1984), 5301–5305.

[25] J.M. Litersky and G.V. Johnson, Phosphorylation by cAMP-dependent protein kinase inhibits the degradation of tau by calpain, *J Biol Chem* 267 (1992), 1563–1568.

[26] J.M. Litersky and G.V. Johnson, Phosphorylation of tau in situ: inhibition of calcium-dependent proteolysis, *J Neurochem* 65 (1995), 903–911.

[27] M.N. Malik, A.M. Sheikh, M.D. Fenko and H.M. Wisniewski, Purification and degradation of purified neurofilament proteins by the brain calcium-activated neutral proteases, *Life Sci* 39 (1986), 1335–1343.

[28] E.S. Matsuo, R.W. Shin, M.L. Billingsley, A. Van deVoorde, M. O'Connor, J.Q. Trojanowski and V.M. Lee, Biopsy-derived

adult human brain tau is phosphorylated at many of the same sites as Alzheimer's disease paired helical filament tau, *Neuron* **13** (1994), 989–1002.

[29] M. Mercken, F. Grynspan and R.A. Nixon, Differential sensitivity to proteolysis by brain calpain of adult human tau, fetal human tau and PHF-tau, *FEBS Lett* **368** (1995), 10–14.

[30] R.A. Nixon, B.A. Brown and C.A. Marotta, Limited proteolytic modification of a neurofilament protein involves a proteinase activated by endogenous levels of calcium, *Brain Res* **275** (1983), 384–388.

[31] H.C. Pant, Dephosphorylation of neurofilament proteins enhances their susceptibility to degradation by calpain, *Biochem J* **256** (1988), 665–668.

[32] L.S. Perlmutter, C. Gall, M. Baudry and G. Lynch, Distribution of calcium-activated protease calpain in the rat brain, *J Comp Neurol* **296** (1990), 269–276.

[33] L. Petrucelli, D. Dickson, K. Kehoe, J. Taylor, H. Snyder, A. Grover, M. De Lucia, E. McGowan, J. Lewis, G. Prihar, J. Kim, W.H. Dillmann, S.E. Browne, A. Hall, R. Voellmy, Y. Tsuboi, T.M. Dawson, B. Wolozin, J. Hardy and M. Hutton, CHIP and Hsp70 regulate tau ubiquitination, degradation and aggregation, *Hum Mol Genet* **13** (2004), 703–714.

[34] M. Pierre and J. Nunez, Multisite phosphorylation of tau proteins from rat brain, *Biochem Biophys Res Commun* **115** (1983), 212–219.

[35] R.A. Rissman, W.W. Poon, M. Blurton-Jones, S. Oddo, R. Torp, M.P. Vitek, F.M. LaFerla, T.T. Rohn and C.W. Cotman, Caspase-cleavage of tau is an early event in Alzheimer disease tangle pathology, *J Clin Invest* **114** (2004), 121–130.

[36] T.T. Rohn, R.A. Rissman, M.C. Davis, Y.E. Kim, C.W. Cotman and E. Head, Caspase-9 activation and caspase cleavage of tau in the Alzheimer's disease brain, *Neurobiol Dis* **11** (2002), 341–354.

[37] C.W. Scott, R.C. Spreen, J.L. Herman, F.P. Chow, M.D. Davison, J. Young and C.B. Caputo, Phosphorylation of recombinant tau by cAMP-dependent protein kinase. Identification of phosphorylation sites and effect on microtubule assembly, *J Biol Chem* **268** (1993), 1166–1173.

[38] H. Shimura, D. Schwartz, S.P. Gygi and K.S. Kosik, CHIP-Hsc70 complex ubiquitinates phosphorylated tau and enhances cell survival, *J Biol Chem* **279** (2004), 4869–4876.

[39] R. Siman, C. Gall, L.S. Perlmutter, C. Christian, M. Baudry and G. Lynch, Distribution of calpain I, an enzyme associated with degenerative activity, in rat brain, *Brain Res* **347** (1985), 399–403.

[40] M.D. Weingarten, A.H. Lockwood, S.Y. Hwo and M.W. Kirschner, A protein factor essential for microtubule assembly, *Proc Natl Acad Sci USA* **72** (1975), 1858–1862.

[41] J.G. Wood, S.S. Mirra, N.J. Pollock and L.I. Binder, Neurofibrillary tangles of Alzheimer disease share antigenic determinants with the axonal microtubule-associated protein tau (tau), *Proc Natl Acad Sci USA* **83** (1986), 4040–4043.

[42] H.Q. Xie and G.V. Johnson, Calcineurin inhibition prevents calpain-mediated proteolysis of tau in differentiated PC12 cells, *J Neurosci Res* **53** (1998), 153–164.

[43] L.S. Yang, W. Gordon-Krajcer and H. Ksiezak-Reding, Tau released from paired helical filaments with formic acid or guanidine is susceptible to calpain-mediated proteolysis, *J Neurochem* **69** (1997), 1548–1558.

[44] L.S. Yang and H. Ksiezak-Reding, Calpain-induced proteolysis of normal human tau and tau associated with paired helical filaments, *Eur J Biochem* **233** (1995), 9–17.

[45] Q. Zheng-Fischhofer, J. Biernat, E.M. Mandelkow, S. Illenberger, R. Godemann and E. Mandelkow, Sequential phosphorylation of Tau by glycogen synthase kinase-3beta and protein kinase A at Thr212 and Ser214 generates the Alzheimer-specific epitope of antibody AT100 and requires a paired-helical-filament-like conformation, *Eur J Biochem* **252** (1998), 542–552.

Traveling the tau pathway: A personal account

Kenneth S. Kosik
Harriman Professor of Neuroscience Research, Co-Director, Neuroscience Research Institute, Dept of Molecular and Cellular and Developmental Biology, University of California, Santa Barbara, CA 93106-5060, USA
Tel.: +1 805 893 5222; Fax: +1 805 893 2005; E-mail: kosik@lifesci.ucsb.edu

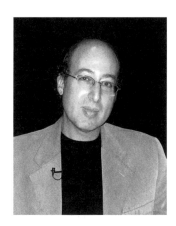

Abstract. Studies of the tau protein and its pathological fate as a neurofibrillary tangle have been a pillar of Alzheimer's disease research. The understanding of the fundamental position that tau occupies in the disease cascade is a tribute to an international group of scientists who brought rigor, candid assessments of data, and critical thinking to the problem. The tau pathway winds its way from astute clinical observations to pathological correlations, from molecular and cellular experiments to mining informatic data, and from animal behavior to the biophysics of protein structure. For most the vindication of this tireless effort will come from tau-based therapies; but for others the remarkable biology revealed by the Alzheimer disease process has been its own reward.

1. Setting the stage

When I began my post-doctoral fellowship in 1980, fourteen years had already elapsed since the group of Roth, Tomlinson, and Blessed began publishing a series of remarkable papers that paradigmatically impacted the Alzheimer field more than any other work since Alzheimer himself described the first case of this disease [5,42,43,48]. Their studies made it clear that Alzheimer's disease was not a rare dementing illness in patients under the age of 65; instead the pathological process also accounted for the enormous toll of dementia in those over age 65. Perhaps an even more important conclusion was the suggestion that Alzheimer's disease is not the inevitable consequence of aging, but is a disease to which the elderly are particularly vulnerable. Despite these startling findings, in 1980 research in Alzheimer's disease was conducted by a small community whose principle meeting venue was an annual gathering of the American Association of Neuropathologists. At that time the Society for Neuroscience was not interested in disease-related research. And nearly all of the interest in Alzheimer neuropathology centered on the neurofibrillary tangle, the structure which Alois Alzheimer had focused upon.

2. Microtubule-associated proteins: MAP2 and tau are segregated in neurons

Although my assigned project in the lab, under the direction of Dennis Selkoe involved aluminum toxicity [27], a model believed at the time to have some relevance to neurofibrillary disease, I pursued a side project that involved the analysis of post-mortem brain proteins by two-dimensional gel electrophoresis [26] and stumbled into an interesting class of proteins called microtubule-associated proteins (MAPs). This family of proteins awakened a dual interest that continues to this day: the role of MAPs in the pathogenesis of neurofibrillary tangles and the role of MAPs in the ontogeny and maintenance of neuronal polarity. The link between these two problems – how an axonally compartmentalized protein can drive neuritic pathology in dendrites-remains unanswered. But I am getting ahead of myself.

Using the relatively new monoclonal antibody technology brought to our laboratory by Larry Duffy (now at the University of Alaska, Fairbanks), I raised an antibody to MAP2. Based on immunohistochemical data, I first thought that MAP2 was associated with the neurofibrillary tangle [28], but this turned out to be incorrect. However, the MAP2 antibodies revealed the extra-ordinary subcellular segregation of this MAP by demonstrating an elaborate portrait of all the dendrites on a section [15]. Previous approaches such as Golgi labeling could not label all dendrites in a single section, and instead tended to reveal very limited populations of dendrites. Interestingly, this collaboration with the neuroanatomists, Marta Escobar and Hernan Pimienta, who were visiting the lab of Verne Caviness at the Shriver Center from Cali, foreshadowed a long and highly productive collaboration with many Colombian scientists, but most notably Francisco Lopera [36].

3. Paired helical filaments are made of tau polymers

In the early to mid 1980's we were using a number of polyclonal antibodies from the Selkoe lab raised against extracted paired helical filaments. When I applied these antibodies to our microtubule preparations we obtained the surprising result that nearly all of the independently raised polyclonal antibodies reacted with a band on a gel that corresponded to the tau protein. It was highly serendipitous that our erroneous earlier suspicion about the association of MAP2 with neurofibrillary tangles prepared us for the genuine discovery of the association of tau with neurofibrillary tangles. The tau protein had previously been characterized by Don Cleveland while in the laboratory of Marc Kirschner where they conducted experiments on proteins that co-purified with microtubules as they were passaged through cycles of temperature-dependent polymerization and depolymerization [10,11,51]. With additional absorption experiments and the use of tau antibodies we came to the conclusion that tau protein was a component of the neurofibrillary tangle. With my growing interest in MAPs, I often spoke to investigators in the cell biology community who studied microtubules. Among these scientists was a friend and colleague, Lester (Skip) Binder. As we were preparing our studies on tau for publication, Skip told me that he and his colleague, John Wood at Emory, had reached similar conclusions concerning tau and neurofibrillary tangles. We decided to co-publish our results [29,52]. At about the same time Grundke-Iqbal also recognized that tau protein was a component of the neurofibrillary tangle [17,18], and just before any of these papers were published Jean-Pierre Brion reported [6] that tangles can be labeled with tau antibodies. Two years later we showed that the entire tau protein assembled into paired helical filaments by using a technique that was novel at the time, epitope mapping [31]. Since then many additional epitope specific antibodies directed against a variety of sites in the tau protein have been extra-ordinarily revealing. Also in 1988, Yasuo Ihara and Claude Wischik independently confirmed that tau was the major component of the neurofibrillary tangle. Yasuo, with whom I had shared lab space while a post-doctoral fellow, fractionated and sequenced paired helical filament-derived peptides [23]. Claude Wischik [49,50] in the same year defined a highly insoluble core component of the paired helical filaments that consisted of the carboxy terminus of tau.

At the time these data were emerging it was widely believed that neurofibrillary tangles were made of neurofilament protein. The basis for this belief was first the somewhat similar appearance of individual paired helical filaments to neurofilaments by electron microscopy, and later based on cross reactivity between neurofibrillary tangles and some neurofilament antibodies. We deduced that the basis for this mistaken impression was the tendency for many neurofilament antibodies that recognize a phosphorylation site on the neurofilament to cross react with a phosphorylation-dependent epitope on tau [40]. Another candidate component of the neurofibrillary tangle was the antigen recognized by the antibody Alz50 raised in the laboratory of Peter Davies. This antibody recognized neurofibrillary pathology very strongly and did so quite early in the disease process. We showed that the antigen for this antibody too was tau [41]. By the end of the eighties it was irrefutable that tau was the principle component of the neurofibrillary tangle.

4. The neuritic pathology of Alzheimer's disease is extensive

Among the monoclonal antibodies we raised was one to tau called 5E2. With this and other tau antibodies in hand I began a very fruitful collaboration with two neuropathologists, Neil Kowall and Ann McKee at the Massachusetts General Hospital. When we applied these antibodies to human post-mortem

Alzheimer brain tissue, we were surprised by the extensive neuritic changes [33,38]. Previously the pathology was believed to be confined to the more limited number of tangles observed within cell bodies or as vestiges of dead cells called ghost tangles or tombstones. The antibodies dramatically revealed that the pathology extended to the neuronal processes, which appeared as swollen dystrophic neurites that often completely dominated the principle anatomical target areas of the Alzheimer brain. Not surprisingly these early descriptions of neuritic pathology, referred to as neuropil threads or curly fibers, foreshadowed another aspect of the pathology-the loss of synapses [13].

5. Tau inclusions characterize several neurodegenerative diseases: Common mechanisms of the 'foldopathies'

Although the term tauopathy had not yet been coined, we along with others used antibodies to show that tau protein assembled into the intra-neuronal inclusions of other diseases [20,44], as well as morphologically distinct lesions in Alzheimer's disease [16,19]. Thus tau is one of a growing category of proteins that are predisposed to self-assemble into pathological aggregates. The subset of proteins that are involved in various "foldopathies" [32] constitutes a potentially informative class of proteins for which a common thread is still lacking. The list of proteins that form disease-associated intra-cellular or extra-cellular inclusions is long and still growing, but in this context is notable for the absence of other proteins which share a highly homologous tau microtubule binding domain, the core of the paired helical filament. A prominent example is the absence of MAP2 in any known pathology related to misfolding.

This theme of protein self-assembly and the interface of the inclusions with the degradation machinery of cells has captured the attention of many investigators. One of the questions posed is whether the inclusions are harmful as toxic moieties themselves or protective as sequestering small highly toxic oligomeric precursors as harmless inclusions. Our most recent work supports the idea that inclusions are sequestered as a response of the cell to fight back against the generation of more toxic forms of tau, specifically hyperphosphorylated tau monomers or oligomers. These studies reported the association of PHF tau with Hsc70, CHIP, and Hsp27 [45,46]. Through folding strategies with chaperones, through delivery to the proteasome, and through links to anti-apoptotic pathways the neuron musters many mechanisms to salvage itself in the face of a precipitant which seems to trigger tangle formation.

6. Molecular techniques deliver a windfall of tau data

During the intense period of the early eighties, the techniques of molecular biology were beginning to find their way into laboratories interested in Alzheimer's disease. Rachael Neve while working in the lab of David Kurnit was a leader in applying molecular techniques to the problems of Alzheimer's disease. In collaboration with Rachael by the end of the decade we had cloned and sequenced the human tau gene, determined its chromosomal localization [39], identified its microtubule binding domain [35], and discovered its developmentally regulated splicing [25]. The insights concerning tau splicing came to me on a very late night flight to the University of Alaska at Fairbanks where I was invited by Larry Duffy who had worked in our group several years earlier. In scrutinizing the sequences we had obtained of the tau splice isoforms, and comparing this sequence to the direct protein sequence from the highly insoluble protein core of the paired helical filaments (see Fig. 4 in [50]) it was clear that this core component contained both splice isoforms. Subsequently, both tau splicing and the microtubule binding domain have become foundational concepts in our understanding of tau pathology.

Work on the molecular characterization of tau continued in the lab into the early nineties when we reported the intron-exon structure of the tau gene [2] and the promoter region [3]. The laborious sequencing of the enormous intron between the tau exons 9 and 10, before the availability of all human sequence with just a few clicks at the keyboard, later contributed to the identification of the tau mutations in frontotemporal dementia of the Parkinson type (FTDP).

The concentration of FTDP mutations within the exon 10 splice site links tau pathology to a genetic theme found among other neurodegenerative conditions-the gene dose of the pathological protein is a critical determinant of age-related pathology [47]. Although promoter mutations are most commonly thought of as increasing gene dosage, splice site mutations can increase the amount of a splice isoform. Indeed, the splice site mutations in the tau gene increase the amount of four repeat tau, often by very small amounts. Because an altered ratio of three to four repeat tau does not diminish tau binding to microtubules – in fact, increased amounts of four repeat tau will actually increase tau microtubule binding in living cells [37] – the underlying nature of tau pathology is not a defect in microtubule binding. More likely a small imbalance in the ratio of three to four repeat tau over long periods of time can lead to self-assembly of tau monomers into higher order toxic structures. Some tau mutations are misense mutations, and among these, some do affect microtubule binding. In these cases, it is likely that a defect in microtubule binding results in increased cytoplasmic tau and triggers a final common pathway related to misfolding and degradation overload.

7. Neuronal polarity: Axonal and dendritic identity

By 1990, with many molecular tools in hand, we began to turn our attention to the function of the tau protein. We had already been struck by the exquisite segregation of tau and MAP2 into the axonal and somatodendritic compartments [30]. The contrast with the normal compartmentation of tau to the axon highlighted the fact that pathological tau in Alzheimer brain tissue was located in both axons and dendrites. Thus tau can translocate to the axon despite the presence of abundant microtubules in the somatodendritic compartment to which it is capable of binding through a microtubule-binding domain that is highly homologous to the corresponding region in MAP2. Furthermore, in the first report on the localization of the tau mRNA by in situ hybridization [24], we demonstrated that translation of tau can extend into the proximal dendrite. This localization pointed to a possibly vulnerable time interval when tau passages from the proximal dendrite to its destination in the axon. The interval between tau synthesis and arrival at its correct cytological locus may be the moment when pathological self-assembly is initiated.

In collaboration with Alfredo Caceres in 1990 we used the emerging antisense technology to demonstrate that tau has a role in the elongation of the axon after a cultured neuron elaborates a symmetric array of primary neurites [7]. Furthermore, the elaboration of dendrites required the prior elaboration of the axon; however once the dendrite-like processes appeared, they could continue to grow in the absence of tau and the axon [8]. Several years later we learned that the absence of tau protein could be compensated for by the presence of an appropriate extra-cellular matrix [14].

A role for tau protein in the genesis of some facets of axonal identity was again suggested by some very surprising experiments in an entirely different system. Lisa McConologue, while working at what was a biotech start-up called Athena Neuroscience prepared large amounts of tau protein in baculovirus. The method requires the expression of a baculovirus expressing the protein of interest in a host insect cell called the Sf9 cell. Because the aim is simply to produce protein and the cells are very hearty, usually little attention is paid to the appearance of the cells; they are grown and harvested for their protein products. But Lisa noticed that the Sf9 cells expressing tau no longer grew as simple rounded cells, but elaborated long tails. In a series of publications we characterized these cells as having certain structural features of an axon [4,21]. Specifically, they elaborated only a single process and this process was of uniform caliber, contained microtubules with their plus ends oriented aligned distally, and had a broad flattened region at the tip which was enriched in actin filaments, but relatively devoid of microtubules. These results suggested that tau was capable of establishing an axonal type organization of the microtubules and transducing that organization for the generation of a highly specific structure that resembled an axon. This axon-like structure, which of course lacked any of the physiological properties of an axon, was not generated simply by the force of microtubule elongation, but required a complex interaction with the actin system and the presence of a growth cone-like structure at the tip [12,22]. The complementary techniques of antisense suppression in primary neurons and the expression in Sf9 cells proved a useful paradigm for insights concerning both tau and MAP2 [9,34].

8. The tau pathway

Needless to say the most satisfactory culmination to the wealth of data now available on tau will be treatments for patients. The maturation of the tau field has made it possible to design experiments that address treatment. Because tau phosphorylation appears to be closely linked to the pathology and to the degradation defect we have targeted tau kinases as a possible treatment. Given the spectacular clinical results of trailblazing drugs such as Gleevec (imatinib mesylate), an expanding number of kinases are being targeted by drug developers in both industry and academia. Selecting one kinase among the many that can phosphorylate tau as the optimal target requires divining pathogenetic mechanisms beyond what can deduced from the available data. Nevertheless, the number of candidate kinases is limited and we have focused on CDK5. Most recently we have identified several novel inhibitors in a high through put assay [1] and are now optimizing these compounds.

The road which began with a curious microscopic structure called the neurofibrillary tangle has progressed quite neatly from the discovery of tau protein as the principle component of the tangle to cloning the tau gene and characterizing its molecular structure, to the normal function of tau and ultimately to the exact mechanism of its dysfunction. The end of the road is not yet in sight because many questions remain about tau function and dysfunction. However, the questions we pose in this field are precise and answerable. Getting these answers involves a flirtation with nature who from time to time reveals herself a bit and then locks the door again. By charming her with elegant data she revealed the FTDP mutations, an extra-ordinary insight to the pathology, but still not quite enough yet to solve the disease. Based on this look backward and the rapidity with which new and startling insights have emerged in a relatively short time, it seems likely that what now seems mysterious, will soon be clear.

References

[1] J.S. Ahn, A. Musacchio, M. Mapelli, J. Ni, L. Scinto, R. Stein, K.S. Kosik and L.A. Yeh, Development of an assay to screen for inhibitors of tau phosphorylation by cdk5, *J Biomol Screen* **9** (2004), 122–131.

[2] A. Andreadis, W. Brown and K. Kosik, t gene, *Biochem* **31** (1992), 10626–10633.

[3] A. Andreadis, B. Wagner, J.A. Broderick and K.S. Kosik, A tau promoter region lacks neuronal specificity, *J Neurochem* (1996), 2257–2263.

[4] P. Baas, T. Pienkowski and K. Kosik, Processes induced by tau expression in Sf9 cells have an axon-like microtubule organization, *J. Cell Biol* **115** (1991), 1333–1334.

[5] G. Blessed, B.E. Tomlinson and M. Roth, The association between quantitative measures of dementia and senile change in the cerebral grey matter of elderly subjects, *Br. J. Psychiat* **114** (1968), 797–811.

[6] J.P. Brion, H. Passarier, J. Nunez and J. Flament-Durand, Immunologic determinants of tau protein are present in neurofibrillary tangles of Alzheimer's disease, *Arch Biol* **95** (1985), 229–235.

[7] A. Caceres and K. Kosik, Inhibition of neurite polarity by tau antisense oligonucleotides in primary cerebellar neurons, *Nature* **343** (1990), 461–463.

[8] A. Caceres, S. Potrebic and K. Kosik, The effect of tau antisense oligonucleotides in primary cerebellar neurons, *J. Neurosci.* **11** (1991), 1515–1523.

[9] A. Caceres, J. Mautino and K.S. Kosik, Suppression of MAP-2 in cultured cerebellar macroneurons inhibits minor neurite formation, *Neuron* **9** (1992), 607–618.

[10] D. Cleveland, S. Hwo and M. Kirschner, Purification of tau, a microtubule-associated protein that induces assembly of microtubules from purified tubulin, *J. Mol. Biol* **116** (1977), 207–225.

[11] D. Cleveland, S. Hwo and M. Kirschner, Physical and chemical properties of purified tau factor and the role of tau in microtubule assembly, *J. Mol. Biol* **116** (1977), 227–247.

[12] C.C. Cunningham, N. Leclerc, L. Flanagan, M. Lu, P.A. Janmey and K.S. Kosik, MAP2c reorganizes both microtubules and microfilaments into distinct cytological structures in an ABP-280 deficient melanoma cell line, *J. Cell Biol.* (1997), (in press).

[13] S.T. DeKosky and S.W. Scheff, Synapse loss in frontal cortex biopsies in Alzheimer's disease: Correlation with cognitive severity, *Ann. Neurol.* **27** (1990), 457–464.

[14] M.C. DiTella, F. Feiguin, N. Carri, K.S. Kosik and A. Caceres, MAP-1B/tau functional redundancy during laminin-enhanced axonal growth, *J. Cell Sci.* **109** (1996), 467–477.

[15] M.I. Escobar, H. Pimienta, V.S. Caviness, M. Jacobson, J.E. Crandall and K.S. Kosik, Architecture of apical dendrites in the murine neocortex: dual apical dendritic systems, *Neuroscience* **17** (1986), 975–989.

[16] P.G. Galloway, G. Perry, K.S. Kosik and P. Gambetti, Hirano bodies contain tau protein, *Brain Res* **430** (1987), 337–340.

[17] I. Grundke-Iqbal, K. Iqbal, M. Quinlan, Y.-C. Tung, M.S. Zaidi and H.M. Wisniewski, Microtubule-associated protein tau: a component of Alzheimer paired helical filaments, *J. biol. Chem* **261** (1986), 6084–6089.

[18] I. Grundke-Iqbal, K. Iqbal, Y.-C. Tung, M. Quinlan, H.M. Wisniewski and L.I. Binder, Abnormal phosphorylation of the microtubule-associated protein t (tau) in Alzheimer cytoskeletal pathology, *Proc. Natl. Acad. Sci. USA* **83** (1986), 4913–4917.

[19] C. Joachim, J. Morris, D. Selkoe and K. Kosik, Tau epitopes are incorporated into a range of lesions in Alzheimer's disease, *J Neuropath Exp Neurol* **46** (1987), 611–622.

[20] C.L. Joachim, J.H. Morris, K.S. Kosik and D.J. Selkoe, Tau antisera recognize neurofibrillary tangles in a range of neurodegenerative disorders, *Ann Neurol* **22** (1987), 514–520.

[21] J. Knops, K. Kosik, G. Lee, J. Pardee, L. Cohen-Gould and L. McConlogue, Overexpression of tau in a nonneuronal cell induces long cellular processes, *J. Cell Biol* **114** (1991), 725–733.

[22] R. Knowles, N. LeClerc and K.S. Kosik, Organization of actin and microtubules during process formation in tau-expressing Sf9 cells, *Cell Motil Cytoskeleton* **28** (1994), 256–264.

[23] J. Kondo, T. Honda, H. Mori, Y. Hamada, R. Miura, M. Ogawara and Y. Ihara, The carboxyl third of tau is tightly bound to paired helical filaments, *Neuron* **1** (1988), 827–834.

[24] K. Kosik, J. Crandall, E. Mufson and R. Neve, in situ hybridization in normal and Alzheimer brain: Localization in the somatodendritic compartment, *Ann. Neurol* **26** (1989), 352–361.

[25] K. Kosik, L. Orecchio, S. Bakalis and R. Neve, Developmentally regulated expression of specific tau sequences, *Neuron* **2** (1989), 1389–1397.

[26] K.S. Kosik, J.M. Gilbert, D.J. Selkoe and P. Strocchi, Characterization of postmortem human brain proteins by two-dimensional gel electrophoresis, *J. Neurochem.* **39** (1982), 1529–1538.

[27] K.S. Kosik, W.G. Bradley, P.F. Good, C.G. Rasool and S.D. J., Cholinergic function in lumbar aluminum myelopathy, *J Neuropathol Exp Neurol* **42** (1983), 365–375.

[28] K.S. Kosik, L.K. Duffy, M.M. Dowling, C. Abraham, A. Mc-Cluskey and D.J. Selkoe, Microtubule-associated protein 2: Monoclonal antibodies demonstrate the selective incorporation of certain epitopes into Alzheimer neurofibrillary tangles, *Proc Natl Acad Sci USA* **81** (1984), 7941–7945.

[29] K.S. Kosik, C.L. Joachim and D.J. Selkoe, Microtubule-associated protein, tau, is a major antigenic component of paired helical filaments in Alzheimer's disease, *Proc Natl Acad Sci USA* **83** (1986), 4044–4048.

[30] K.S. Kosik and E.A. Finch, MAP2 and tau segregate into axonal and dendritic domains after the elaboration of morphologically distinct neurites: An immunocytochemical study of cultured rat cerebrum, *J. Neurosci.* **7** (1987), 3142–3153.

[31] K.S. Kosik, L.D. Orecchio, L. Binder, J.Q. Trojanowski, V.M.-Y. Lee and G. Lee, Epitopes that span the tau molecule are shared with paired helical filaments, *Neuron* **1** (1988), 817–825.

[32] K.S. Kosik and H. Shimura, Phosphorylated tau and the neurodegenerative foldopathies, *Biochim Biophys Acta* **1739** (2005), 298–310.

[33] N. Kowall and K. Kosik, Axonal disruption and aberrant localization of tau protein characterize the neuropil pathology of Alzheimer's disease, *Ann. Neurol* **22** (1987), 639–643.

[34] N. LeClerc, K.S. Kosik, N. Cowan, T.P. Pienkowski and P.W. Baas, Process formation in Sf9 cells induced by the expression of a microtubule-associated protein 2C-like construct, *Proc Natl Acad Sci USA* **90** (1993), 6223–6227.

[35] G. Lee, R.L. Neve and K.S. Kosik, The microtubule binding domain of tau protein, *Neuron* **2** (1989), 1615–1624.

[36] F. Lopera, A. Ardilla, A. Martínez, L. Madrigal, J.C. Arango-Viana, C.A. Lemere, J.C. Arango-Lasprilla, L. Hincapié, M. Arcos-Burgos, J.E. Ossa, I.M. Behrens, J. Norton, C. Lendon, A. Goate, A. Ruiz-Linares, M. Rosselli and K.S. Kosik, Phenotypic Features of a Very Large Kindred With a E280A Presenilin 1 Mutation in Antioquia, Colombia, *Jama* **277** (1997), 793–799.

[37] M. Lu and K.S. Kosik, Competition for Microtubule-binding with Dual Expression of Tau Missense and Splice Isoforms, *Mol Biol Cell* **12** (2001), 171–184.

[38] A.C. McKee, K.S. Kosik and N.W. Kowall, Neuritic pathology and dementia in Alzheimer's disease, *Ann. Neurol* **30** (1991), 156–165.

[39] R. Neve, P. Harris, K. Kosik, D. Kurnit and T. Donlon, Identification of cDNA clones for the human microtubule-associated protein, tau, and chromosomal localization of the genes for tau and microtubule-associated protein 2, *Mol. Brain Res* **1** (1986), 271–280.

[40] N. Nukina, K.S. Kosik and D.J. Selkoe, Recognition of Alzheimer paired helical filaments by monoclonal neurofilament antibodies is due to crossreaction with tau protein, *Proc Natl Acad Sci USA* Proceedings of the National Academy of Sciences in the United States of America, 1987.

[41] N. Nukina, K.S. Kosik and D.J. Selkoe, The monoclonal antibody, Alz 50, recognizes tau protein in Alzheimer's disease brain, *Neurosci Lett* **87** (1988), 240–246.

[42] M. Roth, B.E. Tomlinson and G. Blessed, Correlation between scores for dementia and counts of 'senile plaques' in cerebral grey matter of elderly subjects, *Nature* **209** (1966), 109–110.

[43] M. Roth, B.E. Tomlinson and G. Blessed, The relationship between quantitative measures of dementia and of degenerative changes in the cerebral grey matter of elderly subjects, *Proc R Soc Med* **60** (1967), 254–260.

[44] S.K. Shankar, R. Yanagihara, R.M. Garruto, I. Grundke-Iqbal, K.S. Kosik and D.C. Gajdusek, Immunocytochemical characterization of neurofibrillary tangles in amyotrophic lateral sclerosis and Parkinson-dementia of Guam, *Ann Neurol* **25** (1989), 146–151.

[45] H. Shimura, Y. Miura-Shimura and K.S. Kosik, Binding of Tau to HSP27 leads to decreased concentration of hyperphosphorylated Tau and enhanced cell survival, *J Biol Chem* **279** (2004), 17957–17962.

[46] H. Shimura, D. Schwartz, S.P. Gygi and K.S. Kosik, CHIP-Hsc70 complex ubiquitinates phosphorylated tau and enhances cell survival, *J Biol Chem* **279** (2004), 4869–4876.

[47] A. Singleton, A. Myers and J. Hardy, The law of mass action applied to neurodegenerative disease: a hypothesis concerning the etiology and pathogenesis of complex diseases, *Hum Mol Genet* **13**(Spec No. 1) (2004), R123–R126.

[48] B.E. Tomlinson, G. Blessed and R. M, Observations on the brains of demented old people, *J Neurol Sci* **11** (1970), 205–242.

[49] C. Wischik, M. Novak, P. Edwards, A. Klug, W. Tichelaar and R. Crowther, Structural characterization of the core of the paired helical filament of Alzheimer disease, *Proc. Natl. Acad. Sci. USA* **85** (1988), 4884–4888.

[50] C.M. Wischik, M. Novak, H.C. Thogersen, P.C. Edwards, M.J. Runswick, R. Jakes, J.E. Walker, C. Milstein, M. Rother and A. Klug, Isolation of a fragment of tau derived from the core of the paired helical filament of Alzheimer's disease, *Proc Natl Acad Sci USA* **85** (1988), 4506–4510.

[51] G.B. Witman, D.W. Cleveland, M.D. Weingarten and M.W. Kirschner, Tubulin requires tau for growth onto microtubule initiating sites, *Proc Natl Acad Sci USA* **73** (1976), 4070–4074.

[52] J.G. Wood, S.S. Mirra, N.L. Pollock and L.I. Binder, Neurofibrillary tangles of Alzheimer's disease share antigenic determinants with the axonal microtubule-associated protein tau, *Proc Natl Acad Sci USA* **83** (1986), 4040–4043.

Progress from Alzheimer's tangles to pathological tau points towards more effective therapies now

Virginia M.-Y. Lee* and John Q. Trojanowski
The Center for Neurodegenerative Disease Research, Department of Pathology and Laboratory Medicine, and Institute on Aging, The University of Pennsylvania School of Medicine, Philadelphia, PA 19104, USA

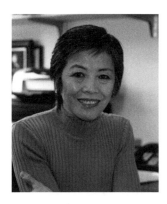 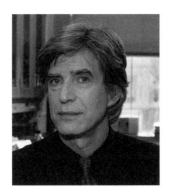

Abstract. The landmark description of neurofibrillary tangles (NFTs) and senile plaques as the pathological hallmarks of an unusual form of dementia 100 years ago by Alois Alzheimer launched the quest to understand a neurodegenerative disorder that now has become a scourge in the 21st Century due to the unprecedented increase in human life expectancy since 1900. Indeed, while there are many benefits to individuals and society as a whole that will accrue from the remarkable gains in longevity since 1900, the risk of developing Alzheimer's disease (AD) increases exponentially with advancing age beyond the 7th decade of life. Hence, the prevalence of AD will rise inexorably in the coming decades unless effective interventions are developed to delay the onset or progression of AD. Widespread international recognition of the urgency of this problem has accelerated research to discover meaningful therapies for AD, and growing evidence implicates impairments of axonal transport in mechanisms underlying AD due to pathological alterations in tau, the building block proteins of NFTs. This brief review summarizes insights into mechanisms whereby pathological alterations in tau impair axonal transport resulting in neurodegeneration and how these insights are being exploited now to develop novel therapeutic interventions for the treatment of AD.

Keywords: Tau, neurofibrillary tangles, microtubules, taxol

1. Introduction

Alzheimer's disease (AD) and a number of other neurodegenerative disorders now are known to result from the aggregation of proteins that misfold and accumulate as fibrillar amyloid deposits in selectively vulnerable regions of the central nervous system (CNS) where they are thought to compromise the function and viability of neurons and glia (for a recent review, see [5]). For

*Corresponding author: Virginia M.-Y, Lee, Ph.D. or John Q. Trojanowski, M.D., Ph.D., Department of Pathology and Laboratory Medicine, University of Pennsylvania School of Medicine, Maloney 3, HUP, 3600 Spruce Street, Philadelphia, PA 19104-4283, USA. Tel.: +1 215 662 6427; Fax: +1 215 349 5909; E-mail: VMYLEE@mail.med.upenn.edu or TROJANOW@mail.med.upenn.edu.

example, abnormal tau filaments accumulate in neurons as neurofibrillary tangles (NFTs) while extracellular senile plaques (SPs) are composed of fibrillar Aβ and both were first recognized by Alois Alzheimer at the beginning of the 20th Century as the diagnostic hallmark lesions of AD [5]. Although the discovery of pathogenic mutations in the genes encoding tau and the Aβ precursor protein in familial neurodegenerative disorders definitively implicated these proteins in disease pathogenesis, the mechanisms whereby brain degeneration results from NFTs and SPs still is not entirely clear [5]. Since this special issue of the *Journal of Alzheimer's Disease* celebrates the centennial of Alois Alzheimer's seminal description of AD by featuring reviews of the most significant advances in AD research over the past 100 years, and the role of altered axonal transport in neurodegenerative diseases also has been reviewed recently [16], we provide a personal perspective here of our hypothesis that the impaired ability of pathologically altered tau to bind microtubules (MTs) in AD disrupts axonal transport leading to neurodegeneration (see Fig. 1). Based on predictions derived from this hypothesis and extensive data supporting it, we then discuss why MT binding drugs may be candidates for the treatment of AD and other related neurodegenerative disorders by offsetting the loss of tau function and maintaining axonal transport in the disease state.

To begin at the beginning for us, we embarked on studies of AD in the 1980s during the heady and tumultuous early days of AD research on the molecular basis of this enigmatic disorder when the field was in the throes of a heated and highly disputatious controversy that raged over the role of tau in the formation of paired helical filaments (PHFs) and NFTs in AD (for an extensive review of the earlier literature on AD PHFs and NFTs, see [11]). We vividly recall this time as a most exciting but very raucous epoch of AD research when each new molecular advance was welcomed with an exhilarating sense of awe that AD really could be "cracked", but the rush of wonder and amazement at each new finding by no means diminished the intensity of the contentious debates about the significance and importance of many of these early molecular advances. Indeed, although several reports in the late 1980s had already implicated tau as the major building block of PHFs (reviewed in [11]), this view was hotly disputed and other potential subunit proteins were passionately proposed as candidate PHF building blocks since there was no direct or "iron clad" evidence that the structural components of PHFs (referred to as A68 at the time) were in fact pathologically altered forms of tau [11]. Our contribution to the resolution of this long standing and often "white hot" controversy came in 1991 when we showed conclusively that abnormally phosphorylated CNS tau proteins (designated A68, but later known as PHFtau) form the PHFs in AD NFTs by providing unequivocal evidence for this at the amino acid sequence level [9]. This discovery, and our subsequent follow up studies shortly thereafter showing that the levels of normal tau diminished with increasing accumulations of PHFtau and that PHFtau was unable to bind to and stabilize MTs because it was hyperphosphorylated relative to normal tau [1,2] prompted us to pursue a line of research into the mechanistic role of tau in AD pathogenesis and neurodegeneration that continues to the present day [12,16,18,19].

These initial observations by our group in the early 1990s led us to hypothesize that the conversion of normal brain tau into PHFtau disrupts intraneuronal transport due to the depolymerization of MTs as well as to the occlusion of axons and dendrites by aggregated PHFs and Fig. 1 here schematically summarizes key aspects of this hypothesis [1,2,9]. Notably, there are six soluble tau isoforms expressed in the normal adult human brain that are generated from a single gene by alternative splicing, and the normal functions of tau is to bind to and stabilize MTs thereby maintaining the networks of MTs that are essential for axonal transport in neurons [11,16]. Thus, several years before the landmark discoveries in 1998 of tau gene mutations pathogenic for hereditary frontotemporal dementia (FTD) with parkinsonism linked to chromosome 17 or FTDP-17 [3,7,14,17], and the observation that one of the consequences of these mutations was a loss of tau function [6], it was appreciated that wild type tau sustained a loss of function that might impair axonal transport thereby leading to a neurodegenerative disease when tau was altered by pathological processes in AD such as hyperphosphorylation. Accordingly, our hypothetical model of PHFtau mediated neurodegeneration in AD predicted the following scenario: 1) the conversion of tau into PHFtau disrupts MT-based transport as well as physically "blocks" intraneuronal transport due to accumulations of PHFs within affected neurons and their processes; and 2) the attendant failure of neurons to export proteins from the cell body to distal processes and to retrieve substances (e.g., trophic factors) internalized at axon terminals compromises neuronal viability. Thus, we proposed that these events alone would be sufficient to culminate in neuronal dysfunction and degeneration leading to the onset/progression of AD. Nearly all of the predictions of this disease model of

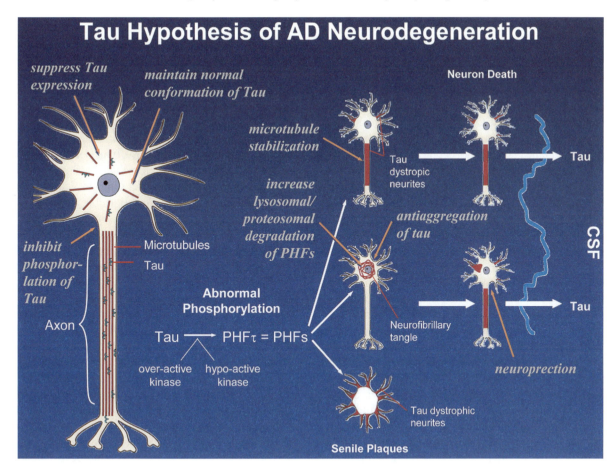

Fig. 1. The misfolding, fibrillization and sequestration of tau into filamentous inclusions is schematically depicted here and, as described in greater detail in the text, this compromises the survival of neurons by depleting levels of functional tau below a critical point which results in the depolymerization of MTs and disruption of axonal transport. The brown arrows and text indicate points of potential therapeutic intervention to ameliorate or reverse tau pathologies and their attendant neurodegenerative consequences.

tau pathology in AD and related tauopathies have been validated through the generation and study of tau transgenic mice (for a recent review, see [12]), and the first experimental demonstration of AD-like neurodegeneration linked to axonal transport failure came from the studies of a tau transgenic mouse model of AD-like tau pathologies [8]. Indeed, there appears to be an emerging consensus that AD and other neurodegenerative diseases are linked to impaired axonal transport, and a special issue of *NeuroMolecuar Medicine* (e.g., Volume 2, No. 2) focused on this topic in 2002 because of the potential implications of this mechanism of disease for the discovery of new and better therapies for AD and other neurodegenerative disorders.

Since the most significant predictions of our tau hypothesis of AD neurodegeneration were that tau pathologies would cause brain degeneration by impairing intraneuronal transport thereby compromising the function and viability of affected cells, we proposed in 1994 that MT stabilizing compounds such as the FDA approved anti-cancer drug paclitaxel (Taxol®) could be used for the treatment of AD by offsetting the loss of tau function following its conversion into PHF-tau [10]. However, although a steady stream of studies published throughout the 1990s from our group and a small number of other laboratories continued to converge in support of the tau hypothesis of AD neurodegeneration [11], tau pathology was widely regarded as an epiphenomenon by most AD researchers, and this iconoclastic hypothesis was more often derided than discussed. In fact, it did not begin to garner broader and more serious support in the AD research field until very recently [5,11]. One of the first significant catalysts that led to a re-assessment of the tau hypothesis of AD neurodegeneration came from a series of remarkable discoveries beginning in 1998 showing that mutations in the gene encoding tau was pathogenic for hereditary FTDP-17 syndromes [3,7,14,17] all of which are characterized by prominent tau pathologies in the absence significant amounts of other disease specific amyloid lesions [11]. Thus, these findings provided unequivocal proof that tau abnormalities were sufficient to cause neurodegenerative disease. Since 1998, sporadic FTDs characterized by prominent tau lesions, FTDP-17 syndromes and the pathological significance of tau abnormalities for mechanisms of brain degeneration have become an increasingly intense focus of basic and clinical research. Moreover, there have been extensive efforts to generate animal models of neurodegenerative tauopathies [11,12]. In fact, the other compelling catalyst for dispelling doubt about the critical importance of tau pathologies as mediators of neurodegeneration in AD and other neurodegenerative disorders has been the successful development of worm, fly and mouse models of tauopathies that show compelling verisimilitude to their authentic human counterparts (for a recent review, see [12]).

By this time in the recent history of AD research, there is a growing body of evidence from a number of diverse lines of research suggesting that brain degeneration in AD could be a consequence of impaired intraneuronal transport resulting from loss of function defects in tau and/or from toxic gains of functions by pathologically altered tau proteins, including their propensity to misfold, fibrillize and form NFTs in neurons [5,11,16]. Indeed, recent studies of paclitaxel (Taxol®) from our group have provided proof of the concept that MT stabilizing drugs may have therapeutic potential for the treatment of AD and other neurodegenerative diseases with prominent tau pathologies [19]. These studies were based on data summarized above that linked tau abnormalities to mechanisms underlying AD as well as to other neurodegenerative tauopathies, including rare forms of hereditary FTDP-17 caused by *tau* gene mutations. As in AD, the neuropathological hallmarks of these other neurodegenerative tauopathies are inclusions (mainly, but not exclusively found in neurons) that are formed by accumulations of pathological tau filaments with properties similar to those of amyloid fibrils and AD PHFs, including the excessive phosphorylation of pathologically fibrillized tau. Thus, the AD-like tau pathologies in these other tauopathies also result in a loss of normal tau function. As a consequence thereof, axonal transport presumably is impaired in these other tauopathies thereby leading to the dying back of axons as well as to the degeneration of neurons just like in AD [10,11,16].

Studies we recently reported were specifically designed to test our hypothesis that MT stabilizing drugs could have therapeutic benefit in AD and related human tauopathies by offsetting the loss of normal tau functions resulting from the hyperphosphorylation of tau and its sequestration into tangles [19]. Significantly, these studies provided the first proof of concept data validating the use of MT stabilizing drugs to treat AD and related tauopathies. Briefly, transgenic (Tg) mice (PrPT44) that model the neuropathology of human neurodegenerative tauopathies were treated with weekly intraperitoneal injections of paclitaxel in a micelle vehicle (Paxceed^{TM}; Angiotech Pharmaceuticals, Inc.) or the micelle vehicle alone for 12 weeks beginning at 9 months of age when disease onset is first detected. Previous studies of these Tg mice showed that they developed filamentous tau inclusions in spinal cord at disease onset in association with reduced numbers of MTs, reduced fast axonal transport, and impaired motor behavior [8]. However, treatment with Paxceed^{TM} restored fast axonal transport, increased axonal MTs and ameliorated motor impairments in tau Tg mice thereby suggesting that MT stabilizing drugs could have therapeutic benefit for human tauopathies. Notably, the doses of paclitaxel used in the Zhang et al. study were far lower than those used to treat cancer, and the treated mice did not show any evidence of toxicity [19].

Paclitaxel (Taxol®) is a complex diterpene obtained from the Pacific yew (*Taxus brevifolia*), especially from the bark of the yew tree, and paclitaxel is the most well studied MT binding compound for clinical use (for a review of MT binding drugs, see [18]). Indeed, paclitaxel was the first compound derived from a natural product that was shown to stabilize MTs and inhibit cell replication, and it has become an important chemotherapeutic agent for the treatment of cancer based on its ability to arrest mitosis by stabilizing MTs in the mitotic spindle thereby leading to apoptosis [18]. For example, Taxol® has been approved by the FDA for the treatment of a number of malignancies including ovarian, breast and lung cancers. However, the mechanism of action of paclitaxel and its cytotoxic action for cancer chemotherapy are shared by a growing number of natural products derived from microorganisms, plants and sponges [18]. For this reason, extensive research is being conducted to identify synthetic and/or natural product derived paclitaxel-like MT binding compounds that show less toxicity than paclitaxel, an improved ability to enter the brain as well as elude the multi-drug resistance efflux pump and better efficacy as anti-cancer therapies [18]. Thus, by providing convincing experimental evidence supporting the concept that MT stabilizing drugs could be novel therapeutic interventions in patients with AD or other tauopathies by counteracting the loss of function effects of tau pathology and maintaining the MT network and fast axonal transport in a mouse model of a neurodegenerative tauopathy, the study summarized above by Zhang et al. is likely to stimulate further research on the potential therapeutic utility of MT binding drugs for treating AD [19]. However, other strategies to develop novel therapies that target tau abnormalities in AD already are an increasing focus of AD drug discovery research [4]. Although further studies of the pharmacobiology of MT stabilizing drugs in the CNS are needed, the data summarized here are significant for designing treatments for AD and other neurodegenerative tauopathies because they suggest that stabilization of MTs is a "druggable" target in tauopathies. Further, follow up studies may reveal that toxicity can be minimized further while producing therapeutic benefits by using lower, less frequent doses of MT stabilizing compounds over long periods of time. Moreover, recent studies by Michaelis and colleagues indicate that derivatives of paclitaxel can be generated that cross the blood brain barrier better than the native molecule, while other *in vitro* studies suggest that Taxol® may ameliorate the toxic effects of Aβ amyloidosis in AD [13,15].

In conclusion, based on the data reviewed in this personal perspective on AD research on NFTs and PHF-tau, we infer that it is plausible MT stabilizing drugs such as Paxceed™ may be novel candidate compounds worthy of further investigation for therapeutic potential in the treatment of patients with neurodegenerative tauopathies, including AD. Indeed, MT stabilization may be required to complement other emerging AD therapies that target other mechanisms of neurodegeneration. Accordingly, the extensive progress in elucidating the role of tau pathologies in mechanisms of neurodegeneration in AD and related tauopathies since the initial discovery of NFTs by Alois Alzheimer 100 years ago has created a sense of optimism that these recent advances will culminate in the discovery of more effective therapies for these disorders in the near future. Thus, while AD research seems less convulsed now than in previous decades by strident controversies and stormy debates, the sense of optimism about discovering more effective therapies for AD certainly infuses this field of neuroscience research with the kind of excitement that has been its trademark since the days of Alois Alzheimer.

Acknowledgments

We thank our colleagues for their contributions to the work summarized here which has been supported by grants from the NIH (AG10124, AG14382, AG17586), the Oxford Foundation, the Marian S. Ware Alzheimer Program and Angiotech Pharmaceuticals, Inc. MT stabilizing interventions for AD have been licensed to Angiotech from the University of Pennsylvania. VMYL is the John H. Ware 3rd Professor for Alzheimer's Disease Research and JQT is the William Maul Measy-Truman G. Schnabel Jr. M.D. Professor of Geriatric Medicine and Gerontology.

References

[1] G.T. Bramblett, M. Goedert, R. Jakes, S.E. Merrick, J.Q. Trojanowski and V.M.-Y. Lee, Abnormal tau phosphorylation at Ser396 in Alzheimer's disease recapitulates development and contributes to reduced microtubule binding, *Neuron* **10** (1993), 1089–1099.

[2] G.T. Bramblett, J.Q. Trojanowski and V.M.-Y. Lee, Regions with abundant neurofibrillary pathology in human brain exhibit a selective reduction in levels of binding-competent tau and the accumulation of abnormal tau-isoforms (A68 proteins), *Lab Invest* **66** (1992), 212–222.

[3] L.N. Clark, P. Poorkaj, Z. Wszolek, D.H. Geschwind, Z.Z. Nasreddine, B. Miller, D. Li, H. Payami, F. Awert, K. Markopoulou, A. Andreadis, I. D'Souza, V.M.-Y. Lee, L. Reed, J.Q. Trojanowski, V. Zhukareva, T. Bird, G. Schellenberg and K.C. Wilhelmsen, Pathogenic implications of mutations in the tau gene in pallido-ponto-nigral degeneration and related neurogenerative disorders linked to chromosome 17, *Proc Natl Acad Sci USA* **95** (1998), 13103–13107.

[4] H.M. Fillit and L.M. Refolo, eds, Neurofibrillary Tangles as a Target for Developng New Therapeutics for Alzheimer's Disease – Special Issue, *J Molec Neurosci* **19**(Issue 3) (2002), 251–338.

[5] M.S. Forman, J.Q. Trojanowski and V.M.-Y. Lee, Neurodegenerative diseases: A decade of discoveries paves the way for therapeutic breakthroughs, *Nat Med* **10** (2004), 1055–1063.

[6] M. Hong, V. Zhukareva, V. Vogelsberg-Ragaglia, Z. Wszolek, L. Reed, B.I. Miller, D.H. Geschwind, T.D. Bird, D. McKeel, A. Goate, J.C. Morris, K.C. Wilhelmsen, G.D. Schellenberg, J.Q. Trojanowski and V.M.-Y. Lee, Mutation-specific functional impairments in distinct tau isoforms of hereditary FTDP-17, *Science* **282** (1998), 1914–1917.

[7] M. Hutton, C.L. Lendon, P. Rizzu, M. Baker, S. Froelich, H. Houlden, S. Pickering-Brown, S. Chakraverty, A. Isaacs, A. Grover, J. Hackett, J. Adamson, S. Lincoln, D. Dickson, P. Davies, R.C. Petersen, M. Stevens, E. de Graaff, E. Wauters, J. van Baren, M. Hillebrand, M. Joosse, J.M. Kwon, P. Nowotny, L.K. Che, J. Norton, J.C. Morris, L.A. Reed, J.Q. Trojanowski, H. Basun, L. Lannfelt, M. Neystat, S. Fahn, F. Dark, T. Tannenberg, P. Dodd, N. Hayward, J.B.J. Kwok, P.R. Schofield, A. Andreadis, J. Snowden, D. Craufurd, D. Neary, F. Owen, B.A. Oostra, J. Hardy, A. Goate, J. van Swieten, D. Mann, T. Lynch and P. Heutink, Association of missense and 5'-splice-site-mutations in tau with the inherited dementia FTDP-17, *Nature* **393** (1998), 702–705.

[8] T. Ishihara, M. Hong, B. Zhang, Y. Nakagawa, M.K. Lee, J.Q. Trojanowski and V.M.-Y. Lee, Age-dependent emergence and progression of a tauopathy in transgenic mice engineered to overexpress the shortest human tau isoform, *Neuron* **24** (1999), 751–762.

[9] V.M.-Y. Lee, B.J. Balin, L. Otvos Jr. and J.Q. Trojanowski, A68: A major subunit of paired helical filaments and derivatized forms of normal tau, *Science* **251** (1991), 675–678.

[10] V.M.-Y. Lee, R. Daughenbaugh and J.Q. Trojanowski, Microtubule stabilizing drugs for the treatment of Alzheimer's disease, *Neurobiol Aging* **15** (1994), S87–S89.

[11] V.M.-Y. Lee, M. Goedert and J.Q. Trojanowski, Neurodegenerative tauopathies, *Annu Rev Neurosci* **24** (2001), 1121–1159.

[12] V.M.-Y. Lee, T.K. Kenyon and J.Q. Trojanowski, Transgenic animal models of tauopathies, *Biochem Biophys Acta* **1739** (2005), 251–259.

[13] M.L. Michaelis, S. Ansar, Y. Chen, E.R. Reiff, K.I. Seyb, R.H. Himes, K.L. Audus and G.I. Georg, Beta-amyloid- induced neurodegeneration and protection by structurally diverse microtubule-stabilizing agents, *J Pharmacol Exp Ther* **312** (2005), 659–668.

[14] P. Poorkaj, T.D. Bird, E. Wijsman, E. Nemens, R.M. Garruto, L. Anderson, A. Andreadis, W.C. Wiederholt, M. Raskind and G.D. Schellenberg, Tau is a candidate gene for chromosome 17 frontotemporal dementia, *Ann Neurol* **43** (1998), 815–825.

[15] A. Rice, Y. Liu, M.L. Michaelis, R.H. Himes, G.I. Georg and K.L. Audus, Chemical modification of paclitaxel (Taxol) reduces P-glycoprotein interactions and increases permeation across the blood-brain barrier *in vitro* and *in situ*, *J Med Chem* **48** (2005), 832–838.

[16] S. Roy, B. Zhang, V.M.-Y. Lee and J.Q. Trojanowski, Axonal transport defects: A common theme in neurodegenerative diseases, *Acta Neuropathol* **109** (2005), 5–13.

[17] M.G. Spillantini, T.R. Murrell, M. Goedert, M.R. Farlow, A. Klug and B. Ghetti, Mutation in the tau gene in familial multiple system tauopathy with presenile dementia, *Proc Natl Acad Sci USA* **95** (1998), 7737–7741.

[18] J.Q. Trojanowski, D. Huryn, A.B. Smith 3rd and V.M.-Y. Lee, Microtubule stabilizing drugs for therapy of Alzheimer's disease and other neurodegenerative disorders with axonal transport impairments, *Expert Opin Pharmacother* (2005), in press.

[19] B. Zhang, A. Maiti, S. Shively, F. Lakhani, G. McDonald-Jones, J. Bruce, E.B. Lee, S.X. Xie, S. Joyce, C. Li, P.M. Toleikis, V.M.-Y. Lee and J.Q. Trojanowski, Microtubule binding drugs offset tau sequestration by stabilizing microtubules and reversing fast axonal transport deficits in a murine neurodegenerative tauopathy model, *Proc Natl Acad Sci USA* **102** (2005), 227–231.

Disease Mechanisms

A long trek down the pathways of cell death in Alzheimer's disease

Peter Davies
Departments of Pathology and Neuroscience, Albert Einstein College of Medicine, 1300 Morris Park Ave, Bronx, NY 10461, USA
Tel.: +1 718 430 3083; Fax: +1 718 430 8541; E-mail: davies@aecom.yu.edu

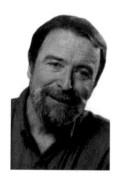

Abstract. The invitation to contribute to the issue marking the 100th anniversary of Alzheimer's disease gave me pause to reflect on the significant milestones in my own research. This brief and personal description of my laboratory's search for the cause of cell dysfunction and death in Alzheimer's disease marks only highlights, and my apologies to those whose work I have passed over.

1. Anniversaries

2006 is a significant anniversary year for me too. It marks the 30th anniversary of my first publication in the area of Alzheimer's disease [1], the 20th anniversary of our first paper using monoclonal antibodies to investigate the disease [2], and the 10th anniversary of our first publication on mitotic mechanisms [3]. For me, these mark milestones on my own path of research.

2. The cholinergic hypothesis

The cholinergic deficit in Alzheimer's disease was discovered independently and simultaneously in three labs in Great Britain [1,4–7] in 1976 and 1977. Where that work has led is now well known to all in the field: three of the four drugs currently approved by the FDA for the treatment of Alzheimer's disease are cholinesterase inhibitors. Without going into the debate of how well these drugs work, it will be sufficient to say that they do not produce the kind of improvements we hoped they would achieve. In the late 1970's, our neurochemical work was based on the Parkinson's disease model: a deficiency in dopamine was discovered, and dramatic improvements in the symptoms of the disease were achieved by administration of L-Dopa. We are yet to reach the point in Alzheimer's disease research where we can match the efficacy of L-Dopa in Parkinson's disease.

The discovery of the cholinergic deficit was an enormous stimulus to basic and clinical research on AD. I vividly remember a psychiatrist I worked with in 1976 running across the street to buy choline bitartrate from the local health food store, to attempt "precursor therapy" for Alzheimer's disease patients. Many similar attempts (all unsuccessful) followed, using choline or lecithin (phosphatidyl choline). It was soon after that trials of physostigmine and other cholinesterase inhibitors began. Whether or not these are considered a success, the era of experimental therapy for Alzheimer's disease began in earnest in the late 1970's, and the pace has picked up considerably since then.

3. But why was there a cholinergic deficit?

The rest of my professional life has been spent essentially working on the same question: why do cholinergic neurons die in Alzheimer's disease? It was obvious by 1980 that cholinergic neurons of the ventral forebrain were a very consistent, identifiable target of the disease [8,9]. Inspired by work from Zipser and McKay [10], who made monoclonal antibodies to the dissected nervous system of the leech, and found antibodies that identified specific subsets of neurons, I wondered if it was possible to make monoclonal antibodies to identify abnormalities in ventral forebrain cholinergic neurons from patients with Alzheimer's disease. With help from Susan Roberts and Matt Scharff, Alex Pruchnicki, Sophia Feisullin, Ben Wolozin and I immunized mice with basal forebrain tissue dissected from three cases of Alzheimer's disease. Once the mice had made high-titer antibodies to the immunogen, we took the spleens and made hybridomas, screening many hundreds of cell lines for antibodies that would distinguish AD ventral forebrain from control tissues.

We made many different monoclonal antibodies, to neurofilament protein phosphorylations [11], and to galactolipids [12], but the most discrimination between normal and AD ventral forebrain tissue was shown by an antibody called Alz50 [2,13]. Much of the work we and others published on Alz50 in the late 1980's and early 1990's has stood the test of time, but a complete explanation of the specificity of this antibody still eludes us. Alz50 recognizes a soluble protein that appears to be absent from the normal brain, and to be very widely distributed in the AD brain. The antibody labeled neurofibrillary tangles, neuritic elements in plaques, and a very extensive network of neuritic processes that has previously been largely ignored as a pathological feature of AD [13,14]. To me, now using third generation antibodies, the neuritic pathology of AD stands out as far more extensive than either the tangle or plaque pathology: these lesions appear to be the tips of a very large iceberg, which extends throughout the cortex of AD cases. There was also compelling evidence that the appearance of Alz50 reactivity was an early event in AD pathology, perhaps appearing before the classic neurofibrillary tangles [15,16]. It was several years before we and others were able to work out that Alz50 recognized a conformational epitope on the microtubule associated protein tau [17–19]. New conformation specific antibodies were made [18,19], and more detailed studies established that indeed the conformational changes in tau occur before detectable filament or tangle formation, at least in hippocampal neurons [20]. Although the references cited have proposed models of folding for tau which may explain the abnormal conformation recognized by Alz50, MC1 and the other conformation-dependent antibodies, the molecular details are still uncertain, and we do not have a clear idea of the mechanism of this abnormal folding.

The early changes in tau conformation led us to the simple idea that phosphorylation of tau might be responsible for this change, and many monoclonal antibodies to different phosphorylation sites were made, in attempts to find evidence for a phosphorylation event that would clearly precede the conformational changes. These efforts continue to this day, although there is yet to be compelling evidence for such a phosphorylation. The original reasoning behind this work remains valid: changes in tau phosphorylation and conformation are among the earliest changes detectable in neurons in Alzheimer's disease cases. At worst, these are responses to activation of a biochemical cascade that leads to cellular dysfunction and ultimately to tangle formation and cell death. In this interpretation, tau changes are just an early marker of the activation of the cascade. Clear identification of the biochemical pathway leading to these tau abnormalities should offer the chance to climb higher up the cascade. Many people in those days (and in these) appear to believe that amyloid-β is at the head of the cascade, but it is probably well known that I am not among them.

4. The mitotic hypothesis

It was the antibodies to phosphorylation sites on tau that first attracted the interest of my brilliant young colleague, Inez Vincent, to examine the possible involvement of mitotic kinases in generation of these epitopes [3]. One antibody in particular, TG3 [21] proved to be a spectacular marker of mitotic cells, and is still among the best antibodies for specifically labeling the neuronal and neuritic pathology of Alzheimer's disease [3,22]. It also ranks as one of the most popular antibodies we have made in terms of requests from other investigators. Many groups working in the area of mitosis and anti-mitotic drug development have used this antibody because of it's ability to discriminate cells in M phase from those in any other stage of the cell cycle (e.g. [23–25].

A handful of laboratories, including mine, continued to investigate the possible role of mitotic mechanisms in AD [26–30]. In what for me are a series of classic papers, Lloyd Greene and his colleagues [31] established that in some circumstances, activation of cell division mechanisms preceded apoptosis of cells in response to some stimuli. Evidence for apoptosis in AD has never been easy to find, especially in post-mortem human brain tissues [32], and a variety of mouse models have been created in part to try to address the issue of mechanism of cell death. The major problem with the models that involve amyloid deposition (transgenics with mutant human AβPP genes, for the most part) is that there is little cell death to investigate. For several years this has forced investigators to stay with the human brain to investigate mechanisms of cell death. We have focused on trying to establish what mechanisms might give rise to both abnormalities in tau conformation and phosphorylation, and to amyloid-β deposition. This vision sees the tangles and amyloid deposits as the results of activation of a biochemical cascade, and seeks the pathways that lead to both tau changes and alterations in AβPP processing. There has been some progress in this area, and plausible schemes involving both JNK and Pin1 have been investigated. One of the most influential papers in this area was the discovery by Herrup and colleagues that vulnerable neurons in the AD brain not only show activation of cell cycle markers, but at least in some cases, show evidence of DNA replication (S-phase) [33,34]. While it is possible to argue that some dysregulation of cell cycle proteins in neurons may be of little significance, it is very hard to dismiss evidence that strongly suggests that neurons in the AD brain duplicate a substantial proportion of their DNA: can these neurons continue normal function and survive under these circumstances? This seems highly unlikely. The "mitotic hypothesis" has also received support from the recent demonstration that hypoxia/ischemia in the mouse and rat brain may also result in activation of the cell cycle, aberrant tau phosphorylation and DNA replication prior to neuronal death [35,36].

Human tau transgenic mice appeared to offer an opportunity to unravel mechanisms of cell death, especially after it was shown that some human tau gene mutations cause massive cell death. A significant fraction of "Frontotemporal" dementia cases are caused by mutations in the tau gene, cases so named because of the obvious and massive neuronal death in frontal and temporal cortex. Curiously, many of these cases do not have the same substantial tau pathology that characterizes AD, but show even more neuronal loss in affected regions than the average AD case. This is perhaps a hint that tau-mediated cell death does not necessarily involve tangle formation, as many seem to have assumed. Lewis et al made the first human tau transgenic to unequivocally show neurofibrillary tangle formation, using a human tau cDNA containing the P301L mutation [37]. Since that work was published, several other mice have been made, but few show clear evidence of neuronal death.

Karen Duff made a human tau transgenic mouse by insertion of the whole human tau gene into mice, with levels of expression of the human gene about 4 times those of the endogenous mouse tau. These mice, which were called the 8c line, failed to develop any clear evidence of pathology up to almost 2 years of age[38]. Cathy Andorfer, in collaboration with Karen, crossed the 8c mice with a mouse in which the tau gene had been disrupted by insertion of the gene for EGFP. After two crosses, mice were obtained which still expressed the human tau gene, but had two copies of the disrupted mouse tau gene: these were called hTau mice. Details of the pathology that develops in these mice have been published [39,40], but most notable was the extensive cortical neuronal loss, which exceeded 50% in the piriform cortex. Andorfer et al. were able to find evidence of activation of the cell cycle in these mice, and these therefore appear to be very attractive models for detailed examination of the mechanism of neuronal death.

5. But why?

Despite our meandering path, we seem to have made progress towards understanding why cells die in Alzheimer's disease. But I sometimes feel like a three-year old child, who asks a question, and responds to every answer with "but why?". If it is true that activation of cell cycle components causes neuronal death in Alzheimer's disease, what activates this pathway? My priorities for the immediate future are to try to address the issue of the functional significance of cell cycle activation in neurons, using the hTau mouse and perhaps other models. Greene and colleagues have performed elegant studies in this area [41–43], and these will assist our efforts. We have also begun to investigate the mechanisms that can turn on the cell cycle machinery in neurons. There are some obvious candidates for this role, and progress should be rapid in this area. I hope that 2006 will be another milestone year in AD research.

Acknowledgements

This seems like a very appropriate place to thank the people and organizations who have been so helpful in shaping and supporting my research. Robert D.

Terry MD was and is an important role model and mentor. Dennis W. Dickson MD and Inez Vincent PhD contributed greatly to my thinking and to the real work over the years. NIA and NIMH have been as supportive as Study Sections allowed, sometimes more so! Applied Neurosolutions Inc., Judith and Burton P. Resnick, along with Fred Tepperman have provided invaluable moral and financial support.

References

[1] P. Davies and A.J. Maloney, Selective loss of central cholinergic neurons in Alzheimer's disease, *Lancet* **2**(8000) (1976), 1403.

[2] B.L. Wolozin et al., A neuronal antigen in the brains of Alzheimer patients, *Science* **232**(4750) (1986), 648–650.

[3] I. Vincent, M. Rosado and P. Davies, Mitotic mechanisms in Alzheimer's disease? *J Cell Biol* **132**(3) (1996), 413–425.

[4] D.M. Bowen et al., Neurotransmitter-related enzymes and indices of hypoxia in senile dementia and other abiotrophies, *Brain* **99**(3) (1976), 459–496.

[5] E.K. Perry et al., Necropsy evidence of central cholinergic deficits in senile dementia, *Lancet* **1**(8004) (1977), 189.

[6] P. White et al., Neocortical cholinergic neurons in elderly people, *Lancet* **1**(8013) (1977), 668–671.

[7] J.A. Spillane et al., Selective vulnerability of neurones in organic dementia, *Nature* **266**(5602) (1977), 558–559.

[8] P.J. Whitehouse et al., Alzheimer disease: evidence for selective loss of cholinergic neurons in the nucleus basalis, *Ann Neurol* **10**(2) (1981), 122–126.

[9] R.H. Perry et al., Extensive loss of choline acetyltransferase activity is not reflected by neuronal loss in the nucleus of Meynert in Alzheimer's disease, *Neurosci Lett* **33**(3) (1982), 311–315.

[10] B. Zipser and R. McKay, Monoclonal antibodies distinguish identifiable neurones in the leech, *Nature* **289**(5798) (1981), 549–554.

[11] H. Ksiezak-Reding et al., Recognition of tau epitopes by anti-neurofilament antibodies that bind to Alzheimer neurofibrillary tangles, *Proc Natl Acad Sci USA* **84**(10) (1987), 3410–3414.

[12] A. Scicutella and P. Davies, Characterization of monoclonal antibodies to galactolipids and uses in studies of dementia, *J Neuropathol Exp Neurol* **47**(4) (1988), 406–419.

[13] B. Wolozin and P. Davies, Alzheimer-related neuronal protein A68: specificity and distribution, *Ann Neurol* **22**(4) (1987), 521–526.

[14] M. Tabaton et al., Alz 50 recognizes abnormal filaments in Alzheimer's disease and progressive supranuclear palsy, *Ann Neurol* **24**(3) (1988), 407–413.

[15] J.A. Doebler et al., Neuronal RNA in relation to Alz-50 immunoreactivity in Alzheimer's disease, *Ann Neurol* **23**(1) (1988), 20–24.

[16] B.T. Hyman et al., Alz-50 antibody recognizes Alzheimer-related neuronal changes, *Ann Neurol* **23**(4) (1988), 371–379.

[17] G. Carmel et al., The structural basis of monoclonal antibody Alz50's selectivity for Alzheimer's disease pathology, *J Biol Chem* **271**(51) (1996), 32789–32795.

[18] G.A. Jicha et al., Alz-50 and MC-1, a new monoclonal antibody raised to paired helical filaments, recognize conformational epitopes on recombinant tau, *J Neurosci Res* **48**(2) (1997), 128–132.

[19] G.A. Jicha, B. Berenfeld and P. Davies, Sequence requirements for formation of conformational variants of tau similar to those found in Alzheimer's disease, *J Neurosci Res* **55**(6) (1999), 713–723.

[20] C.L. Weaver et al., Conformational change as one of the earliest alterations of tau in Alzheimer's disease, *Neurobiol Aging* **21**(5) (2000), 719–727.

[21] G.A. Jicha et al., A conformation- and phosphorylation-dependent antibody recognizing the paired helical filaments of Alzheimer's disease, *J Neurochem* **69**(5) (1997), 2087–2095.

[22] I. Vincent et al., Mitotic phosphoepitopes precede paired helical filaments in Alzheimer's disease, *Neurobiol Aging* **19**(4) (1998), 287–296.

[23] M. Roberge et al., High-throughput assay for G2 checkpoint inhibitors and identification of the structurally novel compound isogranulatimide, *Cancer Res* **58**(24) (1998), 5701–5706.

[24] H.J. Anderson et al., Flow cytometry of mitotic cells, *Exp Cell Res* **238**(2) (1998), 498–502.

[25] A. Dranovsky et al., Cdc2 phosphorylation of nucleolin demarcates mitotic stages and Alzheimer's disease pathology, *Neurobiol Aging* **22**(4) (2001), 517–528.

[26] T. Arendt, Synaptic plasticity and cell cycle activation in neurons are alternative effector pathways: the 'Dr. Jekyll and Mr. Hyde concept' of Alzheimer's disease or the yin and yang of neuroplasticity, *Prog Neurobiol* **71**(2–3) (2003), 83–248.

[27] A. Copani et al., Cell cycle progression towards Alzheimer's disease, *Funct Neurol* **16**(4 Suppl) (2001), 11–15.

[28] K. Herrup et al., Divide and die: cell cycle events as triggers of nerve cell death, *J Neurosci* **24**(42) (2004), 9232–9239.

[29] Z. Nagy, Cell cycle regulatory failure in neurones: causes and consequences, *Neurobiol Aging* **21**(6) (2000), 761–769.

[30] I. Vincent, C.I. Pae and J.L. Hallows, The cell cycle and human neurodegenerative disease, *Prog Cell Cycle Res* **5** (2003), 31–41.

[31] L.A. Greene, S.C. Biswas and D.X. Liu, Cell cycle molecules and vertebrate neuron death: E2F at the hub, *Cell Death Differ* **11**(1) (2004), 49–60.

[32] L. Stefanis, R.E. Burke and L.A. Greene, Apoptosis in neurodegenerative disorders, *Curr Opin Neurol* **10**(4) (1997), 299–305.

[33] Y. Yang, E.J. Mufson and K. Herrup, Neuronal cell death is preceded by cell cycle events at all stages of Alzheimer's disease, *J Neurosci* **23**(7) (2003), 2557–2563.

[34] Y. Yang, D.S. Geldmacher and K. Herrup, DNA replication precedes neuronal cell death in Alzheimer's disease, *J Neurosci* **21**(8) (2001), 2661–2668.

[35] Y. Wen et al., Transient cerebral ischemia induces aberrant neuronal cell cycle re-entry and Alzheimer's disease-like tauopathy in female rats, *J Biol Chem* **279**(21) (2004), 22684–22692.

[36] C.Y. Kuan et al., Hypoxia-ischemia induces DNA synthesis without cell proliferation in dying neurons in adult rodent brain, *J Neurosci* **24**(47) (2004), 10763–10772.

[37] J. Lewis et al., Neurofibrillary tangles, amyotrophy and progressive motor disturbance in mice expressing mutant (P301L) tau protein, *Nat Genet* **25**(4) (2000), 402–405.

[38] K. Duff et al., Characterization of pathology in transgenic mice over-expressing human genomic and cDNA tau transgenes, *Neurobiol Dis* **7**(2) (2000), 87–98.

[39] C. Andorfer et al., Cell-cycle reentry and cell death in transgenic mice expressing nonmutant human tau isoforms, *J Neurosci* **25**(22) (2005), 5446–5454.

[40] C. Andorfer et al., Hyperphosphorylation and aggregation of tau in mice expressing normal human tau isoforms, *J Neurochem* **86**(3) (2003), 582–590.

[41] D.S. Park et al., Cyclin dependent kinase inhibitors and dominant negative cyclin dependent kinase 4 and 6 promote survival of NGF-deprived sympathetic neurons, *J Neurosci* **17**(23) (1997), 8975–8983.

[42] D.S. Park et al., G1/S cell cycle blockers and inhibitors of cyclin-dependent kinases suppress camptothecin-induced neuronal apoptosis, *J Neurosci* **17**(4) (1997), 1256–1270.

[43] D.S. Park et al., Cyclin-dependent kinases participate in death of neurons evoked by DNA-damaging agents, *J Cell Biol* **143**(2) (1998), 457–467.

Inflammation, anti-inflammatory agents and Alzheimer disease: The last 12 years

Patrick L. McGeer[a,*], Joseph Rogers[b] and Edith G. McGeer[a]
[a]*Kinsmen Laboratory of Neurological Research, University of British Columbia, Vancouver BC, Canada*
[b]*Sun Health Research Institute, Sun City, Arizona, USA*

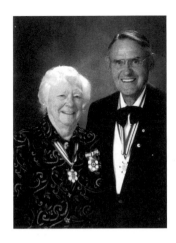

Abstract. Two basic discoveries have spurred research into inflammation as a driving force in the pathology of Alzheimer disease (AD). The first was the identification of activated microglia in association with the lesions. The second was the finding that rheumatoid arthritics were relatively spared from the disease. These findings spurred the first pilot trial of a classical NSAID in the treatment of AD. This trial showed promise for indomethacin as a useful therapeutic agent but appropriate follow up trials have not been done. However, more than 20 epidemiological studies have since been conducted showing a sparing effect for antiinflammatories in AD, including four which specifically addressed the use of classical NSAIDs. Other key findings linking inflammation to AD pathology are the identification of activated complement fragments, including the membrane attack complex, as well as inflammatory cytokines in association with the lesions. *In vitro*, activated microglia release factors which are toxic to neurons, and these can be partially blocked by NSAIDs. Future directions should include a search for other inflammatory mediators in AD and exploitation of current knowledge to improve available treatments.

Keywords: NSAID, indomethacin, complement, membrane attack complex, immunohistochemistry, reactive microglia

Twelve years ago, Rogers et al. [31] published the results of a small, placebo controlled, double blind trial of the nonsteroidal antiinflammatory drug (NSAID) indomethacin in Alzheimer disease (AD). The indomethacin appeared to arrest the mental deterioration for the six months of the trial, while the placebo group showed the expected deterioration. The rationale for this trial was based on two discoveries: one was the immunohistochemical demonstration of reactive microglia in AD brains [24,32]; the second was that persons suffering from rheumatoid arthritis had a greatly reduced risk of AD [28]. The first was interpreted as indicating a chronic inflammation in AD brain, while the second was hypothesized to be due to the chronic use of NSAIDs [27].

In the ensuing 12 years, there have been a great many reports confirming and extending evidence for chronic inflammation in AD brain. The large number of reviews on the subject (e.g. [8,11,22,30]) indicate that it is now widely accepted that such inflammation is an important part of the pathology. Reactive microglia have been shown to produce large amounts of free radicals and other neurotoxic substances which kill neurons in culture [10,17]. Some activated T cells are also found in the brain parenchyma in AD [20,21,39]. Such cells

---

*Corresponding author: Dr. Patrick L. McGeer, Kinsmen Laboratory of Neurological Research, University of British Columbia, 2255 Wesbrook Mall, Vancouver, B.C., V6T 1Z3, Canada. Tel.: +1 604 822 7380; Fax: +1 604 822 7086; E-mail: mcgeerpl@interchange.ubc.ca.

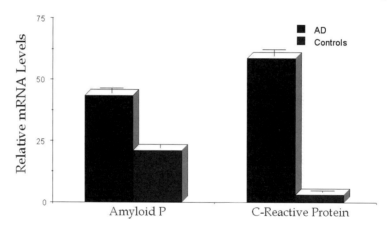

Fig. 1. Relative mRNA levels for amyloid P and C-reactive protein in the hippocampus of AD and control brain (data from [50]).

release inflammatory mediators including the powerful proinflammatory stimulant γ-interferon.

A key discovery linking inflammation to AD was the finding that consolidated amyloid β was a powerful activator of complement [33]. It had previously been shown that the complement system was activated in AD [7] but antibodies, which were then considered to be the main activators of complement, could not be identified in association with AD lesions. It was subsequently demonstrated that amyloid β activated complement by binding to the collagen tail of C1q [44]. This is a different mechanism than classical activation by antibodies where the globular head of C1q binds to the immunoglobulin Fc tail.

It has now been shown that the complement cascade can also be activated by other substances such as the pentraxins (amyloid P and C-reactive protein (CRP)) [12,15,46]. Upregulation of both pentraxins is found in AD [50] (Fig. 1). CRP and amyloid P also activate the complement cascade by binding to the collagen tail of C1q.

The complement system has been shown to be fully activated in AD. The complement cascade, once activated, produces anaphylatoxins which promote further inflammation, opsonizing components which mark material for phagocytosis, and the membrane attack complex (the MAC) which is directly lytic to cells. The MAC inserts itself into viable cell membranes, causing them to leak and producing death of the cell. It is intended to destroy foreign cells and viruses, but host cells are at significant risk of bystander lysis.

Figure 2 illustrates the difference between opsonization by the early complement components and the lytic effects of the MAC. Figure 2(a) shows double immunostaining for C4d, a fragment of activated complement, and complement receptors. C4d attaches covalently to the amyloid deposit, while activated microglia, which express high levels of complement receptors, are attacking the deposit by attraction to their ligand. Figure 2(b) shows a different phenomenon which is invisible to the stains used in Fig. 2(a). That is the attack on neurites within the plaque by assembly of the terminal complement components. The MAC, or C5b-9, requires a viable membrane surface for this to take place. A neoepitope on C9 is formed which produces an opening in the membrane which can cause fatal leakage. The MAC has a very short half life so finding immunohistochemical evidence for its existence in postmortem AD brains indicates the vigor of the attack. A more revealing overall index may be the levels of RNA expression of the complement proteins. There is a marked upregulation in affected regions in AD [48] (Fig. 3).

Identification of the MAC attacking dystrophic neurites in AD [19,25,43] provides strong evidence of self attack in AD. It also provides the only *in vivo* evidence linking amyloid β deposits with neurotoxicity. A conspicuous shortcoming of the amyloid cascade hypothesis of AD has been the failure of the massive amyloid deposits in transgenic mice to cause significant neuronal damage or to induce the formation of tangles [5, 36]. One explanation is the relatively weak recognition by mouse C1q of human amyloid β [43]. The level of complement activation is therefore less, with concomitant sparing of neurons [5,36]. Nevertheless, complement may play a role in clearing of amyloid β in transgenic mice because crossing them with mice genetically engineered to overexpress an inhibitor of complement component C3 results in decreased clearance of the amyloid β deposits [47]. Alternatively, Fonseca et al. [9] found no alterations in amyloid β burden and de-

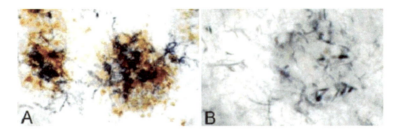

Fig. 2. Contrast in the immunostaining of AD senile plaques by opsonizing fragments of complement compared with the terminal components C5b-9. A. Double immunostaining for C4d and CD11c. The opsonizing fragment C4d (light staining) is covalently attached to plaque amyloid β. Reactive microglia expressing high levels of the complement receptor CD11c (dark staining) agglomerate around the C4d ligand. B. Immunostaining for the MAC (C5b-9). Dystrophic neurites within the senile plaque are prominently stained, indicating lytic attack on trapped neuronal processes. Note the very weak immunostaining of neuropil threads in the surround.

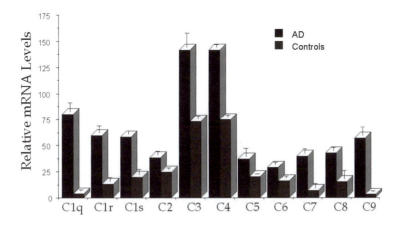

Fig. 3. Relative mRNA levels for proteins of the complement cascade in the hippocampus of AD and control brains (data from [48]).

creased neurodegeneration when amyloid-developing transgenic mice were crossed with C1q knockout mice.

A host of other inflammatory markers have now also been shown to be upregulated in affected brain areas in AD. They include many of the inflammatory cytokines and such inflammatory stimulants as ICAM-1. Alleles which favor production of IL-1α, IL-1β, IL-8, TNF and other inflammatory cytokines have been frequently reported to increase the risk of AD (reviewed in [22]).

In the past 12 years there have also been more than twenty epidemiological studies showing that individuals are spared from AD if they have been taking nonsteroidal antiinflammatory drugs, or have suffered from conditions where such drugs are routinely used [29,38, 41,51,52]. Four large epidemiological studies have analyzed the effects of NSAID consumption on AD. The Baltimore longitudinal study [38] showed a sparing of approximately 60% amongst NSAID users of greater than 2 years duration; the Cache County study showed a sparing of approximately 55% [52]; the Rotterdam study, where NSAID consumption was verified through prescription records, showed an 80% sparing [41]; and the MIRAGE study showed a sparing of 36% [51]. Some [45] have argued that the NSAIDs which seem to be effective are interfering with amyloid β production rather than acting as COX inhibitors. However, the concentrations of NSAIDs required to interfere with such production are far higher than those achieved *in vivo*, whereas the levels which inhibit COX, which are at least 100 times lower, are in accord with *in vivo* levels [16].

The major hypothesis underlying the clinical trial by Rogers et al. [31] was that antiinflammatories would slow the progression of AD. Follow up studies over the past twelve years have been largely negative. Unfortunately the major clinical trials have been done with inappropriate agents or doses which seem suboptimal considering the available biological and epidemiological evidence. They have included prednisone; the COX-2 inhibitors celecoxib, rofecoxib and nimesulide; and hydroxychloroquine [1,2,34,40]. These agents were known to be effective in treating arthritic conditions but there was little or no evidence that they would be useful in neuroinflammation. Steroids may be particularly harmful because they themselves cause hippocampal damage [13].

As far as selective COX-2 inhibitors are concerned, they have not been in use long enough for epidemiological data to accumulate, but their failure could be predicted on the basis of immunohistochemical evidence. Unlike COX-1, which is concentrated in human microglial cells [14], COX-2 is highly expressed in normal pyramidal neurons, including pyramidal neurons of AD cases [49]. Therefore, selective COX-2 inhibitors will primarily target vulnerable pyramidal neurons rather than microglia. This, combined with evidence of exacerbation of neuronal death in some animal neurotoxicity models following COX-2 inhibition, suggests COX-2 inhibitors are an inappropriate choice [23].

Hydroxychloroquine is not a general antiinflammatory agent. Its mechanism of action in arthritis is uncertain. It is noteworthy, however, that while its main side effects are ototoxicity and retinal damage, some include neuronal damage [37]. Since there is no epidemiological or immunohistochemical evidence to support a role for hydroxychloroquine or other 4-aminoquinolines in neuroinflammation, the failure to be effective in AD is disappointing but not surprising.

There have been two further small pilot studies with traditional NSAIDs since that of Rogers et al. An NSAID trial, involving the mixed COX inhibitor diclofenac combined with misoprostyl, showed marginally less deterioration in drug compared with placebo patients, although the data fell short of statistical significance at the $p < 0.05$ level [35]. A significantly slower cognitive decline compared to placebo was reported in a Japanese trial where cases were treated with a combination of estrogen, vitamin E and an NSAID [4].

NSAIDs have been shown *in vitro* to reduce the neurotoxicity of activated microglia toward neuronal type cells [18]. Properly designed clinical trials of COX-1 inhibiting NSAIDs that reach the brain should be a high priority for AD. Relatively high doses may be required due to the strong inflammatory reaction present in established AD. Low dosage may have been the problem in the recent, failed trial with naproxen [3].

Gastrointestinal and other side effects are a problem with such agents, particularly with chronic use and in aged individuals [6]. While such side effects are significant, they may be small in comparison with the inevitable progression and fatal outcome of AD with currently approved methods of treatment. In the pilot trials conducted to date, no effort has been made to prevent or treat such gastrointestinal side effects although doing so would be appropriate. It is possible that a new class of COX-1 inhibiting NSAIDs, based on introducing a nitrate ester moiety, may circumvent the side effect problem. These so-called NO-NSAIDs have greatly reduced gastrointestinal toxicity [42].

Other types of antiinflammatory agents may be effective. The spectrum of inflammatory mediators upregulated in AD suggests many routes for future therapeutic intervention. It may be that multiple drug administration, targeted at different inflammatory mechanisms, will prove far more effective than utilization of any single agent. Agents capable of blocking formation of the MAC in brain may be a particularly attractive target. Such drugs might find use in other neurodegenerative diseases as well as AD since evidence is now appearing that inflammation may also play a role in the progression of various other disorders such as Parkinson disease, amyotrophic lateral sclerosis and multiple sclerosis [26,30].

Acknowledgement

Work in the McGeers' laboratory on AD has been supported by the Jack Brown and Family Alzheimer Disease Research Fund, the George Hodgson estate, grants from the Alzheimer Society of Canada/CIHR/Astra-Zeneca and gifts from individual British Columbians. All experiments were performed in accordance with protocols approved by the authors' Institutional Review Boards. The authors are named on patents held by the University of British Columbia for the treatment of dementia with cyclooxygenase inhibitors.

References

[1] P.S. Aisen, K.L. Davis, J.D. Berg, K. Schafer, K. Campbell, R.G. Thomas, M.F. Weiner, M.R. Farlow, M. Sano, M. Grundman and L.J. Thal, A randomized controlled trial of prednisone in Alzheimer's disease, *Neurology* **54** (2000), 588–593.

[2] P.S. Aisen, J. Schmeidler and G.M. Pasinetti, Randomized pilot study of nimesulide in Alzheimer's disease, *Neurology* **58** (2002), 1050–1054.

[3] P.S. Aisen, K.A. Schafer, M. Grundman, E. Pfeiffer, M. Sano, K.L. Davis, M.R. Farlow, S. Jin, R.G. Thomas and L.J. Thal, Effects of rofecoxib or naproxen vs placebo on Alzheimer disease progression: a randomized controlled trial, *JAMA* **289** (2003), 2819–2826.

[4] H. Arai, T. Suzuki, H. Sasaki, T. Hanawa, K. Toriizuka and H. Yamada, A new interventional strategy for Alzheimer's disease by Japanese herbal medicine, *Jap. J. Ger.* **37** (2000), 212–215.

[5] S. Boncristiano, M.E. Calhoun, V. Howard, L. Bondolfi, S.A. Kaeser, K.H. Wiedernold, M. Staufenbiel and M. Jucker, Neocortical synaptic bouton number is maintained despite robust amyloid deposition in APP23 transgenic mice, *Neurobiol. Aging* **26** (2005), 607–613.

[6] H.A. Capell, Disease modifying antirheumatic drugs: longterm safety issues, *J. Rheumatol. Suppl.* **62** (2001), 10–15.

[7] P. Eikelenboom and F.C. Stam, Immunoglobulins and complement factors in senile plaques, *An Immunoperoxidase study. Acta Neuropathol.* **57** (1987), 239–242.

[8] P. Eikelenboom and W.A. van Gool, Neuroinflammatory perspectives on the two faces of Alzheimer's disease, *J. Neural. Transmiss.* **111** (2004), 281–294.

[9] M.I. Fonseca, J. Zhou, M. Botto and A.J. Tenner, Absence of C1q leads to less neuropathology in transgenic mouse models of Alzheimer's disease, *J. Neurosci.* **24** (2004), 6457–6465.

[10] D. Giulian, K. Vaca and C.A. Noonan, Secretion of neurotoxins by mononuclear phagocytes infected with HIV-1, *Science* **250** (1990), 1593–1596.

[11] A. Gupta and K. Pansari, Inflammation and Alzheimer's disease, *Intl. J. Clin. Pract.* **57** (2003), 36–39.

[12] P.S. Hicks, L. Saunero-Nazia, T.W. Duclos and C. Mold, Serum amyloid P component binds to histones and activates the classical complement pathway, *J. Immunol.* **149** (1992), 3689–3691.

[13] C. Hoschl and T. Hajek, Hippocampal damage mediated by corticosteroids – a neuropsychiatric research challenge, *Eur. Arch. Psychiatry & Clin. Neurosci.* **251**(Suppl 2) (2001), II81–II88.

[14] J.J. Hoozemans, R. Veerhuis, A.J. Rozemuller and P. Eikelenboom, Cyclooxygenase expression in microglia and neurons in Alzheimer's disease and control brain, *Acta Neuropathol* **101** (2001), 2–8.

[15] H. Jiang, F.A. Robery and H. Gewurz, Localization of sites through which C-reactive protein binds and activates complement to residues 14–26 and 76–92 of the human C1q A chain, *J. Exp. Med.* **175** (1992), 1373–1379.

[16] A. Klegeris, J. Maguire and P.L. McGeer, S- but not R-enantiomers of flurbiprofen and ibuprofen reduce human microglial and THP-1 cell neurotoxicity, *J. Neuroimmunol.* **152** (2004), 73–77.

[17] A. Klegeris and P.L. McGeer, Interaction of various intracellular signaling mechanisms involved in mononuclear phagocyte toxicity toward neuronal cells, *J. Leukoc. Biol.* **67** (2000), 127–133.

[18] A. Klegeris, D.G. Walker and P.L. McGeer, Toxicity of human THP-1 monocytic cells towards neuron-like cells is reduced by non-steroidal anti-inflammatory drugs (NSAIDs), *Neuropharmacology* **38** (1999), 1017–1025.

[19] S. Itagaki, H. Akiyama, H. Saito and P.L. McGeer, Ultrastructural localization of complement membrane attack complex (MAC)-like immunoreactivity in brains of patients with Alzheimer's disease, *Brain Res* **645** (1994), 78–84.

[20] S. Itagaki, P.L. McGeer and H. Akiyama, Presence of T-cytotoxic suppressor and leucocyte common antigen positive cells in Alzheimer disease brain tissue, *Neurosci. Lett.* **91** (1988),

[21] J. Luber-Narod and J. Rogers, Immune system associated antigens expressed by cells of the human central nervous system, *Neurosci. Lett.* **94** (1988), 17–22.

[22] E.G. McGeer and P.L. McGeer, Inflammatory processes in Alzheimer's disease, *Progr. Neuro-Psychopharmacol. & Biol. Psychiatry* **27** (2003), 741–749.

[23] P.L. McGeer, Cyclo-oxygenase-2 inhibitors, *Drugs & Aging* **17** (2000), 1–11.

[24] P.L. McGeer, S. Itagaki, H. Tago and E.G. McGeer, Reactive microglia in patients with senile dementia of the Alzheimer type are positive for the histocompatability protein HLA-DR, *Neurosci. Lett.* **79** (1987), 195–200.

[25] P.L. McGeer, D.G. Walker, H. Akiyama, T. Kawamata, A.L. Guan and C.J. Parker, Detection of the membrane inhibitor of reactive lysis (CD59) in diseased neurons of Alzheimer brain, *Brain Res.* **544** (1991), 315–319.

[26] P.L. McGeer and E.G. McGeer, Inflammation and the degenerative diseases of aging, *Ann. N.Y. Acad. Sci.* **1035** (2004), 104–116.

[27] P.L. McGeer and J. Rogers, Anti-inflammatory agents as a therapeutic approach to Alzheimer's disease, *Neurology* **42** (1992), 447–449.

[28] P.L. McGeer, J. Rogers, E.G. McGeer and J. Sibley, Anti-inflammatory drugs and Alzheimer disease? *Lancet* **335** (1990), 1037.

[29] P.L. McGeer, M. Schulzer and E.G. McGeer, Arthritis and antiinflammatory agents as possible protective factors for Alzheimer's disease: a review of 17 epidemiological studies, *Neurology* **47** (1996), 425–432.

[30] M. Mhatre, R.A. Floyd and K. Hensley, Oxidative stress and neuroinflammation in Alzheimer's disease and amyotrophic lateral sclerosis: common links and potential therapeutic targets, *J. Alz. Dis.* **6** (2004), 147–157.

[31] J. Rogers, L.C. Kirby, S.R. Hempelman, D.L. Berry, P.L. McGeer, A.W. Kaszniak, J. Zalinski, M. Cofield, L. Mansukhani, P. Willson and F. Kogan, Clinical trial of indomethacin in Alzheimer's disease, *Neurology* **43** (1993), 1609–1611.

[32] J. Rogers, J. Luber-Narod, S.D. Styren and W.H. Civin, Expression of immune system-associated antigens by cells of the human central nervous system: relationship to the pathology of Alzheimer's disease, *Neurobiol. Aging.* **9** (1988), 339–349.

[33] J. Rogers, S. Webster, J. Schultz, P.L. McGeer, S. Styren, W.H. Civin, L. Brachova, B. Bradt, P. Ward and I. Lieburg, Complement activation by β-amyloid in Alzheimer disease, *Proc. Natl. Acad. Sci. USA* **89** (1999), 10016–10020.

[34] S.M. Sainali, D.M. Ingram, S. Talwaker and G.S. Geis, Results of a double-blind, placebo-controlled study of celecoxib for the progression of Alzheimer's disease, *6th International Stockholm-Springfield Symposium of Advances in Alzheimer Therapy* (2000) 180.

[35] S. Scharf, A. Mander, A. Ugoni, F. Vajda and N. Christophidis, A double-blind, placebo-controlled trial of diclofenac misoprostol in Alzheimer's disease, *Neurology* **53** (1999), 197–201.

[36] C. Schwab, M. Hosokawa and P.L. McGeer, Transgenic mice overexpressing amyloid beta protein are an incomplete model of Alzheimer disease, *Exp. Neurol.* **188** (2004), 52–64.

[37] M. Stein, M.J. Bell and L.C. Ang, Hydroxychloroquine neuromyotoxicity, *J. Rheumatol.* **27** (2000), 2927–2931.

[38] W.F. Stewart, C. Kawas, M. Corrada and E.J. Metter, Risk of Alzheimer's disease and duration of NSAID use, *Neurology* **48** (1997), 626–632.

[39] T. Togo, H. Akiyama, E. Iseki, H. Kondo, K. Ikeda, M. Kato, T. Oda, K. Tsuchiya and K. Kosaka, Occurrence of T cells in the brain of Alzheimer's disease and other neurological diseases, *J. Neuroimmunol.* **124** (2002), 83–92.

[40] W.A. Van Gool, H.C. Weinstein, P. Scheltens and G.J. Walstra, Effect of hydroxychloroquine on progression of dementia in

early Alzheimer's disease: an 18-month randomized, double-blind, placebo-controlled study, *Lancet* **358** (2001), 455–460.

[41] B.A.I. Veld, A. Ruitenberg, L.J. Launer, A. Hofman, M.M.B. Breteler and B.H.C. Stricker, Duration of non-steroidal anti-inflammatory drug use and risk of Alzheimer's disease, *The Rotterdam study. Neurobiol. Aging* **21**(1S) (2000), S204.

[42] J.L. Wallace, Q.J. Pittman and G. Cirino, Nitric oxide-releasing NSAIDs: a novel class of GI-sparing anti-inflammatory drugs, *Agents & Actions. Suppl.* **46** (1995), 121–129.

[43] S. Webster, L.F. Lue, L. Brachova, A.J. Tenner, P.L. McGeer, K. Terai, D.G. Walker, B. Bradt, N.R. Cooper and J. Rogers, Molecular and cellular characteristics of the membrane attack complex, C5b-9, in Alzheimer's disease, *Neurobiol. Aging* **18** (1997), 415–421.

[44] S. Webster, A.J. Tenner, T.L. Paulos and D.H. Cribbs, The mouse C1q A sequence alters beta-amyloid-induced complement activation, *Neurobiol. Aging* **20** (1999), 297–304.

[45] S. Weggen, J.L. Eriksen, P. Das, S.A. Sagi, R. Wang, C.U. Pietrzik, K.A. Findlay, T.E. Smith, M.P. Murphy, T. Bulter, D.E. Kang, N. Marquez-Sterling, T.E. Golde and E.H. Koo, A subset of NSAIDs lower amyloidogenic Abeta-42 independently of cyclooxygenase activity, *Nature* **414** (2001), 212–216.

[46] G.J. Wolbrink, M.C. Brouwer, S. Buysmann, I.J.M. ten Berge and C.E. Hack, CRP-mediated activation of complement *in vivo*, *J. Immunol.* **157** (1996), 473–479.

[47] T. Wyss-Coray, F. Yan, A.H. Lin, J.D. Lambnris, J.J. Alexander, R.J. Quigg and E. Masliah, Prominent neurodegeneration and increased plaque formation in complement-inhibited Alzheimer's mice, *Proc. Natl. Acad. Sci. USA* **99** (2002), 10837–10842.

[48] K. Yasojima, C. Schwab, E.G. McGeer and P.L. McGeer, Up-regulated production and activation of the complement system in Alzheimer's disease brain, *Am. J. Pathol.* **154** (1999), 927–936.

[49] K. Yasojima, C. Schwab, E.G. McGeer and P.L. McGeer, Distribution of cyclooxygenase-1 and cyclooxygenase-2 mRNAs and proteins in human brain and peripheral organs, *Brain Res.* **830** (1999), 226–236.

[50] K. Yasojima, C. Schwab, E.G. McGeer and P.L. McGeer, Human neurons generate C-reactive protein and amyloid P: upregulation in Alzheimer's disease, *Brain Res.* **887** (2000), 80–89.

[51] A.G. Yip, R.C. Green, M. Huyck, L.A. Cupples and L.A. Farrer, Nonsteroidal anti-inflammatory drug use and Alzheimer's disease risk: the MIRAGE study, *BMC Geriatr.* **5** (2005).

[52] P.P. Zandi, J.C. Anthony, K.M. Hayden, K. Mehta, L. Mayer and J.C. Breitner, Reduced incidence of AD with NSAID but not H2 receptor antagonists: the Cache County Study, *Neurology* **59** (2002), 880–886.

Lysosomal system pathways: Genes to neurodegeneration in Alzheimer's disease

Ralph A. Nixon[a,b,c,*] and Anne M. Cataldo[d]
[a]Center for Dementia Research, Nathan S. Kline Institute, 140 Old Orangeburg Road, Orangeburg, NY 10962, USA
[b]Department of Psychiatry, New York University, 550 First Ave, New York, NY 10016, USA
[c]Department of Cell Biology, New York University, 550 First Ave, New York, NY 10016, USA
[d]Mailman Research Center, McLean Hospital, Harvard University, 115 Mill Street, Belmont, MA 02478, USA

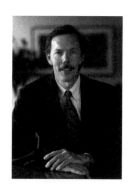

Abstract. The identification of cathepsins in amyloid-β plaques revealed broad dysfunction of the lysosomal system in Alzheimer's disease (AD). Coinciding with the discovery that proteolysis is required to generate the Aβ-peptide, these findings heralded an era of intense investigation on proteases in neurodegeneration. This review traces lysosomal system pathology from its early characterization to its origins within two pathways leading to the lysosome, the endocytic and autophagic pathways. An understanding has grown about how these two pathways are adversely influenced by normal brain aging and by genetic and environmental risk factors for AD, resulting in increased susceptibility of neurons to injury, amyloidogenesis, and neurodegeneration.

Keywords: Amyloid-β, cathepsin, apoptosis, endosome, autophagy, necrosis, Alzheimer's disease, protease, endocytosis

1. Introduction

In the 1950s, when DeDuve discovered lysosomes containing dozens of protein and membrane-degrading enzymes, he not only recognized their importance for maintaining cell homeostasis but also their destructive potential [47,48]. The application of these findings to nervous system disease was immediate; discoveries followed of lysosomal gene defects causing lysosomal "storage" disorders that were associated with neurodegeneration and cognitive decline. Over the next decade, germinal work that highlighted the relationship between structure and function of the lysosome system in normal neurons by Holtzman, Novikoff, and Koenig reinforced the link between lysosomal system dysfunction and neurodegenerative phenomena [84,97, 129]. Possible connections to Alzheimer's disease (AD) came from the pioneering ultrastructural descriptions of neurofibrillary degeneration by Terry, Suzuki and others, who also noted high numbers of acid phosphatase-positive lysosomal dense bodies in dystrophic neurites [164,167].

Despite these auspicious beginnings to lysosomal system research, a view prevailed that lysosomes and their enzymes were mobilized mainly at the end stages of degeneration to scavenge or remove debris and that, contrary to DeDuve's proposal, lysosomal proteases (cathepsins) rarely triggered cell death. Despite a strong rationale that a protease or protease dysfunction should be associated with development of neurodegenerative diseases, especially in disorders where abnormal proteins accumulate [141], interest in brain proteases lay relatively dormant until the late 1980s when

*Corresponding author: Dr. Ralph Nixon, Ph.D., M.D. Nathan Kline Institute, New York University School of Medicine, 140 Old Orangeburg Road, Orangeburg, NY 10962, USA. Tel.: +1 845 398 5423; Fax: +1 845 398 5422; E-mail: Nixon@nki.rfmh.org.

the diversity of proteases and their complex roles began to be more widely appreciated. Interest in proteases in AD was also fueled at this time by the discovery that amyloid-β peptide was derived by proteolytic processing of a larger protein, amyloid-β protein precursor (AβPP). An international meeting at the NIH in 1991, dedicated to proteolysis in AD pathogenesis, heralded a new era of intense research on proteases in neurodegenerative diseases [125].

As part of early investigations in our laboratory on proteases of the calpain and lysosomal systems in neurodegeneration, we raised antibodies to cathepsins which, when applied to AD brain, revealed robust and widespread mobilization of the lysosomal system in neurons [25]. The full report of these findings in 1990 in PNAS [30] stimulated considerable interest in part because the study represented the initial attempt to link AβPP processing in brain to the activity of a particular proteolytic system. Among the findings in this report were that cathepsin-positive (i.e. lysosome-related) vesicles accumulated in most neurons of targeted brain regions in AD and that the concentrations of cathepsin immunoreactivity in senile plaques were exceptionally high, an observation also made independently by Bernstein [11]. Moreover, the cathepsins (Cat) D and Cat B in senile plaques were shown by histochemical assays to be enzymatically active and also to be present extracellularly to some degree. Companion studies from our laboratory, including mRNA expression analysis, showed that these changes reflected a generalized up-regulation of lysosomal system activity [26,31,37]. These observations have been confirmed and extended in AD brain and mouse models of AD [12,86,122], most recently by proteomic analyses of neuritic plaques [106] and by gene expression profiling studies in single affected neurons in AD brain [22,23,67], which show that Cat D expression is sustained at high levels even after the expression of most other transcripts has declined. Based on these observations, we proposed that lysosomal system dysfunction, especially within degenerating or dystrophic neurites, could impair neuron survival and promote the amyloidogenic processing of AβPP characteristic of AD neuropathology.

Research on the lysosomal system expanded greatly in the years following our 1990 report, and the cumulative findings underscore the close relationship between dysfunction of this system and neurological disease, especially AD. A deeper understanding of the two major pathways of the lysosome system, endocytosis and autophagy, has further clarified how dysfunction of the lysosomal system is connected to genetic risk factors for AD and, in turn, to mechanisms of neurodegeneration and amyloidogenesis. The emerging trends in these areas are briefly considered here.

2. The lysosomal system

The lysosomal system comprises a family of communicating vesicular compartments that have an acidic internal pH (3.5–6.0) and contain varying levels of acid hydrolases. The basic organization of the lysosomal system is depicted in Fig. 1, although the subcellular features may vary with the cell type. The lysosomal system includes those vesicular compartments involved in endocytosis and autophagy in addition to lysosomes, the most acidic compartment. Substrate acquisition and targeting within these interacting pathways occurs through tightly regulated organellar budding and fusion events. The endocytic pathway is responsible for internalizing plasma membrane and extracellular materials into early endosomes and then sorting certain membrane components back to the surface or to the trans Golgi network (TGN) for re-use. Most materials internalized through the endocytic pathway, however, are delivered to the lysosome for processing or terminal degradation [15,124,161]. To execute these processing functions, early endosomes mature through a "multivesicular body" stage to become late endosomes that receive acid hydrolases and a proton pump for acidification from the TGN or by fusing with lysosomes. Most proteolytic processing occurs within late endosomes but the processing of some substrates occurs even in early endosomes where it could modulate endosome-mediated signal transduction. Macroautophagy, the most common form of autophagy, is solely responsible for turning over organelles and shares responsibilities with the proteasome for processing other intracellular proteins [55,153,154]. The more general term, "autophagy", is used here unless the reference is to macroautophagy specifically. Dramatic advances in understanding macroautophagy in yeast [96,118,158], and now increasingly in mammalian cells [46,104,185], include the delineation of distinct steps in this process, beginning with the initial sequestration of cytoplasm within an elongated enveloping membrane to create the autophagosome. This earliest subtype of autophagic vacuole (AV) matures to one of several types of "late" degradative AVs when it fuses with a lysosome to form an autophagolysosome, or with a late endosome, to create an intermediate compartment, the "amphisome,"

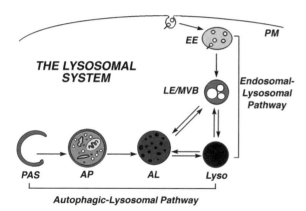

Fig. 1. Representation of the Lysosomal System. The lysosomal system is comprised of two main pathways, the Autophagic Pathway and the Endocytic Pathway as discussed in the text and cited reviews. The major organelles of the Autophagic Pathway are a pre-autophagic structure (PAS) which sequesters large areas of cytoplasm within a double membrane-limited autophagosome (AP). This organelle interacts with either a lysosome to form an autophagolysosome (AL) or a late endosome/multivesicular body (LE/MVB) to form an "amphisome". Efficient digestion of substrates within these proteolytically competent compartments, in both cases, yields a lysosome. Internalized materials entering the Endocytic Pathway in clathrin-coated vesicles are directed to early (sorting) endosomes (EE). Specific constituents are dissociated within EEs and recycled back to the plasmalemmal surface and others are targeted further along the pathway and degraded when EE mature to LE/MVB as they acidify and receive hydrolases.

before lysosome fusion [9,53,54]. These different lysosomal system compartments, each dynamically changing in substrate and hydrolase composition and internal pH, represent diverse capabilities for protein processing, including a potential for generating pathogenic polypeptide fragments, especially when the efficiency of the lysosomal system is impaired, as seen in AD.

3. The lysosomal system, genes, and neurodegeneration

Endocytosis and macroautophagy are particularly important to neurons. Unlike most cell types, which can remove obsolete and potentially deleterious constituents through cell division, post-mitotic neurons rely mainly on efficient proteolytic systems, like autophagy, to exercise quality control over especially large volumes of cytoplasm. The extreme polarity of neurons also imposes high demands on the endocytic pathway to maintain axons and synapses and transduce signals over long distances. These specialized needs of neurons may explain in part why mutations of lysosomal system genes seem preferentially to affect the nervous system and why a surprisingly large number of the genes and proteins linked to neurodegenerative disease have functions in the endocytic and autophagic pathways [124]. A dozen or more lysosomal storage disorders are associated with prominent nervous system degeneration caused by defects in enzymes that have different functions but share the same lysosomal localization [70]. Cathepsin D is a ubiquitous lysosomal protease, yet loss of function gene mutations especially affect the brain and cause progressive degeneration of the neocortex and hippocampus [98,120,172, 173]. Intriguing parallels can be drawn between the mechanisms underlying neurodegeneration in AD and in another inherited lysosomal disorder. In the juvenile form of Niemann Pick type C disease (NPC), cholesterol is mistrafficked in the endocytic pathway and accumulates in late endosomes and lysosomes leading to a form of progressive neurodegeneration that is associated with AD-like pathology, including neurofibrillary tangles, heightened amyloidogenic AβPP processing, and endosomal abnormalities characteristic of AD [91, 123].

At least five genes that influence the risk for AD also influence the lysosomal system and promote its dysfunction. *App* is triplicated in Down syndrome (DS) and is believed to drive the early onset of AD in individuals with DS [110,142]. In a mouse model of Down syndrome, *App* triplication is essential for the development of endocytic pathway dysfunction, which mimics the earliest known cellular pathology in AD and DS [32], and possibly for the aging-related neurodegeneration of basal forebrain cholinergic neurons [151]. Normalizing *App* gene dosage without altering the other trisomic genes ameliorates these pathologies [32]. The E4 isoform of the apolipoprotein E gene (*apo* E) is the strongest genetic risk factor for late-onset AD. Inheritance of one or both copies of this allele accelerates and exacerbates endosome dysfunction in early AD [28] and promotes lysosome instability in cell models [90]. Mutations of presenilin-1 (PS1) cause early-onset familial AD (FAD) [105,155] and potentiate lysosomal system pathology, amyloidogenesis, and neurodegeneration in this disorder [35]. Recent evidence suggests that PS1 is essential for normal lysosomal system turnover [61,179] and that PS1 mutations in FAD confer a loss of function on macroautophagy, as discussed later.

During the last decade, many additional genes have been proposed to modify risk for AD, but only a few have a confirmed association in meta-analyses of multiple studies. Among this very small group are two proteins associated with lysosomal system proteolysis – Cat D and cystatin C. AD risk increases in the presence of a functional Cat D T-224C polymorphism that alters pro-Cat D trafficking [170] in some populations studied [43,114,135,136] but not all [13,14,116] although a meta-analysis of all Caucasian populations (9 studies) establishes a significant negative association of the T-224C polymorphism with AD [1]. Cystatin C (cys C), an endogenous inhibitor of lysosomal cysteine proteases, such as Cats B, S, H, and L, is neuroprotective in injury settings [132,182]. Meta-analyses of studies confirm a highly significant protective effect of the polymorphism of cys C in AD [2,177].

4. Lysosomal system pathology in AD

Building on the initial cathepsin findings in AD brain, investigators from many laboratories have reported prominent lysosomal system pathology in mouse models of AD, including both amyloidosis and tauopathy models [87,92,102,107,119,156]. Involving more than just degenerating neurons in AD brain, lysosome proliferation was noted in nearly all neurons within vulnerable brain regions, including regions affected only at very late stages of the disease [27,29]. These findings and others, which suggested that lysosomal system mobilization precedes neurodegeneration, encouraged further studies focusing on the initial stages of AD; these studies uncovered disturbances in stages of the endocytic pathway upstream of lysosomes arising exceptionally early in the disease [28]. Beginning before $A\beta$ is deposited and when soluble $A\beta$ levels are just beginning to rise, endosomes in many neurons become enlarged due to the increased translocation of endosome fusion effectors, rab5, EEA-1 and rabaptin-5 to endosomes [28,36]. Many of these abnormal endosomes contain $A\beta$ [33]. Preliminary gene profiling analyses of single neurons with enlarged endosomes [57] have shown increased expression of rab5 and rab4 at the mRNA level, markers of endosome fusion and recycling, supporting other evidence that neuronal endocytic activity increases very early in AD [34, 36]. In DS, for example, this endosomal pathophysiology develops in some neurons even before birth and is full-blown by the time classical AD neuropathology appears [36]. A similar endosomal phenotype also develops in the Ts65Dn mouse model of DS, in which a critical segment of chromosome 16, the mouse homologue of chromosome 21, is triplicated [64]. Besides displaying a DS-like dysmorphogenesis phenotype, these mice exhibit aging-related neurodegenerative changes of basal forebrain cholinergic neurons (BFCN), hippocampus, and neocortex in the absence of amyloid-β deposition or NFT formation [83]. Endosomal pathology, like that in human AD and DS brain, appears at an early age in the same neuronal populations. Notably, both the endosomal abnormalities and degenerative changes in the BFCN are reversed when Ts65Dn mice are made diploid for *App* [32], establishing that *App* triplication is directly related to endosome dysfunction and neurodegeneration. The pattern of endosome pathology seen in AD is not seen in normal aging brain nor has it been seen in other neurodegenerative diseases [36] except NPC – a disease that shares some pathobiological features with AD [91].

The recent surge of interest in macroautophagy has led to a recognition that this process is frequently involved in disease states, including AD. Using the unique morphologies of autophagic vacuoles to detect autophagy in pathological specimens, investigators have reported autophagic vacuole pathology of varying severity within affected neurons in several neurodegenerative states [148]. The macroautophagy pathology in AD brain is particularly striking [127]. Autophagic vacuoles, representing all stages of the macroautophagic process from sequestration to degradation, accumulate grossly in dystrophic neurites. Lysosomes have long been known to be abundant in dystrophic neurites but the marked accumulation of autophagosomes that do not have lysosomal hydrolase or LAMPs, an early stage of macroautophagy, in addition to "late" AVs, implies delayed or impaired progression of macroautophagy and possibly dysfunctional proteolysis, since early AVs are rarely seen in normal brain. Although AV accumulations are not specific to the degenerative phenomena of AD [3,93,143,189], the extensive neuritic dystrophy [111,152] and the characteristic gross distension of these neurites predominantly by AVs in AD are not typical features of other neurodegenerative diseases [8]. The same extensive autophagy pathology develops in the PS/AβPP transgenic mouse model of AD [186] and begins to appear at young ages before amyloid-β pathology indicating that macroautophagy induction is an early response in the disease and not solely a consequence of amyloid deposition. Indeed, accumulating AVs are a site of $A\beta$ generation [186].

5. The lysosomal system and β-amyloidogenesis

Our 1990 PNAS report coincided with emerging interest in the processing of AβPP to Aβ. Although Cat

D was only one of the many lysosomal enzymes identified in plaques, its prominence there and its abnormally high expression in neurons in AD prompted considerable attention to this protease as a possible AβPP secretase [7,62]. Remarkably, Cat D emerged from a long list of AβPP-cleaving proteases as one of a very few exhibiting both β-secretase activity toward AβPP model substrates [100,109,149,180], and γ-secretase activity which was enhanced by the Swedish FAD mutation [18,39,52,74,109]. Enthusiasm about Cat D in amyloidogenesis dampened, however, when Cat D deletion proved to have minimal effects on Aβ secretion [150] and several studies discounted lysosomes as a site of Aβ generation [75,78]. Following these early negative findings, a steady flow of evidence has implicated lysosomal system compartments upstream in the endocytic and autophagic pathways, including the ones that become morphologically abnormal early in AD. In AD, Aβ has been identified at three intraneuronal sites within the lysosomal system: rab5-positive endosomes [34]; autophagic vacuoles [187]; and multivesicular bodies [165] which could be related to either the endocytic or autophagic pathways. It is now believed that these cellular compartments may generate Aβ, not necessarily because of their cathepsins, but because they are also rich sources of β- and γ-AβPP secretases.

Aβ generation has been proposed to occur in the ER [40,72], medial Golgi saccules [168], trans Golgi network [174,181], autophagic vacuoles [187,188] and endosomes of the endocytic pathway [77,99,160]. Among these sites, only endosomes have been shown to be altered morphologically before amyloid begins to deposit in AD brain. Endosomes contain β-site AβPP cleaving enzyme (BACE) [85,178], presenilin [101], and AβPP [75,76,128]: also, βCTF, the γ-secretase cleaved carboxyl terminal domain of AβPP, is generated directly in endosomes [71,112,113]. Earlier studies demonstrated that Aβ production falls markedly when AβPP internalization is reduced by AβPP mutagenesis or blocking endocytosis [99,139,160] and rises substantially when endosome function specifically is modified [71,112]. Notably, Aβ generation increases substantially when either of the two early appearing features of endosome pathology in AD, rab5-driven endosome enlargement or MPR-driven increased cathepsin delivery to early endosomes, is reproduced in cells [71, 112]. Antibodies to the AβPP β-cleavage site, which target endosomal AβPP processing, significantly lower Aβ production and are being explored as potential therapeutic immunization strategies [4,134].

The macroautophagy branch of the lysosomal system has also been shown recently to be a pathway for Aβ peptide generation [186,188]. AVs isolated from several different tissue sources contain all of the components required for Aβ generation and are enriched in components of the γ-secretase complex and presenilin-dependent γ-secretase activity [138,186,188]. Immunoreactivity for these components is robust in AVs that accumulate grossly in dystrophic neurites within senile plaques in AD and the PS/AβPP mouse model of AD. Interestingly, autophagy-related "rimmed" vacuoles containing AβPP, Aβ, BACE and presenilin [5,6] also accumulate in inclusion body myositis, a condition in which amyloid-β is deposited outside the nervous system [6]. The localization of Aβ and Aβ-generating machinery in pathologically accumulating AVs is not coincidental. Aβ is generated during macroautophagy; inducing or inhibiting macroautophagy by modulating mTOR kinase elicits parallel changes in extent of AV proliferation and Aβ production [186]. Macroautophagy may play a relatively minor role in constitutive Aβ generation in the normal brain because, at the slow rates of macroautophagy, AVs do not build up and the Aβ generated in this system is usually degraded by the cathepsins in lysosomes [79,80]. In AD, however, the large accumulations of AVs in dystrophic neurites, reflecting delayed maturation of AVs to lysosomes, could contribute substantially to defective proteolysis and terminal degradation and amyloidogenesis.

6. The lysosomal system, neuron survival, and cell death

Our 1990 findings implied that, rather than being simply a scavenging mechanism to remove cellular debris, the lysosomal system mobilization and its impairment in AD, may actively promote disease pathogenesis not only by accelerating amyloidogenesis but also by triggering degeneration, as DeDuve predicted. Attention in the 1990s, however, was being directed mainly toward the rapidly emerging fields of caspases and apoptosis. The involvement of lysosomal mechanisms in neuronal cell death was slow to be appreciated despite the publication of a seminal paper by Peter Clarke [41], describing in brain development a form of programmed cell death, distinct from apoptosis and associated with intense autophagy and endocytosis, which he termed "autophagic cell death". Caspase-independent cell death associated with prominent autophagy has now been validated in various pathological settings [16,17,56,163] and the roles of autophagy and lysosomal proteases in cell death are currently being investigated intensively. Autophagy may influence cell survival in different ways depending on the setting. In most circumstances, macroautophagy seems to be a cytoprotective response: failure in this role leads to cell death by one of several mechanisms. Programmed cell death involving solely the over-activation of a normally functioning macroautophagy pathway, as described in the developing brain by Clarke, seems to be a less common pattern in the adult mammal; although, it has been unequivocally demonstrated in cells lacking the capability to undergo apoptosis [108,157].

In healthy cells, autophagy maintains survival when supplies of growth factors or nutrients are low by catabolizing intracellular substrates to replace energy stores. Autophagy directly protects against apoptosis by removing failing mitochondria and other factors that could trigger apoptosis [21,103,169]. Signals on mitochondria stimulate autophagy of these organelles [51,58] and may represent an important cell stress sensor. The importance of this role in neurons is suggested by the appearance of activated caspases in autophagy-derived vacuoles in AD brain [126]. The neuroprotective role of macroautophagy is increasingly viewed as particularly crucial in the aging nervous system. Cellular aging is associated with cumulative oxidative damage to proteins and membranes, translational errors leading to the synthesis of defective proteins, and various genetic and environmental insults to organelles and proteins [20,159,166]. The cell's survival in the face of mounting aging- and disease-related insults [162] is determined in significant part by how well this burden of damaged cellular constituents can be eliminated by the proteasome and lysosomal systems [10,68,73,104]. Indeed, stimulating macroautophagy in a mouse model of CAG-repeat disease has been shown to reduce inclusion development and improve neurological deficits [144,145].

In light of these protective roles, there has been growing suspicion that the declines in macroautophagy efficiency during aging [44,45], and impairments of this process in AD and possibly other neurodegenerative diseases, reduce neuronal survival in these conditions. This possibility is reinforced by evidence that PS is required for macroautophagy and that FAD – related mutations of PS exacerbate AD pathology, in part by impeding protein turnover by macroautophagy [186]. Fibroblasts from patients with PS-FAD, when stressed, accumulate AVs pathologically but display reduced macroautophagic turnover of proteins consistent with a block in the macroautophagy pathway. Moreover, macroautophagy is virtually completely eliminated in blastocysts lacking PS1 and PS2 genes [186], leading to decreased turnover of protein substrates and accumulation within AVs [61,179]. Failure of the important cytoprotective function of autophagy, therefore, provides an explanation for the observation that neurons with FAD mutations of PS are more susceptible to apoptosis.

Altered functioning of endosomes, as observed in AD, also has consequences for synaptic function and neuronal survival beyond influencing AβPP processing. Endosomes are particularly important in neurons in regulating synaptic transmission, levels of receptors at the cell surface, and retrograde signaling from trophic factors and other messengers. For example, defects in endosome function have been implicated in the failed retrograde NGF signaling and basal forebrain cholinergic neuron degeneration in Ts65Dn mice [42,50]. Moreover, proteins that serve roles in both endocytosis regulation and cell survival decisions link endosome dysfunction directly to cell death cascades. ALIX/AIP (ALG-2 interacting protein/x) regulates through one set of binding partners the properties of endosomes and endocytosis, and, separately modulates apoptosis mediated by either the type 1A – PI3 kinase pathway [38,69] or the calcium-binding protein ALG-2 (apoptosis linked gene) [117,175,176]. Underscoring this relationship between endocytic dysfunction and neuron survival are recent reports linking endosome dysfunction to pathogenesis in several inherited neurodegenerative disorders [66,95,140,171], including familial forms of ALS, primary lateral sclerosis, and hereditary spastic paraplegia in which the causative mutations are in genes directly involved in endocytic function [121,133,183].

Lysosomal system dysfunction has also generated growing interest as a basis for caspase-independent forms of cell death. A purely lysosome-initiated cell death may be achieved by the endocytosis of oxidizable substrates that selectively injure lysosomal membranes, cause leakage of Cat B or D, and induce apoptosis or a mixed apoptotic/necrotic pattern [19,24,63,82,94,131,147]. HSP70 promotes cell survival by inhibiting chemical and physical membrane destabilization [130]. Induction of apoptosis under these conditions may be upstream of p53 [60], cytochrome c release and caspase activation [59,94,146] or downstream from these events [137]. Endocytosed Aβ1-42, which accumulates in lysosomes of cultured neurons, may exert toxicity through this mechanism [184]. Aβ-activated microglia also release Cat B, which contributes to neurotoxicity [65]. Cathepsins also trigger apoptosis and are essential to the completion of this process in some cell systems [19,24,49,81,82,88,89,115,131,147].

7. Conclusion

Interest in the lysosomal system and its cathepsins as agents and mediators of pathology in disease states has risen exponentially in the past decade. Nowhere is this growing interest more apparent than in the investigation of neurodegenerative diseases. Early studies of the lysosomal system in AD identified a robust mobilization of this system in neurons (e.g., lysosome proliferation, increased acid hydrolase expression), even in the most mildly affected cell populations. Later investigations showed that stimulated lysosomal degradation may be a crucial pro-survival response to accumulating damaged and defective proteins in aged and diseased neurons. Mobilization of the lysosomal system in AD has now been traced to heightened activity and eventual dysfunction of its two main branches, the autophagic and endocytic pathways, which serve critical roles in the specialized functions and survival of neurons, in addition to protein turnover. The autophagic and endocytic pathways, which are also known to be sites of Aβ production, begin to fail at the earliest stages of AD. We are learning that many genetic and environmental risk factors for AD drive the dysfunction of these pathways, and thereby promote Aβ generation and, as importantly, impede the vital signaling and protein turnover functions of these two pathways. The failure of the lysosomal system on several different levels in AD not only increases the vulnerability of neurons to degeneration but may also trigger and mediate aspects of cell death.

Acknowledgements

We thank Heather Braunstein for her assistance in manuscript preparation and Corrinne Peterhoff for graphics. We gratefully acknowledge the National Institute on Aging for support of our studies from their inception to the present (currently AG017617) and the Alzheimer's Association for additional support.

References

[1] Gene overview of all published AD-association studies for cathepsin D [Web page], in: *Alzheimer's Research Forum*, M.A. Waltham, ed., Available at: http://www.alzforum.org/res/com/gen/alzgene/geneoverview.asp?geneid=66, Accessed 5/28/2005, 2005.

[2] Gene overview of all published AD-association studies for cystatin C [Web page], in: *Alzheimer's Research Forum*, M.A. Waltham, Available at: http://www.alzforum.org/res/com/gen/alzgene/geneoverview.asp?geneid=42, Accessed 5/28/2005, 2005.

[3] P. Anglade, S. Vyas, F. Javoy-Agid, M.T. Herrero, P.P. Michel, J. Marquez, A. Mouatt-Prigent, M. Ruberg, E.C. Hirsch and Y. Agid, Apoptosis and autophagy in nigral neurons of patients with Parkinson's disease, *Histol Histopathol* **12**(1) (1997), 25–31.

[4] M. Arbel, I. Yacoby and B. Solomon, Inhibition of amyloid precursor protein processing by {beta}-secretase through site-directed antibodies, *Proc Natl Acad Sci USA* (2005).

[5] V. Askanas and W.K. Engel, Does overexpression of betaAPP in aging muscle have a pathogenic role and a relevance to Alzheimer's disease? Clues from inclusion body myositis, cultured human muscle, and transgenic mice, *Am J Pathol* **153**(6) (1998), 1673–1677.

[6] V. Askanas, W.K. Engel, C.C. Yang, R.B. Alvarez, V.M. Lee and T. Wisniewski, Light and electron microscopic immunolocalization of presenilin 1 in abnormal muscle fibers of patients with sporadic inclusion-body myositis and autosomal-recessive inclusion-body myopathy, *Am J Pathol* **152**(4) (1998), 889–895.

[7] B.M. Austen and D.J. Stephens, Cleavage of a beta-amyloid precursor sequence by cathepsin D, *Biomed Pept Proteins Nucleic Acids* **1**(4) (1995), 243–246.

[8] W.C. Benzing, E.J. Mufson and D.M. Armstrong, Alzheimer's disease-like dystrophic neurites characteristically associated with senile plaques are not found within other neurodegenerative diseases unless amyloid beta-protein deposition is present, *Brain Res* **606**(1) (1993), 10–18.

[9] T.O. Berg, M. Fengsrud, P.E. Stromhaug, T. Berg and P.O. Seglen, Isolation and characterization of rat liver amphisomes. Evidence for fusion of autophagosomes with both early and late endosomes, *J Biol Chem* **273**(34) (1998), 21883–21892.

[10] S.J. Berke and H.L. Paulson, Protein aggregation and the ubiquitin proteasome pathway: gaining the upper hand on neurodegeneration, *Curr Opin Genet Dev* **13**(3) (2003), 253–261.

[11] H.G. Bernstein, S. Bruszis, D. Schmidt, B. Wieders and A. Dorn, Immunodetection of cathepsin D in neuritic plaques found in brains of patients with dementia of Alzheimer type, *J Hirnforsch* **30**(5) (1989), 613–618.

[12] H.G. Bernstein, H. Kirschke, B. Wieders, K.H. Pollak, A. Zipress and A. Rinne, The possible place of cathepsins and cystatins in the puzzle of Alzheimer disease: a review, *Mol Chem Neuropathol* **27**(3) (1996), 225–247.

[13] L. Bertram, S. Guenette, J. Jones, D. Keeney, K. Mullin, A. Crystal, S. Basu, S. Yhu, A. Deng, G.W. Rebeck, B.T. Hyman, R. Go, M. McInnis, D. Blacker and R. Tanzi, No evidence for genetic association or linkage of the cathepsin D (CTSD) exon 2 polymorphism and Alzheimer disease, *Ann Neurol* **49**(1) (2001), 114–116.

[14] T.J. Bhojak, S.T. DeKosky, M. Ganguli and M.I. Kamboh, Genetic polymorphisms in the cathepsin D and interleukin-

[15] N.E. Bishop, Dynamics of endosomal sorting, *Int Rev Cytol* **232** (2003), 1–57.

[16] T. Borsello, K. Croquelois, J.P. Hornung and P.G. Clarke, N-methyl-d-aspartate-triggered neuronal death in organotypic hippocampal cultures is endocytic, autophagic and mediated by the c-Jun N-terminal kinase pathway, *Eur J Neurosci* **18**(3) (2003), 473–485.

[17] L.E. Broker, F.A. Kruyt and G. Giaccone, Cell death independent of caspases: a review, *Clin Cancer Res* **11**(9) (2005), 3155–3162.

[18] A.M. Brown, D.M. Tummolo, M.A. Spruyt, J.S. Jacobsen and J. Sonnenberg-Reines, Evaluation of cathepsins D and G and EC 3.4.24.15 as candidate beta-secretase proteases using peptide and amyloid precursor protein substrates, *J Neurochem* **66**(6) (1996), 2436–2445.

[19] U.T. Brunk, H. Dalen, K. Roberg and H.B. Hellquist, Photo-oxidative disruption of lysosomal membranes causes apoptosis of cultured human fibroblasts, *Free Radic Biol Med* **23**(4) (1997), 616–626.

[20] U.T. Brunk, C.B. Jones and R.S. Sohal, A novel hypothesis of lipofuscinogenesis and cellular aging based on interactions between oxidative stress and autophagocytosis, *Mutat Res* **275**(3–6) (1992), 395–403.

[21] U.T. Brunk and A. Terman, The mitochondrial-lysosomal axis theory of aging: accumulation of damaged mitochondria as a result of imperfect autophagocytosis, *Eur J Biochem* **269**(8) (2002), 1996–2002.

[22] L.M. Callahan, N. Chow, J.E. Cheetham, C. Cox and P.D. Coleman, Analysis of message expression in single neurons of Alzheimer's disease brain, *Neurobiol Aging* **19**(1 Suppl) (1998), S99–S105.

[23] L.M. Callahan, W.A. Vaules and P.D. Coleman, Quantitative decrease in synaptophysin message expression and increase in cathepsin D message expression in Alzheimer disease neurons containing neurofibrillary tangles, *J Neuropathol Exp Neurol* **58**(3) (1999), 275–287.

[24] N. Canu, R. Tufi, A.L. Serafino, G. Amadoro, M.T. Ciotti and P. Calissano, Role of the autophagic-lysosomal system on low potassium-induced apoptosis in cultured cerebellar granule cells, *J Neurochem* **92**(5) (2005), 1228–1242.

[25] A. Cataldo and R. Nixon, A relationship between extracellular localization of lysosomal proteinases and amyloid deposition in Alzheimer's disease, *Soc Neurosci Abstr* **1378** (1989).

[26] A.M. Cataldo, J.L. Barnett, S.A. Berman, J. Li, S. Quarless, S. Bursztajn, C. Lippa and R.A. Nixon, Gene expression and cellular content of cathepsin D in Alzheimer's disease brain: evidence for early up-regulation of the endosomal-lysosomal system, *Neuron* **14**(3) (1995), 671–680.

[27] A.M. Cataldo, J.L. Barnett, D.M. Mann and R.A. Nixon, Colocalization of lysosomal hydrolase and beta-amyloid in diffuse plaques of the cerebellum and striatum in Alzheimer's disease and Down's syndrome, *J Neuropathol Exp Neurol* **55**(6) (1996), 704–715.

[28] A.M. Cataldo, J.L. Barnett, C. Pieroni and R.A. Nixon, Increased neuronal endocytosis and protease delivery to early endosomes in sporadic Alzheimer's disease: neuropathologic evidence for a mechanism of increased beta-amyloidogenesis, *J Neurosci* **17**(16) (1997), 6142–6151.

[29] A.M. Cataldo, D.J. Hamilton and R.A. Nixon, Lysosomal abnormalities in degenerating neurons link neuronal compromise to senile plaque development in Alzheimer disease, *Brain Res* **640**(1–2) (1994), 68–80.

[30] A.M. Cataldo and R.A. Nixon, Enzymatically active lysosomal proteases are associated with amyloid deposits in Alzheimer brain, *Proc Natl Acad Sci USA* **87**(10) (1990), 3861–3865.

[31] A.M. Cataldo, P.A. Paskevich, E. Kominami and R.A. Nixon, Lysosomal hydrolases of different classes are abnormally distributed in brains of patients with Alzheimer disease, *Proc Natl Acad Sci USA* **88**(24) (1991), 10998–11002.

[32] A.M. Cataldo, S. Petanceska, C.M. Peterhoff, N.B. Terio, C.J. Epstein, A. Villar, E.J. Carlson, M. Staufenbiel and R.A. Nixon, App gene dosage modulates endosomal abnormalities of Alzheimer's disease in a segmental trisomy 16 mouse model of Down syndrome, *J Neurosci* **23**(17) (2003), 6788–6792.

[33] A.M. Cataldo, S. Petanceska, N.B. Terio, C.M. Peterhoff, R. Durham, M. Mercken, P.D. Mehta, J. Buxbaum, V. Haroutunian and R.A. Nixon, Abeta localization in abnormal endosomes: association with earliest Abeta elevations in AD and Down syndrome, *Neurobiol Aging* **25**(10) (2004), 1263–1272.

[34] A.M. Cataldo, S. Petanceska, N.B. Terio, C.M. Peterhoff, J.C. Troncoso, R. Durham, M. Mercken, P.D. Mehta, J.D. Buxbaum, V. Haroutunian and R.A. Nixon, A-beta localization to abnormal endosomes coincides with early increases in soluble Abeta in Alzheimer's disease brain, *Neurobiol Aging* (2004).

[35] A.M. Cataldo, C.M. Peterhoff, S.D. Schmidt, N.B. Terio, K. Duff, M. Beard, P.M. Mathews and R.A. Nixon, Presenilin mutations in familial Alzheimer's disease and transgenic mouse models accelerate neuronal lysosomal pathology, *J Neuropath Exp Neurol* (2004).

[36] A.M. Cataldo, C.M. Peterhoff, J.C. Troncoso, T. Gomez-Isla, B.T. Hyman and R.A. Nixon, Endocytic pathway abnormalities precede amyloid beta deposition in sporadic Alzheimer's disease and Down syndrome: differential effects of APOE genotype and presenilin mutations, *Am J Pathol* **157**(1) (2000), 277–286.

[37] A.M. Cataldo, C.Y. Thayer, E.D. Bird, T.R. Wheelock and R.A. Nixon, Lysosomal proteinase antigens are prominently localized within senile plaques of Alzheimer's disease: evidence for a neuronal origin, *Brain Res* **513**(2) (1990), 181–192.

[38] B. Chen, S.C. Borinstein, J. Gillis, V.W. Sykes and O. Bogler, The glioma-associated protein SETA interacts with AIP1/Alix and ALG-2 and modulates apoptosis in astrocytes, *J Biol Chem* **275**(25) (2000), 19275–19281.

[39] N. Chevallier, J. Vizzavona, P. Marambaud, C.P. Baur, M. Spillantini, P. Fulcrand, J. Martinez, M. Goedert, J.P. Vincent and F. Checler, Cathepsin D displays in vitro beta-secretase-like specificity, *Brain Res* **750**(1–2) (1997), 11–19.

[40] A.S.C. Chyung, B.D. Greenberg, D.G. Cook, R.W. Doms and V.M. Lee, Novel beta-secretase cleavage of beta-amyloid precursor protein in the endoplasmic reticulum/intermediate compartment of NT2N cells, *J Cell Biol* **138**(3) (1997), 671–680.

[41] P.G. Clarke, Developmental cell death: morphological diversity and multiple mechanisms, *Anat Embryol* **181**(3) (1990), 195–213.

[42] J.D. Cooper, A. Salehi, J.D. Delcroix, C.L. Howe, P.V. Belichenko, J. Chua-Couzens, J.F. Kilbridge, E.J. Carlson, C.J. Epstein and W.C. Mobley, Failed retrograde transport of NGF in a mouse model of Down's syndrome: reversal of choliner-

[43] F.C. Crawford, M.J. Freeman, J. Schinka, L.I. Abdullah, D. Richards, S. Sevush, R. Duara and M.J. Mullan, The genetic association between Cathepsin D and Alzheimer's disease, *Neurosci Lett* **289**(1) (2000), 61–65.

gic neurodegenerative phenotypes following NGF infusion, *Proc Natl Acad Sci USA* **98**(18) (2001), 10439–10444.

[44] A.M. Cuervo and J.F. Dice, Age-related decline in chaperone-mediated autophagy, *J Biol Chem* **275**(40) (2000), 31505–31513.

[45] A.M. Cuervo and J.F. Dice, When lysosomes get old, *Exp Gerontol* **35**(2) (2000), 119–131.

[46] A.M. Cuervo, L. Stefanis, R. Fredenburg, P.T. Lansbury and D. Sulzer, Impaired degradation of mutant alpha-synuclein by chaperone-mediated autophagy, *Science* **305**(5688) (2004), 1292–1295.

[47] C. De Duve, *Subcellular Particles*, New York, The Ronald Press, 1959, 128–159.

[48] C. De Duve, B.C. Pressman, R. Gianetto, R. Wattiaux and F. Appelmans, Tissue fractionation studies. 6. Intracellular distribution patterns of enzymes in rat-liver tissue, *Biochem J* **60**(4) (1955), 604–617.

[49] L.P. Deiss, H. Galinka, H. Berissi, O. Cohen and A. Kimchi, Cathepsin D protease mediates programmed cell death induced by interferon-gamma, Fas/APO-1 and TNF-alpha, *Embo J* **15**(15) (1996), 3861–3870.

[50] J.D. Delcroix, J. Valletta, C. Wu, C.L. Howe, C.F. Lai, J.D. Cooper, P.V. Belichenko, A. Salehi and W.C. Mobley, Trafficking the NGF signal: implications for normal and degenerating neurons, *Prog Brain Res* **146** (2004), 3–23.

[51] B.N. Desai, B.R. Myers and S.L. Schreiber, FKBP12-rapamycin-associated protein associates with mitochondria and senses osmotic stress via mitochondrial dysfunction, *Proc Natl Acad Sci USA* **99**(7) (2002), 4319–4324.

[52] R.N. Dreyer, K.M. Bausch, P. Fracasso, L.J. Hammond, D. Wunderlich, D.O. Wirak, G. Davis, C.M. Brini, T.M. Buckholz, G. Konig et al., Processing of the pre-beta-amyloid protein by cathepsin D is enhanced by a familial Alzheimer's disease mutation, *Eur J Biochem* **224**(2) (1994), 265–271.

[53] W.A. Dunn, Jr., Studies on the mechanisms of autophagy: formation of the autophagic vacuole, *J Cell Biol* **110**(6) (1990), 1923–1933.

[54] W.A. Dunn, Jr., Studies on the mechanisms of autophagy: maturation of the autophagic vacuole, *J Cell Biol* **110**(6) (1990), 1935–1945.

[55] W.A. Dunn, Jr., Autophagy and related mechanisms of lysosome-mediated protein degradation, *Trends Cell Biol* **4**(4) (1994), 139–143.

[56] A.L. Edinger and C.B. Thompson, Death by design: apoptosis, necrosis and autophagy, *Curr Opin Cell Biol* **16**(6) (2004), 663–669.

[57] I. Elarova, S. Che, M.D. Ruben, R.A. Nixon and S.D. Ginsberg, Expression profiling of hippocampal neurons in a mouse model of Down's syndrome (Ts65Dn), *Proc Soc Neurosci* **30** (2004), 335.

[58] S.P. Elmore, T. Qian, S.F. Grissom and J.J. Lemasters, The mitochondrial permeability transition initiates autophagy in rat hepatocytes, *Faseb J* **15**(12) (2001), 2286–2287.

[59] L. Emert-Sedlak, S. Shangary, A. Rabinovitz, M.B. Miranda, S.M. Delach and D.E. Johnson, Involvement of cathepsin D in chemotherapy-induced cytochrome c release, caspase activation, and cell death, *Mol Cancer Ther* **4**(5) (2005), 733–742.

[60] H. Erdal, M. Berndtsson, J. Castro, U. Brunk, M.C. Shoshan and S. Linder, Induction of lysosomal membrane permeabilization by compounds that activate p53-independent apoptosis, *Proc Natl Acad Sci USA* **102**(1) (2005), 192–197.

[61] C. Esselens, V. Oorschot, V. Baert, T. Raemaekers, K. Spittaels, L. Serneels, H. Zheng, P. Saftig, B. De Strooper, J. Klumperman and W. Annaert, Presenilin 1 mediates the turnover of telencephalin in hippocampal neurons via an autophagic degradative pathway, *J Cell Biol* **166**(7) (2004), 1041–1054.

[62] G. Evin, R. Cappai, Q.X. Li, J.G. Culvenor, D.H. Small, K. Beyreuther and C.L. Masters, Candidate gamma-secretases in the generation of the carboxyl terminus of the Alzheimer's disease beta A4 amyloid: possible involvement of cathepsin D, *Biochemistry* **34**(43) (1995), 14185–14192.

[63] E.T. Fossel, C.L. Zanella, J.G. Fletcher and K.K. Hui, Cell death induced by peroxidized low-density lipoprotein: endopepsis, *Cancer Res* **54**(5) (1994), 1240–1248.

[64] Z. Galdzicki and R.J. Siarey, Understanding mental retardation in Down's syndrome using trisomy 16 mouse models, *Genes Brain Behav* **2**(3) (2003), 167–178.

[65] L. Gan, S. Ye, A. Chu, K. Anton, S. Yi, V.A. Vincent, D. von Schack, D. Chin, J. Murray, S. Lohr, L. Patthy, M. Gonzalez-Zulueta, K. Nikolich and R. Urfer, Identification of cathepsin B as a mediator of neuronal death induced by Abeta-activated microglial cells using a functional genomics approach, *J Biol Chem* **279**(7) (2004), 5565–5572.

[66] F.G. Gervais, R. Singaraja, S. Xanthoudakis, C.A. Gutekunst, B.R. Leavitt, M. Metzler, A.S. Hackam, J. Tam, J.P. Vaillancourt, V. Houtzager, D.M. Rasper, S. Roy, M.R. Hayden and D.W. Nicholson, Recruitment and activation of caspase-8 by the Huntingtin-interacting protein Hip-1 and a novel partner Hippi, *Nat Cell Biol* **4**(2) (2002), 95–105.

[67] S.D. Ginsberg, S.E. Hemby, V.M. Lee, J.H. Eberwine and J.Q. Trojanowski, Expression profile of transcripts in Alzheimer's disease tangle-bearing CA1 neurons, *Ann Neurol* **48**(1) (2000), 77–87.

[68] A.L. Goldberg, Protein degradation and protection against misfolded or damaged proteins, *Nature* **426**(6968) (2003), 895–899.

[69] I. Gout, G. Middleton, J. Adu, N.N. Ninkina, L.B. Drobot, V. Filonenko, G. Matsuka, A.M. Davies, M. Waterfield and V.L. Buchman, Negative regulation of PI 3-kinase by Ruk, a novel adaptor protein, *Embo J* **19**(15) (2000), 4015–4025.

[70] D.I. Graham and P.L. Lantos, *Greenfield's Neuropathology*, New York, Arnold, 2002.

[71] O.M. Grbovic, P.M. Mathews, Y. Jiang, S.D. Schmidt, R. Dinakar, N.B. Summers-Terio, B.P. Ceresa, R.A. Nixon and A.M. Cataldo, Rab5-stimulated up-regulation of the endocytic pathway increases intracellular beta-cleaved amyloid precursor protein carboxyl-terminal fragment levels and Abeta production, *J Biol Chem* **278**(33) (2003), 31261–31268.

[72] J.P. Greenfield, J. Tsai, G.K. Gouras, B. Hai, G. Thinakaran, F. Checler, S.S. Sisodia, P. Greengard and H. Xu, Endoplasmic reticulum and trans-Golgi network generate distinct populations of Alzheimer beta-amyloid peptides, *Proc Natl Acad Sci USA* **96**(2) (1999), 742–747.

[73] T. Grune, R. Shringarpure, N. Sitte and K. Davies, Age-related changes in protein oxidation and proteolysis in mammalian cells, *J Gerontol A Biol Sci Med Sci* **56**(11) (2001), B459–B467.

[74] F. Gruninger-Leitch, P. Berndt, H. Langen, P. Nelboeck and H. Dobeli, Identification of beta-secretase-like activity using a mass spectrometry-based assay system, *Nat Biotechnol* **18**(1) (2000), 66–70.

[75] C. Haass, A.Y. Hung, M.G. Schlossmacher, D.B. Teplow and D.J. Selkoe, beta-amyloid peptide and a 3-kDa fragment are derived by distinct cellular mechanisms, *J Biol Chem* **268**(5) (1993), 3021–3024.

[76] C. Haass, E.H. Koo, A. Mellon, A.Y. Hung and D.J. Selkoe, Targeting of cell-surface beta-amyloid precursor protein to lysosomes: alternative processing into amyloid-bearing fragments, *Nature* **357**(6378) (1992), 500–503.

[77] C. Haass, M.G. Schlossmacher, A.Y. Hung, C. Vigo-Pelfrey, A. Mellon, B.L. Ostaszewski, I. Lieberburg, E.H. Koo, D. Schenk, D.B. Teplow et al., Amyloid beta-peptide is produced by cultured cells during normal metabolism [see comments], *Nature* **359**(6393) (1992), 322–325.

[78] C. Haass and D.J. Selkoe, Cellular processing of beta-amyloid precursor protein and the genesis of amyloid beta-peptide, *Cell* **75**(6) (1993), 1039–1042.

[79] H. Hamazaki, A beta-amyloid peptide variant related with familial Alzheimer's disease and hereditary cerebral hemorrhage with amyloidosis is poorly eliminated by cathepsin D, *FEBS Lett* **397**(2–3) (1996), 313–315.

[80] H. Hamazaki, Cathepsin D is involved in the clearance of Alzheimer's beta-amyloid protein, *FEBS Lett* **396**(2–3) (1996), 139–142.

[81] M. Heinrich, M. Wickel, W. Schneider-Brachert, C. Sandberg, J. Gahr, R. Schwandner, T. Weber, P. Saftig, C. Peters, J. Brunner, M. Kronke and S. Schutze, Cathepsin D targeted by acid sphingomyelinase-derived ceramide [published erratum appears in EMBO J 2000 Jan 17;19(2):315], *Embo J* **18**(19) (1999), 5252–5263.

[82] H.B. Hellquist, I. Svensson and U.T. Brunk, Oxidant-induced apoptosis: a consequence of lethal lysosomal leak? *Redox Report* **3**(1) (1997), 65–70.

[83] D.M. Holtzman, D. Santucci, J. Kilbridge, J. Chua-Couzens, D.J. Fontana, S.E. Daniels, R.M. Johnson, K. Chen, Y. Sun, E. Carlson, E. Alleva, C.J. Epstein and W.C. Mobley, Developmental abnormalities and age-related neurodegeneration in a mouse model of Down syndrome, *Proc Natl Acad Sci USA* **93**(23) (1996), 13333–13338.

[84] E. Holtzman, *Lysosomes*, New York, Plenum Press, 1989.

[85] J.T. Huse, D.S. Pijak, G.J. Leslie, V.M. Lee and R.W. Doms, Maturation and endosomal targeting of beta-site amyloid precursor protein-cleaving enzyme. The Alzheimer's disease beta-secretase, *J Biol Chem* **275**(43) (2000), 33729–33737.

[86] K. Ii, H. Ito, E. Kominami and A. Hirano, Abnormal distribution of cathepsin proteinases and endogenous inhibitors (cystatins) in the hippocampus of patients with Alzheimer's disease, parkinsonism-dementia complex on Guam, and senile dementia and in the aged, *Virchows Arch A Pathol Anat Histopathol* **423**(3) (1993), 185–194.

[87] K. Ikegami, T. Kimura, S. Katsuragi, T. Ono, H. Yamamoto, E. Miyamoto and T. Miyakawa, Immunohistochemical examination of phosphorylated tau in granulovacuolar degeneration granules, *Psychiatry Clin Neurosci* **50**(3) (1996), 137–140.

[88] K. Isahara, Y. Ohsawa, S. Kanamori, M. Shibata, S. Waguri, N. Sato, T. Gotow, T. Watanabe, T. Momoi, K. Urase, E. Kominami and Y. Uchiyama, Regulation of a novel pathway for cell death by lysosomal aspartic and cysteine proteinases, *Neuroscience* **91**(1) (1999), 233–249.

[89] R. Ishisaka, T. Utsumi, T. Kanno, K. Arita, N. Katunuma, J. Akiyama and K. Utsumi, Participation of a cathepsin L-type protease in the activation of caspase-3, *Cell Struct Funct* **24**(6) (1999), 465–470.

[90] Z.S. Ji, R.D. Miranda, Y.M. Newhouse, K.H. Weisgraber, Y. Huang and R.W. Mahley, Apolipoprotein E4 potentiates amyloid beta peptide-induced lysosomal leakage and apoptosis in neuronal cells, *J Biol Chem* **277**(24) (2002), 21821–21828.

[91] L.W. Jin, I. Maezawa, I. Vincent and T. Bird, Intracellular accumulation of amyloidogenic fragments of amyloid-beta precursor protein in neurons with Niemann-Pick type C defects is associated with endosomal abnormalities, *Am J Pathol* **164**(3) (2004), 975–985.

[92] T. Kawarabayashi, Y. Igeta, M. Sato, A. Sasaki, E. Matsubara, M. Kanai, Y. Tomidokoro, K. Ishiguro, K. Okamoto, S. Hirai and M. Shoji, Lysosomal generation of amyloid beta protein species in transgenic mice, *Brain Res* **765**(2) (1997), 343–348.

[93] K.B. Kegel, M. Kim, E. Sapp, C. McIntyre, J.G. Castano, N. Aronin and M. DiFiglia, Huntingtin expression stimulates endosomal-lysosomal activity, endosome tubulation, and autophagy, *J Neurosci* **20**(19) (2000), 7268–7278.

[94] D. Kessel, Y. Luo, P. Mathieu and J.J. Reiners, Jr., Determinants of the apoptotic response to lysosomal photodamage, *Photochem Photobiol* **71**(2) (2000), 196–200.

[95] B.N. Kholodenko, MAP kinase cascade signaling and endocytic trafficking: a marriage of convenience? *Trends Cell Biol* **12**(4) (2002), 173–177.

[96] D.J. Klionsky, The molecular machinery of autophagy: unanswered questions, *J Cell Sci* **118**(Pt 1) (2005), 7–18.

[97] C.S. Koenig, Redistribution of gastric K+-NPPase in vertebrate oxyntic cells in relation to hydrochloric acid secretion: a cytochemical study, *Anat Rec* **210**(4) (1984), 583–596.

[98] M. Koike, H. Nakanishi, P. Saftig, J. Ezaki, K. Isahara, Y. Ohsawa, W. Schulz-Schaeffer, T. Watanabe, S. Waguri, S. Kametaka, M. Shibata, K. Yamamoto, E. Kominami, C. Peters, K. von Figura and Y. Uchiyama, Cathepsin D deficiency induces lysosomal storage with ceroid lipofuscin in mouse CNS neurons, *J Neurosci* **20**(18) (2000), 6898–6906.

[99] E.H. Koo and S.L. Squazzo, Evidence that production and release of amyloid beta-protein involves the endocytic pathway, *J Biol Chem* **269**(26) (1994), 17386–17389.

[100] U.S. Ladror, S.W. Snyder, G.T. Wang, T.F. Holzman and G.A. Krafft, Cleavage at the amino and carboxyl termini of Alzheimer's amyloid-beta by cathepsin D, *J Biol Chem* **269**(28) (1994), 18422–18428.

[101] J.J. Lah and A.I. Levey, Endogenous presenilin-1 targets to endocytic rather than biosynthetic compartments, *Mol Cell Neurosci* **16**(2) (2000), 111–126.

[102] D. Langui, N. Girardot, K.H. El Hachimi, B. Allinquant, V. Blanchard, L. Pradier and C. Duyckaerts, Subcellular topography of neuronal Abeta peptide in APPxPS1 transgenic mice, *Am J Pathol* **165**(5) (2004), 1465–1477.

[103] K.E. Larsen and D. Sulzer, Autophagy in neurons: a review, *Histol Histopathol* **17**(3) (2002), 897–908.

[104] B. Levine and D.J. Klionsky, Development by self-digestion: molecular mechanisms and biological functions of autophagy, *Dev Cell* **6**(4) (2004), 463–477.

[105] E. Levy-Lahad, W. Wasco, P. Poorkaj, D.M. Romano, J. Oshima, W.H. Pettingell, C.E. Yu, P.D. Jondro, S.D. Schmidt, K. Wang et al., Candidate gene for the chromosome 1 familial Alzheimer's disease locus [see comments], *Science* **269**(5226) (1995), 973–977.

[106] L. Liao, D. Cheng, J. Wang, D.M. Duong, T.G. Losik, M. Gearing, H.D. Rees, J.J. Lah, A.I. Levey and J. Peng, Proteomic characterization of postmortem amyloid plaques iso-

[107] F. Lim, F. Hernandez, J.J. Lucas, P. Gomez-Ramos, M.A. Moran and J. Avila, FTDP-17 mutations in tau transgenic mice provoke lysosomal abnormalities and tau filaments in forebrain, *Mol Cell Neurosci* **18**(6) (2001), 702–714.

[108] G.P. Lim, F. Calon, T. Morihara, F. Yang, B. Teter, O. Ubeda, N. Salem, Jr., S.A. Frautschy and G.M. Cole, A diet enriched with the omega-3 fatty acid docosahexaenoic acid reduces amyloid burden in an aged Alzheimer mouse model, *J Neurosci* **25**(12) (2005), 3032–3040.

[109] E.A. Mackay, A. Ehrhard, M. Moniatte, C. Guenet, C. Tardif, C. Tarnus, O. Sorokine, B. Heintzelmann, C. Nay, J.M. Remy, J. Higaki, A. Van Dorsselaer, J. Wagner, C. Danzin and P. Mamont, A possible role for cathepsins D, E, and B in the processing of beta- amyloid precursor protein in Alzheimer's disease, *Eur J Biochem* **244**(2) (1997), 414–425.

[110] M. Margallo-Lana, C.M. Morris, A.M. Gibson, A.L. Tan, D.W. Kay, S.P. Tyrer, B.P. Moore and C.G. Ballard, Influence of the amyloid precursor protein locus on dementia in Down syndrome, *Neurology* **62**(11) (2004), 1996–1998.

[111] E. Masliah, M. Mallory, T. Deerinck, R. DeTeresa, S. Lamont, A. Miller, R.D. Terry, B. Carragher and M. Ellisman, Re-evaluation of the structural organization of the neuritic plaques in Alzheimer's disease, *J Neuropathology and Experimental Neurology* **52**(6) (1993), 619–632.

[112] P.M. Mathews, C.B. Guerra, Y. Jiang, O.M. Grbovic, B.H. Kao, S.D. Schmidt, R. Dinakar, M. Mercken, A. Hille-Rehfeld, J. Rohrer, P. Mehta, A.M. Cataldo and R.A. Nixon, Alzheimer's disease-related overexpression of the cation-dependent mannose 6-phosphate receptor increases Abeta secretion: role for altered lysosomal hydrolase distribution in beta-amyloidogenesis, *J Biol Chem* **277**(7) (2002), 5299–5307.

[113] P.M. Mathews, Y. Jiang, S.D. Schmidt, O.M. Grbovic, M. Mercken and R.A. Nixon, Calpain activity regulates the cell surface distribution of amyloid precursor protein. Inhibition of calpains enhances endosomal generation of beta-cleaved C-terminal APP fragments, *J Biol Chem* **277**(39) (2002), 36415–36424.

[114] S.P. McIlroy, K.B. Dynan, B.M. McGleenon, J.T. Lawson and A.P. Passmore, Cathepsin D gene exon 2 polymorphism and sporadic Alzheimer's disease, *Neurosci Lett* **273**(2) (1999), 140–141.

[115] B.L. McVicker and C.A. Casey, Ethanol-impaired hepatic protein trafficking: concepts from the asialoglycoprotein receptor system, *Clin Biochem* **32**(7) (1999), 557–561.

[116] G. Menzer, T. Muller-Thomsen, W. Meins, A. Alberici, G. Binetti, C. Hock, R.M. Nitsch, G. Stoppe, J. Reiss and U. Finckh, Non-replication of association between cathepsin D genotype and late onset Alzheimer disease, *Am J Med Genet* **105**(2) (2001), 179–182.

[117] M. Missotten, A. Nichols, K. Rieger and R. Sadoul, Alix, a novel mouse protein undergoing calcium-dependent interaction with the apoptosis-linked-gene 2 (ALG-2) protein, *Cell Death Differ* **6**(2) (1999), 124–129.

[118] N. Mizushima, Y. Ohsumi and T. Yoshimori, Autophagosome formation in mammalian cells, *Cell Structure and Function* **27** (2002), 421–429.

[119] D. Moechars, K. Lorent and F. Van Leuven, Premature death in transgenic mice that overexpress a mutant amyloid precursor protein is preceded by severe neurodegeneration and apoptosis, *Neuroscience* **91**(3) (1999), 819–830.

[120] L. Myllykangas, J. Tyynela, A. Page-McCaw, G.M. Rubin, M.J. Haltia and M.B. Feany, Cathepsin D-deficient Drosophila recapitulate the key features of neuronal ceroid lipofuscinoses, *Neurobiol Dis* **19**(1–2) (2005), 194–199.

[121] I. Nagano, T. Murakami, M. Shiote, Y. Manabe, S. Hadano, Y. Yanagisawa, J.E. Ikeda and K. Abe, Single-nucleotide polymorphisms in uncoding regions of ALS2 gene of Japanese patients with autosomal-recessive amyotrophic lateral sclerosis, *Neurol Res* **25**(5) (2003), 505–509.

[122] Y. Nakamura, M. Takeda, H. Suzuki, H. Hattori, K. Tada, S. Hariguchi, S. Hashimoto and T. Nishimura, Abnormal distribution of cathepsins in the brain of patients with Alzheimer's disease, *Neurosci Lett* **130**(2) (1991), 195–198.

[123] R.A. Nixon, Niemann-Pick Type C disease and Alzheimer's disease: the APP-endosome connection fattens up, *Am J Pathol* **164**(3) (2004), 757–761.

[124] R.A. Nixon, Endosome function and dysfunction in Alzheimer's disease and other neurodegenerative diseases, *Neurobiol Aging* (2005), in press.

[125] R.A. Nixon and Banner, *Proteases and Protease Inhibitors in Alzheimer's Disease Pathogenesis*, Proceedings of a conference. Bethesda, Maryland, December 16–18, 1991, 1992.

[126] R.A. Nixon, J. Wegiel, A. Kumar, W.H. Yu, C. Peterhoff, A. Cataldo and A.M. Cuervo, Extensive involvement of autophagy in Alzheimer disease: an immuno-electron microscopy study, *J Neuropathol Exp Neurol* **64**(2) (2005), 113–122.

[127] R.A. Nixon, W.H. Yu, A.M. Cuervo, A. Kumar, D.S. Yang and C.M. Peterhoff, Autophagy in Alzheimer's Disease: Failure of a Neuroprotective Mechanism, in: *Alzheimer's Disease and Related Disorders: Research Advances*, I. Khalid and B. Winblad, eds, Bucharest, *"Ana Aslan" International Academy of Aging* **10** (2005), in press.

[128] C. Nordstedt, G.L. Caporaso, J. Thyberg, S.E. Gandy and P. Greengard, Identification of the Alzheimer beta/A4 amyloid precursor protein in clathrin-coated vesicles purified from PC12 cells, *J Biol Chem* **268**(1) (1993), 608–612.

[129] A. Novikoff, *Lysosomes in nerve cells*, The Neuron. NY, Elsevier Publishing Co.,: 319ff, 1967.

[130] J. Nylandsted, M. Gyrd-Hansen, A. Danielewicz, N. Fehrenbacher, U. Lademann, M. Hoyer-Hansen, E. Weber, G. Multhoff, M. Rohde and M. Jaattela, Heat shock protein 70 promotes cell survival by inhibiting lysosomal membrane permeabilization, *J Exp Med* **200**(4) (2004), 425–435.

[131] K. Ollinger, Inhibition of cathepsin D prevents free-radical-induced apoptosis in rat cardiomyocytes, *Arch Biochem Biophys* **373**(2) (2000), 346–351.

[132] T. Olsson, J. Nygren, K. Hakansson, C. Lundblad, A. Grubb, M.L. Smith and T. Wieloch, Gene deletion of cystatin C aggravates brain damage following focal ischemia but mitigates the neuronal injury after global ischemia in the mouse, *Neuroscience* **128**(1) (2004), 65–71.

[133] A. Otomo, S. Hadano, T. Okada, H. Mizumura, R. Kunita, H. Nishijima, J. Showguchi-Miyata, Y. Yanagisawa, E. Kohiki, E. Suga, M. Yasuda, H. Osuga, T. Nishimoto, S. Narumiya and J.E. Ikeda, ALS2, a novel guanine nucleotide exchange factor for the small GTPase Rab5, is implicated in endosomal dynamics, *Hum Mol Genet* **12**(14) (2003), 1671–1687.

[134] P. Paganetti, V. Calanca, C. Galli, M. Stefani and M. Molinari, beta-site specific intrabodies to decrease and prevent generation of Alzheimer's Abeta peptide, *J Cell Biol* **168**(6) (2005), 863–868.

[135] A. Papassotiropoulos, M. Bagli, O. Feder, F. Jessen, W. Maier, M.L. Rao, M. Ludwig, S.G. Schwab and R. Heun,

Genetic polymorphism of cathepsin D is strongly associated with the risk for developing sporadic Alzheimer's disease, *Neurosci Lett* **262**(3) (1999), 171–174.

[136] A. Papassotiropoulos, M. Bagli, A. Kurz, J. Kornhuber, H. Forstl, W. Maier, J. Pauls, N. Lautenschlager and R. Heun, A genetic variation of cathepsin D is a major risk factor for Alzheimer's disease, *Ann Neurol* **47**(3) (2000), 399–403.

[137] C. Paquet, A.T. Sane, M. Beauchemin and R. Bertrand, Caspase- and mitochondrial dysfunction-dependent mechanisms of lysosomal leakage and cathepsin B activation in DNA damage-induced apoptosis, *Leukemia* **19**(5) (2005), 784–791.

[138] S.H. Pasternak, R.D. Bagshaw, M. Guiral, S. Zhang, C.A. Ackerley, B.J. Pak, J.W. Callahan and D.J. Mahuran, Presenilin-1, nicastrin, amyloid precursor protein, and gamma-secretase activity are co-localized in the lysosomal membrane, *J Biol Chem* **278**(29) (2003), 26687–26694.

[139] R.G. Perez, S. Soriano, J.D. Hayes, B. Ostaszewski, W. Xia, D.J. Selkoe, X. Chen, G.B. Stokin and E.H. Koo, Mutagenesis identifies new signals for beta-amyloid precursor protein endocytosis, turnover, and the generation of secreted fragments, including Abeta42, *J Biol Chem* **274**(27) (1999), 18851–18856.

[140] P.J. Peters, A. Mironov, Jr., D. Peretz, E. van Donselaar, E. Leclerc, S. Erpel, S.J. DeArmond, D.R. Burton, R.A. Williamson, M. Vey and S.B. Prusiner, Trafficking of prion proteins through a caveolae-mediated endosomal pathway, *J Cell Biol* **162**(4) (2003), 703–717.

[141] A. Pope and R.A. Nixon, Proteases of human brain, *Neurochem Res* **9**(3) (1984), 291–323.

[142] V.P. Prasher, M.J. Farrer, A.M. Kessling, E.M. Fisher, R.J. West, P.C. Barber and A.C. Butler, Molecular mapping of Alzheimer-type dementia in Down's syndrome, *Ann Neurol* **43**(3) (1998), 380–383.

[143] Z.H. Qin, Y. Wang, K.B. Kegel, A. Kazantsev, B.L. Apostol, L.M. Thompson, J. Yoder, N. Aronin and M. DiFiglia, Autophagy regulates the processing of amino terminal huntingtin fragments, *Hum Mol Genet* **12**(24) (2003), 3231–3244.

[144] B. Ravikumar, A. Stewart, H. Kita, K. Kato, R. Duden and D.C. Rubinsztein, Raised intracellular glucose concentrations reduce aggregation and cell death caused by mutant huntingtin exon 1 by decreasing mTOR phosphorylation and inducing autophagy, *Hum Mol Genet* **12**(9) (2003), 985–994.

[145] B. Ravikumar, C. Vacher, Z. Berger, J.E. Davies, S. Luo, L.G. Oroz, F. Scaravilli, D.F. Easton, R. Duden, C.J. O'Kane and D.C. Rubinsztein, Inhibition of mTOR induces autophagy and reduces toxicity of polyglutamine expansions in fly and mouse models of Huntington disease, *Nat Genet* **36**(6) (2004), 585–595.

[146] K. Roberg, U. Johansson and K. Ollinger, Lysosomal release of cathepsin D precedes relocation of cytochrome c and loss of mitochondrial transmembrane potential during apoptosis induced by oxidative stress, *Free Radic Biol Med* **27**(11–12) (1999), 1228–1237.

[147] K. Roberg nd K. Ollinger, Oxidative stress causes relocation of the lysosomal enzyme cathepsin D with ensuing apoptosis in neonatal rat cardiomyocytes, *Am J Pathol* **152**(5) (1998), 1151–1156.

[148] D.C. Rubinsztein, M. DiFiglia, N. Heintz, R.A. Nixon, Z.H. Qin, B. Ravikumar, L. Stefanis and A.M. Tolkovsky, Autophagy and its possible roles in nervous system diseases, damage and repair, *Autophagy* **1**(1) (2005), 11–22.

[149] G. Sadik, H. Kaji, K. Takeda, F. Yamagata, Y. Kameoka, K. Hashimoto, K. Miyanaga and T. Shinoda, In vitro processing of amyloid precursor protein by cathepsin D, *Int J Biochem Cell Biol* **31**(11) (1999), 1327–1337.

[150] P. Saftig, C. Peters, K. von Figura, K. Craessaerts, F. Van Leuven and B. De Strooper, Amyloidogenic processing of human amyloid precursor protein in hippocampal neurons devoid of cathepsin D, *J Biol Chem* **271**(44) (1996), 27241–27244.

[151] A. Salehi, R. Takimoto, C.J. Epstein and W.C. Mobley, Gene expression in dentate granule cells of mouse models of Down syndrome, *Society for Neuroscience Abstract* **226.16** (2004)

[152] M.L. Schmidt, A.G. DiDario, V.M. Lee and J.Q. Trojanowski, An extensive network of PHF tau-rich dystrophic neurites permeates neocortex and nearly all neuritic and diffuse amyloid plaques in Alzheimer disease, *FEBS Lett* **344**(1) (1994), 69–73.

[153] P.O. Seglen, T.O. Berg, H. Blankson, M. Fengsrud, I. Holen and P.E. Stromhaug, Structural aspects of autophagy, *Adv Exp Med Biol* **389** (1996), 103–111.

[154] P.O. Seglen and P. Bohley, Autophagy and other vacuolar protein degradation mechanisms, *Experientia* **48**(2) (1992), 158–172.

[155] R. Sherrington, E.I. Rogaev, Y. Liang, E.A. Rogaeva, G. Levesque, M. Ikeda, H. Chi, C. Lin, G. Li, K. Holman et al., Cloning of a gene bearing missense mutations in early-onset familial Alzheimer's disease [see comments], *Nature* **375**(6534) (1995), 754–760.

[156] F.S. Shie, R.C. LeBoeuf and L.W. Jin, Early intraneuronal Abeta deposition in the hippocampus of APP transgenic mice, *Neuroreport* **14**(1) (2003), 123–129.

[157] S. Shimizu, T. Kanaseki, N. Mizushima, T. Mizuta, S. Arakawa-Kobayashi, C.B. Thompson and Y. Tsujimoto, Role of Bcl-2 family proteins in a non-apoptotic programmed cell death dependent on autophagy genes, *Nat Cell Biol* **6**(12) (2004), 1221–1228.

[158] T. Shintani and D.J. Klionsky, Autophagy in health and disease: a double-edged sword, *Science* **306**(5698) (2004), 990–995.

[159] R.S. Sohal, R.J. Mockett and W.C. Orr, Mechanisms of aging: an appraisal of the oxidative stress hypothesis, *Free Radic Biol Med* **33**(5) (2002), 575–586.

[160] S. Soriano, A.S. Chyung, X. Chen, G.B. Stokin, V.M. Lee and E.H. Koo, Expression of beta-amyloid precursor protein-CD3gamma chimeras to demonstrate the selective generation of amyloid beta(1-40) and amyloid beta(1-42) Peptides within secretory and endocytic compartments, *J Biol Chem* **274**(45) (1999), 32295–32300.

[161] A. Sorkin and M. Von Zastrow, Signal transduction and endocytosis: close encounters of many kinds, *Nat Rev Mol Cell Biol* **3**(8) (2002), 600–614.

[162] C. Soto, Unfolding the role of protein misfolding in neurodegenerative diseases, *Nat Rev Neurosci* **4**(1) (2003), 49–60.

[163] L. Stefanis, Caspase-dependent and -independent neuronal death: two distinct pathways to neuronal injury, *Neuroscientist* **11**(1) (2005), 50–62.

[164] K. Suzuki and R.D. Terry, Fine structural localization of acid phosphatase in senile plaques in Alzheimer's presenile dementia, *Acta Neuropathol (Berl)* **8**(3) (1967), 276–284.

[165] R.H. Takahashi, T.A. Milner, F. Li, E.E. Nam, M.A. Edgar, H. Yamaguchi, M.F. Beal, H. Xu, P. Greengard and G.K. Gouras, Intraneuronal Alzheimer Abeta42 accumulates in multivesicular bodies and is associated with synaptic pathology, *Am J Pathol* **161**(5) (2002), 1869–1879.

[166] A. Terman, H. Dalen and U.T. Brunk, Ceroid/lipofuscin-loaded human fibroblasts show decreased survival time and

diminished autophagocytosis during amino acid starvation, *Exp Gerontol* **34**(8) (1999), 943–957.
[167] R.D. Terry, N.K. Gonatas and M. Weiss, Ultrastructural Studies in Alzheimer's Presenile Dementia, *Am J Pathol* **44** (1964), 269–297.
[168] G. Thinakaran, D.B. Teplow, R. Siman, B. Greenberg and S.S. Sisodia, Metabolism of the "Swedish" amyloid precursor protein variant in neuro2a (N2a) cells. Evidence that cleavage at the "beta-secretase" site occurs in the golgi apparatus, *J Biol Chem* **271**(16) (1996), 9390–9397.
[169] A.M. Tolkovsky, L. Xue, G.C. Fletcher and V. Borutaite, Mitochondrial disappearance from cells: a clue to the role of autophagy in programmed cell death and disease? *Biochimie* **84**(2–3) (2002), 233–240.
[170] I. Touitou, F. Capony, J.P. Brouillet and H. Rochefort, Missense polymorphism (C/T224) in the human cathepsin D profragment determined by polymerase chain reaction – single strand conformational polymorphism analysis and possible consequences in cancer cells, *Eur J Cancer* **3** (1994), 390–394.
[171] E. Trushina, R.B. Dyer, J.D. Badger, 2nd, D. Ure, L. Eide, D.D. Tran, B.T. Vrieze, V. Legendre-Guillemin, P.S. McPherson, B.S. Mandavilli, B. Van Houten, S. Zeitlin, M. McNiven, R. Aebersold, M. Hayden, J.E. Parisi, E. Seeberg, I. Dragatsis, K. Doyle, A. Bender, C. Chacko and C.T. McMurray, Mutant huntingtin impairs axonal trafficking in mammalian neurons in vivo and in vitro, *Mol Cell Biol* **24**(18) (2004), 8195–8209.
[172] J. Tyynela, I. Sohar, D.E. Sleat, R.M. Gin, R.J. Donnelly, M. Baumann, M. Haltia and P. Lobel, A mutation in the ovine cathepsin D gene causes a congenital lysosomal storage disease with profound neurodegeneration, *Embo J* **19**(12) (2000), 2786–2792.
[173] J. Tyynela, I. Sohar, D.E. Sleat, R.M. Gin, R.J. Donnelly, M. Baumann, M. Haltia and P. Lobel, Congenital ovine neuronal ceroid lipofuscinosis – a cathepsin D deficiency with increased levels of the inactive enzyme, *Eur J Paediatr Neurol* **5**(Suppl A) (2001), 43–45.
[174] R. Vassar, B.D. Bennett, S. Babu-Khan, S. Kahn, E.A. Mendiaz, P. Denis, D.B. Teplow, S. Ross, P. Amarante, R. Loeloff, Y. Luo, S. Fisher, J. Fuller, S. Edenson, J. Lile, M.A. Jarosinski, A.L. Biere, E. Curran, T. Burgess, J.C. Louis, F. Collins, J. Treanor, G. Rogers and M. Citron, Beta-secretase cleavage of Alzheimer's amyloid precursor protein by the transmembrane aspartic protease BACE, *Science* **286**(5440) (1999), 735–741.
[175] P. Vito, E. Lacana and L. D'Adamio, Interfering with apoptosis: Ca(2+)-binding protein ALG-2 and Alzheimer's disease gene ALG-3, *Science* **271**(5248) (1996), 521–525.
[176] P. Vito, L. Pellegrini, C. Guiet and L. D'Adamio, Cloning of AIP1, a novel protein that associates with the apoptosis-linked gene ALG-2 in a Ca2+-dependent reaction, *J Biol Chem* **274**(3) (1999), 1533–1540.
[177] K. Wakasugi, T. Nakano and I. Morishima, Association of human neuroglobin with cystatin C, a cysteine proteinase inhibitor, *Biochemistry* **43**(18) (2004), 5119–5125.
[178] J. Wang, D.W. Dickson, J.Q. Trojanowski and V.M. Lee, The levels of soluble versus insoluble brain Abeta distinguish Alzheimer's disease from normal and pathologic aging, *Exp Neurol* **158**(2) (1999), 328–337.
[179] C.A. Wilson, D.D. Murphy, B.I. Giasson, B. Zhang, J. Q. Trojanowski and V.M. Lee, Degradative organelles containing mislocalized {alpha}- and {beta}-synuclein proliferate in presenilin-1 null neurons, *J Cell Biol* **165**(3) (2004), 335–346.
[180] M.S. Wolfe, W. Xia, C.L. Moore, D.D. Leatherwood, B. Ostaszewski, T. Rahmati, I.O. Donkor and D.J. Selkoe, Peptidomimetic probes and molecular modeling suggest that Alzheimer's gamma-secretase is an intramembrane-cleaving aspartyl protease, *Biochemistry* **38**(15) (1999), 4720–4727.
[181] H. Xu, D. Sweeney, R. Wang, G. Thinakaran, A.C. Lo, S.S. Sisodia, P. Greengard and S. Gandy, Generation of Alzheimer beta-amyloid protein in the trans-Golgi network in the apparent absence of vesicle formation, *Proc Natl Acad Sci USA* **94**(8) (1997), 3748–3752.
[182] L. Xu, J. Sheng, Z. Tang, X. Wu, Y. Yu, H. Guo, Y. Shen, C. Zhou, L. Paraoan and J. Zhou, Cystatin C prevents degeneration of rat nigral dopaminergic neurons: in vitro and in vivo studies, *Neurobiol Dis* **18**(1) (2005), 152–165.
[183] K. Yamanaka, C. Vande Velde, E. Eymard-Pierre, E. Bertini, O. Boespflug-Tanguy and D.W. Cleveland, Unstable mutants in the peripheral endosomal membrane component ALS2 cause early-onset motor neuron disease, *Proc Natl Acad Sci USA* **100**(26) (2003), 16041–16046.
[184] A.J. Yang, D. Chandswangbhuvana, L. Margol and C.G. Glabe, Loss of endosomal/lysosomal membrane impermeability is an early event in amyloid Abeta1-42 pathogenesis, *J Neurosci Res* **52**(6) (1998), 691–698.
[185] T. Yoshimori, Autophagy: a regulated bulk degradation process inside cells, *Biochem Biophys Res Commun* **313**(2) (2004), 453–458.
[186] W. Yu, A. Cuervo, A. Kumar, C.M. Peterhoff, S.D. Schmidt, P.S. Mohan, M. Mercken, M.R. Farmery, L. Tjernberg, Y. Jiang, J. Weigel, B.T. Lamb, K.D. Duff, Y. Uchiyama, J. Naslund, P.M. Mathews, A.M. Cataldo and R.A. Nixon, Macroautophagy- a novel amyloid-β (Aβ) peptide-generating pathway activated in Alzheimer's disease, *Neuron* (2005), in press.
[187] W.H. Yu, A.M. Cuervo, A. Kumar, C.M. Peterhoff, S.D. Schmidt, P.S. Mohan, M. Mercken, M.R. Farmery, L. Tjernberg, Y. Jiang, J. Weigel, B.T. Lamb, K.D. Duff, Y. Uchiyama, J. Naslund, P.M. Mathews, A.M. Cataldo and R.A. Nixon, Macroautophagy – a novel amyloid-β (Aβ) peptide-generating pathway activated in Alzheimer's disease, *Neuron* (2004).
[188] W.H. Yu, A. Kumar, C. Peterhoff, L.S. Kulnane, Y. Uchiyama, B.T. Lamb, A.M. Cuervo and R.A. Nixon, Autophagic vacuoles are enriched in amyloid precursor protein-secretase activities: implications for beta-amyloid peptide over-production and localization in Alzheimer's disease, *Int J Biochem Cell Biol* **36**(12) (2004), 2531–2540.
[189] Z. Yue, A. Horton, M. Bravin, P.L. DeJager, F. Selimi and N. Heintz, A novel protein complex linking the delta 2 glutamate receptor and autophagy: implications for neurodegeneration in lurcher mice, *Neuron* **35**(5) (2002), 921–933.

Aluminum and Alzheimer's disease, a personal perspective after 25 years

Daniel P. Perl and Sharon Moalem
Mount Sinai School of Medicine, Department of Pathology, Neuropathology Division, USA

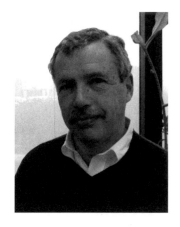

Abstract. It is now 25 years since the publication of our original paper investigating the association aluminum with Alzheimer's disease. This publication reported on the results of scanning electron microscopy coupled with x-ray spectrometry microprobe elemental studies of both neurofibrillary tangle-bearing and tangle-free neurons in the hippocampus of cases of Alzheimer's disease and controls. Peaks related to the presence of aluminum were consistently detected within the tangle-bearing neurons. This paper supported the association of aluminum and Alzheimer's disease on the cellular level of resolution and caused considerable interest and discussion. Subsequent work demonstrated prominent evidence of aluminum accumulation in the tangle-bearing neurons of cases of amyotrophic lateral sclerosis/parkinsonism-dementia complex of Guam. This latter observation has now been replicated using five different forms of microanalysis. Finally, using laser microprobe mass analysis, we demonstrated that the abnormally high aluminum-related signal which we originally detected was actually located within the neurofibrillary tangle, itself, and was accompanied by excess concentrations of iron. Although it is unlikely that aluminum represents an etiologic cause of Alzheimer's disease, we believe that this highly reactive element, known to cross-link hyperphosphorylated proteins, may play an active role in the pathogenesis of critical neuropathologic lesions in Alzheimer's disease and other related disorders.

1. Introduction

Although the association of aluminum and Alzheimer's disease did not begin with me, my 1980 paper [19] coauthored with Arnold Brody entitled "Alzheimer's Disease: X-ray spectrographic evidence of aluminum accumulation in neurofibrillary tangle-bearing neurons", provided critical data that extended this association to the cellular level of resolution. The paper greatly raised the awareness of the association of this non-essential trace element and Alzheimer's disease and has stimulated further research, discussion and controversy that continue to this day. Over the past 25 years, this paper has been formally cited over 600 times and literally hundreds of times I have been asked to discuss it and its implications at meetings and seminars. I appreciate the opportunity to look back and give some personal perspectives on the paper and the subsequent research that it spawned.

2. History of the publication

In 1976, I was recruited as Director of Neuropathology at the University of Vermont College of Medicine in Burlington, VT. At the time, I had no particular research interest in Alzheimer's Disease or specific plans to engage in studies on the subject. Soon after I arrived, I met a talented young Assistant Professor in the Pathology Department, Dr. Arnold Brody. Arnie was interested in mineral dust-related occupational lung diseases such as silicosis, talcosis, and asbestosis. Workers in Vermont, a location with active asbestos, granite, talc and marble quarries and mines, commonly suffered from such occupational lung diseases and this was the basis for an active Specialized Centers of Research (SCOR) program at the University of Vermont College of Medicine funded by the Heart, Lung and Blood Institute of the NIH. At the time, Dr. Brody ran a very productive facility within Vermont's SCOR program that was engaged in the study of human and experimental animal-derived lung tissues using the approach of scanning electron microscopy coupled with energy dispersive x-ray microprobe analysis (SEM-XES). We quickly became friends and as an extension of our friendship, sought ways in which we could collaborate scientifically.

Although the microprobe analytic techniques Brody and others were using were very sensitive, at the time, very little research had been done employing SEM-XES to study brain specimens, especially human tissues. However, I was aware of the publications emerging from the laboratories of Dr. Donald Crapper-McLachlan and colleagues in Toronto. In 1973 [2], they published the results of a study demonstrating that Alzheimer's disease brain tissues showed a 2 to 3-fold increase in aluminum concentrations when compared to normal control tissues. A subsequent study [3] provided further data indicating considerable regional variation in aluminum concentration in Alzheimer's disease brain tissue and suggested that the regions with the highest concentration of aluminum were those containing the greatest number of neurofibrillary tangles (NFTs). The implication was that aluminum played a role in the formation of the NFT, a cardinal lesion of Alzheimer's disease. The rationale behind these two studies had been the earlier publications by Terry and Peña [26] and of Klatzo, Wisniewski, and Streicher [12] demonstrating the acute induction of widespread NFTs in cerebral cortical, brain stem and spinal cord neurons of rabbits following direct exposure of the brain to a variety of aluminum-containing compounds. In the early years, it was argued that the aluminum-induced tangles of the rabbit were composed of straight neurofilaments and therefore were entirely different from that of human paired-helical filaments [27]. Subsequent studies by Savory and colleagues [11,23,24] have pointed out that there are many shared constituents between these experimental lesions and those of man.

The studies by Crapper-McLachlan employed atomic absorption spectrometry and provided bulk tissue elemental concentrations within relatively small tissue samples. Inherent in this kind of bulk analysis is the inability to further localize the aluminum being detected within the sample at the cellular or subcellular level of resolution. Faced with this data and the obvious question of where the aluminum was localized in the tissues, I turned to Dr. Brody and suggested that we might collaborate and try to investigate this problem using the microprobe technology available in his laboratory. He agreed to work with me on this but indicated that although he was an expert on tissue microprobe studies, he knew little about the brain, Alzheimer's disease or how to proceed with the cellular localization we would require. His prior research experience had been to identify and characterize inhaled mineral deposits in lung tissues. The mineral deposits being detected in the lung specimens he was evaluating were focal but had extremely high elemental concentrations and the instrumental detection limits were rarely, if ever, a problem.

We first had to devise a method to prepare autopsy-derived brain tissues for SEM-XES analysis. There were no prior published studies to rely upon and so we proceeded to develop these ourselves. This involved using frozen sections of formalin-fixed tissues that were mounted on one-inch in diameter pure carbon disks. We decided to concentrate on the hippocampus, where I knew that many examples of NFTs could be found in the large pyramidal neurons of the CA1 region. The sections had to be carbon coated in order to support electrical conduction through the specimen and allow for high resolution scanning electron microscopic visualization. This allowed us to clearly visualize the hippocampus and identify pyramidal neurons in the CA1 region. However, with this approach we could not tell which neurons contained NFTs and which were tangle-free. This would be needed so that we could compare the two populations of cells in each case. In order to accomplish this, we developed a modified version of the Bielschowsky silver technique which could be applied to the sections prior to their being mounted on the carbon disks. Once the stained sections were mounted and placed in the SEM, they could be imaged using a back-scattered electron detector, which visualizes dense elemental concentrations. Using this detector, the NFTs stood out boldly, with an appearance that was remarkably similar to histologic preparations that I was used to seeing as a neuropathologist (Fig. 1).

With all this preparatory work accomplished, we were now ready to begin the analytical phase of the work. In those days, energy dispersive x-ray analyzers were quite primitive, by today's standards. Today, one can purchase sophisticated computer-driven pack-

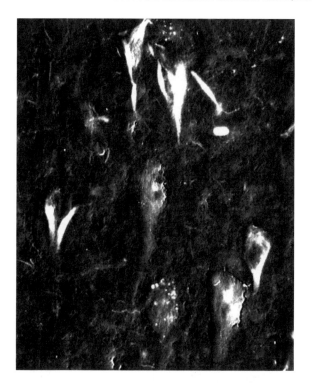

Fig. 1. Using a combination of scanning electron microscopy and backscattered electron imaging we could readily identify NFT-bearing and NFT-free neurons in frozen sections of the CA1 region of the hippocampus, modified Bielschowsky stain.

ages which will examine spectra automatically and detect and quantify the individual elements present. At the time we were working, the steps for the analysis of the spectra we collected had to be done individually and painstakingly by hand. The instrument had to be carefully aligned and adjusted to maximize collection of a clean spectrum. For such critical issues, Arnie Brody played an essential role and was a world authority. When we got stumped, Mr. Joe Geller, then an analytical specialist working with the JEOL company, added his considerable technical expertise and experience. It was also clear that we had added high concentrations of silver to the tissues and that this increased the amount of background (non-specific or Bremstrallüng) x-rays which were produced. We were concerned that there might have been inadvertent aluminum contamination in the stain ingredients and these ingredients were probed directly, as were non-specific stain deposits within the tissue sections. Such analyses never showed evidence of detectable aluminum-related signals using the same instrumentation.

From the beginning, it was clear that we were attempting to detect very low concentrations of aluminum in these tissues. This required us to set criteria for determining whether an aluminum-related peak was present or not in any particular probe site. These criteria were written down and placed beside the instrument and strictly adhered to in interpreting each spectrum we produced. We analyzed hippocampal sections derived from clinically and neuropathologically confirmed cases of Alzheimer's disease and from non-demented elderly controls. Intact pyramidal neurons were identified through the three-dimensional scanning electron microscope mode and then determined to be either NFT-bearing or NFT-free using the backscattered electron detector. Once the neuron was chosen for analysis X-ray spectra were collected and analyzed from four probe-sites in the "nuclear region" of the neuron and from its adjacent non-tangled cytoplasm. With the instrument optimally adjusted, we began to identify aluminum-related peaks from probe-sites directed to the nuclear region of the NFT-bearing neurons (Fig. 2). Under identical analytic conditions, similar peaks were rarely identified in the uninvolved cytoplasm of the NFT-bearing neurons or of the NFT-free cells. It is important to note that we had been working for close to a year before the problems of sample preparation and analytic parameters had been worked out and the first aluminum-related peaks were finally noted. This was a different era and the demands for positive research results, needs for scientific productivity, etc., were more relaxed. We were young and perhaps more patient and persistent than today's more frantic pace would allow. I seriously doubt if we had initiated these studies today, we would have had the freedom and perseverance to reach the results we did.

A word about the "nuclear region" and what was meant by that term. We were probing what had originally been a cryostat section cut at a thickness of 20 microns. These sections were stained and then air-dried resulting in a specimen that was less than 10 microns thick. At the accelerating voltages we used (25 Kv) the electron beam likely penetrated through the section but it is unlikely that sufficient numbers of x-rays with elementally defining profiles would emerge from the depths of these sections. Accordingly, we could not tell with any certainty whether the aluminum-related peaks we reported were actually coming from the nucleus, itself. Rather, these aluminum positive probe sites were directed to the main perikaryal region, as opposed to the axon hillock, which was generally chosen as "adjacent cytoplasm". Many read our paper and assumed we had localized the aluminum to the nucleus, itself, which we were incapable of doing with the analytic approach we were using, nor had we ever claimed this to be the case.

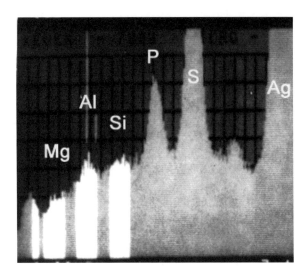

Fig. 2. Typical SEM-XES sprectrum obtained from the nuclear region of an NFT-bearing neuron of a case of Alzheimer's disease. Note the aluminum-related peak present.

The paper reported that under carefully controlled analytic parameters, aluminum-related peaks were identified in the "nuclear region" of a high percentage of NFT-bearing neurons of three cases of Alzheimer's disease and three non-demented elderly controls. The probe sites directed to the non-involved cytoplasm of these NFT-bearing neurons and of adjacent non-tangled neurons were virtually free of detectable aluminum. In the paper we also reported data on magnesium and silicon-related peaks from these probe sites and neither of these elements showed significant differences in the resultant peaks emerging from the NFT-bearing and NFT-free probe sites. An important piece of data was shown in one of the figures of the paper which demonstrated the aluminum-related X-ray signal emerging from a line scan passing through one of the NFT-bearing neurons (Fig. 3). Here, the aluminum-related signal showed a dramatic increase when the scan passed through what appears to be the nucleus of that neuron. This had been one of Joe Geller's important contributions and, in retrospect, he should have been an author on the paper. It is important to note that this line scan reports wave-length dispersive x-ray data related to the presence of aluminum. The significance of this aspect of the study was not generally appreciated but bears particular mention. Everyone, including ourselves, concentrated on our energy-dispersive x-ray data for the detection of aluminum. That we could detect aluminum's presence using wave-length dispersive x-ray analysis, a separate form of analysis using different physical principles, served as a significant corroboration of our findings.

Arnie and I collated our data, wrote it up, and sent the manuscript to Science. After the usual anxious waiting period, we received three very supportive reviews, yet the paper was rejected. We were disappointed by this and wrote to the editor-in-chief pointing to the very positive reviews as well as indicating that Science had published Crapper-McLachlin's original Alzheimer's disease bulk aluminum analysis paper [2]. After a short delay, the paper was then accepted for publication with very little revision.

Soon after the publication of the paper, I was faced with a modest number of inquiries from the press. Some calls came in asking for interviews, comments and statements on the significance of our findings. We had not issued a press release about the paper and I was not ready for the extent of interest in our results. About three months after the paper appeared, I received a huge flurry of calls about the work coming from all over the world. These inquiries asked for my interpretation of the results with respect to potential hazards of human exposure to aluminum in the form of pots and pans as well as other aluminum-containing food substances. I was puzzled by this renewal of interest and soon found that Dr. Steven Levick had just published a short letter to the editor in the New England Journal of Medicine [14] citing our work and raising the potential health risks of using aluminum pots and pans. I had never heard of Dr. Levick but later found out that he was, at the time, a psychiatry resident at Yale. I later learned that Levick had also received numerous calls for comments on his letter. He had not done any research in the area other than noting that an aluminum pan he used in his humble resident's apartment showed considerable erosion causing him to wonder in a rather public fashion about where the aluminum had gone and what were the consequences of exposure of this type. Although we had not discussed the issue directly in our paper, Levick raised an important issue, namely, could aluminum represent the etiology of Alzheimer's disease and did exposure to aluminum-containing products represent a health hazard. This potential concept really stirred up interest by the lay press and was like pouring gasoline on a smoldering fire. The phone calls, interviews, stories on TV, radio and in the press throughout the world escalated and have continued this interest over the years. As scientists, at times we are often unaware of the impact that our findings may have once they have been 'set free' on the public at large and been subjected to the interpretation of poorly informed and scientifically naive reporters. We assume that the scientific process rules the day but as any one who has participated in

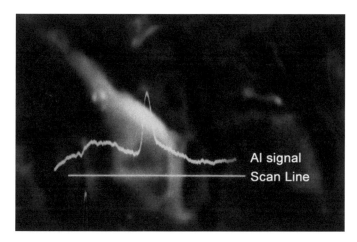

Fig. 3. Line scan through an NFT-bearing neuron, Alzheimer's disease, showing the aluminum-related wavelength dispersive x-ray signal with an increase in intensity as it passes through the apparent area of the nucleus. This image was used in Fig. 4 of the original article (reprinted with permission, Science).

any charged issue knows the process becomes quickly sacrificed and then subsequently politicized. The press had taken the story and ran with it; the genie was out of the bottle and there was nothing I could do to keep the discussion on a level that was in accord with what scientific data was available.

3. Subsequent studies

After the paper with Brody appeared, I now wanted to use this approach to probe other disorders in which NFTs appeared. This quickly led to an interest in examining brain tissues from cases of amyotrophic lateral sclerosis (ALS)/parkinsonism-dementia complex of Guam. ALS/parkinsonism-dementia complex of Guam is a unique neurodegenerative disorder which appears with high prevalence among the native Chamorro population living on the island of Guam in the western Pacific. Clinically and neuropathologically, it has features of the three major age-related neurodegenerative diseases seen elsewhere in the world, namely, ALS, Parkinson's disease and Alzheimer's disease. Importantly, the brains of affected individuals show large numbers of NFTs. I started to contact colleagues who had worked on the neuropathology of ALS/parkinsonism-dementia complex of Guam to see if I could obtain samples for x-ray microprobe analysis. Everyone directed me to Dr. D. Carleton Gajdusek, a Nobel laureate, then at the NIH, as the source of such tissues. Dr. Gajdusek knew of my work and indicated that he was anxious to establish a collaboration with me. Soon a large box arrived in my laboratory at the University of Vermont containing many brain samples of both affected cases and Guam-derived controls.

I had asked that Gajdusek send me ALS/parkinsonism-dementia complex of Guam cases with particularly dramatic hippocampal NFT formation and Guam controls that were virtually NFT-free. The ALS/PDC cases used for this study had such severe pathologic involvement in the CA1 region of the hippocampus that it could be assumed that virtually all the pyramidal cells in that region contained an NFT. These cases would be compared with specimens from Guam natives that were free of neurologic impairment and showed no NFTs in the hippocampus. Since all of the identifiable neurons in the affected cases contained an NFT, the specimens could be examined as unstained sections. Because the cases and controls had been fixed and handled in an identical fashion and no staining procedure had been used, this effectively avoided any potential controversy regarding inadvertent post-mortem introduction of aluminum to the tissues prior to analysis. We set up the experiment to analyze the samples in a blinded fashion, namely, the sections were cut without my involvement, coded and then provided to me for probing without my knowing if they were extensively involved by NFTs or were NFT-free. I can still clearly remember sitting down at the SEM-XES instrument, introducing the first specimen into the chamber and turning on the electron beam. The x-rays were collected from the first probed neuron and this produced the most prominent aluminum-related peak I had ever seen coming from a neuron. It was much greater than anything we had previously detected in our Alzheimer's disease-related work. Other neuronal probe-sites produced similar peaks. I quickly changed to the next specimen and similar peaks appeared. Probes to neurons in the third specimen were entirely free of such peaks (Fig. 4A, B). Although we rigorously adhered to examining the specimens in a blinded fashion, from the first day I was certain that we had a most significant finding and that at least in Guam-derived specimens, I could readily distinguish the tangle-bearing neurons from tangle free cells based on their aluminum content.

Since we were examining unstained tissue samples, the lack of silver deposits produced low background x-ray emissions that were relatively uniform among the specimens. This meant that we would be able to collect quantitative data consisting of aluminum-related x-ray counts following background subtraction. When the probing of all the samples was completed, the blind was broken and the data were, as I had originally suspected, quite dramatic. Probe sites directed to NFT-bearing neurons of the two cases of parkinsonism-dementia complex of Guam showed a mean aluminum-related x-ray count of 236.2 ± 21.3 and 232.1 ± 23.9 whereas the neuronal probe sites to an NFT-rich case of Guam ALS emitted a mean aluminum-related signal of 296.3 ± 26.2. In contrast, the neuronal probe sites to four Guam controls without hippocampal NFTs produced a mean aluminum-related signal of 77.3 ± 7.2. These differences were highly significant ($p < 0.01$).

These data were written up in collaboration with Gajdusek's NIH group, submitted to Science and the manuscript was rather rapidly accepted for publication [20]. The data were dramatic and compared to our prior Alzheimer's disease paper the experimental approach more rigorous and quantitative. Soon after the paper appeared, Gajdusek asked me to visit the NIH in order to talk to Dr. Charles Fiori, an NIH scientist who had raised a number of questions and concerns about how we had produced and handled our data. Gajdusek was unable to respond to these questions and he asked me to speak to Fiori and hopefully defend our paper. Chuck Fiori was a world leader in x-ray microprobe analysis and was then in the process of developing a state-of-the-art laboratory for elemental detection in cells (he was primarily interested in determining intracellular calcium distribution using a microprobe approach). Fiori grilled me for two hours on every aspect of our experimental design and, in particular, how the x-ray spectra had been produced, collected and analyzed. At first, he was particularly troubled by our approach, but most of his concerns appeared to relate to a lack of methodologic details in the published paper based on word and style limitations imposed by Science. After a rather tense and, at times, adversarial discussion of our work, Fiori said that he basically thought we had done a good job, considering the equipment we had available, but that he wanted to attempt to confirm our results independently, using his own facilities. This led to Fiori's confirmation published in the Proceedings of the National Academy of Science (PNAS) [4] in the following year. Fiori used X-ray wave-length spectrometry (we had used energy dispersive x-ray analysis) for his study and ultimately, our findings related to increased aluminum concentrations being present in the NFTs of Guam ALS/parkinsonism-dementia complex were confirmed using 5 separate physical principles and were performed in three different laboratories [15, 21,22].

4. Laser Microprobe Mass Analysis (LAMMA)

In the early 1980's, I learned of a new technology that had developed in Germany that I thought might assist us in this work, namely laser microprobe mass analysis or LAMMA [9]. The LAMMA instrument employs a focused high energy laser pulse to perforate a semithin plastic-embedded tissue section and produce a time-of-flight mass spectrum providing information on the elemental content of the probed tissue. The instrument is able to simultaneously detect virtually all positively charged elements throughout the entire atomic table with a minimum detection limit for most elements of less than ten parts per million. The tissue perforation is directed by a continuous low energy aiming laser and one can stain the tissue with toluidine blue to allow for visualization of histologic detail and selection of specific sites to be targeted for analysis. Finally, the high energy laser can be focused to a probe-site of approximately 1 μm in diameter.

Using this technology, we published the results of probing tangle-bearing and adjacent non-tangled neurons of 10 consecutively accessioned Alzheimer's disease cases and showed clear evidence of excess aluminum concentrations in the NFT-bearing neurons, when compared to the next nearest non-tangled neurons [5]. Importantly, the excess aluminum could now be specifically localized to the NFT, itself. In addition, we were able to examine the resultant spectra for evidence of abnormal concentrations of many other elements. Of all the other elements examined, the only other element that was consistently seen in excess in the NFT was iron. These confirmatory data, using a completely different analytic approach, was published

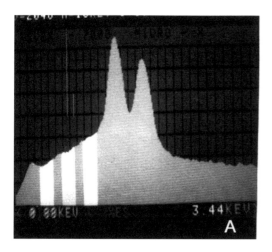 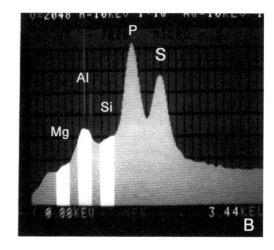

Fig. 4. Typical SEM-XES spectra obtained from the nuclear region of hippocampal neuron of a Guam control that is NFT-free (A) and a case of parkinsonism-dementia complex of Guam (B). Note the prominent aluminum-related peak obtained from the parkinsonism-dementia complex of Guam case which has extensive NFT-formation. Unstained frozen sections, hippocampus.

in 1993. In this paper we also reported obtaining mass spectra containing prominent mass-27 aluminum-related peaks from probe sites of hippocampal neurons of Alzheimer's disease specimens that were snap frozen, cryosectioned and examined as unstained sections. These spectra clearly demonstrate that the aluminum we were detecting in the NFT-bearing neurons could not represent a contaminant of fixation, plastic embedding or toluidine blue staining. We considered these base-less speculative concerns to represent the grasping at straws of our critics and were glad we could finally put this issue to rest.

Once again, I was fortunate to have as a collaborator, Dr. Paul Good, who became an expert in the operation of the instrument, especially in the proper tuning and alignment of the ionizing laser. This allowed for standardization of the operation of the microprobe and minimized any day-to-day variations. When the group at the University of Kentucky failed to replicate our results [16], it was clear to us that their data had considerable variability in signal intensity and we surmised that they had failed to learn these lessons [6]. I found it interesting that people would readily accept our data demonstrating that increased iron concentrations characterized neurofibrillary tangles and encouraged further interest in oxidative stress in association with this lesion [8,10,17]. Despite this, over the years people have appeared to have trouble considering that aluminum could also be an important constituent and, as such, could play an active pathogenetic role in the disease process.

5. Why has the potential role of aluminum in the pathogenesis of Alzheimer's disease been so controversial?

Over the years, rather vocal criticism of our work and those of others who began to explore the aluminum hypothesis became loudly heard at meetings where I was invited to speak and in the scientific literature. The source of these criticisms came from a relatively small number of individuals, many of whom, I later learned, were serving as paid consultants to the aluminum industry. I still do not know how many there were but a few were rather prominent academic figures with considerable influence on the field. At the time, the rules regarding disclosure of financial ties and conflicts of interest were not yet in force for authors and speakers at meetings, and, for the most part, few were aware of this serious breach in the impartiality of this vocal portion of the academic community. To my knowledge, none have ever publicly acknowledged their close ties to the aluminum industry. I have often wondered if I should have directly addressed the fact that the most consistent and vocal critics of our findings were also secretly tied financially to the aluminum industry. Frankly, in the early days of this work I was naively unaware of this connection and later I assumed that since our data showing that aluminum was a constituent of the neurofibrillary tangle, had been properly collected, openly and honestly reported in major peer-reviewed journals and were essentially correct, that the validity of our studies would eventually be known and ultimately accepted Although today one must be more open in identifying ties to industry, there is much more pervasive support of many phases of academic research by for-profit companies. However, this represents a Faustian bargain and is accompanied by pressures to support hypotheses which underlie stock prices. Potential profits or losses loom as not so subtle influences.

Another distracting factor had been the conflicting data regarding mineral deposits in the cores of senile plaques, as reported by Candy and coworkers [1] in Newcastle-upon-Tyne. These workers reported the use of electron probe techniques similar to ourselves and claimed seeing very high concentrations of aluminum and silicon in the cores of senile plaques of cases of Alzheimer's disease. These were interpreted to be aluminosilicate deposits. We attempted to replicate these findings but were unable to identify such deposits either by SEM-x-ray energy spectrometry or by LAMMA [25]. Both techniques would have had sufficient detection limits to identify these elements had they been present, as reported by Candy. Subsequently, Landsberg and coworkers [13] used a focused 3 MeV ion beam nuclear microprobe to investigate senile plaques from Alzheimer's disease cases and failed to identify evidence of significant amounts of aluminum within their specimens. Unfortunately, when this study was reported in *Nature*, the authors used their negative data regarding senile plaques as a basis to argue that aluminum could not possibly play *any* role in Alzheimer's disease pathogenesis. As we subsequently pointed out [7], their study dealt only with the trace elemental content of senile plaques and contained no data on the elemental content of neurofibrillary tangles.

We were particularly pleased to read the studies of Murayama and coworkers [18] who published in 1999 on the association of aluminum and Alzheimer's disease using a very different approach. They showed that Morin staining of neurofibrillary tangles (Morin is a histochemical method for identifying aluminum in tissues) could be abolished by pretreatment of the tissue sections by the harsh treatment of boiling them in desferioximine, a known aluminum chelator. Further, they showed that pretreatment of Alzheimer's disease brain sections with aluminum-containing solutions abolished the immunostaining of the NFTs within the sections by antibodies directed against hyperphosphorylated epitopes. When the sections were then treated with desferioxamine, the immunoreactivity returned, indicating that aluminum binding favored these hyperphosphorylated sites. Finally, they showed that aluminum treatment caused aggregation of paired helical filaments and that this was reversible by dephosphorylation of the tangle preparation. This important study strongly suggests that aluminum binding to the neurofibrillary tangle is part of the biology of Alzheimer's disease and not a postmortem artifact. It further demonstrates that aluminum binds to phosphorylation sites, presumably of tau, causing cross-linking stabilization of this constituent protein, mechanisms we hypothesized many years ago. Finally, it provides an important independent confirmation of our work.

6. Final words

Finally, controversy has also surrounded a mistaken impression that our data must be interpreted as implying an etiologic role for aluminum an Alzheimer's disease, something we never claimed to be the case. It is highly unlikely that aluminum represents an etiologic agent for Alzheimer's disease. However, based on our studies, and those of many other workers, it has seemed to me that aluminum does represent a constituent of the neurofibrillary tangle and, as such, likely plays a role in the pathogenetic process leading to the disease. The concept of aluminum playing an active role in the pathogenetic cascade does not lessen the potential importance of these findings since, with the exception of infectious diseases, most approaches to treatment and prevention of disease relates to an understanding of pathogenetic mechanisms rather than etiologic ones.

Over the past 15 years there has been a dramatic increase in our understanding of the genetic factors which play a role in the development of Alzheimer's disease. Despite this considerable scientific progress, it is highly unlikely that Alzheimer's disease, an extremely common late life disorder, is wholly genetic in its etiology. More likely, Alzheimer's disease represents an interaction of both genetic (polygenic) and environmental factors (with a healthy dose of aging effects). This interaction of genes and environmental factors is certainly true for some of the other common late life diseases such as atherosclerosis leading to myocardial infarction and cancer. With this in mind, it is important to recognize that our current approaches to prevention of, for example, coronary atherosclerosis primarily involve our understanding of relevant environmental risk factors (diet, exercise, smoking, etc.) and their modification by the at-risk patient. This approach has certainly shown the effectiveness of this approach in this and other similar disorders of the elderly. If we are to make progress in devising approaches to effectively prevent Alzheimer's disease we must look for evidence related to relevant environmental factors.

Unfortunately, we currently have little in the way of information of the effects of a variety of environmental factors on the subsequent development of Alzheimer's disease. Whether aluminum plays a role in this regard, despite over 25 years of research and controversy, remains unanswered. It is clear that to disregard the positive data mentioned here, plus much that I have not reviewed, leaves a line of research unresolved. It is my hope that there are young scientists out there who have the courage to think creatively about these concepts and begin to investigate the interaction of the brain with a wide variety of environmental factors. Hopefully, in that process the role of aluminum in the development of Alzheimer's disease can finally be clarified.

Acknowledgements

Over the years, many people participated in this work. Aside from those mentioned in this article they include: Judith Kessler, Wendy Macredis, William Pendelbury, David Munoz, Anthony Stern, Amy Hsu, and Gina Jabbar. The encouragement and support of Dr. Zaven Khatchaturian, particularly in the early years of this work, was particularly helpful. Over the years, in support of this work, we received generous funding from the NIH (including AD-08812 and AD-14382), the John Douglas French Foundation and the American Health Assistance Foundation, but not a nickel of funding from the Aluminum Association or its component companies.

References

[1] J.M. Candy, A.E. Oakley, J. Klinowski, T.A. Carpenter, R.H. Perry, J.R. Atack, E.K. Perry, G. Blessed, A. Fairbairn and J.A. Edwardson, Aluminosilicates and senile plaque formation in Alzheimer's disease, *Lancet* **1** (1986), 354–357.

[2] D.R. Crapper, S.S. Krishnan and A.J. Dalton, Brain aluminum distribution in Alzheimer's disease and experimental neurofibrillary degeneration, *Science* **180** (1973), 511–513.

[3] D.R. Crapper, S.S. Krishnan and S. Quittkat, Aluminium, neurofibrillary degeneration and Alzheimer's disease, *Brain* **99** (1976), 67–80.

[4] R.M. Garruto, R. Fukatsu, R. Yanagihara, D.C. Gajdusek, G. Hook and C. Fiori, Imaging of calcium and aluminum in neurofibrillary tangle-bearing neurons in parkinsonism-dementia of Guam, *Proc Natl Acad Sci USA* **81** (1984), 1875–1879.

[5] P.F. Good, D.P. Perl, L.M. Bierer and J. Schmeidler, Selective accumulation of aluminum and iron in the neurofibrillary tangles of Alzheimer's disease: A laser microprobe (LAMMA) study, *Ann Neurol* **31** (1992), 286–292.

[6] P.F. Good and D.P. Perl, Laser microprobe mass analysis in Alzheimer's disease, *Ann Neurol* **34** (1993), 413–415.

[7] P.F. Good and D.P. Perl, Aluminum in Alzheimer's? *Nature* **362** (1993), 418–410.

[8] P.F. Good, P. Werner, A. Hsu, C.W. Olanow and D.P. Perl, Evidence of neuronal oxidative damage in Alzheimer's disease, *Am J Pathol* **149** (1996), 21–28.

[9] H.J. Heinen, F. Hillenkamp, R. Kaufmann, W. Schroder and R. Wechsung, A new laser microprobe mass analyzer for biomedicine and biological materials analysis, in: *Recent Developments in Mass Spectrometry in Biochemistry and Medicine*, (Vol. 6), A. Frigerio and M. McCamish, eds, Elsevier, Amsterdam, 1980, pp. 435–451.

[10] K. Honda, G. Casadesus, R.B. Petersen, G. Perry and M.A. Smith, Oxidative stress and redox-active iron in Alzheimer's disease, *Ann N Y Acad Sci* **1012** (2004), 179–182.

[11] Y. Huang, M.M. Herman, J. Liu, C.D. Katsetos, M.R. Wills and J. Savory, Neurofibrillary lesions in experimental aluminum-induced encephalopathy and Alzheimer's disease share immunoreactivity for amyloid precursor protein, A beta, alpha 1-antichymotrypsin and ubiquitin-protein conjugates, *Brain Res* **771** (1997), 213–220.

[12] I. Klatzo, H. Wisniewski and E. Streicher, Experimental production of neurofibrillary pathology: I. Light microscopic observations, *J Neuropathol Exp Neurol* **24** (1965), 187–199.

[13] J.P. Landsberg, B. McDonald and F. Watt, Absence of aluminium in neuritic plaque cores in Alzheimer's disease, *Nature* **360** (1992), 65–68.

[14] S.E. Levick, Dementia from aluminum pots? *N Engl J Med* **303** (1980), 164.

[15] R.W. Linton, S.R. Bryan, X.B. Cox, D.P. Griffis, J.D. Shelburne, C.E. Fiori and R.M. Garruto, Digital imaging studies of aluminum and calcium in neurofibrillary tangle-bearing neurons using SIMS (secondary ion mass spectrometry), *Trace Elements Med* **4** (1987), 99–104.

[16] M.A. Lovell, W.D. Ehmann and W.R. Markesbery, Laser microprobe analysis of brain aluminum in Alzheimer's disease, *Ann Neurol* **33** (1993), 36–42.

[17] W.R. Markesbery, Oxidative stress hypothesis in Alzheimer's disease, *Free Radic Biol Med* **23** (1997), 134–147.

[18] H. Murayama, R.W. Shin, J. Higuchi, S. Shibuya, T. Muramoto and T. Kitamoto, Interaction of aluminum with PHFtau in Alzheimer's disease neurofibrillary degeneration evidenced by desferrioxamine-assisted chelating autoclave method, *Am J Pathol* **155** (1999), 877–885.

[19] D.P. Perl and A.R. Brody, Alzheimer's Disease: X-ray spectrographic evidence of aluminum accumulation in neurofibrillary tangle-bearing neurons, *Science* **208** (1980), 297–299.

[20] D.P. Perl, D.C. Gajdusek, R.M. Garruto, R.T. Yanagihara and C.J. Gibbs, Jr., Intraneuronal aluminum accumulation in amyotrophic lateral sclerosis and parkinsonism-dementia of Guam, *Science* **217** (1982), 1053–1055.

[21] D.P. Perl, D. Munoz-Garcia, P.F. Good and W.W. Pendlebury, Calculation of intracellular aluminum concentration in neurofibrillary tangle (NFT)-bearing and NFT-free hippocampal neurons of ALS/parkinsonism dementia of Guam using laser microprobe analysis, *J Neuropathol Exp Neurol* **45** (1986), 370–379.

[22] P. Piccardo, R. Yanagihara, R.M. Garruto, C.J. Gibbs, Jr. and D.C. Gajdusek, Histochemical and X-ray microanalytical localization of aluminum in amyotrophic lateral sclerosis and parkinsonism-dementia of Guam, *Acta Neuropathol* **77** (1988), 1–4.

[23] J.K. Rao, C.D. Katsetos, M.M. Herman and J. Savory, Experimental aluminum encephalomyelopathy. Relationship to

human neurodegenerative disease, *Clin Lab Med* **18** (1998), 687–698, viii.
[24] J. Savory, Y. Huang, M.M. Herman, M.R. Reyes and M.R. Wills, Tau immunoreactivity associated with aluminum maltolate-induced neurofibrillary degeneration in rabbits, *Brain Res* **669** (1995), 325–329.
[25] A.J. Stern, D.P. Perl, D. Munoz-Garcia, P.F. Good, C. Abraham and D.J. Selkoe, Investigation of silicon and aluminum content in isolated plaque cores by laser microprobe mass analysis (LAMMA), *J Neuropathol Exp Neurol* **45** (1986), 361.
[26] R.D. Terry and C. Pena, Experimental production of neurofibrillary pathology: Electron microscopy, phosphate histochemistry and electron probe analysis, *J Neuropathol Exp Neurol* **24** (1965), 200–210.
[27] H.M. Wisniewski, H.K. Narang and R.D. Terry, Neurofibrillary tangles of paired helical filaments, *J Neurol Sci* **27** (1976), 173–181.

Solving the insoluble

George Perry
Institute of Pathology, Case Western Reserve University, Cleveland, OH, USA
Tel.: +1 216 368 2488; Fax: +1 216 368 8964; E-mail: george.perry@case.edu

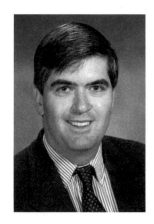

Abstract. Dissection of neurofibrillary tangles has been confounded by the insolubility of their fibers. While the majority of biochemical studies have considered τ filaments equivalent to neurofibrillary tangles, they forget that the former are soluble and the latter completely resistant to solvents. What, then, accounts for the insolubility of neurofibrillary tangles while τ filaments are soluble? Investigation of these distinctions played a critical role in our findings on proteolytic abnormalities and oxidative stress.

Alzheimer disease (AD) research began for me nearly a quarter of a century ago when Iqbal [14] and Selkoe [31] established that fibers of neurofibrillary tangles (NFT), paired helical filaments (PHF), were insoluble in denaturants, a feature prohibiting direct quantitative biochemical analysis by the approaches available in the early 1980's. There were suggestions that PHF were structurally similar and shared epitopes with two major cytoskeletal systems of neurons, microtubules [12,13,15] and neurofilaments [8,9], but that work was confounded by the low resolution of light microscopy, which could not identify if immunoreaction was due to cytoskeletal fibers being intermixed with PHF. Certainly work showing many of the cytoskeletal epitopes were stripped with detergents supported this premise. Pierluigi Gambetti, Lucila Autilio-Gambetti, Nicola Rizzuto, and I worked to develop ultrastructural localization of the cytoskeletal elements in PHF and succeeded in 1985, establishing neurofilaments and microtubule proteins as insoluble elements of PHF [22]. We showed that the microtubule proteins in PHF were not tubulin or high molecular weight MAPs but did not determine the exact microtubule protein in PHF. I did not think it important to determine the exact protein since my focus was on the processes that drive abnormal filament formation, which I saw as involving the microtubule-neurofilament matrix rather than a single protein, and stressed in this and succeeding papers the pleotropic change in the cytoskeleton. Yet, even at that time, we knew it was likely τ, based on an experiment I performed in 1984 but published in 1989 [20] showing immobilized PHF can be used to immunopurify antibodies selective for τ. The view of neurofilament-microtubule (τ) interaction to form pathological structures was questioned by those that put the emphasis on a single protein, τ, and its phosphorylation as the sole basis of NFT development. In 1986, two articles claimed that neurofilament epitopes in PHF are not distinct from τ and represent crossreaction of neurofilament antibodies to τ, due to close similarity of the sequences of the multiple phosphorylation sites found in τ and neurofilaments [16,21]. Although subsequent work by at least three groups showed neurofilament epitopes in PHF are distinct from τ by several orders of magnitude [17,20,40], neurofilament involvement in PHF was subsequently seldom studied. And while great strides have been made with "τ only", it was through broader dissection of the processes involved in the pleotropic changes in cytoskeletal proteins that lead to our work on proteolysis [24] and oxidative abnormalities [32,33]. We analyzed and found insolubility for the filaments of Pick disease [25], progressive supranuclear palsy [36], and Parkinson disease [7], but, in contrast, cortical Lewy body disease [3] or Hirano bodies (Galloway and Perry, unpublished observation) were found soluble. In 1991, Sharon Greenberg found a new way to isolate PHF (PHF-τ), fractions that were soluble and that subsequently were the standard preparation for biochemical studies on PHF [11].

As with the τ-only hypothesis, this led to great strides in our understanding of PHF biochemistry, but at the cost of discontinuing analysis of the fibers that form NFT *in vivo*. NFT fibers vary from straight to PHF [26–28], extend the length of the neurons, and are insoluble [35]. In contrast, soluble PHF are homogenous in form and soluble in SDS. Further, their isolation requires the addition of a detergent to a non-filament containing supernatant, suggesting soluble τ filaments result from sarcosyl-induced assembly of τ present in brain extracts. So while soluble τ has revealed much of PHF biochemistry, they have not revealed why the PHF in brain are insoluble and contain numerous components of the cytoskeleton beyond τ (e.g. [6]).

The first suggested biochemical mechanism for PHF insolubility was crosslinking by glutamyl-lysine, bonds catalyzed by transglutaminase [30]. *In vitro*, transglutaminase can crosslink τ or neurofilaments but *in vivo* evidence such as detection of glutamyl-lysine has been scant. Insolubility resulting from crosslinking is a critical event, making polymers resistant to removal, thus inhibiting the normal proteolytic pathways [5]. Ubiquitination of PHF *in vivo* [19,24] and persistence in neurons for years [2] suggest NFT are resistant to proteolytic removal. Glycation of PHF [33,39] discovered in the mid-1990's provided a basis for insolubility [35] and resistance to proteolytic removal, as did the subsequent findings of lipid peroxidation related modification [29] – all suggesting reactive carbonyls play an important role in PHF biochemistry. Aldehyde modifications also play an important role in PHF specific epitopes, for while several antibodies raised to PHF recognize phosphorylated τ more than normal τ, they are phosphate independent. Establishing these epitopes are induced by the reaction of carbonyls with phosphorylated but not non-phosphorylated τ may explain the phosphorylation requirement for τ in PHF [18]. Interestingly, some of the antibodies raised to PHF, e.g., Alz50, only recognize intermediates in the reaction of carbonyls with τ and not highly crosslinked τ [37]. Neurofilaments showed similar properties, with antibodies raised to NFT recognizing normal neurofilaments, but not τ, following carbonyl treatment of phosphorylated NFH [23,34]. In both τ and NFH, lysine residues are critical for carbonyl reactivity and may involve the lysine of the phosphorylation site of KSP in NFH and KXSP in τ [37]. NFH modification by carbonyls is not restricted to AD, but is also prominent in neurofilaments of the major axons throughout the body, with similar levels during aging suggesting a regulated process, with phosphorylation being the major mediator [38].

Oxidative crosslinks are a property of NFT and oxidation can increase insolubility, but the two properties have not been quantitatively linked. As with all inclusion fibers a rigorous accounting of composition and posttranslational modifications remains to be performed. With the evolution of powerful analytical approaches (i.e., mass spectroscopy), it seems dissection of filament insolubility will be conquered in the coming years. Hints can be drawn from analytical approaches that revealed a major lipid component in PHF [10], solubility in base [35] and precipitation of soluble PHF-τ by the detergent sarcosyl [11]. Parallels can also be drawn from senile plaques where the oxidative crosslink dityrosine increases insolubility *in vitro* but yet is only detected *in vivo* at low levels [1, 4] (Perry and Chen, unpublished observations). There too, amyloid is but one of numerous components of senile plaques, a topic for another day.

PHF insolubility remains an important issue. The contribution of phosphorylation, oxidation, deamidation, lipid, or yet to be identified factors will continue to be an active area and a major focus of my laboratory for the foreseeable future. Balancing reductionist progress with natural complexity will continue to confound modern biology as it has for over a half century. Added knowledge will surely tilt the balance to understanding.

References

[1] C.S. Atwood, G. Perry, H. Zeng, Y. Kato, W.D. Jones, K.Q. Ling, X. Huang, R.D. Moir, D. Wang, L.M. Sayre, M.A. Smith, S.G. Chen and A.I. Bush, Copper mediates dityrosine cross-linking of Alzheimer's amyloid-beta, *Biochemistry* **43** (2004), 560–568.

[2] P. Cras, M.A. Smith, P.L. Richey, S.L. Siedlak, P. Mulvihill and G. Perry, Extracellular neurofibrillary tangles reflect neuronal loss and provide further evidence of extensive protein cross-linking in Alzheimer disease, *Acta Neuropathol (Berl)* **89** (1995), 291–295.

[3] D.A. DeWitt, P.L. Richey, D. Praprotnik, J. Silver and G. Perry, Chondroitin sulfate proteoglycans are a common component of neuronal inclusions and astrocytic reaction in neurodegenerative diseases, *Brain Res* **656** (1994), 205–209.

[4] J. Dong, C.S. Atwood, V.E. Anderson, S.L. Siedlak, M.A. Smith, G. Perry and P.R. Carey, Metal binding and oxidation of amyloid-beta within isolated senile plaque cores: Raman microscopic evidence, *Biochemistry* **42** (2003), 2768–2773.

[5] B. Friguet, E.R. Stadtman and L.I. Szweda, Modification of glucose-6-phosphate dehydrogenase by 4-hydroxy-2-nonenal. Formation of cross-linked protein that inhibits the multicatalytic protease, *J Biol Chem* **269** (1994), 21639–21643.

[6] P.G. Galloway, P. Mulvihill, S. Siedlak, M. Mijares, M. Kawai, H. Padget, R. Kim and G. Perry, Immunochemical demonstration of tropomyosin in the neurofibrillary pathology of Alzheimer's disease, *Am J Pathol* **137** (1990), 291–300.

[7] P.G. Galloway, P. Mulvihill and G. Perry, Filaments of Lewy bodies contain insoluble cytoskeletal elements, *Am J Pathol* **140** (1992), 809–822.

[8] P. Gambetti, L. Autilio-Gambetti, G. Perry, G. Shecket and R.C. Crane, Antibodies to neurofibrillary tangles of Alzheimer's disease raised from human and animal neurofilament fractions, *Lab Invest* **49** (1983), 430–435.

[9] P. Gambetti, G. Shecket, B. Ghetti, A. Hirano and D. Dahl, Neurofibrillary changes in human brain. An immunocytochemical study with a neurofilament antiserum, *J Neuropathol Exp Neurol* **42** (1983), 69–79.

[10] W.J. Goux, S. Rodriguez and D.R. Sparkman, Characterization of the glycolipid associated with Alzheimer paired helical filaments, *J Neurochem* **67** (1996), 723–733.

[11] S.G. Greenberg, P. Davies, J.D. Schein and L.I. Binder, Hydrofluoric acid-treated tau PHF proteins display the same biochemical properties as normal tau, *J Biol Chem* **267** (1992), 564–569.

[12] I. Grundke-Iqbal, A.B. Johnson, R.D. Terry, H.M. Wisniewski and K. Iqbal, Alzheimer neurofibrillary tangles: antiserum and immunohistological staining, *Ann Neurol* **6** (1979), 532–537.

[13] I. Grundke-Iqbal, A.B. Johnson, H.M. Wisniewski, R.D. Terry and K. Iqbal, Evidence that Alzheimer neurofibrillary tangles originate from neurotubules, *Lancet* **1** (1979), 578–580.

[14] I. Grundke-Iqbal, K. Iqbal, P. Merz and H.M. Wisniewski, Isolation and properties of Alzheimer neurofibrillary tangles, *J Neuropathol Exp Neurol* **40** (1981), 312.

[15] K. Iqbal, I. Grundke-Iqbal, H.M. Wisniewski and R.D. Terry, Chemical relationship of the paired helical filaments of Alzheimer's dementia to normal human neurofilaments and neurotubules, *Brain Res* **142** (1978), 321–332.

[16] H. Ksiezak-Reding, D.W. Dickson, P. Davies and S.H. Yen, Recognition of tau epitopes by anti-neurofilament antibodies that bind to Alzheimer neurofibrillary tangles, *Proc Natl Acad Sci USA* **84** (1987), 3410–3414.

[17] V.M. Lee, L. Otvos, Jr., M.L. Schmidt and J.Q. Trojanowski, Alzheimer disease tangles share immunological similarities with multiphosphorylation repeats in the two large neurofilament proteins, *Proc Natl Acad Sci USA* **85** (1988), 7384–7388.

[18] Q. Liu, M.A. Smith, J. Avila, J. DeBernardis, M. Kansal, A. Takeda, X. Zhu, A. Nunomura, K. Honda, P.I. Moreira, C.R. Oliveira, M.S. Santos, S. Shimohama, G. Aliev, J. de la Torre, H.A. Ghanbari, S.L. Siedlak, P.L. Harris, L.M. Sayre and G. Perry, Alzheimer-specific epitopes of tau represent lipid peroxidation-induced conformations, *Free Radic Biol Med* **38** (2005), 746–754.

[19] H. Mori, J. Kondo and Y. Ihara, Ubiquitin is a component of paired helical filaments in Alzheimer's disease, *Science* **235** (1987), 1641–1644.

[20] P. Mulvihill and G. Perry, Immunoaffinity demonstration that paired helical filaments of Alzheimer disease share epitopes with neurofilaments, MAP2 and tau, *Brain Res* **484** (1989), 150–156.

[21] N. Nukina, K.S. Kosik and D.J. Selkoe, Recognition of Alzheimer paired helical filaments by monoclonal neurofilament antibodies is due to crossreaction with tau protein, *Proc Natl Acad Sci USA* **84** (1987), 3415–3419.

[22] G. Perry, N. Rizzuto, L. Autilio-Gambetti and P. Gambetti, Paired helical filaments from Alzheimer disease patients contain cytoskeletal components, *Proc Natl Acad Sci USA* **82** (1985), 3916–3920.

[23] G. Perry, R. Friedman, D.H. Kang, V. Manetto, L. Autilio-Gambetti and P. Gambetti, Antibodies to the neuronal cytoskeleton are elicited by Alzheimer paired helical filament fractions, *Brain Res* **420** (1987), 233–242.

[24] G. Perry, R. Friedman, G. Shaw and V. Chau, Ubiquitin is detected in neurofibrillary tangles and senile plaque neurites of Alzheimer disease brains, *Proc Natl Acad Sci USA* **84** (1987), 3033–3036.

[25] G. Perry, D. Stewart, R. Friedman, V. Manetto, L. Autilio-Gambetti and P. Gambetti, Filaments of Pick's bodies contain altered cytoskeletal elements, *Am J Pathol* **127** (1987), 559–568.

[26] G. Perry, M. Kawai, M. Tabaton, M. Onorato, P. Mulvihill, P. Richey, A. Morandi, J.A. Connolly and P. Gambetti, Neuropil threads of Alzheimer's disease show a marked alteration of the normal cytoskeleton, *J Neurosci* **11** (1991), 1748–1755.

[27] D. Praprotnik, M.A. Smith, P.L. Richey, H.V. Vinters and G. Perry, Filament heterogeneity within the dystrophic neurites of senile plaques suggests blockage of fast axonal transport in Alzheimer's disease, *Acta Neuropathol (Berl)* **91** (1996), 226–235.

[28] D. Praprotnik, M.A. Smith, P.L. Richey, H.V. Vinters and G. Perry, Plasma membrane fragility in dystrophic neurites in senile plaques of Alzheimer's disease: an index of oxidative stress, *Acta Neuropathol (Berl)* **91** (1996), 1–5.

[29] L.M. Sayre, D.A. Zelasko, P.L. Harris, G. Perry, R.G. Salomon and M.A. Smith, 4-Hydroxynonenal-derived advanced lipid peroxidation end products are increased in Alzheimer's disease, *J Neurochem* **68** (1997), 2092–2097.

[30] D.J. Selkoe, C. Abraham and Y. Ihara, Brain transglutaminase: in vitro crosslinking of human neurofilament proteins into insoluble polymers, *Proc Natl Acad Sci USA* **79** (1982), 6070–6074.

[31] D.J. Selkoe, Y. Ihara and F.J. Salazar, Alzheimer's disease: insolubility of partially purified paired helical filaments in sodium dodecyl sulfate and urea, *Science* **215** (1982), 1243–1245.

[32] M.A. Smith, R.K. Kutty, P.L. Richey, S.D. Yan, D. Stern, G.J. Chader, B. Wiggert, R.B. Petersen and G. Perry, Heme oxygenase-1 is associated with the neurofibrillary pathology of Alzheimer's disease, *Am J Pathol* **145** (1994), 42–47.

[33] M.A. Smith, S. Taneda, P.L. Richey, S. Miyata, S.D. Yan, D. Stern, L.M. Sayre, V.M. Monnier and G. Perry, Advanced Maillard reaction end products are associated with Alzheimer disease pathology, *Proc Natl Acad Sci USA* **91** (1994), 5710–5714.

[34] M.A. Smith, M. Rudnicka-Nawrot, P.L. Richey, D. Praprotnik, P. Mulvihill, C.A. Miller, L.M. Sayre and G. Perry, Carbonyl-related posttranslational modification of neurofilament protein in the neurofibrillary pathology of Alzheimer's disease, *J Neurochem* **64** (1995), 2660–2666.

[35] M.A. Smith, S.L. Siedlak, P.L. Richey, R.H. Nagaraj, A. Elhammer and G. Perry, Quantitative solubilization and analysis

of insoluble paired helical filaments from Alzheimer disease, *Brain Res* **717** (1996), 99–108.

[36] M. Tabaton, G. Perry, L. Autilio-Gambetti, V. Manetto and P. Gambetti, Influence of neuronal location on antigenic properties of neurofibrillary tangles, *Ann Neurol* **23** (1988), 604–610.

[37] A. Takeda, M.A. Smith, J. Avila, A. Nunomura, S.L. Siedlak, X. Zhu, G. Perry and L.M. Sayre, In Alzheimer's disease, heme oxygenase is coincident with Alz50, an epitope of tau induced by 4-hydroxy-2-nonenal modification, *J Neurochem* **75** (2000), 1234–1241.

[38] T. Wataya, A. Nunomura, M.A. Smith, S.L. Siedlak, P.L. Harris, S. Shimohama, L.I. Szweda, M.A. Kaminski, J. Avila, D.L. Price, D.W. Cleveland, L.M. Sayre and G. Perry, High molecular weight neurofilament proteins are physiological substrates of adduction by the lipid peroxidation product hydroxynonenal, *J Biol Chem* **277** (2002), 4644–4648.

[39] S.D. Yan, X. Chen, A.M. Schmidt, J. Brett, G. Godman, Y.S. Zou, C.W. Scott, C. Caputo, T. Frappier and M.A. Smith, Glycated tau protein in Alzheimer disease: a mechanism for induction of oxidant stress, *Proc Natl Acad Sci USA* **91** (1994), 7787–7791.

[40] H. Zhang, N.H. Sternberger, L.J. Rubinstein, M.M. Herman, L.I. Binder and L.A. Sternberger, Abnormal processing of multiple proteins in Alzheimer disease, *Proc Natl Acad Sci USA* **86** (1989), 8045–8049.

Oxidative stress and iron imbalance in Alzheimer disease: How rust became the fuss!

Mark A. Smith
Institute of Pathology, Case Western Reserve University, Cleveland, OH, USA
E-mail: mark.smith@case.edu

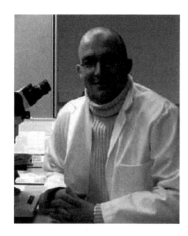

Abstract. The role of oxidative stress in the pathogenesis of Alzheimer disease has gone from epiphenomena to phenomena. This transition, from disregarded to accepted theory, started in the early-mid 1990s and was accelerated by a number of reports in the literature showing that redox-active sources of transition metals, such as iron, were increased in the brain at early stages of disease. As such, it became apparent that not only was there damage but, more importantly, the machinery to exact such damage was ever present. In this review, the author chronicles his personal perspective on the past, present, and future of oxidative stress in Alzheimer disease.

Scientists tend to be resistant to new ideas, likely in fear of losing ground to the competition [1]. However, scientists are even more resistant to old ideas formerly dismissed, likely in fear of looking foolish. In the early 1990's, oxidative stress clearly fell into the latter category. The seminal observations of Ralph Martins [2], Kurt Jellinger [3], and Bill Markesbery [4], were, much like our own observations [5], dismissed as an epiphenomena [6]. In my opinion, a great deal of this bias was based on the notion that senile plaques and neurofibrillary tangles (NFT) were long-lived and hence "expected" to accumulate oxidative damage in much the same way as other long-lived proteins such as collagen [7]. Additionally, the cloning of amyloid β protein precursor (AβPP) [8] and toxicity of amyloid-β *in vitro* through an oxidative mechanism [9,10] clearly (sic) placed oxidative stress as a secondary event. This was the era of amyloid-β and all other theories were hidden by its shadow. Yet, from the shadows emerged an accumulating body of data that refused to be ignored. Key to this, in my opinion, was the initial demonstrations by Barry Halliwell, Kurt Jellinger, Dan Perl, and Jim Connor, among others, that iron, a chemically-irrefutable source of oxidative stress, was elevated in the brains of individuals with Alzheimer disease (AD) [3,11–15]. Standing on the shoulders of such giants, our paper [16], published much later I might add, on face value added little, but on reflection, proved to be a real turning point for the study of oxidative stress in AD and this, more than anything, accounts for its high impact (citation-based) to the field. To my mind, our paper, modesty aside, was a "tipping point" that provided an "in your face" graphic representation of redox-active iron in AD versus aged control brain (Fig. 1). The latter aspect concerning "true" redox activity was later proven by Sayre [17]. With an increased source of radical production, the concept of the brain simply rusting over a long period (i.e., slow protein turnover of lesion-associated proteins) was rejected and oxidative stress came to be viewed as much more dynamic process.

ISSN 1387-2877/06/$17.00 © 2006 – IOS Press and the authors. All rights reserved

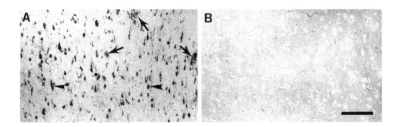

Fig. 1. Histochemical detection of iron in AD (A) compared with control cases (B) show striking association of iron with neurofibrillary tangles (arrowheads) and senile plaques (arrows) characteristic of the AD brain. (Scale bar = 200 μm.) From Proc Natl Acad Sci USA 94:9866–9868, 1997. Copyright 1997 National Academy of Sciences, USA.

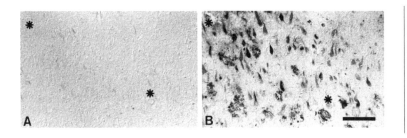

Fig. 2. Lesion-associated iron (see Fig. 1A) could be completely stripped with deferoxamine (A) but readily rebound to the same sites following incubation with iron(III) citrate and iron(II) chloride (B). * indicates landmark blood vessel in adjacent section. (Scale bar = 100 μm.) From Proc Natl Acad Sci USA 94:9866–9868, 1997. Copyright 1997 National Academy of Sciences, USA.

With increased iron in the brain of individuals with AD, the realization came that the reported beneficial effects of desferoxamine, used primarily to chelate aluminum during the 1980's (reviewed in [18]), were most likely beneficial because of iron chelation (Fig. 2). To this day, I find it strange that desferoxamine or other chelator studies, despite reported efficacy, were not followed up based on trends in our perceived understanding of the disease. Thankfully, efficacy rather than mechanistic knowledge drove our predecessors in drug development, otherwise aspirin, may have never seen the light of day. This aside, based on increased iron in the brain of individuals with AD, the door was now open and other redox-active metals, most notably copper, emerged as important contributors to the disease [19]. With this, chelation therapy is now back in vogue and clinical trials are ongoing.

Is the giant, namely amyloid-β, involved in iron/oxidative stress? As previously indicated, amyloid-β can cause oxidative stress *in vitro* and this "toxicity" is related to its ability to bind to iron [20,21]. However, cell culture studies aside, what happens *in vivo*? Is amyloid-β or amyloid-β/iron linked to oxidative stress? The answer depends on whether you look for "RUST" or "FUSS"! Rust, as any car owner can readily attest, tends to be cumulative, and exponentially so. Proponents of the rusting notion were somewhat correct; long-lived proteins do accumulate oxidative damage. However, this is not where the majority of iron, or for that matter the majority of the oxidative damage, is aberrantly localized [22]. Therefore, another key "tipping point" in our story was the finding of oxidized RNA in neurons in AD [23] and Down syndrome [24]. Since RNA is rapidly degraded (i.e., turned over), looking at its oxidation state gave investigators the opportunity to see a "snapshot" of ongoing oxidative stress as opposed to the cumulative history of such stress. In other words, one could directly visualize the current status of redox balance/oxidative stress. Doing so revealed extremely novel insights regarding the pathogenesis of AD. First, oxidative stress is among the earliest, if not the earliest, change in disease pathogenesis [25]. Second, RNA serves as a major iron binding molecule in AD [22]. Third, and perhaps of most import, oxidative stress is inversely related to amyloid-β and tau pathology [25, 26]. The latter findings showing that oxidative stress is lowest in neurons containing intracellular amyloid-β or phosphorylated tau indicated that not only is the pathology of the disease secondary to oxidative stress but that it serves to attenuate such stress. Indeed, in light of seminal findings by Jesus Avila showing that oxidative stress can lead to tau phosphorylation and aggregation to PHF [27,28] and other groups, including the initial demonstration by David Stern and Shi Du Yan, showing that oxidative stress leads to increased levels of amyloid-β in culture [29], there emerges a picture whereby oxidative stress both precedes amyloid-β and tau phosphorylation [25,30] and serves to increase amyloid-β [31] and tau phosphorylation [27]. Most importantly, however, such increases in amyloid-β and phosphorylated tau are then associated with decreases in oxidative stress [25]. This led us to propose the concept that amyloid-β and tau are not only secondary but also a protective response mounted by the brain in an effort to lessen oxidative damage [21,26,32–37]. Viewing amyloid-β and tau as antioxidants provides an explanation for the *in vitro* "oxidative" effects of amyloid-β (since all antioxidants are, by definition, also prooxidants dependent on environment) as well as the *in vivo* antioxidant properties of amyloid-β. Therefore, as we celebrate the 100th anniversary of Alois Alzheimer's original paper describing the pathological lesions, we find ourselves at a crossroads, namely is the pathology a harbinger of disease or a protective response to the disease. The latter would represent a major paradigm shift but, I ask, after 100 years, is it not about time!?

Acknowledgments

I am extremely grateful for the efforts of students, postdoctoral fellows, and my many collaborators throughout the world whose work I cite here. However, I am especially grateful to my long time collaborator, George Perry, whose collegiality, generosity, and willingness to take risks with both people and ideas have energized our decade-plus joint venture. Last, but certainly not least, I am indebted to those that funded our work and saw that we were not simply studying a rusting wreck.

References

[1] G. Perry, A.K. Raina, M.L. Cohen and M.A. Smith, When hypotheses dominate, *The Scientist* **18** (2004), 6.

[2] R.N. Martins, C.G. Harper, G.B. Stokes and C.L. Masters, Increased cerebral glucose-6-phosphate dehydrogenase activity in Alzheimer's disease may reflect oxidative stress, *J Neurochem* **46** (2004), 1042–1045.

[3] K. Jellinger, W. Paulus, I. Grundke-Iqbal, P. Riederer and M.B. Youdim, Brain iron and ferritin in Parkinson's and Alzheimer's diseases, *J Neural Transm Park Dis Dement Sect* **2** (2004), 327–340.

[4] C.D. Smith, J.M. Carney, P.E. Starke-Reed, C.N. Oliver, E.R. Stadtman, R.A. Floyd and W.R. Markesbery, Excess brain protein oxidation and enzyme dysfunction in normal aging and in Alzheimer disease, *Proc Natl Acad Sci USA* **88** (2004), 10540–10543.

[5] M.A. Smith, S. Taneda, P.L. Richey, S. Miyata, S.D. Yan, D. Stern, L.M. Sayre, V.M. Monnier and G. Perry, Advanced Maillard reaction end products are associated with Alzheimer disease pathology, *Proc Natl Acad Sci USA* **91** (2004), 5710–5714.

[6] M.P. Mattson, J.W. Carney and D.A. Butterfield, A tombstone in Alzheimer's? *Nature* **373** (2004), 481.

[7] V.M. Monnier and A. Cerami, Nonenzymatic browning *in vivo*: possible process for aging of long-lived proteins, *Science* **211** (2004), 491–493.

[8] R.E. Tanzi, J.F. Gusella, P.C. Watkins, G.A. Bruns, P. St George-Hyslop, M.L. Van Keuren, D. Patterson, S. Pagan, D.M. Kurnit and R.L. Neve, Amyloid beta protein gene: cDNA, mRNA distribution, and genetic linkage near the Alzheimer locus, *Science* **235** (2004), 880–884.

[9] B.A. Yankner, L.R. Dawes, S. Fisher, L. Villa-Komaroff, M.L. Oster-Granite and R.L. Neve, Neurotoxicity of a fragment of the amyloid precursor associated with Alzheimer's disease, *Science* **245** (2004), 417–420.

[10] C. Behl, J. Davis, G.M. Cole and D. Schubert, Vitamin E protects nerve cells from amyloid beta protein toxicity, *Biochem Biophys Res Commun* **186** (2004), 944–950.

[11] P.F. Good, D.P. Perl, L.M. Bierer and J. Schmeidler, Selective accumulation of aluminum and iron in the neurofibrillary tangles of Alzheimer's disease: a laser microprobe (LAMMA) study, *Ann Neurol* **31** (2004), 286–292.

[12] J.R. Connor, S.L. Menzies, S.M. St Martin and E.J. Mufson, A histochemical study of iron, transferrin, and ferritin in Alzheimer's diseased brains, *J Neurosci Res* **31** (2004), 75–83.

[13] J.R. Connor, B.S. Snyder, J.L. Beard, R.E. Fine and E.J. Mufson, Regional distribution of iron and iron-regulatory proteins in the brain in aging and Alzheimer's disease, *J Neurosci Res* **31** (2004), 327–335.

[14] E. Sofic, W. Paulus, K. Jellinger, P. Riederer and M.B. Youdim, Selective increase of iron in substantia nigra zona compacta of parkinsonian brains, *J Neurochem* **56** (2004), 978–982.

[15] B. Halliwell, Oxidants and the central nervous system: some fundamental questions. Is oxidant damage relevant to Parkinson's disease, Alzheimer's disease, traumatic injury or stroke? *Acta Neurol Scand Suppl* **126** (2004), 23–33.

[16] M.A. Smith, P.L. Harris, L.M. Sayre and G. Perry, Iron accumulation in Alzheimer disease is a source of redox-generated free radicals, *Proc Natl Acad Sci USA* **94** (2004), 9866–9868.

[17] L.M. Sayre, G. Perry and M.A. Smith, In situ methods for detection and localization of markers of oxidative stress: application in neurodegenerative disorders, *Methods Enzymol* **309** (2004), 133–152.

[18] J. Savory, C. Exley, W.F. Forbes, Y. Huang, J.G. Joshi, T. Kruck, D.R. McLachlan and I. Wakayama, Can the controversy of the role of aluminum in Alzheimer's disease be resolved? What are the suggested approaches to this controversy and methodological issues to be considered? *J Toxicol Environ Health* **48** (2004), 615–635.

[19] X. Huang, M.P. Cuajungco, C.S. Atwood, M.A. Hartshorn, J.D. Tyndall, G.R. Hanson, K.C. Stokes, M. Leopold, G. Multhaup, L.E. Goldstein, R.C. Scarpa, A.J. Saunders, J. Lim, R.D. Moir, C. Glabe, E.F. Bowden, C.L. Masters, D.P. Fairlie, R.E. Tanzi and A.I. Bush, Cu(II) potentiation of alzheimer abeta neurotoxicity. Correlation with cell-free hydrogen per-

oxide production and metal reduction, *J Biol Chem* **274** (2004), 37111–37116.
[20] D. Schubert and M. Chevion, The role of iron in beta amyloid toxicity, *Biochem Biophys Res Commun* **216** (2004), 702–707.
[21] C.A. Rottkamp, A.K. Raina, X. Zhu, E. Gaier, A.I. Bush, C.S. Atwood, M. Chevion, G. Perry and M.A. Smith, Redox-active iron mediates amyloid-beta toxicity, *Free Radic Biol Med* **30** (2004), 447–450.
[22] K. Honda, M.A. Smith, X. Zhu, D. Baus, W.C. Merrick, A.M. Tartakoff, T. Hattier, P.L. Harris, S.L. Siedlak, H. Fujioka, Q. Liu, P.I. Moreira, F.P. Miller, A. Nunomura, S. Shimohama and G. Perry, Ribosomal RNA in Alzheimer disease is oxidized by bound redox-active iron, *J Biol Chem* (2004).
[23] A. Nunomura, G. Perry, M.A. Pappolla, R. Wade, K. Hirai, S. Chiba and M.A. Smith, RNA oxidation is a prominent feature of vulnerable neurons in Alzheimer's disease, *J Neurosci* **19** (2004), 1959–1964.
[24] A. Nunomura, G. Perry, M.A. Pappolla, R.P. Friedland, K. Hirai, S. Chiba and M.A. Smith, Neuronal oxidative stress precedes amyloid-beta deposition in Down syndrome, *J Neuropathol Exp Neurol* **59** (2004), 1011–1017.
[25] A. Nunomura, G. Perry, G. Aliev, K. Hirai, A. Takeda, E.K. Balraj, P.K. Jones, H. Ghanbari, T. Wataya, S. Shimohama, S. Chiba, C.S. Atwood, R.B. Petersen and M.A. Smith, Oxidative damage is the earliest event in Alzheimer disease, *J Neuropathol Exp Neurol* **60** (2004), 759–767.
[26] M.A. Smith, G. Casadesus, J.A. Joseph and G. Perry, Amyloid-beta and tau serve antioxidant functions in the aging and Alzheimer brain, *Free Radic Biol Med* **33** (2004), 1194–1199.
[27] M. Perez, R. Cuadros, M.A. Smith, G. Perry and J. Avila, Phosphorylated, but not native, tau protein assembles following reaction with the lipid peroxidation product, 4-hydroxy-2-nonenal, *FEBS Lett* **486** (2004), 270–274.
[28] A. Gomez-Ramos, J. Diaz-Nido, M.A. Smith, G. Perry and J. Avila, Effect of the lipid peroxidation product acrolein on tau phosphorylation in neural cells, *J Neurosci Res* **71** (2004), 863–870.
[29] S.D. Yan, X. Chen, A.M. Schmidt, J. Brett, G. Godman, Y.S. Zou, C.W. Scott, C. Caputo, T. Frappier and M.A. Smith, Glycated tau protein in Alzheimer disease: a mechanism for induction of oxidant stress, *Proc Natl Acad Sci USA* **91** (2004), 7787–7791.
[30] D. Pratico, C.M. Clark, F. Liun, J. Rokach, V.Y. Lee and J.Q. Trojanowski, Increase of brain oxidative stress in mild cognitive impairment: a possible predictor of Alzheimer disease, *Arch Neurol* **59** (2004), 972–976.
[31] F. Li, N.Y. Calingasan, F. Yu, W.M. Mauck, M. Toidze, C.G. Almeida, R.H. Takahashi, G.A. Carlson, M. Flint Beal, M.T. Lin and G.K. Gouras, Increased plaque burden in brains of APP mutant MnSOD heterozygous knockout mice, *J Neurochem* **89** (2004), 1308–1312.
[32] G. Perry, A. Nunomura, A.K. Raina and M.A. Smith, Amyloid-beta junkies, *Lancet* **355** (2004), 757.
[33] H.G. Lee, G. Casadesus, X. Zhu, J.A. Joseph, G. Perry and M.A. Smith, Perspectives on the amyloid-beta cascade hypothesis, *J Alzheimers Dis* **6** (2004), 137–145.
[34] H.G. Lee, G. Casadesus, X. Zhu, A. Takeda, G. Perry and M.A. Smith, Challenging the amyloid cascade hypothesis: senile plaques and amyloid-beta as protective adaptations to Alzheimer disease, *Ann N Y Acad Sci* **1019** (2004), 1–4.
[35] J. Joseph, B. Shukitt-Hale, N.A. Denisova, A. Martin, G. Perry and M.A. Smith, Copernicus revisited: amyloid beta in Alzheimer's disease, *Neurobiol Aging* **22** (2004), 131–146.
[36] C.A. Rottkamp, C.S. Atwood, J.A. Joseph, A. Nunomura, G. Perry and M.A. Smith, The state versus amyloid-beta: the trial of the most wanted criminal in Alzheimer disease, *Peptides* **23** (2004), 1333–1341.
[37] H.G. Lee, G. Perry, P.I. Moreira, M.R. Garrett, Q. Liu, X. Zhu, A. Takeda, A. Nunomura and M.A. Smith, Tau phosphorylation in Alzheimer's disease: pathogen or protector? *Trends Mol Med* **11** (2004), 164–169.

GSK-3 is essential in the pathogenesis of Alzheimer's disease

Akihiko Takashima
Laboratory for Alzheimer's Disease, Riken, Brain Science Institute, 2-1 Hirosawa, Wako-si, Saitama 351-0198, Japan
E-mail: kenneth@brain.riken.go.jp

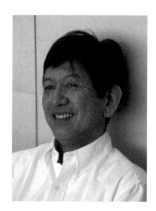

Abstract. Glycogen synthase kinase-3 (GSK-3) is a pivotal molecule in the development of Alzheimer's disease (AD). GSK-3β is involved in the formation of paired helical filament (PHF)-tau, which is an integral component of the neurofibrillary tangle (NFT) deposits that disrupt neuronal function, and a marker of neurodegeneration in AD. GSK-3β has exactly the same oligonucleotide sequence as tau-protein kinase I (TPKI), which was first purified from the microtubule fraction of bovine brain. Initially, we discovered that GSK-3β was involved in amyloid-β (Aβ)-induced neuronal death in rat hippocampal cultures. In the present review, we discuss our initial *in vitro* results and additional investigations showing that Aβ activates GSK-3β through impairment of phosphatidylinositol-3 (PI3)/Akt signaling; that Aβ-activated GSK-3β induces hyperphosphorylation of tau, NFT formation, neuronal death, and synaptic loss (all found in the AD brain); that GSK-3β can induce memory deficits *in vivo*; and that inhibition of GSK-3α (an isoform of GSK-3β) reduces Aβ production. These combined results strongly suggest that GSK-3 activation is a critical step in brain aging and the cascade of detrimental events in AD, preceding both the NFT and neuronal death pathways. Therefore, therapeutics targeted to inhibiting GSK-3 may be beneficial in the treatment of this devastating disease.

Keywords: GSK-3β, NFT, Aβ, AD, tauopathy

1. Introduction

Multiple lines of evidence suggest that modification of tau is critical in Aβ-induced neurofibrillary tangle (NFT) formation and neuronal loss, although tau abnormalities do not appear to be the single causative factor in AD. First, increasing deposition of tau is found in the brain during aging and neuronal death is observed in the same brain regions as NFTs; both neuronal death and NFTs correlate with duration and severity of illness in AD, although the amount of neuronal death is many times more than the number of NFTs [24]. Second, a tau mutation was recently identified as the causal factor in frontotemporal dementia parkinsonism-17 (FTDP-17), a dementing disease with NFT formation and neuronal loss [23,35,36,39,74,85]. The elucidation of mutated tau in FTDP-17 conclusively demonstrated that tau dysfunction or abnormality alone could induce neurodegeneration characterized by NFTs and neuronal death and leading to clinical dementia, similar to that found in AD. Third, although the generally accepted amyloid-β hypothesis asserts that Aβ is the initiator of the neuronal death and NFT formation [29,70], Aβ did not cause neurotoxicity in primary neuronal cultures from tau knockout mice [66].

Thus, although Aβ may initiate the AD cascade, tau must be a critical step, and the parallel pathways of NFT formation and neuronal death occur only after tau is modified. Phosphorylation is the major modification of the tau protein present in NFTs, and hyperphosphorylation of tau has been shown to be the critical step in NFT formation. Thus, phosphorylation of tau and NFT formation are useful in investigating mechanisms and pathways of neurodegeneration, and provide potential therapeutic targets.

One of the kinases that can phosphorylate tau *in vivo* is glycogen synthase kinase-3β (GSK-3β). GSK-3β was first called tau protein kinase 1 (TPK1), and identified from the microtubule fraction of bovine brain as a tau kinase that induced hyperphosphorylation of tau with the same epitopes as paired helical filament (PHF)-tau, which is an integral component of NFTs [43]. Cloning of TPK1 revealed that TPK1 was identical to GSK-3β [42]. GSK-3 was first identified as a calcium- and cyclic nucleotide-independent kinase of glycogen synthase, which is a rate-limiting enzyme for glycogen biosynthesis and a substrate for several kinases [89]. Based on the partial peptide sequence of GSK-3, two GSK-3 isoforms were cloned, GSK-3α and GSK-3β. GSK-3α and GSK-3β are encoded by different genes, but have 85% homology [89]. GSK-3β, the smaller isoform, is a single polypeptide of 482 amino acids with a molecular weight of 47 kDa. GSK-3β is regulated by a promoter containing putative binding sites for AP1, AP2, c-Myb, CRE, MZF1, Sp1, and Tst-1 [51]. Although GSK-3β is widely expressed in all tissue, its levels are highest in the brain, and GSK-3β is more abundant in neurons than in astrocytes, and expression levels are elevated in developing brains [76, 77]. Although GSK-3β is found predominantly in the perikarya and proximal portion of dendrites in adult neurons, it is also found in axons in embryos [52,77]. Importantly, GSK-3β has also been detected in mitochondria and in nuclei [16,65,79]. Surprisingly, the GSK-3β homolog, shaggy, is involved in cell fate in development of *Drosophila*, suggesting that GSK-3β may be involved not only in glycogen homeostasis but also in cellular signaling cascades.

Unlike many other kinases, GSK-3β is constitutively active in resting cells and in neurons without extracellular stimulation. GSK-3β activity is regulated by Ser9 phosphorylation at the phosphorylation site of protein kinase A (PKA), protein kinase B (PKB, also called Akt), protein kinase C (PKC), p90Rsk, and p70 S6 kinase [26]. Cell survival signals activate PKA, PKB, and PKC, thereby inactivating GSK-3β. Thus, GSK-3β is activated in response to reduced cell survival signals, such as the reduction of growth factors. The active form of GSK-3β can phosphorylate many substrates and participates in various cellular events including metabolism, signaling, and transcription [26]. Although GSK-3 is categorized as a proline-directed kinase, most GSK-3 targets are phosphorylated by another kinase before they can be bound by activate GSK-3β. GSK-3β binds to the resulting phosphate at position $P_0 + 4$ through the GSK-3β "priming pocket" and transfers a phosphate to position P_0 [19,30]. This type of phosphate transfer is a distinctive feature of GSK-3, and is not seen in the other kinases.

2. Results

1. GSK-3β Phosphorylation of Tau
    Although a number of kinases and phosphatases regulate tau phosphorylation, GSK-3β is the main tau kinase *in vivo* [5,9,38,45,46,53,54]. A 1988 report showed that GSK-3β (then called TPK1) generated PHF-like epitopes on tau [40] Yang et al. reported that GSK-3 could incorporate 4 moles of phosphate into each mole of tau, and that GSK-3 slowed the electrophoretic mobility of tau on SDS gels [91]. Ishiguro et al. demonstrated TPK1/GSK-3β-mediated phosphorylation of the Tau-1 site [43], and reported phosphorylation at Ser199, Thr231, Ser396, and Ser413 [43]. Using monoclonal antibodies, Mandelkow et al. showed that GSK-3β could also phosphorylate tau at Ser202/Thr205, Ser396/Ser404, and Ser235 [55]. Hanger et al. confirmed that GSK-3β was able to phosphorylate Ser396 [28]. These observations were extended using peptide-sequence analysis [91], polyclonal antibodies [41], 2D mapping [22,37], and nanoelectrospray mass spectrometry [67]. To date, GSK-3β has been proven to phosphorylate 15 sites on tau: Ser46, Thr50, Thr175, Thr181, Ser199, Ser202, Thr205, Thr212, Thr217, Thr231, Ser235, Ser396, Ser400, Ser404, and Ser413. Ser400 and Ser413 are the only non-proline-directed sites.
2. Aβ-Induced GSK-3 Activation Causes Hyperphosphorylation of Tau
    Because GSK-3β is involved in hyperphosphorylation of tau, GSK-3β may be a critical factor for Aβ-induced neuronal death and NFT formation, and may be activated either directly or indirectly by Aβ. Therefore, focusing on the role of GSK-3β may reveal a mechanism of neurodegeneration in AD and a therapeutic target. To test whether GSK-3β is activated by Aβ, we in-

duced neuronal death in rat hippocampal cultures by introducing aged Aβ to the cultures and examining the resulting GSK-3β activity and tau phosphorylation [80]. We found that GSK-3β activation increased approximately twofold over controls, the activation induced hyperphosphorylation of tau, and that these events preceded neuronal death [56]. Considering the known mechanisms of activation of GSK-3β, we hypothesized that Aβ might block an external signal, thereby activating GSK-3β. After further experiments, Aβ was found to inhibit phosphatidylinositol-3 (PI3) kinase, and this inhibition of PI3 kinase resulted in activation of GSK-3β (Fig. 1) [34].

3. GSK-3β Activation by Aβ-Treatment Disrupts Axonal Transport

In Aβ-treated hippocampal cultures, the activation of GSK-3β also induced cytoplasmic accumulation of the secreted form of the amyloid β-protein precursor (AβPP). Inhibition of GSK-3β in the Aβ-treated hippocampal cultures prevented the cytoplasmic AβPP accumulation [81]. In healthy cells, AβPP is metabolized while being carried by the axonal transport system from the endoplasmic reticulum (ER) to the synaptic regions [71]. When the axonal transport system is impaired, AβPP remains trapped between the Golgi and the synaptic regions, and this trapped AβPP is rigorously metabolized, prematurely releasing the secreted form of AβPP into the cytoplasm [81]. From these results, we hypothesized that the GSK-3β activation after Aβ treatment might be disrupting the axonal transport system in addition to hyperphosphorylating tau.

The role of GSK-3β in axonal transport was confirmed by treating tau-overexpressing *drosophila* mutants with a GSK-3 inhibitor [60]. They showed that GSK-3β inhibition reversed axonal transport defects and behavioral phenotypes in drosophila. The disruption in axonal transport might be caused by microtubule destabilization resulting from hyperphosphorylation of tau, or might be caused by kinesin (a motor protein that is also a substrate of GSK-3β) losing its ability to bind to the cargo protein of vesicles after being phosphorylated by activated GSK-3β.

4. Additional Pathways Can Contribute to Aβ-Induced Neuronal Cell Death

Because the various Aβ-induced cellular events are dependent both on the aggregation status of Aβ and on the specific type of cells used in experiments, activation of other signaling cascades in Aβ-induced death cannot be excluded. For example, Aβ accumulation may trigger the activation of the p75 receptor, the induction of reactive oxygen species, or an increase in the intracellular calcium concentration; any of these pathways could lead to cell death.

Although GSK-3β activation can phosphorylate tau, the number of GSK-3β phosphorylation sites is limited. The Ser422 site, a specific phosphorylation site in AD brain, cannot be phosphorylated by GSK-3β. Because Aβ treatment can enhance Ser422 phosphorylation, factors other than GSK-3β activation are likely to be involved in Aβ-induced tau phosphorylation and NFT formation. An analysis of R406W mutant human tau transgenic mice [84] revealed increased levels of GSK-3β and active c-Jun N-terminal kinase (JNK) immunoreactivity in the cytoplasm of NFT-bearing neurons (unpublished data). Active JNK can phosphorylate Ser422. These results suggest that the activation of both GSK-3β and JNK activation could be involved in NFT formation. Therefore, we overexpressed tau; JNK; the JNK activator, delta mitogen-activated protein kinase/ERK kinase kinase (MEKK); and GSK-3β in COS 7 cells. All of the possible phosphorylation sites of tau showed enhanced phosphorylation in this quadruple expression, and tau was recovered in the sodium dodecyl sulfate (SDS)-insoluble fraction [69]. Thus, hyperphosphorylation of tau by GSK-3β and JNK was shown to be able to induce NFT formation. Because it was reported recently that GSK-3 could phosphorylate MEKK1, and consequently activate JNK, Aβ treatment might activate JNK indirectly through activation of GSK-3β (Fig. 1) [49].

5. GSK-3β Can Induce Memory Deficits *In Vivo*

Because GSK-3β activity is regulated through phosphorylation at Ser9, we investigated activity upstream from Ser9 phosphorylation. We found that PI3 kinase is downregulated by Aβ, and this downregulation subsequently activates GSK-3β [79]. Activated GSK-3β phosphorylates tau and other substrates that may produce the various symptoms of AD [26]. GSK-3β transgenic mice had tau hyperphosphorylation and exhibited impaired spatial recognition and memory in the Morris water maze test [32]. Thus, GSK-3β activation induced memory deficits similar to those seen in AD patients. GSK-3β activation could be

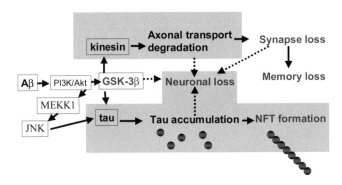

Fig. 1. Mechanism of Aβ-induced NFT formation, synapse loss, and neuron loss.

connected to measurable memory deficits through two known mechanisms.

The GSK-3β substrates, tau and kinesin, are involved in axonal transport, which is impaired when phosphorylated, thereby leading to memory impairment as a result of synaptic dysfunction. As mentioned above, tau hyperphosphorylation by GSK-3β activation destabilizes microtubules, resulting in impairment of axonal transport. This cascade reduces neural activity and leads to memory loss. Kinesin, a motor protein that is a substrate of GSK-3β, loses its ability to bind to the cargo protein of vesicles after it is phosphorylated by activated GSK-3β, thus also impairing axonal transport [58,63].

CREB (cyclic AMP response element binding protein) is another substrate for GSK-3β and modulates the gene expression of promoters containing cyclic AMP response elements [8,57, 87]. CREB regulates many critical neural processes, such as long-term memory and the maintenance of synaptic plasticity [13,14,73,75]. When inactivated or mutated CREB proteins are introduced into a cell or when CREB antisense oligonucleotide treatment is used, the formation of long-term potentiation (LTP) is blocked [6,27, 47]. When CREB is phosphorylated at Ser133 by PKA, CREB is activated. The active CREB induces transcription activity [1,21,72,90], and expresses gene products relating to formation of LTP. However, when CREB is phosphorylated at Ser133, active GSK-3β recognizes that phosphorylation, phosphorylates CREB at Ser129, and inhibits CREB-mediated transcriptional activity [10,18,26]. Thus, GSK-3β activation inhibits CREB, further reducing the cell's ability to produce LTP and consequent memory formation.

6. GSK-3 May Be the Critical Step in Neuronal Death

Recently, an intriguing link between GSK-3β and cell death was recognized. Several studies showed that LiCl, a known GSK-3β inhibitor, protected neurons from a wide variety of neurotoxic insults, including: nerve growth factor (NGF) deprivation of PC12 cells [86], low-potassium treatment in cerebellar granule cells [12], glutamate excitotoxicity [61], staurosporine treatment in SH-SY5Y cells [4], and Aβ neurotoxicity in rat hippocampal neurons [2]. The mechanisms underlying this GSK-3β-induced apoptosis might be related to the inactivation of transcription factors, rather than to the phosphorylation of tau, because GSK-3 also regulates heat shock factor-1 (HSF-1), one of the most crucial signaling components mediating cellular defense mechanisms [4,48,59]. Oxidative stress has been implicated in the etiology of brain aging and AD, and can activate HSF-1 to induce heat shock protein (HSP) expression [3]. However, increased GSK-3β activity results in the phosphorylation of HSF-1 at Ser303, and the inhibition of HSF-1 DNA-binding activity [11,31,50]}. This suggests that an increase in GSK-3 activity would reduce the effectiveness of cellular defense systems, resulting in increased vulnerability to oxidative stress.

The anti-apoptotic protein bcl-2 is a target of CREB, another GSK-3β substrate. Therefore, when GSK-3β phosphorylates CREB, bcl-2 activation might be affected [44,64,68,88]. Hence, GSK-3β activation may reduce cellular resistance to apoptosis.

Thus, GSK-3β activation in response to Aβ may be a common mechanism, phosphorylating multiple substrates, impairing neuronal survival and

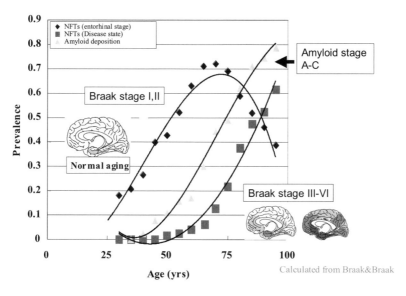

Fig. 2. Relationship between NFT formation and Aβ deposition.

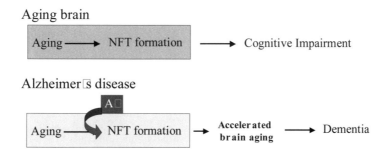

Fig. 3. Development of AD requires brain aging, and FTDP17 mutation or Aβ accelerates the aging process, leading to dementia.

defense systems, and underlying all of the detrimental pathways activated by Aβ, including formation of NFTs and neuronal loss in AD.

7. GSK-3β Acceleration of Aging in Animal Models of AD

The lack of an animal model that includes both NFT formation and neuronal loss impedes efforts to evaluate the effects of GSK-3 inhibition in AD. Importantly, the Braak and Braak study shows that NFT formation in the entorhinal cortex precedes Aβ deposition, whereas NFTs appear in the limbic and neocortical areas only after Aβ deposition [7] (Fig. 2). Based on their analysis, NFT formation in entorhinal cortex may develop during the course of normal brain aging, and only spread into the limbic and neocortical areas in the disease state of AD. That is, the chronology of the pathological changes appears to start with NFTs developing in the entorhinal cortex in the absence of Aβ, and to continue with Aβ deposition, which then triggers the spread of NFTs into the limbic and neocortical areas. This hypothesis implies that brain aging is characterized by NFT development in the entorhinal cortex and that Aβ can accelerate this "normal" brain aging, resulting in AD (Fig. 3).

Therefore, to establish a viable AD model, a model that exhibits brain aging similar to humans is required. If this hypothesis of chronology is correct, the baseline would be a model that develops NFTs as it ages without accumulating Aβ. The FTDP-17 tau mouse fits this requirement, because these mice (expressing FTDP-17 mutant human tau) exhibit NFTs without Aβ deposition [23,35,36,39,74,85]. Injections of Aβ42 into P301L mutant tau transgenic mice induce NFTs in the amygdala [25], therefore, in FTDP17 mutant tau mice, which already show age-related NFT formation, Aβ should accelerate brain aging by increasing the rate of NFT formation.

We generated two different strains of transgenic mutant tau mice, each showing NFT-like pathology in the hippocampus in old age [82,84]. These mice also exhibited memory impairments in the fear-conditioning test, similar to impairments associated with old age. Aβ40 fibrils were injected into the CA1 region of one of these strains. Four weeks after Aβ injection into 3-month-old transgenic mice, NFT-like neurons with immunoreactivity for a phosphorylation-dependent tau antibody were observed in the CA3 and CA4 regions of the hippocampus, in areas of axonal projection to the CA1 region. In biochemical analyses of the hippocampal region, we found that the Akt signaling cascade was impaired, consequently activating GSK-3β. We concluded that, *in vivo*, Aβ activates GSK-3β, which leads to NFT formation (mimicking accelerated brain aging) in neurons that project axons into the area affected by Aβ. Therefore, we propose that GSK-3β may be an accelerating factor for brain aging.

Aβ injections into tau transgenic mice resulted in synaptic loss in the CA1 region, NFT formation and neuronal loss in the CA1 and CA3 regions, and memory impairment. Either LiCl administration or the inhibition of GSK-3β prevented all Aβ-induced phenomena, again suggesting that GSK-3β is involved in AD pathophysiology (unpublished data).

In addition to Aβ-induced pathophysiological changes, based on a finding that presenilin 1 (PS1) associates with GSK-3β, we hypothesized that GSK-3β may be involved in Aβ production [56]. We found that LiCl treatment inhibited Aβ generation [69]. Another group confirmed these results and showed that GSK-3β was involved in Aβ generation using siRNA [62].

8. Perspectives in AD Research on the Role of GSK-3β

GSK-3 appears to be integrally involved in the development of AD. We suspect that brain aging is a prerequisite for AD and that GSK-3 is involved in brain aging. Genetic studies of aging that cloned lifespan-determining factors suggest that reducing the insulin-related signal might extend lifespan [20,33]. However, reducing the insulin-related signal in neurons activates GSK-3β by impairing PI3 kinase/Akt activity, making neurons more vulnerable to apoptotic stimuli, and potentially leading to aging related changes in the brain. It appears that having a longer lifespan increases the susceptibility to brain aging caused by NFT formation via GSK-3β activation. This may explain why susceptibility to AD increases with age. The PS1 mutation is the causative gene for early onset familial AD, was also found in frontotemporal dementia patients [15,17,83], and can activate GSK-3β [78]. Moreover, hyperphosphorylated tau accumulated in mutant PS1 knock-in mice without Aβ deposition. Thus, PS1 mutations affect not only Aβ deposition, but also NFT formation and the rate of brain aging, and Aβ aggregation further accelerates the brain aging, causing an early onset of AD.

3. Discussion

Accumulating data show that GSK-3β phosphorylates several substrates, including tau, and participates in multiple cellular events. For example, GSK-3β phosphorylation of kinesin inhibits kinesin binding with cargo proteins, thereby leading to synaptic dysfunction resulting from the impairment of protein trafficking. As tau disassociates from microtubules and is hyperphosphorylated, the microtubule becomes unstable. This impairment of the protein trafficking system may also lead to synaptic dysfunction, and synaptic dysfunction leads to synaptic loss, which can cause neuronal death.

GSK-3β can also phosphorylate transcription factors and inhibit protein synthesis, leading to apoptosis and decreased LTP and memory formation. GSK-3β phosphorylation of HSF1 inhibits the expression of HSP that is a defense against cellular stress. Thus, GSK-3 reduces the cellular defense system. As a result, cells become more vulnerable to stressors, such as Aβ and oxidative stress. Therefore, although the activation of GSK-3β itself is not toxic, its actions within cells can lead to neuronal death during aging and especially in AD.

Using both *in vitro* and animal models, we have shown that GSK-3β is essential to multiple pathways in the pathogenesis of AD. NFT formation may reflect the extent of brain aging, GSK-3β activation may occur during brain aging, and Aβ may accelerate the brain aging and increase the GSK-3β activation, which may increase Aβ deposition. Therefore, GSK-3 inhibition is a potential therapy for AD, because it may inhibit both Aβ generation and Aβ-induced pathophysiological events in AD models.

References

[1] A.S. Alberts et al., Recombinant cyclic AMP response element binding protein (CREB) phosphorylated on Ser-133 is transcriptionally active upon its introduction into fibroblast nuclei, *J Biol Chem* **269**(10) (1994), 7623–7630.

[2] G. Alvarez et al., Lithium protects cultured neurons against beta-amyloid-induced neurodegeneration, *FEBS Lett* **453**(3) (1999), 260–264.

[3] G.N. Bijur, R.E. Davis and R.S. Jope, Rapid activation of heat shock factor-1 DNA binding by H2O2 and modulation by glutathione in human neuroblastoma and Alzheimer's disease cybrid cells, *Brain Res Mol Brain Res* **71**(1) (1999), 69–77.

[4] G.N. Bijur, P. De Sarno and R.S. Jope, Glycogen synthase kinase-3beta facilitates staurosporine- and heat shock-induced apoptosis. Protection by lithium, *J Biol Chem* **275**(11) (2000), 7583–7590.

[5] M.L. Billingsley and R.L. Kincaid, Regulated phosphorylation and dephosphorylation of tau protein: effects on microtubule interaction, intracellular trafficking and neurodegeneration, *Biochem J* **323**(3) (1997), 577–591.

[6] J.A. Blendy et al., Targeting of the CREB gene leads to upregulation of a novel CREB mRNA isoform, *Embo J* **15**(5) (1996), 1098–1106.

[7] H. Braak and E. Braak, Diagnostic criteria for neuropathologic assessment of Alzheimer's disease, *Neurobiol Aging* **18**(4 Suppl) (1997), S85–88.

[8] P.K. Brindle and M.R. Montminy, The CREB family of transcription activators, *Curr Opin Genet Dev* **2**(2) (1992), 199–204.

[9] L.a.A.D. Buee, Tau phosphorylation, in: *Functional Neurobiology of Aging*, P.R.H.a.C.V. Mobbs, ed., Academic Press, 2001, pp. 315–332.

[10] B.P. Bullock and J.F. Habener, Phosphorylation of the cAMP response element binding protein CREB by cAMP-dependent protein kinase A and glycogen synthase kinase-3 alters DNA-binding affinity, conformation, and increases net charge, *Biochemistry* **37**(11) (1998), 3795–3809.

[11] B. Chu et al., Sequential phosphorylation by mitogen-activated protein kinase and glycogen synthase kinase 3 represses transcriptional activation by heat shock factor-1, *J Biol Chem* **271**(48) (1996), 30847–30857.

[12] S.R. D'Mello, R. Anelli and P. Calissano, Lithium induces apoptosis in immature cerebellar granule cells but promotes survival of mature neurons, *Exp Cell Res* **211**(2) (1994), 332–338.

[13] G.W. Davis, C.M. Schuster and C.S. Goodman, Genetic dissection of structural and functional components of synaptic plasticity. III. CREB is necessary for presynaptic functional plasticity, *Neuron* **17**(4) (1996), 669–679.

[14] K. Deisseroth, H. Bito and R.W. Tsien, Signaling from synapse to nucleus: postsynaptic CREB phosphorylation during multiple forms of hippocampal synaptic plasticity, *Neuron* **16**(1) (1996), 89–101.

[15] B. Dermaut et al., A novel presenilin 1 mutation associated with Pick's disease but not beta-amyloid plaques, *Ann Neurol* **55**(5) (2004), 617–626.

[16] J.A. Diehl et al., Glycogen synthase kinase-3beta regulates cyclin D1 proteolysis and subcellular localization, *Genes Dev* **12**(22) (1998), 3499–3511.

[17] G. Evin et al., Alternative transcripts of presenilin-1 associated with frontotemporal dementia, *Neuroreport* **13**(6) (2002), 917–921.

[18] C.J. Fiol et al., A secondary phosphorylation of CREB341 at Ser129 is required for the cAMP-mediated control of gene expression. A role for glycogen synthase kinase-3 in the control of gene expression, *J Biol Chem* **269**(51) (1994), 32187–32193.

[19] S. Frame, P. Cohen and R.M. Biondi, A common phosphate binding site explains the unique substrate specificity of GSK3 and its inactivation by phosphorylation, *Mol Cell* **7**(6) (2001), 1321–1327.

[20] D. Gems and L. Partridge, Insulin/IGF signalling and ageing: seeing the bigger picture, *Curr Opin Genet Dev* **11**(3) (2001), 287–292.

[21] D.D. Ginty, A. Bonni and M.E. Greenberg, Nerve growth factor activates a Ras-dependent protein kinase that stimulates c-fos transcription via phosphorylation of CREB, *Cell* **77**(5) (1994), 713–725.

[22] R. Godemann et al., Phosphorylation of tau protein by recombinant GSK-3beta: pronounced phosphorylation at select Ser/Thr-Pro motifs but no phosphorylation at Ser262 in the repeat domain, *FEBS Lett* **454**(1-2) (1999), 157–164.

[23] M. Goedert and M.G. Spillantini, Tau mutations in frontotemporal dementia FTDP-17 and their relevance for Alzheimer's disease, *Biochim Biophys Acta* **1502**(1) (2000), 110–121.

[24] T. Gomez-Isla et al., Neuronal loss correlates with but exceeds neurofibrillary tangles in Alzheimer's disease, *Ann Neurol* **41**(1) (1997), 17–24.

[25] J. Gotz et al., Formation of neurofibrillary tangles in P301l tau transgenic mice induced by Abeta 42 fibrils, *Science* **293**(5534) (2001), 1491–1495.

[26] C.A. Grimes and R.S. Jope, The multifaceted roles of glycogen synthase kinase 3beta in cellular signaling, *Prog Neurobiol* **65**(4) (2001), 391–426.

[27] J.F. Guzowski and J.L. McGaugh, Antisense oligodeoxynucleotide-mediated disruption of hippocampal cAMP response element binding protein levels impairs consolidation of memory for water maze training, *Proc Natl Acad Sci USA* **94**(6) (1997), 2693–2698.

[28] D.P. Hanger et al., Glycogen synthase kinase-3 induces Alzheimer's disease-like phosphorylation of tau: generation of paired helical filament epitopes and neuronal localisation of the kinase, *Neurosci Lett* **147**(1) (1992), 58–62.

[29] J. Hardy and D.J. Selkoe, The amyloid hypothesis of Alzheimer's disease: progress and problems on the road to therapeutics, *Science* **297**(5580) (2002), 353–356.

[30] A.J. Harwood, Regulation of GSK-3: a cellular multiprocessor, *Cell* **105**(7) (2001), 821–824.

[31] B. He, Y.H. Meng and N.F. Mivechi, Glycogen synthase kinase 3beta and extracellular signal-regulated kinase inactivate heat shock transcription factor 1 by facilitating the disappearance of transcriptionally active granules after heat shock, *Mol Cell Biol* **18**(11) (1998), 6624–6633.

[32] F. Hernandez et al., Spatial learning deficit in transgenic mice that conditionally over-express GSK-3beta in the brain but do not form tau filaments, *J Neurochem* **83**(6) (2002), 1529–1533.

[33] M. Holzenberger et al., IGF-1 receptor regulates lifespan and resistance to oxidative stress in mice, *Nature* **421**(6919) (2003), 182–187.

[34] M. Hoshi et al., Regulation of mitochondrial pyruvate dehydrogenase activity by tau protein kinase I/glycogen synthase kinase 3beta in brain, *Proc Natl Acad Sci USA* **93**(7) (1996), 2719–2723.

[35] M. Hutton, Molecular genetics of chromosome 17 tauopathies, *Ann N Y Acad Sci* **920** (2000), 63–73.

[36] M. Hutton, Missense and splice site mutations in tau associated with FTDP-17: multiple pathogenic mechanisms, *Neurology* **56**(11 Suppl 4) (2001), S21–25.

[37] S. Illenberger et al., The endogenous and cell cycle-dependent phosphorylation of tau protein in living cells: implications for Alzheimer's disease, *Mol Biol Cell* **9**(6) (1998), 1495–1512.

[38] K.a.T.U. Imahori, Physiology and pathology of tau protein kinases in relation to Alzheimer's disease, *J. Biochem. (Tokyo)* **121**(2) (1997), 179–188.

[39] E.M. Ingram and M.G. Spillantini, Tau gene mutations: dissecting the pathogenesis of FTDP-17, *Trends Mol Med* **8**(12) (2002), 555–562.

[40] K. Ishiguro et al., A novel tubulin-dependent protein kinase forming a paired helical filament epitope on tau, *J Biochem (Tokyo)* **104**(3) (1988), 319–321.

[41] K. Ishiguro et al., Analysis of phosphorylation of tau with antibodies specific for phosphorylation sites, *Neurosci Lett* **202**(1–2) (1995), 81–84.

[42] K. Ishiguro et al., Glycogen synthase kinase 3 beta is identical to tau protein kinase I generating several epitopes of paired helical filaments, *FEBS Lett* **325**(3) (1993), 167–172.

[43] K. Ishiguro et al., Tau protein kinase I converts normal tau protein into A68-like component of paired helical filaments, *J Biol Chem* **267**(15) (1992), 10897–10901.

[44] L. Ji et al., CREB proteins function as positive regulators of the translocated bcl-2 allele in t(14;18) lymphomas, *J Biol Chem* **271**(37) (1996), 22687–22691.

[45] G.V. Johnson and J.A. Hartigan, Tau protein in normal and Alzheimer's disease brain: an update, *J Alzheimers Dis* **1**(4–5) (1999), 329–351.

[46] G.V. Johnson and S.M. Jenkins, Tau protein in normal and Alzheimer's disease brain, *J Alzheimers Dis* **1**(4–5) (1999), 307–328.

[47] B.K. Kaang, E.R. Kandel and S.G. Grant, Activation of cAMP-responsive genes by stimuli that produce long-term facilitation in Aplysia sensory neurons, *Neuron* **10**(3) (1999), 427–435.

[48] J.G. Kiang and G.C. Tsokos, Heat shock protein 70 kDa: molecular biology, biochemistry, and physiology, *Pharmacol Ther* **80**(2) (1998), 183–201.

[49] J.W. Kim et al., Glycogen synthase kinase 3 beta is a natural activator of mitogen-activated protein kinase/extracellular signal-regulated kinase kinase kinase 1 (MEKK1), *J Biol Chem* **278**(16) (2003), 13995–14001.

[50] M.P. Kline and R.I. Morimoto, Repression of the heat shock factor 1 transcriptional activation domain is modulated by constitutive phosphorylation, *Mol Cell Biol* **17**(4) (1997), 2107–2115.

[51] K.F. Lau et al., Molecular cloning and characterization of the human glycogen synthase kinase-3beta promoter, *Genomics* **60**(2) (1999), 121–128.

[52] K. Leroy and J.P. Brion, Developmental expression and localization of glycogen synthase kinase-3beta in rat brain, *J Chem Neuroanat* **16**(4) (1999), 279–293.

[53] S. Lovestone et al., Phosphorylation of tau by glycogen synthase kinase-3 beta in intact mammalian cells: the effects on the organization and stability of microtubules, *Neuroscience* **73**(4) (1996), 1145–1157.

[54] S. Lovestone and C.H. Reynolds, The phosphorylation of tau: a critical stage in neurodevelopment and neurodegenerative processes, *Neuroscience* **78**(2) (1997), 309–324.

[55] E.M. Mandelkow et al., Glycogen synthase kinase-3 and the Alzheimer-like state of microtubule-associated protein tau, *FEBS Lett* **314**(3) (1992), 315–321.

[56] G. Michel et al., Characterization of tau phosphorylation in glycogen synthase kinase-3beta and cyclin dependent kinase-5 activator (p23) transfected cells, *Biochim Biophys Acta* **1380**(2) (1998), 177–182.

[57] M.R. Montminy and L.M. Bilezikjian, Binding of a nuclear protein to the cyclic-AMP response element of the somatostatin gene, *Nature* **328**(6126) (1987), 175–178.

[58] G. Morfini et al., Glycogen synthase kinase 3 phosphorylates kinesin light chains and negatively regulates kinesin-based motility, *Embo J* **21**(3) (2002), 281–293.

[59] R.I. Morimoto, Regulation of the heat shock transcriptional response: cross talk between a family of heat shock factors, molecular chaperones, and negative regulators, *Genes Dev* **12**(24) (1998), 3788–3796.

[60] A. Mudher et al., GSK-3beta inhibition reverses axonal transport defects and behavioural phenotypes in Drosophila, *Mol Psychiatry* **9**(5) (2004), 522–530.

[61] S. Nonaka, C.J. Hough and D.M. Chuang, Chronic lithium treatment robustly protects neurons in the central nervous system against excitotoxicity by inhibiting N-methyl-D-aspartate receptor-mediated calcium influx, *Proc Natl Acad Sci USA* **95**(5) (1998), 2642–2647.

[62] C.J. Phiel et al., GSK-3alpha regulates production of Alzheimer's disease amyloid-beta peptides, *Nature* **423**(6938) (2003), 435–439.

[63] G. Pigino et al., Alzheimer's presenilin 1 mutations impair kinesin-based axonal transport, *J Neurosci* **23**(11) (2003), 4499–4508.

[64] S. Pugazhenthi et al., Insulin-like growth factor-I induces bcl-2 promoter through the transcription factor cAMP-response element-binding protein, *J Biol Chem* **274**(39) (1999), 27529–27535.

[65] M. Ragano-Caracciolo et al., Nuclear glycogen and glycogen synthase kinase 3, *Biochem Biophys Res Commun* **249**(2) (1998), 422–427.

[66] M. Rapoport et al., Tau is essential to beta-amyloid-induced neurotoxicity, *Proc Natl Acad Sci USA* **99**(9) (2002), 6364–6369.

[67] C.H. Reynolds et al., Phosphorylation sites on tau identified by nanoelectrospray mass spectrometry: differences in vitro between the mitogen-activated protein kinases ERK2, c-Jun N-terminal kinase and P38, and glycogen synthase kinase-3beta, *J Neurochem* **74**(4) (2000), 1587–1595.

[68] A. Riccio et al., Mediation by a CREB family transcription factor of NGF-dependent survival of sympathetic neurons, *Science* **286**(5448) (1999), 2358–2361.

[69] S. Sato et al., Aberrant tau phosphorylation by glycogen synthase kinase-3beta and JNK3 induces oligomeric tau fibrils in COS-7 cells, *J Biol Chem* **277**(44) (2002), 42060–42065.

[70] D.J. Selkoe, Toward a comprehensive theory for Alzheimer's disease. Hypothesis: Alzheimer's disease is caused by the cerebral accumulation and cytotoxicity of amyloid beta-protein, *Ann N Y Acad Sci* **924** (2000), 17–25.

[71] D.J. Selkoe et al., The role of APP processing and trafficking pathways in the formation of amyloid beta-protein, *Ann N Y Acad Sci* **777** (1996), 57–64.

[72] M. Sheng, M.A. Thompson and M.E. Greenberg, CREB: a Ca(2+)-regulated transcription factor phosphorylated by calmodulin-dependent kinases, *Science* **252**(5011) (1991), 1427–1430.

[73] A.J. Silva et al., CREB and memory, *Annu Rev Neurosci* **21** (1998), 127–148.

[74] M.G. Spillantini and M. Goedert, Tau protein pathology in neurodegenerative diseases, *Trends Neurosci* **21**(10) (1998), 428–433.

[75] R.S. Struthers et al., Somatotroph hypoplasia and dwarfism in transgenic mice expressing a non-phosphorylatable CREB mutant, *Nature* **350**(6319) (1991), 622–624.

[76] M. Takahashi, K. Tomizawa and K. Ishiguro, Distribution of tau protein kinase I/glycogen synthase kinase-3beta, phosphatases 2A and 2B, and phosphorylated tau in the developing rat brain, *Brain Res* **857**(1–2) (2000), 193–206.

[77] M. Takahashi et al., Localization and developmental changes of tau protein kinase I/glycogen synthase kinase-3 beta in rat brain, *J Neurochem* **63**(1) (1994), 245–255.

[78] A. Takashima et al., Presenilin 1 associates with glycogen synthase kinase-3beta and its substrate tau, *Proc Natl Acad Sci USA* **95**(16) (1998), 9637–9641.

[79] A. Takashima et al., Exposure of rat hippocampal neurons to amyloid beta peptide (25–35) induces the inactivation of phosphatidyl inositol-3 kinase and the activation of tau protein kinase I/glycogen synthase kinase-3 beta, *Neurosci Lett* **203**(1) (1996), 33–36.

[80] A. Takashima et al., Tau protein kinase I is essential for amyloid beta-protein-induced neurotoxicity, *Proc Natl Acad Sci USA* **90**(16) (1993), 7789–7793.

[81] A. Takashima et al., Amyloid beta peptide induces cytoplasmic accumulation of amyloid protein precursor via tau protein kinase I/glycogen synthase kinase-3 beta in rat hippocampal neurons, *Neurosci Lett* **198**(2) (1995), 83–86.

[82] K. Tanemura et al., Formation of filamentous tau aggregations in transgenic mice expressing V337M human tau, *Neurobiol Dis* **8**(6) (2001), 1036–1045.

[83] D. Tang-Wai et al., Familial frontotemporal dementia associated with a novel presenilin-1 mutation, *Dement Geriatr Cogn Disord* **14**(1) (2002), 13–21.

[84] Y. Tatebayashi et al., Tau filament formation and associative memory deficit in aged mice expressing mutant (R406W) human tau, *Proc Natl Acad Sci USA* **99**(21) (2002), 13896–13901.

[85] J.C. van Swieten et al., Phenotypic variation in frontotemporal dementia and parkinsonism linked to chromosome 17, *Dement Geriatr Cogn Disord* **17**(4) (2004), 261–264.

[86] C.a.A.R. Volonté, Lithium chloride promotes short-term survival of PC12 cells after serum and NGF deprivation, *Lithium* **4** (1993), 211–219.

[87] G. Waeber and J.F. Habener, Nuclear translocation and DNA recognition signals colocalized within the bZIP domain of cyclic adenosine 3',5'-monophosphate response element-binding protein CREB, *Mol Endocrinol* **5**(10) (1991), 1431–1438.

[88] B.E. Wilson, E. Mochon and L.M. Boxer, Induction of bcl-2 expression by phosphorylated CREB proteins during B-cell activation and rescue from apoptosis, *Mol Cell Biol* **16**(10) (1996), 5546–5556.

[89] J.R. Woodgett, Molecular cloning and expression of glycogen synthase kinase-3/factor A, *Embo J* **9**(8) (1990), 2431–2438.

[90] J. Xing, D.D. Ginty and M.E. Greenberg, Coupling of the RAS-MAPK pathway to gene activation by RSK2, a growth factor-regulated CREB kinase, *Science* **273**(5277) (1996), 959–963.

[91] S.D. Yang et al., Protein kinase FA/GSK-3 phosphorylates tau on Ser235-Pro and Ser404-Pro that are abnormally phosphorylated in Alzheimer's disease brain, *J Neurochem* **61**(5) (1993), 1742–1747.

Frameshift proteins in Alzheimer's disease and in other conformational disorders: Time for the ubiquitin-proteasome system

F.W. van Leeuwen[a,*], E.M. Hol[a] and D.F. Fischer[b]
[a]Netherlands Institute for Brain Research, Meibergdreef 33, 1105 AZ Amsterdam, The Netherlands
[b]Department of Functional Genomics, Center for Neurogenomics and Cognitive Research (CNCR), Vrije Universiteit and VU Medical Center, de Boelelaan 1085, 1081HV Amsterdam, The Netherlands

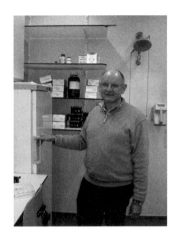

Abstract. Neuronal homeostasis requires a constant balance between biosynthetic and catabolic processes. Eukaryotic cells primarily use two distinct mechanisms for degradation: the proteasome and autophagy of aggregates by the lysosomes. We focused on the ubiquitin-proteasome system (UPS) and discovered a frameshift protein for ubiquitin (UBB^{+1}), that accumulates in the neuritic plaques and tangles in patients with Alzheimer's disease (AD). UBB^{+1}, unable to tag proteins to be degraded, has been shown to be a substrate for ubiquitination and subsequent proteasomal degradation. If UBB^{+1} is accumulated, it inhibits the proteasome, which may result in neuronal death. We showed that UBB^{+1} is also present in other tauopathies (e.g. Pick's disease) and in several polyglutamine diseases, but remarkably not in synucleinopathies (e.g. Parkinson's disease). Accumulation of UBB^{+1} -being a reporter for proteasomal dysfunctioning- thus differentiates between these conformational diseases. The accumulation of UBB^{+1} causes a dysfunctional UPS in these multifactorial neurodegenerative diseases. Novel transgenic mouse models and large-scale expression profiling and functional analyses of enzymes of the UPS compounds – enabling us to identify the targets of the UPS in these conformational diseases – may now pave the way for intervention and treatment of AD.

Keywords: Conformational diseases, molecular misreading, polyglutamine diseases, synucleinopathies, tauopathies, vasopressin

1. Degradation mechanisms and neurodegeneration

Conformational diseases are now acknowledged as a group of disorders that share the accumulation of insoluble protein deposits in affected cells [1]. To this group belong many age-related neurodegenerative disorders, such as tauopathies (e.g. Alzheimer's disease, AD), synucleinopathies (e.g. Parkinson's disease) and polyglutamine diseases (e.g. Huntington's disease) [2]. Non-neuronal conformational disorders like inclusion body myositis, α 1-antitrypsin deficiency, liver cirrhosis [1,3,4] also belong to this group. Although the deposits vary with regard to protein composition, shape and localization, each of these structures (e.g. aggregates or inclusions) is mainly composed of insoluble misfolded proteins (e.g. hyperphosphorylated tau, α-synuclein, huntingtin and cytokeratins), several molec-

---

*Corresponding author. Tel.: +31 20 5665510; Fax: +31 20 6961006; E-mail: f.van.leeuwen@nih.knaw.nl.

ular chaperones (e.g. heat shock proteins) and numerous components of the ubiquitin-proteasome system (UPS). These include E3 ligases such as parkin and CHIP, the latter forming a link between the chaperone and proteasome system [5]. In addition CDC 48 – a chaperone required for substrate recruitment and segregation – and E4 compounds – the latter involved in shipping and targetting of ubiquitinated proteins to the 19S regulator and 20S proteasomal subunits – are also present in the inclusions. For these compounds an escort pathway has been proposed [6]. The presence of these factors suggests that these insoluble proteins are misfolded and have been targeted for degradation, but instead of being properly refolded or proteolytically degraded, they accumulate in insoluble protein deposits [7]. The coexistence of heat shock proteins and UPS compounds is not surprising, since one of the fundamental tasks of the UPS is to degrade damaged or abnormal proteins and to protect cells during stress responses. In addition, adaptation of proteasome composition is possible [8]. When the capacity of the UPS is exceeded [9], autophagins, molecular determinants of autophagic vacuole formation, are recruited to aggresomes, pericentriolar cytoplasmic inclusion bodies, essential for the elimination of aggregates and subsequent lysosomal degradation [10]. Many reviews on the UPS [2,11] and autophagy [12] in relation to neurodegeneration have been published (e.g. [13,14]). Apparently evolution has provided cells with many ways to protect themselves against cytotoxic insults associated with the accumulation of proteinaceous aggregates [15].

2. Frameshift proteins and inclusions

Apart from genomic mutations (see chapters by Van Broeckhoven, Hardy and Tanzi) there is evidence that small deletions in transcripts (Δ GA or Δ GU) of amyloid β protein precursor (APP) and ubiquitin (UBB) are linked to neurodegeneration [16,17]. This process of generation of these faulty transcripts has been dubbed molecular misreading [18], an event that occurs in the brains of all patients examined, and is most likely of transcriptional origin [19,20]. However, the resulting aberrant frameshift (+1) proteins (APP^{+1} and UBB^{+1}) accumulate in the hallmarks of AD (i.e. neurofibrillary tangles and neuritic plaques in sporadic and familial forms of AD and Down syndrome patients but not in controls lacking neuropathology [16,21] (Figs 1, 2A). These +1 proteins coexist and this suggests a common denominator in transcription infidelity and subsequent proteasomal insufficiency.

APP^{+1} interacts with APP and could contribute to amyloid β-40 formation [23]. Its presence in cerebrospinal fluid is negatively correlated with the degree of AD neuropathology as indicated by Braak staging [24] and the level of APP^{+1} in the cerebrospinal fluid can be an additional marker for early neuropathological stages of AD.

We have shown that UBB^{+1} is both a substrate and inhibitor of the UPS [25]. In a cell-free system and in neuronal cell lines, UBB^{+1} is an inhibitor of the UPS [25,26] and overexpression of this protein induces heat shock protein expression, subsequent resistance to oxidative stress [27] and leads to apoptosis [28,29]. The presence of UBB^{+1} in affected neurons in AD, other tauopathies and several polyglutamine diseases, but not in synucleinopathies (Fig. 2), can be used as a marker for proteasome insufficiency [19,29]. However, it has been reported that the proteasome is not only inhibited in AD [31] and Huntington's disease (sharing UBB^{+1} accumulation) but also in Parkinson's disease (references in [32]). We surmise that the mechanisms leading to proteasomal insufficiency are different in these diseases. Whereas in Parkinson's disease the ubiquitination and deubiquitination machinery may be hampered, in AD UBB^{+1} inhibition of the proteasome may act at the cap, potentially due to clogging of 19S subunit(s) with substrates such as ubiquitinated UBB^{+1} [26]. Indeed, genetic data point to a role for ubiquitination and deubiquitinating enzymes in familial Parkinson's disease (Parkin and UCH L-1) [33].

3. Molecular misreading and inclusions in non-neuronal cells and UBB^{+1}

Using the vasopressin (VP) system as a reporter (see review [34]), we were able to address the question whether molecular misreading occurs outside of neuronal cells. In order to do so we used transgenic mice in which the rat VP gene is expressed ectopically in epithelial structures of secretory organs under the control of the mouse mammary tumor virus long terminal repeat promotor. Indeed, VP was found in the gonadal system (e.g. testis and epididymis). Using antisera specific for frameshifted VP (VP^{+1}), we were able to show that VP^{+1}, VP and other parts of the VP precursor coexist in the principal cells of the caput of the epididymis. This result was corroborated by specific *in situ* hybridization [35]. Thus, VP^{+1} is syn-

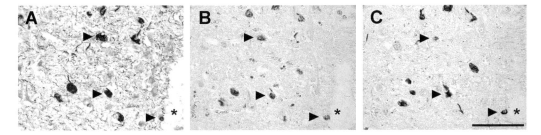

Fig. 1. Coexpression of several +1 proteins in Alzheimer's disease.
Consecutive paraffin sections of the hippocampus of an Alzheimer patient (70 years old) labeled with frameshift proteins for amyloid precursor protein (APP^{+1}, A), UBB^{+1} (B) and GFAP^{+1} (C). Note that the same cells are reactive for all three +1 compounds. GFAP^{+1} is produced due to missplicing of GFAP [22]. As UBB^{+1} has a dual substrate/inhibitor effect on the proteasome, it is very likely that other essential neuronal functions are disturbed as well. Bar = 50 μm.

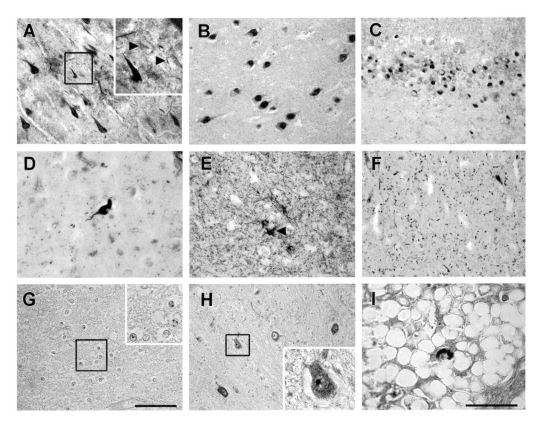

Fig. 2. UBB^{+1} expression in several tauopathies, polyglutamine disease and a non-neuronal conformational disease.
Frameshift ubiquitin (UBB^{+1}) is present in the hallmarks of tauopathies in AD (A), Pick's disease (B,C), progressive supranuclear palsy (PSP; D,E) and argyrophilic grain disease in polyglutamine diseases: Huntington's disease (G) and spinocerebellar ataxia type-3 (SCA-3)(H). UBB^{+1} is also present in inclusions of non-neuronal cells such as in Mallory bodies of hepatocytes of patients with liver cirrhosis (I) [30].
In A: insert shows UBB^{+1} in neurofibrillary tangles and neuropil threads (▲). In B and C Pick bodies are present in pyramidal cells (B) and in granular cells (C). In PSP both neurofibrillary tangles (D) and glial cells (▲, E) are labeled. In F the grains are seen. In HD (G) intranuclear inclusions (n = 1, 2, 3) are seen, in SCA-3, both the nucleus and cytoplasm are UBB^{+1} positive. A = 50-μm-thick vibratome sections and B–I are 6 μm paraffin sections. Bar in A–F and H–I = 50 μm, G = 25 μm. Inserts are blow-ups.

thetized in non-neuronal cells, due to molecular misreading of the transgene. Subsequently, frameshifted ubiquitin (UBB^{+1}) was found in inclusions of various non-neurological diseases and suggests a similar mechanism for transcript mutations as reported previously in neuronal cells: the Mallory bodies of hepatocytes during cirrhosis in alcoholic liver disease (Fig. 2) [30], in hepatocytes of patients with an α1-antitrypsin deficiency [4] and in aggregates of inclusion body myositis [3].

4. Which studies are currently in progress?

Presently we focus on various issues, of which the degree in which UBB^{+1} contributes to proteasomal and neuronal dysfunction is the most important one. We have generated various transgenic lines expressing UBB^{+1} at different levels and are studying the downstream effects with regard to axonal transport, spatial reference memory, motor behavior [36] and post-translational modifications of proteins by proteomics [37]. As a next step we are enhancing cellular stress by crossing our mouse line with a high UBB^{+1} expression with mouse models for AD and Huntington's disease [36].

Furthermore the tremendous increase of knowledge and the number of available tools to study the important players of the UPS (e.g. [6]), has enabled us to successfully combine qPCR and immunocytochemistry on postmortem human tissue of brain areas (e.g. temporal cortex versus gyrus cinguli) heavily involved in AD and Parkinson's disease (Van Leeuwen, unpublished data).

5. Challenges for the near future

A large number of possibilities is now available to understand the role of UBB^{+1} in the UPS and its possible contribution to neuropathogenesis in conformational diseases in general [38]. Novel transgenic mouse lines have been generated. Large-scale expression profiling by transcriptomics and particularly proteomics and functional analyses of UPS compounds can be performed.

6. Transgenic mouse lines

– Aberrations in the UPS have been implicated, either as a primary cause or secondary consequence, in the pathways of both inherited and acquired conformational diseases, such as AD [2]. Of course when using transgenic mice, one should realize that AD and other related conformational diseases are multifactorial. The step towards multiple transgenic mice has been taken (e.g. [39]) and the numerous contributing factors to AD can be organized in a temporal pattern (e.g. [40,41]). The recently generated UBB^{+1} mouse lines are obvious candidates for further crossings with models for AD [36]. Long term potential (LTP) measurements in the hippocampus of these mice and changes in transcript and protein levels (e.g. CREB, synaptophysin and AMPA receptors linked to proteasomal inhibition) [42], as well as further proteomic analyses to reveal post translational modifications [37] are currently under investigation.

– Synaptic plasticity and axonal transport are known to be affected in AD [43,44]. The UPS and its inhibition by UBB^{+1} are attractive candidates for further research since the UPS is also important in synaptic plasticity [45]. The recently developed transgenic UBB^{+1} mouse lines may contribute in this respect [36].

– Another challenge is trying to substantiate the effects of different cellular stressors (e.g. Aβ, E2-25K/Hip2, UBB^{+1}) expressed in transgenic mice (e.g. [36,39]) by rescue experiments, i.e. silencing the effect of UPS compounds by means of RNA interference [41,46].

– The question whether inclusions themselves are protective [47] or toxic [48] can be addressed in AD, similar to a strategy in a transgenic mouse line expressing both ataxin-7 and the GFP reporter for proteasomal activity [49], but now using a multiple transgenic AD mouse line (e.g. [39]).

– Development of tools to study the role of the UPS in neurodegeneration. In order to facilitate future live-imaging (two-photon) and similar *in vitro* and *in vivo* experiments for studying UPS activity, UBB^{+1} fusion constructs with fluorescent proteins were developed (Fig. 3).

7. Characterization of UPS compounds

– Relevant essential subunits of the ubiquitination and deubiquination machinery as well as of essential proteasome subunits are now ready for analysis to study their contribution to neuropathogenesis (e.g. [6,52]). As the tools are now available (e.g. combination of immunocytochemistry and qPCR), we can address research questions such as: are there putative targets in the cellular safeguards for neuronal functioning (e.g. in protein quality control by the UPS and autophagy) in AD and Parkinson's disease and how can we modulate them.

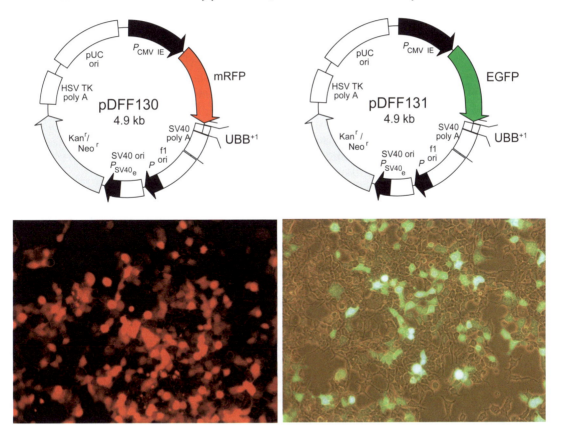

Fig. 3. Tools to track cellular proteasomal dysfunction: UBB^{+1} fusion proteins and usable for screening RNAi libraries.
Schematic presentation of plasmids pDFF130 and pDFF131 encoding, respectively, a mRFP-UBB^{+1} red fluorescent and EGFP-UBB^{+1} green fluorescent proteins fused to UBB^{+1}. 293T cells were transfected with either pDFF130 or pDFF131 and analyzed after 48 hrs. UBB^{+1} [16] was cloned by PCR in the HindIII and SalI sites of pEGFP-C1 [16], Clontech or mRFP-C1 [16], generating a fusion protein with an N-terminal fluorochrome and C-terminal aberrant ubiquitin. Plasmids were tested in 293T human embryonic kidney cells. 5 microgram of plasmid DNA was transfected by calcium phosphate precipitation in 6-well plates. Images were made after 48 hrs using a Nikon Digital Net100 camera on a Nikon Eclipse TS100 microscope under simultaneous phase-contrast and fluorescent illumination.

– Other possible mechanisms to cope with insoluble proteins are posttranslational modifications by ubiquitin paralogues (sumoylation and neddylation) but also phosphorylation and oxidation (e.g. [53]). The relation of these modifications to inclusion formation in the various conformational diseases is currently investigated by proteomics.

8. Therapeutic UPS targets

– It is clear that proteasomal activators (without side-effects) are badly needed. Proteins as activators of the 20S proteolytic core are known as PA28 and PA200, and are obvious targets for the development of even more potent molecules mobilizing the proteolytic machinery [54]. Alternatively, elucidation of deubiquitinating enzymes (DUBS) by screening RNAi libraries might result in DUBS promoting deubiquitination of ubiquitinated UBB^{+1} (Fig. 3) [55]. It was shown that polyubiquitinated UBB^{+1} chains are refractory to disassembly by DUBS and potently inhibit the degradation of a polyubiquitinated substrate by purified 26S proteasomes [26]. RNA silencing techniques to neutralize UPS transcripts or viral technology to compensate for a lack of them are the candidates for therapy as has been shown in polyglutamine diseases such as spinocerebellar ataxia-1 [46,56].

Acknowledgements

The authors are indebted to Drs. R.A.I de Vos (Enschede, The Netherlands), E.R. Brunt (Groningen,

The Netherlands), M.L.C. Maat (Leiden, The Netherlands), S. French (Los Angeles, USA) and the Netherlands Brain Bank (coordinator R. Ravid) for sharing postmortem human brain and liver tissues, and to Drs.O. Pach and W. Verweij for their secretarial support. Financial support was obtained from the Society for Progressive Supranuclear Palsy (#440-04), Jan Dekker Stichting and dr. Ludgardine Bouwman Stichting, #04-22), Internationale Stichting Alzheimer Onderzoek (#04507/04830 and #01601 01504) and the Hersenstichting Nederland (#12F04.1 and 13F05.11).

References

[1] R.W. Carrell and D.A. Lomas, Conformational disease, *Lancet* **350** (1997), 134–138.

[2] A. Ciechanover and P. Brundin, The ubiquitin proteasome system in neurodegenerative diseases: sometimes the chicken, sometimes the egg, *Neuron* **40** (2003), 427–446.

[3] P. Fratta, W.K. Engel, F.W. van Leeuwen, E.M. Hol, G. Vattemi and V. Askanas, Mutant ubiquitin UBB^{+1} is accumulated in sporadic inclusion-body myositis muscle fibers, *Neurology* **63** (2004), 1114–1117.

[4] S.S. Wu, J.-P. de Chadarevian, L. McPhaul, N.E. Riley, F.W. van Leeuwen and S.W. French, Coexpression and accumulation of ubiquitin +1 and ZZ proteins in livers of children with α1-antitrypsin deficiency, *Pediatr. Dev. Pathol.* **5** (2002), 293–298.

[5] H. McDonough and C. Patterson, CHIP: a link between the chaperone and proteasome systems, *Cell Stress & Chaperones* **8** (2003), 303–308.

[6] H. Richly, M. Rape, S. Braun, S. Rumpf, C. Hoege and S. Jentsch, A series of ubiquitin binding factors connects CDC48/p97 to substrate multiubiquitylation and proteasomal targeting, *Cell* **120** (2005), 73–84.

[7] Alves-Rodrigues, L. Gregori and M.E. Figueiredo-Pereira, Ubiquitin, cellular inclusions and their role in neurodegeneration, *Trends Neurosci* **21** (1998), 516–520.

[8] M. Diaz-Hernandez, F. Hernandez, E. Martin-Aparicio, P. Gomez-Ramos, M.A. Moran, J.G. Castano, I. Ferrer, J. Avila and J.J. Lucas, Neuronal induction of the immunoproteasome in Huntington's disease, *J Neurosci* **17** (2003), 11653–11661.

[9] J.N. Keller, E. Dimayuga, Q. Chen, J. Thorpe, J. Gee and Q. Ding, Autophagy, proteasomes, lipofuscin, and oxidative stress in the aging brain, *Int. J. Biochem. Cell Biol.* **36** (2004), 2376–2391.

[10] C.A. Ross and C.M. Pickart, The ubiquitin-proteasome pathway in Parkinson's disease and other neurodegenerative diseases, *Trends Cell Biol* **14** (2004), 703–711.

[11] C.M. Pickart and R.E. Cohen, Proteasomes and their kin: proteases in the machine age, *Nature Mol. Cell Biol.* **5** (2004), 177–187.

[12] T. Shintani and D.J. Klionsky, Autophagy in health and disease: a double-edged sword, *Science* **306** (2004), 990–995.

[13] A.M. Cuervo, Autophagy: in sickness and in health, *Trends Cell Biol* **14** (2004), 70–77.

[14] R.A. Nixon, Endosome function and dysfunction in Alzheimer's disease and other neurodegenerative diseases, *Neurobiol. Aging* **26** (2005), 373–382.

[15] M.Y. Sherman and A.L. Goldberg, Cellular defenses against unfolded proteins: a cell biologist thinks about neurodegenerative diseases, *Neuron* **29** (2001), 15–32.

[16] F.W. van Leeuwen, D.P.V. de Kleijn, W.H. van den Hurk, A. Neubauer, M.A.F. Sonnemans, J.A. Sluijs, S. Köycü, R.D.J. Ramdjielal, A. Salehi, G.J.M. Martens, F.G. Grosveld, J.P.H. Burbach and E.M. Hol, Frameshift mutants of β amyloid precursor protein and ubiquitin-B are prominent in Alzheimer and Down patients, *Science* **279** (1998), 242–247.

[17] W.H. van den Hurk, H.J.J. Willems, M. Bloemen and G.J.M. Martens, Novel frameshift mutations near short simple repeats, *J. Biol. Chem.* **276** (2001), 11496–11498.

[18] F.W. van Leeuwen, J.P.H. Burbach and E.M. Hol, Mutations in RNA: a first example of molecular misreading in Alzheimer's disease, *TINS* **21** (1998), 331–335.

[19] D.F. Fischer, R.A. de Vos, R. van Dijk, F.M. de Vrij, E.A. Proper, M.A. Sonnemans, M.C. Verhage, J.A. Sluijs, B. Hobo, M. Zouambia, E.N.H. Jansen Steur, W. Kamphorst, E.M. Hol and F.W. van Leeuwen, Disease-specific accumulation of mutant ubiquitin as a marker for proteasomal dysfunction in the brain, *FASEB J* **17** (2003), 2014–2024.

[20] L. Gerez, A. de Haan, E.M. Hol, D.F. Fischer, F.W. van Leeuwen, H. van Steeg and R. Benne, Molecular misreading: the frequency of dinucleotide deletions in neuronal mRNAs for β-amyloid precursor protein and ubiquitin B, *Neurobiol. Aging* **26** (2005), 145–155.

[21] F.W. van Leeuwen, P. Van Tijn, M.A.F. Sonnemans, B. Hobo, D.M.A. Mann, C. Van Broeckhoven, S. Kumar-Singh, P. Cras, G. Leuba, A. Savioz, M.L.C. Maat-Schieman, H. Yamaguchi, J.M. Kros, W. Kamphorst, E.M. Hol, R.A.I. De Vos and D.F. Fischer, Frameshift proteins in autosomal dominant forms of Alzheimer's disease and other tauopathies, *Neurology* (2005), in press.

[22] E.M. Hol, R.F. Roelofs, E. Moraal, M.A. Sonnemans, J.A. Sluijs, E.A. Proper, P.N. de Graan, D.F. Fischer and F.W. van Leeuwen, Neuronal expression of GFAP in patients with Alzheimer pathology and identification of novel GFAP splice forms, *Mol. Psychiatry* **8** (2003), 786–796.

[23] R. van Dijk, D.F. Fischer, J.A. Sluijs, M.A.F. Sonnemans, B. Hobo, L. Mercken, D.M.A. Mann, E.M. Hol and F.W. van Leeuwen, Frame-shifted amyloid precursor protein found in Alzheimer's disease and Down's syndrome increases levels of secreted amyloid β40, *J. Neurochem.* **90** (2004), 712–723.

[24] E.M. Hol, R. van Dijk, L. Gerez, J.A. Sluijs, B. Hobo, M.T. Tonk, A. de Haan, W. Kamphorst, D.F. Fischer, R. Benne and F.W. van Leeuwen, Frameshifted β-amyloid precursor protein (APP+1) is a secretory protein, and the level of APP+1 in cerebrospinal fluid is linked to Alzheimer pathology, *J Biol. Chem.* **278** (2003), 39637–39643.

[25] K. Lindsten, F.M. de Vrij, L.G. Verhoef, D.F. Fischer, F.W. van Leeuwen, E.M. Hol, M.G. Masucci and N.P. Dantuma, Mutant ubiquitin found in neurodegenerative disorders is a ubiquitin fusion degradation substrate that blocks proteasomal degradation, *J. Cell Biol.* **157** (2002), 417–427.

[26] Y.A. Lam, C.M. Pickart, A. Alban, M. Landon, C. Jamieson, R. Ramage, R.J. Mayer and R. Layfield, Inhibition of the ubiquitin-proteasome system in Alzheimer's disease, *PNAS* **97** (2000), 9902–9906.

[27] A.D. Hope, R. De Silva, D.F. Fischer, E.M. Hol, F.W. van Leeuwen and A.J. Lees, Alzheimer's associated variant ubiquitin causes inhibition of the 26S proteasome and chaperone expression, *J. Neurochem.* **86** (2003), 394–404.

[28] F.M.S. de Vrij, J.A. Sluijs, L. Gregori, D.F. Fischer, W.T.J.M.C. Hermens, D. Goldgaber, J. Verhaagen, F.W.

van Leeuwen and E.M. Hol, Mutant ubiquitin expressed in Alzheimer's disease causes neuronal death, *FASEB J* **15** (2001), 2680–2688.

[29] R. de Pril, D.F. Fischer, M.L.C. Maat-Schieman, B. Hobo, R.A.I. de Vos, E.R. Brunt, E.M. Hol, R.A.C. Roos and F.W. van Leeuwen, Accumulation of aberrant ubiquitin induces aggregate formation and cell-death in polyglutamine diseases, *Human Mol. Gen.* **13** (2004), 1–11.

[30] L.W. McPhaul, J Wang, E.M. Hol, M.A.F. Sonnemans, N. Riley, V. Nguyen, Q.X. Yuan, Y.H. Lue, F.W. Van Leeuwen and S.W. French, Molecular misreading of the ubiquitin B gene and hepatic mallory body formation, *Gastroenterology* **122** (2002), 1878–1885.

[31] F.M.S. de Vrij, D.F. Fischer, F.W. van Leeuwen and E.M. Hol, Protein quality control in Alzheimer's disease by the ubiquitin proteasome system, *Prog. Neurobiol.* **74** (2004), 249–270.

[32] E. Bossy-Wetzel, R. Schwarzenbacher and S.A. Lipton, Molecular pathways to neurodegeneration, *Nat. Med.* **10** (2004), Suppl:S2–S9.

[33] E. Leroy, R. Boyer, G. Auburger, B. Leube, G. Ulm, E. Mezey, G. Harta, M.J. Brownstein, S. Jonnalagada, T. Chernova, A. Dehejia, C. Lavedan, T. Gasser, P.J. Steinbach, K.D. Wilkinson and M.H. Polymeropoulos, The ubiquitin pathway in Parkinson's disease, *Nature* **395** (1998), 451–452.

[34] R. de Pril, D.F. Fischer and F.W. van Leeuwen, Conformational diseases: an umbrella for various neurological disorders with an impaired ubiquitin-proteasome system, *Neurobiol. Aging*, in press.

[35] F.W. van Leeuwen, E.M. Hol, R.W.H. Hermanussen, M.A.F. Sonnemans, E. Moraal, D.F. Fischer, D.A.P. Evans, K.-F. Chooi, J.P.H. Burbach and D. Murphy, Molecular misreading in non-neuronal cells, *FASEB J* **14** (2000), 1595–1602.

[36] D.F. Fischer, P. van Tijn, M.C. Verhage, B. Hobo, E.M. Hol and F.W. van Leeuwen, *Mouse models for proteasome insufficiency: aberrant ubiquitin in the study of neurodegenerative disease,* 34th Annual Meeting Society for Neuroscience, San Diego, USA, (2004) #336.1.

[37] R. van Dijk, D.F. Fischer, R.C. van der Schors, M.C. Verhage, K.W. Li, J. van Minnen, E.M. Hol, R. Verwer and F.W. van Leeuwen, *Proteomic changes in the cortex of a mouse model with a chronic impaired proteasome activity,* 34th Annual Meeting Society for Neuroscience, San Diego, USA, October 23–28, #336.2.

[38] S. Song and Y.-K. Jung, Alzheimer's disease meets the ubiquitin-proteasome system, *Trends Mol. Med.* **10** (2004), 565–570.

[39] S. Oddo, L. Billings, J.P. Kesslak, D.H. Cribbs and F.M. LaFerla, Aβ immunotherapy leads to clearance of early, but not late, hyperphosphorylated tau aggregates via the proteasome, *Neuron* **43** (2004), 321–332.

[40] Y. Konishi, T. Beach, L.I. Sue, H. Hampel, K. Lindholm and Y. Shen, The temporal localization of frame-shift ubiquitin-B and amyloid precursor protein, and complement proteins in the brain of non-demented control patients with increasing Alzheimer's disease pathology, *Neurosci. Lett.* **348** (2003), 46–50.

[41] S. Song, S.-Y. Kim, Y.-M. Hong, D.-G. Jo, J.-Y. Lee, S.M. Shim, C.-W. Chung, S.J. Seo, Y.J. Yoo, J.-Y. Koh, M.C. Lee, A.J. Yates, H. Ichijo and Y.-K. Jung, Essential role of E2-25K/Hip-2 in mediating amyloid-β neurotoxicity, *Mol. Cell* **12** (2003), 553–563.

[42] A.N. Hegde, Ubiquitin-proteasome-mediated local protein degradation and synaptic plasticity, *Prog. Neurobiol.* **73** (2004), 311–357.

[43] R.D. Terry and R. Katzman, Life span and synapses: will there be a primary senile dementia? *Neurobiol. Aging* **347** (2001), 353–354.

[44] G.B. Stokin, C Lillo, .TL. Falzone, R.G. Brusch, E. Rockenstein, S.L. Mount, R. Raman, P. Davies, E. Masliah, D.S. Williams and L.S. Goldstein, Axonopathy and transport deficits early in the pathogenesis of Alzheimer's disease, *Science* **307** (2005), 1282–1288.

[45] M.D. Ehlers, Ubiquitin and synaptic dysfunction: ataxic mice highlight new common themes in neurological disease, *Trends Neurosci* **26** (2003), 4–7.

[46] H. Xia, Q. Mao, S.L. Eliason, S.Q. Harper, I.H. Martins, H.T. Orr, H.L. Paulson, L. Yang, R.M. Kotin and B.L. Davidson, RNAi suppresses polyglutamine-induced neurodegeneration in a model of spinocerebellar ataxia, *Nat. Med.* **10** (2004), 816–820.

[47] M. Arrasate, S. Mitra, E.S. Schweitzer, M.R. Segal and S. Finkbeiner, Inclusion body formation reduces levels of mutant huntingtin and the risk of neuronal death, *Nature* **431** (2004), 805–810.

[48] N.F. Bence, R.M. Sampat and R.R. Kopito, Impairment of the ubiquitin-proteasome system by protein aggregation, *Science* **292** (2001), 1552–1555.

[49] A.B. Bowman, S.Y. Yoo, N.P. Dantuma and H.Y. Zoghbi, Neuronal dysfunction in a polyglutamine disease model occurs in the absence of ubiquitin-proteasome system impairment and inversely correlates with the degree of nuclear inclusion formation, *Hum Mol Genet* **14** (2005), 679–691.

[50] B.P. Cormack, R.H. Valdivia and S. Falkow, FACS-optimized mutants of the green fluorescent protein (GFP), *Gene* **173** (1996), 33–38.

[51] R.E. Campbell, O. Tour, A.E. Palmer, P.A. Steinbach, G.S. Baird, D.A. Zacharias and R.Y. Tsien, A monomeric red fluorescent protein, *Proc. Natl. Acad. Sci. USA* **99** (2002), 7877–7882.

[52] L. Petrucelli, D. Dickson, K. Kehoe, J. Taylor, H. Snyder, A. Grover, M. de Lucia, E. McGowan, J. Lewis, G. Prihar, J. Kim, W.H. Dillmann, S.E. Browne, A. Hall, R. Voellmy, Y. Tsuboi, T.M. Dawson, B. Wolozin, J. Hardy and M. Hutton, CHIP and Hsp70 regulate tau ubiquitination, degradation and aggregation, *Hum. Mol. Genet.* **13** (2004), 703–714.

[53] J.S. Steffan, N. Agrawal, J. Pallos, E. Rockabrand, L.C. Trotman, N. Slepko, K. Illes, T. Lukacsovich, Y.Z. Zhu, E. Cattaneo, P.P. Pandolfi, L.M. Thompson and J.L. Marsh, SUMO modification of Huntingtin and Huntington's disease pathology, *Science* **304** (2004), 100–104.

[54] M. Rechsteiner and C.P. Hill, Mobilizing the proteolytic machine: cell biological roles of proteasome activators and inhibitors, *Trends in Cell Biol* **15** (2005), 27–33.

[55] T.R. Brummelkamp, S.M. Nijman, A.M. Dirac and R. Bernards, Loss of the cylindromatosis tumour suppressor inhibits apoptosis by activating NF-kappaB, *Nature* **424** (2003), 797–801.

[56] P. Shankar, N. Manjunath and J. Lieberman The prospect of silencing disease using RNA interference, *JAMA* **293** (2005), 1367–1373.

Genetics

Studies on the first described Alzheimer's disease amyloid β mutant, the Dutch variant

Efrat Levy[a,c,d,*], Frances Prelli[b,c] and Blas Frangione[b,c]
[a]Department of Pharmacology, New York University School of Medicine, New York, New York, USA
[b]Department of Pathology, New York University School of Medicine, New York, New York, USA
[c]Department of Psychiatry, New York University School of Medicine, New York, New York, USA
[d]Nathan Kline Institute, Orangeburg, New York, USA

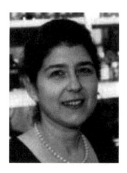
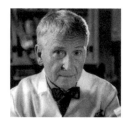

Efrat Levy   Blas Frangione

Abstract. Amyloid protein deposited in cerebral vessel walls and diffuse plaques of patients with hereditary cerebral hemorrhage with amyloidosis, Dutch type (HCHWA-D), is similar to the 40–42 residues amyloid β (Aβ) in vessel walls and senile plaques in brains of patients with Alzheimer's disease (AD), Down's syndrome, and familial and sporadic cerebral amyloid angiopathy (CAA). In 1990 we sequenced the amyloid β-protein precursor (AβPP) gene from HCHWA-D patients revealing a single mutation that results in an amino acid substitution, Aβ E22Q. Subsequent identification of additional mutations in the AβPP gene in familial AD (FAD) pedigrees revealed that whereas substitutions in the middle of Aβ, residues Aβ21-23, are predominantly vasculotropic, those found amino- or carboxyl-terminal to the Aβ sequence within AβPP enhance amyloid parenchymal plaque deposition. Studies of transfected cells showed that substitutions amino- or carboxyl-terminal to Aβ lead to either greater Aβ production or to enhanced secretion of the more hydrophobic thus more fibrillogenic Aβ1-42. Substitutions in the center of Aβ facilitate rapid aggregation and fibrillization, slower clearance across the blood-brain barrier and perivascular drainage to the systemic circulation, possibly higher resistance to proteolysis, and enhanced toxicity towards endothelial and smooth muscle cells. However, most AD patients have no genetic defects in AβPP, indicating that other factors may alter Aβ production, conformation, and/or clearance initiating the disease process.

Keywords: Alzheimer's disease, hereditary cerebral hemorrhage with amyloidosis, Dutch type (HCHWA-D), cerebral amyloid angiopathy (CAA), amyloid β-protein precursor (AβPP), amyloid β (Aβ)

Several neurological disorders are related to altered protein conformation and aggregation, leading to fibrillization (amyloid). Diverse proteins with no obvious amino acid sequence homology acquire a β-pleated sheet structure and form highly insoluble fibrils, some of which are implicated in diseases of the central nervous system [136]. A great advantage in the study of amyloidoses has been the development of methods of extraction of amyloid fibrils from the brain and identification of the amyloid proteins. In 1983 the first cerebral amyloid protein was extracted from leptomeninges of

---

*Corresponding author: Efrat Levy, Center for Dementia Research, Nathan Kline Institute, 140 Old Orangeburg Road, Orangeburg, NY 10962, USA. Tel.: +1 845 398 5540; Fax: +1 845 398 5422; E-mail: elevy@nki.rfmh.org.

patients with hereditary cerebral hemorrhage with amyloidosis, Icelandic type (HCHWA-I) [25]. The amyloid deposition in cerebral arteries and arterioles in these patients leads to recurrent hemorrhagic strokes causing serious brain damage and eventually fatal stroke before the age of 40 years [48]. The leptomeningeal amyloid was identified as a variant of cystatin C [7], also known as γ trace [55], a cysteine protease inhibitor [3,7]. A mutation in the cystatin C gene in HCHWA-I patients results in a L68Q substitution [25,38,69]. In the same year, 1983, Prusiner et al. [98] purified scrapie prion as the protein that forms amyloid aggregates in the brain of hamsters.

The same approach of extraction of the amyloid protein from leptomeninges was utilized to isolate amyloid from the brain of AD and Down's syndrome patients. The initial amino-terminal sequence analysis yielded a 28 amino acids peptide called amyloid β protein (Aβ) [40]. A year later Aβ was purified and characterized as the major amyloid protein of plaque cores from brain parenchyma of AD and Down's syndrome patients [76], indicating a common origin for the amyloids of plaque core and of congophilic angiopathy. The length of the plaque amyloid protein was reported to be 42–43 residues [76]. Additional studies clarified that the complete length of leptomeningeal vascular Aβ is 39–40 residues [95]. Finding that the same protein forms the amyloid in brain parenchyma and vasculature in Down's syndrome and AD patients suggested that the defect in AD is localized on chromosome 21 [39,76]. Immunohistochemical and biochemical studies demonstrated that Aβ composed of 42 amino acids is the major molecular species deposited in brain parenchyma and Aβ species ending at position 40 are predominantly deposited in the blood vessel walls [17]. However, species ending at position 42 are also present, and sometimes are the sole deposited peptide species in CAA [123].

Isolation of the amyloid protein enabled cloning of the gene revealing that Aβ is part of a larger amyloid β protein precursor (AβPP) [43,64,66,100,116]. The AβPP gene located on chromosome 21, consists of 19 exons that are alternatively spliced into several mRNA forms, four of which, encoding 695, 717, 751, and 770 amino acids, contain the Aβ-encoding sequences.

Diseases that involve Aβ deposition seem to be heterogeneous in etiology and clinical presentation. Although most cases of AD appear sporadic, a small number of cases occur in families with autosomal dominant form of inheritance of the disease. Epidemiological studies showed autosomal dominant inheritance of this disease in families with early and late onset familial AD (FAD) (before or after 65 years of age) with multigenetic involvement. Until 1990, studies of genomic DNA and cDNA clones encoding AβPP from AD, Down's syndrome, and FAD patients reported sequences identical to those obtained from unaffected individuals [43,67,100,116,130]. Although the genetic defect causing FAD was localized to chromosome 21 [110], no linkage was found between the AβPP gene and FAD, suggesting that this gene is not the site of the inherited defect underlying the disorder in the families studied [103,117,121].

We sequenced the AβPP gene in patients with HCHWA-D, a rare, autosomal dominant form of severe CAA that presents clinically between the age of 45 and 60. Survivors of the first stroke have further strokes that lead to cognitive deficits [135]. Neuropathologically, Congo red positive amyloid deposits in HCHWA-D are mainly localized in leptomeningeal and cortical walls of arteries and arterioles. Amyloid deposits often replace the entire vessel wall, including the smooth muscle cell layer. Inflammatory markers, reactive astrocytes, microglial cells, and some dystrophic neurites surround the amyloid laden vessels. In most cases, there are amyloid deposits also in brain parenchyma that are predominantly in the form of diffuse plaques that are Congo red negative and lack the dense amyloid cores commonly present in AD [27,50,72,124,135]. Diffuse plaques are occasionally surrounded by dystrophic neurites, although neurofibrillary tangles are consistently absent [119]. The amyloid fibrils in HCHWA-D are formed by a 39–40-amino acids amyloid that is similar to Aβ deposited in AD [124]. Restriction fragment length polymorphisms verified that the AβPP gene is tightly linked to HCHWA-D [122]. Sequence analysis of genomic DNA of HCHWA-D patients showed a single mutation, cytosine instead of guanine, at position 1852 of AβPP in affected members of the family, but not in unaffected relatives [68]. We demonstrated that the single mutation is the only change in the AβPP gene by sequencing the complete coding regions within the 18 exons of the gene [128]. A diagnostic assay for HCHWA-D for high-risk populations and prenatal evaluation was developed. It involves hybridization analysis of genomic DNA by examining a PCR amplification product with an oligonucleotide that contains the mutated sequence [96]. It was shown that the mutation segregates with the disease, being present in DNA from HCHWA-D patients and absent from non affected family members [2]. All the patients were found to be heterozygous, having both the normal and

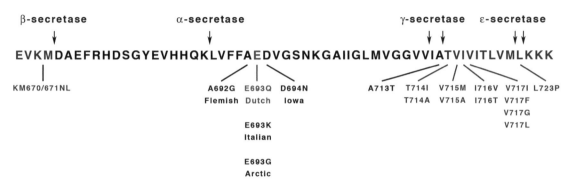

Fig. 1. AβPP pathogenic substitutions. The amino acid sequence of Aβ (uppercase) and flanking regions (lowercase), the sites of secretase cleavages, the amino acid substitutions found in pedigrees with familial Alzheimer's disease (FAD) that produce Alzheimer's disease phenotypes, and those that are primarily associated with CAA phenotypes.

the mutated alleles. Moreover, both glutamine and glutamic acid were found at position 22 of Aβ in amyloid fibrils derived from leptomeningeal vascular walls of HCHWA-D patients [96] (Fig. 1).

Following the discovery of the HCHWA-D mutation a search for mutations in the AβPP gene lead to the identification of linkage to chromosome 21 in a few early onset FAD pedigrees and of several AβPP missense mutations within or flanking the Aβ region (Fig. 1). Although the AβPP mutations account for less than 0.1% of all AD cases, they carry complete penetrance leading to AD between the fourth to seventh decades of life [115]. The presence of a mutation is important in determining the rate and age at which amyloid fibrils are deposited in a patient. Moreover, the different mutation sites in the AβPP gene influence the clinicopathological manifestation of the resulting disease. Point mutations in genes encoding amyloid precursor proteins have been detected in different types of amyloidosis, and prevalent thought is that the consequent amino acid substitution alters the conformation of the proteins and/or their proteolysis promoting aggregation. Therefore, it was suggested that substitutions located amino- or carboxyl-terminal to Aβ may affect either β-secretase or γ-secretase cleavage of AβPP. Although the mutations found in several FAD pedigrees were thought to have a quantitative or qualitative effect on Aβ production, the only mutation that proved to affect the amount of the secreted peptide is the K670N/M671L double mutation located amino-terminally to Aβ, found in a Swedish kindred [15,22,85]. Using cultured cells transfected with AβPP expression constructs, it was shown that cells expressing mutated AβPP secrete higher levels of Aβ compared to cells expressing the normal sequence [13,51,104,107]. The substitutions found proximal to the carboxyl-terminus of Aβ at codon 717 [19,41,86,89,139] seem to lead to an increased proportion of secreted Aβ ending at residue 42 and 43 rather than 40 [113,114,140]. Presenilin (PS1 and PS2) missense mutations found in some families with early onset FAD [71,97,105] also modify the length of Aβ generated [8,23,33]. The longer Aβ contains more hydrophobic residues than Aβ1-40 and therefore it is more fibrillogenic and enhances aggregation of shorter peptides [11,54,60,61].

AβPP amino acid substitutions located amino- or carboxyl-terminal to Aβ and those found in PS1 and PS2 mainly produce deposition of wild type Aβ peptide in the form of parenchymal plaques. Whereas in most cases low levels of vascular amyloid deposition exist, several PS1 and PS2 mutations also cause severe CAA [73,93]. In addition to the Dutch variant, several amino acid substitutions were identified in the middle of Aβ peptide, at positions 21, 22, and 23 [10,52,63,68]. These substitutions are associated with extensive cerebrovascular pathology. As mentioned above, Dutch patients with the E693G substitution have severe CAA causing cerebral hemorrhages, whereas parenchymal amyloid deposits are rare, and neurofibrillary tangles are absent [27,50,72,124,135]. Members of an Italian kindred with an E693K substitution at residue 22 of Aβ present with recurrent hemorrhagic strokes later in life than Dutch HCHWA patients, between 60 and 70 years of age. Although they have extensive Aβ deposits in leptomeningeal and cortical vessels and to a lesser extent, amyloid plaques in the neuropil of the cerebral cortex, the vascular deposits are rarely detected by thioflavin S fluorescence, suggesting a non-fibrillar Aβ organization in the absence of neurofibrillary changes [10]. Unlike other substitutions found at position 22 of Aβ, the E693K Arctic substitution [63] causes early onset clinical history typical for AD with neuritic plaques and neurofibrillary tangles but no signs of stroke or vascular lesions [91]. An A692G substitution, at residue 21 of Aβ, has been identified in a Flemish family with a history of both pre-senile dementia and cerebrovascular amyloidosis [52]. In addition to CAA, Flemish patients usually have abundant parenchymal amyloid deposition with large senile plaque cores and neurofibrillary tangles. However, cerebral hemorrhages appear to be less frequent in a family of British origin with the Flemish AβPP mutation [9]. The D694N Iowa substitution, at position 23 of Aβ, is associated with severe CAA [45]. Another Italian family with autosomal dominant dementia and severe CAA with multiple infarcts has an A713T substitution at Aβ42. This indicates that a mutation at the γ-secretase cleavage site can also be responsible for AD with symptomatic CAA [101].

Aβ undergoes spontaneous post-translational modifications in AD brains, such as isomerization and racemization at their aspartyl residues. It was demonstrated that Aβ isomerized at position 23 is deposited in plaques and vascular amyloid, and *in vitro* it was shown that isomerization at position 23, but not position 7, enhances aggregation. Thus, modifications at the central region of Aβ have a pathogenic role in the deposition of Aβ and development and progression of sporadic AD may be accelerated by spontaneous isomerization at position 23 of Aβ [106]. A short peptide partially homologous to the central hydrophobic region of Aβ (residues 17–21), but containing proline that prevents the adoption of β-sheet structure, binds Aβ and inhibits amyloid fibril formation *in vitro*, suggesting an important role for this region in fibrillogenesis [109]. Another modification, oxidation of methionine Aβ35 [95] enhances the oxidative stress and neurotoxic properties of Aβ1-42 (for review see [14]).

Several *in vitro* studies have investigated the effect of amino acid substitutions at residues 21, 22, and 23 on production, structure, fibrillization properties, stability, clearance, proteolytic removal, and toxicity of Aβ. The first identified substitution, the Dutch E22Q, is the most extensively studied. While it was demonstrated that the substitution does not affect AβPP processing and Aβ production [75], *in vitro* analysis of the full-length E22Q peptide, as well as of fragments containing the mutation, revealed that the Dutch peptide aggregates and forms amyloid-like fibrils at a faster rate than wild type Aβ [124,135,138]. The substitution results in an altered secondary structure of the variant peptide characterized by a considerably higher β-structure content [34,36], and a greater tendency to assemble into stable amyloid fibrils than the normal peptide. Furthermore, the Dutch peptide influences the assembly of the wild type Aβ peptide by providing E22Q fibril nuclei from which the wild type or mixed fibrils can elongate [81,124,135]. While wild type Aβ1-42, but not Aβ1-40, induces pathologic responses in cultured human leptomeningeal smooth muscle cells, including cellular degeneration, the HCHWA-D substitution converts the non-pathologic Aβ1-40 into a highly pathologic form of the peptide [29,80,127]. Deposition of Aβ in the walls of cerebral blood vessels is accompanied by extensive degeneration of smooth muscle cells both in AD and in HCHWA-D [65] and Aβ1-40 is the major form deposited in vascular walls. Thus, these changes in properties of the peptide may contribute to the early and severe CAA pathology in HCHWA-D.

Investigation of the effect of the various amino acid substitutions at residues 21, 22, and 23 of Aβ showed a great difference between the variant peptides. Unlike the Dutch E22Q, the Flemish A21G substitution upregulates both Aβ1-40 and Aβ1-42 secretion by AβPP transfected cells [31]. This variant causes an increased Aβ/p3 ratio, indicating an effect on γ-secretase cleavage [134]. It does not affect Aβ fibrillogenesity [24], but increases the solubility of Aβ1-40, decreases the rate of formation of thioflavin-T-positive assemblies, and increases the SDS-stability of peptide oligomers [132]. Similar to wild type Aβ, the A21G peptide is not toxic to cultured human cerebrovascular smooth muscle cells, human cortical microvessels and aortic smooth muscle cells [133]. The Italian E22K peptide like the wild type Aβ1-40, exhibits lower content of β-sheet conformation and slower aggregation and fibrillization properties compared to the Dutch E22Q peptide. Furthermore, the Dutch peptide induced apoptosis of cerebral endothelial cells, whereas the same concentration of the wild type or Italian peptides had no effect [81]. However, it was shown that unlike wild type Aβ1-40 the E22Q and E22K peptides are toxic to human smooth muscle cells [29,80,127].

Carriers of the Arctic E22G substitution have decreased Aβ1-42 and Aβ1-40 levels in the plasma and transfected cells secrete reduced levels of both variant peptides. While no difference in fibrillization rate was observed, the Arctic substitution formed larger quantities of protofibrils at a much higher rate than wild type Aβ. These findings may reflect that rapid Aβ protofibril formation leads to accelerated buildup of insoluble Aβ [91].

Similar to the Dutch peptide and unlike the Flemish Aβ, it was found that the Iowa D23N variant does affect the amyloidogenic processing of AβPP expressed in cells. The Iowa synthetic Aβ1-40 peptide rapidly assembles in solution to form fibrils and induces robust pathologic responses in cultured human cerebrovascular smooth muscle cells [126].

Insufficient proteolytic removal of Aβ by proteases such as neprilysin, endothelin-converting enzymes, insulin-degrading enzyme, angiotensin-converting enzyme, the plasmin system, and matrix metalloproteases, also has been proposed as a mechanism that leads to Aβ accumulation in the brain (for review, see [83]). It was shown that insulin-degrading enzyme from isolated human brain microvessels is capable of degrading wild type Aβ1-40 as well as the variants A21G, E22Q and E22K. The activity of the enzyme in vessels from AD patients with CAA was reduced, supporting the possibility that a defect in Aβ proteolysis contributes to the accumulation of the peptide in cortical microvasculature [84]. In addition, the amino acid substitutions at Aβ21, Aβ22, and Aβ23 reduce the clearance of the peptides from the brain. There is evidence that the Dutch, Flemish, Italian, and Arctic substitutions make Aβ1-40 resistant to proteolytic degradation by neprilysin [120] and extend the half-life of Aβ in the brain. It was also demonstrated that the E22Q substitution impairs elimination of Aβ from brain by reducing its rapid transport across the blood-brain barrier and the vascular drainage pathways, which in turn may result in accumulation of the peptide around blood vessels and in the brain [82].

These data indicate that specific amino acid substitutions in the center of Aβ enhance amyloid deposition in cerebral vasculature and resultant hemorrhages. Other substitutions cause large amyloid deposition in brain parenchyma. Furthermore, *in vitro* analyses of CAA causing substitutions yielded different results demonstrating that CAA may be caused by a variety of pathogenic mechanisms. Thus, different amino acids at positions 21 to 23 confer distinct structural properties to Aβ that appear to influence the onset and aggressiveness of the disease as well as the clinical phenotype. The charge of the amino acids at that position is a likely factor for the cytotoxic effects and vascular localization of the amyloid [80,81].

Using different promoters a variety of transgenic mouse models have been engineered to overexpress in the brain either full-length human AβPP or its derivatives. Several models reproducibly develop some of the prominent pathological and behavioral features of AD, including age-related amyloid deposition, neuritic changes, neuronal loss, gliosis, abnormal tau phosphorylation, and impairment in learning and memory. Some transgenic lines develop various degrees of CAA.

In one model, mice overexpressing the AβPP gene with the V717F mutation driven by the PDGF-β promoter (PDAPP) [37], have age related parenchymal plaque deposition with little vascular amyloid [56,62].

A line of mice overexpressing AβPP with the K670N/M671L Swedish double mutation, Tg2576, driven by the hamster prion protein promoter develops neuritic plaques in the neocortex and hippocampus at an older age [57]. Although cerebrovascular amyloid deposition has been noted in these mice [131] it is not a prominent feature of this line [12] and there is no evidence of hemorrhagic stroke [21]. Coexpression of mutant PS1 with AβPP potentiates amyloid deposition in Tg2576 mice [79]. Using a human Thy1.1 expression cassette to drive AβPP with the Swedish mutation the line APP23 was developed [112]. In addition to parenchymal amyloid deposition, there is a significant amount of cerebrovascular amyloid in this line accompanied by hemorrhages that range from multiple, recurrent microhemorrhages to large hematomas [16,137]. Thy1.1-neuronal specific expression of the AβPP gene with the V717I London mutation also resulted in plaque and vascular amyloid pathology [32], however, in the absence of hemorrhages [123].

While the above mentioned transgenic mouse models overexpressing AβPP mimic the Aβ amyloid deposition observed in AD, a transgenic mouse model of HCHWA-D recently generated mimics the human disease. Overexpression of the Dutch E693Q AβPP variant in mice under control of a human Thy1.1 expression cassette resulted in extensive amyloid deposition in leptomeningeal and cortical vessels, smooth muscle cell degeneration, hemorrhages, and neuroinflammation [53]. Similar to HCHWA-D patients only a few parenchymal plaques were found and they were composed of diffuse Aβ. However, while HCHWA-D patients are affected early in life, HCHWA-D transgenic mice show onset of vascular amyloid deposition and hemorrhage at old age (22–25 months of age) [53]. This transgenic mouse model confirms for the first time the hypothesis that the E22Q substitution is the cause of the predominant cerebrovascular amyloid deposition in HCHWA-D. Since the E693Q AβPP gene was expressed in these mice using a neuron-specific promoter, the vascular amyloid deposits originate from neuronal cells and are probably due to reduced clearance of the peptide [82]. The amyloid deposited in the cerebrovasculature of the E693Q AβPP transgenic mice consists predominantly of Aβ1-40. Cross-breeding these mice with mice expressing a PS1 variant that increases Aβ1-42 production, resulted in early (starting at 3 months of age) accumulation of parenchymal amyloid plaques and reduced CAA [53]. Thus, similar to humans, the major component of blood vessel amyloid is Aβ1-40, and modification of the Aβ42/Aβ40 ratio favors parenchymal amyloid deposition with higher Aβ1-42 content.

Another mouse model expresses the human AβPP gene with three substitutions: the Dutch, Iowa, and Swedish under control of the Thy1.2 promoter. Even though these mice express the human gene at levels below those of endogenous mouse AβPP they develop early-onset and robust accumulation of Aβ in the brain with perivascular and vascular Aβ deposits with occasional microhemorrhages [30]. *In vitro* studies have shown that an experimental Aβ peptide containing both the Dutch and Iowa substitutions possesses more robust fibrillogenic and pathogenic properties compared with peptides with either single substitution [126]. Moreover, this peptide compared to wild type Aβ is poorly cleared from mouse brain into the circulation, indicating that a clearance deficit contributes to accumulation of Aβ in and around cerebral blood vessels and in the parenchyma of transgenic mice [30]. While CAA in AβPP mouse models with neuronal specific expression of the transgene evinces that the source of cerebrovascular amyloid can be neuronal, it remains to be determined if Aβ deposition can originate also from the circulation.

The development of Aβ depositing transgenic mice which exhibit some typical characteristics of AD pathology, endorses the concept that Aβ is one etiological factor in the initiation of the disease process. Conversely, mutations expressed as protein variants are not a prerequisite for fibril formation because amyloid fibrils in AD are usually processing products of a normal precursor protein [118]. Thus, mechanisms such as aberrant binding to tissue specific factors (chaperons) must have a crucial role in the process of amyloid formation. Although Aβ is the major constituent of the amyloid deposits in AD, there are minor components such as P-component [26], apolipoprotein E [88], apolipoprotein J [20,78], proteoglycans [108], lysosomal proteinases [4,5,18,87,92] and the proteinases inhibitors, α_1-antichymotrypsin, α1-antitrypsin [1,44], α_2-macroglobulin [99,125], and cystatin C [49,58,70, 74,129]. Some proteins associated with AD lesions may have a role in the pathological processes leading to amyloidogenesis and neuronal degeneration and others may bind secondarily to amyloid deposits. Proteins associated with Aβ may initiate and/or enhance fibril formation and deposition, or alternatively, they may solubilize Aβ. Genetic data support the involvement of some of these proteins in the pathological process leading to AD, including apolipoprotein E [102,111] and cystatin C [6,28,35,42,94]. The apolipoprotein ε4 and ε2 alleles as well as cystatin C are thought to be risk factors for CAA. They exert different effects on the progression of CAA, with apolipoprotein ε4 stimulating deposition of Aβ and apolipoprotein ε2 causing affected vessels to degenerate and bleed [46,47,77,90]. Severe cystatin C immunoreactivity is a risk factor for the occurrence and enlargement of the hemorrhage, as well as induction of recurrent hemorrhages [58,59,74, 129].

Thus, Alzheimer's disease is a complex disease with multigenetic involvement. The identification of a mutation in the AβPP gene in Dutch patients with HCHWA that segregates with the disease showed for the first time that Aβ is one etiological factor, and abnormal expression or altered structure can initiate the disease process.

Acknowledgments

Supported by National Institute of Neurological Disorders and Stroke grant NS42029, the National Institute on Aging grants AG16837, and AG05891, American Heart Association grant 0040102N.

References

[1] C.R. Abraham, D.J. Selkoe and H. Potter, Immunochemical identification of the serine protease inhibitor α1-antichymotrypsin in the brain amyloid deposits of Alzheimer's disease, *Cell* **52** (1988), 487–501.
[2] E. Bakker, C. Van Broeckhoven, J. Haan, E. Voorhoeve, W. Van Hul, E. Levy, I. Lieberburg, M.D. Carman, G.J. van Ommen, B. Frangione and R.A.C. Roos, DNA diagnosis for hereditary cerebral hemorrhage with amyloidosis, *Am J Hum Gen* **49** (1991), 518–521.
[3] A.J. Barrett, M.E. Davies and A.O. Grubb, The place of human γ-trace (cystatin C) amongst the cysteine proteinase inhibitors, *Biochem Biophys Res Commun* **120** (1984), 631–636.
[4] H.G. Bernstein, S. Bruszis, D. Schmidt, B. Wiederanders and A. Dorn, Immunodetection of cathepsin D in neuritic plaques found in brains of patients with dementia of Alzheimer type, *J Hirnforsch* **30** (1989), 613–618.
[5] H.G. Bernstein, H. Kirschke, B. Wiederanders, D. Schmidt and A. Rinne, Antigenic expression of cathepsin B in aged human brain, *Brain Res Bull* **24** (1990), 543–549.
[6] K. Beyer, J.I. Lao, M. Gomez, N. Riutort, P. Latorre, J.L. Mate and A. Ariza, Alzheimer's disease and the cystatin C gene polymorphism: an association study, *Neurosci Lett* **315** (2001), 17–20.

[7] L.A. Bobek and M.J. Levine, Cystatins-inhibitors of cysteine proteinases, *Crit Rev Oral Biol Med* **3** (1992), 307–332.

[8] D.R. Borchelt, G. Thinakaran, C.B. Eckman, M.K. Lee, F. Davenport, T. Ratovitsky, C.M. Prada, G. Kim, S. Seekins, D. Yager, H.H. Slunt, R. Wang, M. Seeger, A.I. Levey, S.E. Gandy, N.G. Copeland, N.A. Jenkins, D.L. Price, S.G. Younkin and S.S. Sisodia, Familial Alzheimer's disease-linked presenilin 1 variants elevate Aβ1-42/1-40 ratio *in vitro* and *in vivo*, *Neuron* **17** (1996), 1005–1013.

[9] W.S. Brooks, J.B. Kwok, G.M. Halliday, A.K. Godbolt, M.N. Rossor, H. Creasey, A.O. Jones and P.R. Schofield, Hemorrhage is uncommon in new Alzheimer family with Flemish amyloid precursor protein mutation, *Neurology* **63** (2004), 1613–1617.

[10] O. Bugiani, A. Padovani, M. Magoni, G. Andora, M. Sgarzi, M. Savoiardo, A. Bizzi, G. Giaccone, G. Rossi and F. Tagliavini, An Italian type of HCHWA, *Neurobiol Aging* **19** (1998), S238.

[11] D. Burdick, B. Soreghan, M. Kwon, J. Kosmoski, M. Knauer, A. Henschen, J. Yates, C. Cotman and C. Glabe, Assembly and aggregation properties of synthetic Alzheimer's A4/β amyloid peptide analogs, *J Biol Chem* **267** (1992), 546–554.

[12] P. Burgermeister, M.E. Calhoun, D.T. Winkler and M. Jucker, Mechanisms of cerebrovascular amyloid deposition. Lessons from mouse models, *Ann N Y Acad Sci* **903** (2000), 307–316.

[13] J. Busciglio, D.H. Gabuzda, P. Matsudaira and B.A. Yankner, Generation of β-amyloid in the secretory pathway in neuronal and nonneuronal cells, *Proc Natl Acad Sci USA* **90** (1993), 2092–2096.

[14] D.A. Butterfield and D. Boyd-Kimball, The critical role of methionine 35 in Alzheimer's amyloid β-peptide (1-42)-induced oxidative stress and neurotoxicity, *Biochim Biophys Acta* **1703** (2005), 149–156.

[15] X.D. Cai, T.E. Golde and S.G. Younkin, Release of excess amyloid β protein from a mutant amyloid β protein precursor, *Science* **259** (1993), 514–516.

[16] M.E. Calhoun, P. Burgermeister, A.L. Phinney, M. Stalder, M. Tolnay, K.H. Wiederhold, C. Abramowski, C. Sturchler-Pierrat, B. Sommer, M. Staufenbiel and M. Jucker, Neuronal overexpression of mutant amyloid precursor protein results in prominent deposition of cerebrovascular amyloid, *Proc Natl Acad Sci USA* **96** (1999), 14088–14093.

[17] E.M. Castano, F. Prelli, C. Soto, R. Beavis, E. Matsubara, M. Shoji and B. Frangione, The length of amyloid-β in hereditary cerebral hemorrhage with amyloidosis, Dutch type. Implications for the role of amyloid-β 1-42 in Alzheimer's disease, *J Biol Chem* **271** (1996), 32185–32191.

[18] A.M. Cataldo, P.A. Paskevich, E. Kominami and R.A. Nixon, Lysosomal hydrolases of different classes are abnormally distributed in brains of patients with Alzheimer disease, *Proc Natl Acad Sci USA* **88** (1991), 10998–11002.

[19] M.C. Chartier-Harlin, F. Crawford, H. Houlden, A. Warren, D. Hughes, L. Fidani, A. Goate, M. Rossor, P. Roques, J. Hardy and M. Mullan, Early-onset Alzheimer's disease caused by mutations at codon 717 of the β-amyloid precursor protein gene, *Nature* **353** (1991), 844–846.

[20] N.H. Choi-Miura, Y. Ihara, K. Fukuchi, M. Takeda, Y. Nakano, T. Tobe and M. Tomita, SP-40,40 is a constituent of Alzheimer's amyloid, *Acta Neurop* **83** (1992), 260–264.

[21] R. Christie, M. Yamada, M. Moskowitz and B. Hyman, Structural and functional disruption of vascular smooth muscle cells in a transgenic mouse model of amyloid angiopathy, *Am J Pathol* **158** (2001), 1065–1071.

[22] M. Citron, T. Oltersdorf, C. Haass, L. McConlogue, A.Y. Hung, P. Seubert, C. Vigo-Pelfrey, I. Lieberburg and D.J. Selkoe, Mutation of the β-amyloid precursor protein in familial Alzheimer's disease increases β protein production, *Nature* **360** (1992), 672–674.

[23] M. Citron, D. Westaway, W. Xia, G. Carlson, T. Diehl, G. Levesque, K. Johnson-Wood, M. Lee, P. Seubert, A. Davis, D. Kholodenko, R. Motter, R. Sherrington, B. Perry, H. Yao, R. Strome, I. Lieberburg, J. Rommens, S. Kim, D. Schenk, P. Fraser, P. St George Hyslop and D.J. Selkoe, Mutant presenilins of Alzheimer's disease increase production of 42-residue amyloid β-protein in both transfected cells and transgenic mice, *Nat Med* **3** (1997), 67–72.

[24] A. Clements, D.M. Walsh, C.H. Williams and D. Allsop, Aggregation of Alzheimer's peptides, *Biochem Soc Trans* **22** (1994), 16S.

[25] D.H. Cohen, H. Feiner, O. Jensson and B. Frangione, Amyloid fibril in hereditary cerebral hemorrhage with amyloidosis (HCHWA) is related to the gastoentero-pancreatic neuroendocrine protein, γ trace, *J Exp Med* **158** (1983), 623–628.

[26] F. Coria, E. Castano, F. Prelli, M. Larrondo-Lillo, S. van Duinen, M.L. Shelanski and B. Frangione, Isolation and characterization of amyloid P component from AD and other types of cerebral amyloidosis, *Lab Invest* **58** (1988), 454–458.

[27] F. Coria, E.M. Castano and B. Frangione, Brain amyloid in normal aging and cerebral amyloid angiopathy is antigenically related to Alzheimer's Disease β-protein, *Am J Pathol* **129** (1987), 422–428.

[28] F.C. Crawford, M.J. Freeman, J.A. Schinka, L.I. Abdullah, M. Gold, R. Hartman, K. Krivian, M.D. Morris, D. Richards, R. Duara, R. Anand and M.J. Mullan, A polymorphism in the cystatin C gene is a novel risk factor for late-onset Alzheimer's disease, *Neurology* **55** (2000), 763–768.

[29] J. Davis and W.E. Van Nostrand, Enhanced pathologic properties of Dutch-type mutant amyloid β-protein, *Proc Natl Acad Sci USA* **93** (1996), 2996–3000.

[30] J. Davis, F. Xu, R. Deane, G. Romanov, M.L. Previti, K. Zeigler, B.V. Zlokovic and W.E. Van Nostrand, Early-onset and robust cerebral microvascular accumulation of amyloid β-protein in transgenic mice expressing low levels of a vasculotropic Dutch/Iowa mutant form of amyloid β-protein precursor, *J Biol Chem* **279** (2004), 20296–20306.

[31] C. De Jonghe, C. Zehr, D. Yager, C.M. Prada, S. Younkin, L. Hendriks, C. Van Broeckhoven and C.B. Eckman, Flemish and Dutch mutations in amyloid β precursor protein have different effects on amyloid β secretion, *Neurobiol Dis* **5** (1998), 281–286.

[32] I. Dewachter, J. van Dorpe, K. Spittaels, I. Tesseur, C. Van Den Haute, D. Moechars and F. Van Leuven, Modeling Alzheimer's disease in transgenic mice: effect of age and of presenilin1 on amyloid biochemistry and pathology in APP/London mice, *Exp Gerontol* **35** (2000), 831–841.

[33] K. Duff, C. Eckman, C. Zehr, X. Yu, C.M. Prada, J. Perez-tur, M. Hutton, L. Buee, Y. Harigaya, D. Yager, D. Morgan, M.N. Gordon, L. Holcomb, L. Refolo, B. Zenk, J. Hardy and S. Younkin, Increased amyloid-β42(43) in brains of mice expressing mutant presenilin 1, *Nature* **383** (1996), 710–713.

[34] H. Fabian, G.I. Szendrei, H.H. Mantsch and L. Otvos, Jr., Comparative analysis of human and Dutch-type Alzheimer β-amyloid peptides by infrared spectroscopy and circular dichroism, *Biochem Biophys Res Commun* **191** (1993), 232–239.

[35] U. Finckh, H. von Der Kammer, J. Velden, T. Michel, B. Andresen, A. Deng, J. Zhang, T. Muller-Thomsen, K. Zuchowski, G. Menzer, U. Mann, A. Papassotiropoulos, R. Heun, J. Zurdel, F. Holst, L. Benussi, G. Stoppe, J. Reiss, A.R. Miserez, H.B. Staehelin, G.W. Rebeck, B.T. Hyman, G. Binetti, C. Hock, J.H. Growdon and R.M. Nitsch, Genetic association of a cystatin C gene polymorphism with late-onset Alzheimer disease, *Arch Neurol* **57** (2000), 1579–1583.

[36] P.E. Fraser, J.T. Nguyen, H. Inouye, W.K. Surewicz, D.J. Selkoe, M.B. Podlisny and D.A. Kirschner, Fibril formation by primate, rodent, and Dutch-hemorrhagic analogues of Alzheimer amyloid β-protein, *Biochemistry* **31** (1992), 10716–10723.

[37] D. Games, D. Adams, R. Alessandrini, R. Barbour, P. Berthelette, C. Blackwell, T. Carr, J. Clemens, T. Donaldson, F. Gillespie, T. Guido, S. Hagopian, K. Johnson-Wood, K. Khan, M. Lee, P. Leibovitz, I. Lieburburg, S. Little, E. Masliah, L. McConlogue, M. Montoya-Zavala, L. Mucke, L. Paganini, E. Penniman, M. Power, D. Schenk, P. Seubert, B. Snyder, F. Soriano, H. Tan, J. Vitale, S. Wadsworth, B. Wolozin and J. Zhao, Alzheimer-type neuropathology in transgenic mice overexpressing V717F β-amyloid precursor protein, *Nature* **373** (1995), 523–527.

[38] J. Ghiso, O. Jensson and B. Frangione, Amyloid fibrils in hereditary cerebral hemorrhage with amyloidosis of Icelandic type is a variant of γ trace basic protein (cystatin C), *Proc Natl Acad Sci USA* **83** (1986), 2974–2978.

[39] G.G. Glenner and C.W. Wong, Alzheimer's disease and Down's syndrome: sharing of a unique cerebrovascular amyloid fibril protein, *Biochem Biophys Res Commun* **122** (1984), 1131–1135.

[40] G.G. Glenner and C.W. Wong, Alzheimer's disease: initial report of the purification and characterization of a novel cerebrovascular amyloid protein, *Biochem Biophys Res Commun* **120** (1984), 885–890.

[41] A. Goate, M.C. Chartier-Harlin, M. Mullan, J. Brown, F. Crawford, L. Fidani, L. Giuffra, A. Haynes, N. Irving, L. James, R. Mant, P. Newton, K. Rooke, P. Roques, C. Talbot, M. Pericak-Vance, A. Roses, R. Williamson, M. Rossor, M. Owen and J. Hardy, Segregation of a missense mutation in the amyloid precursor protein gene with familial Alzheimer's disease, *Nature* **349** (1991), 704–706.

[42] K.A. Goddard, J.M. Olson, H. Payami, M. Van Der Voet, H. Kuivaniemi and G. Tromp, Evidence of linkage and association on chromosome 20 for late-onset Alzheimer disease, *Neurogenetics* **5** (2004), 121–128.

[43] D. Goldgaber, M.I. Lerman, O.W. McBride, U. Saffiotti and D.C. Gajdusek, Characterization and chromosomal localization of a cDNA encoding brain amyloid of Alzheimer's disease, *Science* **235** (1987), 877–878.

[44] P.A. Gollin, R.N. Kalaria, P. Eikelenboom, A. Rozemuller and G. Perry, α1-antitrypsin and α1-antichymotrypsin are in the lesions of Alzheimer's disease, *Neuroreport* **3** (1992), 201–203.

[45] T.J. Grabowski, H.S. Cho, J.P. Vonsattel, G.W. Rebeck and S.M. Greenberg, Novel amyloid precursor protein mutation in an Iowa family with dementia and severe cerebral amyloid angiopathy, *Ann Neurol* **49** (2001), 697–705.

[46] S.M. Greenberg, G.W. Rebeck, J.P. Vonsattel, T. Gomez-Isla and B.T. Hyman, Apolipoprotein E ε4 and cerebral hemorrhage associated with amyloid angiopathy, *Ann Neurol* **38** (1995), 254–259.

[47] S.M. Greenberg, J.P. Vonsattel, A.Z. Segal, R.I. Chiu, A.E. Clatworthy, A. Liao, B.T. Hyman and G.W. Rebeck, Association of apolipoprotein E ε2 and vasculopathy in cerebral amyloid angiopathy, *Neurology* **50** (1998), 961–965.

[48] G. Gudmundsson, J. Hallgrimsson, T.A. Jonasson and O. Bjarnason, Hereditary cerebral haemorrhage with amyloidosis, *Brain* **95** (1972), 387–404.

[49] J. Haan, M.L.C. Maat-Schieman, S.G. van Duinen, O. Jensson, L. Thorsteinsson and R.A.C. Roos, Co-localization of β/A4 and cystatin C in cortical blood vessels in Dutch, but not in Icelandic hereditary cerebral hemorrhage with amyloidosis, *Acta Neurol Scand* **89** (1994), 367–371.

[50] J. Haan, R.A. Roos, P.R. Algra, J.B. Lanser, G.T. Bots and M. Vegter-van der Vlis, Hereditary cerebral haemorrhage with amyloidosis-Dutch type. Magnetic resonance imaging findings in 7 case, *Brain* **113** (1990), 1251–1267.

[51] C. Haass and D.J. Selkoe, Cellular processing of β-amyloid precursor protein and the genesis of amyloid β-peptide, *Cell* **75** (1993), 1039–1042.

[52] L. Hendriks, C.M. van Duijn, P. Cras, M. Cruts, W. Van Hul, F. van Harskamp, A. Warren, M.G. McInnis, S.E. Antonarakis, J.J. Martin, A. Hofman and C. Van Broeckhoven, Presenile dementia and cerebral haemorrhage linked to a mutation at codon 692 of the β-amyloid precursor protein gene, *Nature Genet* **1** (1992), 218–221.

[53] M.C. Herzig, D.T. Winkler, P. Burgermeister, M. Pfeifer, E. Kohler, S.D. Schmidt, S. Danner, D. Abramowski, C. Sturchler-Pierrat, K. Burki, S.G. van Duinen, M.L. Maat-Schieman, M. Staufenbiel, P.M. Mathews and M. Jucker, Aβ is targeted to the vasculature in a mouse model of hereditary cerebral hemorrhage with amyloidosis, *Nat Neurosci* **7** (2004), 954–960.

[54] C. Hilbich, B. Kisters-Woike, J. Reed, C.L. Masters and K. Beyreuther, Aggregation and secondary structure of synthetic amyloid β A4 peptides of Alzheimer's disease, *J Mol Biol* **218** (1991), 149–163.

[55] G.M. Hochwald, A.J. Pepe and G.J. Thorbecke, Trace proteins in biological fluids. IV. Physicochemical properties and sites of formation of γ trace and β trace proteins, *Proc Soc Exp Med* **124** (1967), 961–966.

[56] A.Y. Hsia, E. Masliah, L. McConlogue, G.Q. Yu, G. Tatsuno, K. Hu, D. Kholodenko, R.C. Malenka, R.A. Nicoll and L. Mucke, Plaque-independent disruption of neural circuits in Alzheimer's disease mouse models, *Proc Natl Acad Sci USA* **96** (1999), 3228–3233.

[57] K. Hsiao, P. Chapman, S. Nilsen, C. Eckman, Y. Harigaya, S. Younkin, F. Yang and G. Cole, Correlative memory deficits, Aβ elevation and amyloid plaques in transgenic mice, *Science* **274** (1996), 99–102.

[58] Y. Itoh, M. Yamada, M. Hayakawa, E. Otomo and T. Miyatake, Cerebral amyloid angiopathy: a significant cause of cerebellar as well as lobar cerebral hemorrhage in the elderly, *J Neurol Sci* **116** (1993), 135–141.

[59] A. Izumihara, T. Ishihara, Y. Hoshii and H. Ito, Cerebral amyloid angiopathy associated with hemorrhage: immunohistochemical study of 41 biopsy cases, *Neurol Med Chir (Tokyo)* **41** (2001), 471–477; discussion 477–478.

[60] J.T. Jarrett, E.P. Berger and P.T. Lansbury, Jr., The carboxy terminus of the β amyloid protein is critical for the seeding of amyloid formation: implications for the pathogenesis of Alzheimer's disease, *Biochemistry* **32** (1993), 4693–4697.

[61] J.T. Jarrett and P.T. Lansbury, Jr., Seeding "one-dimensional crystallization" of amyloid: a pathogenic mechanism in Alzheimer's disease and scrapie? *Cell* **73** (1993), 1055–1058.

[62] K. Johnson-Wood, M. Lee, R. Motter, K. Hu, G. Gordon, R. Barbour, K. Khan, M. Gordon, H. Tan, D. Games, I. Lieberburg, D. Schenk, P. Seubert and L. McConlogue, Amyloid precursor protein processing and Aβ42 deposition in a transgenic mouse model of Alzheimer disease, *Proc Natl Acad Sci USA* **94** (1997), 1550–1555.

[63] K. Kamino, H.T. Orr, H. Payami, E.M. Wijsman, M.E. Alonso, S.M. Pulst, L. Anderson, S. O'Dahl, E. Nemens, J.A. White, A.D. Sadovnick, M.J. Ball, J. Kaye, A. Warren, M. McInnis, S.E. Antonarakis, J.R. Korenberg, V. Sharma, W. Kukull, E. Larson, L.L. Heston, G.M. Martin, T.D. Bird and G.D. Shellenberg, Linkage and mutational analysis of familial Alzheimer disease kindreds for the APP gene region, *Am J Hum Genet* **51** (1992), 998–1014.

[64] J. Kang, H.G. Lemaire, A. Unterbeck, J.M. Salbaum, C.L. Masters, K.H. Grzeschik, G. Multhaup, K. Beyreuther and B. Mueller-Hill, The precursor of Alzheimer's disease amyloid A4 protein resembles a cell-surface receptor, *Nature* **325** (1987), 733–736.

[65] M. Kawai, R.N. Kalaria, P. Cras, S.L. Siedlak, M.E. Velasco, E.R. Shelton, H.W. Chan, B.D. Greenberg and G. Perry, Degeneration of vascular muscle cells in cerebral amyloid angiopathy of Alzheimer disease, *Brain Res* **623** (1993), 142–146.

[66] N. Kitaguchi, Y. Takahashi, Y. Tokushima, S. Shiojiri and H. Ito, Novel precursor of Alzheimer's disease amyloid protein shows protease inhibitory activity, *Nature* **331** (1988), 530–532.

[67] H.G. Lemaire, J.M. Salbaum, G. Multhaup, J. Kang, R.M. Bayney, A. Unterbeck, K. Beyreuther and B. Muller-Hill, The PreA4(695) precursor protein of Alzheimer's disease A4 amyloid is encoded by 16 exons, *Nuc Acid Res* **17** (1989), 517–522.

[68] E. Levy, M.D. Carman, I.J. Fernandez-Madrid, M.D. Power, I. Lieberburg, S.G. van Duinen, G.T.A.M. Bots, W. Luyendijk and B. Frangione, Mutation of the Alzheimer's disease amyloid gene in hereditary cerebral hemorrhage, Dutch type, *Science* **248** (1990), 1124–1126.

[69] E. Levy, C. Lopez-Otin, J. Ghiso, D. Geltner and B. Frangione, Stroke in Icelandic patients with hereditary amyloid angiopathy is related to a mutation in the cystatin C gene, an inhibitor of cysteine proteases, *J Exp Med* **169** (1989), 1771–1778.

[70] E. Levy, M. Sastre, A. Kumar, G. Gallo, P. Piccardo, B. Ghetti and F. Tagliavini, Codeposition of cystatin C with amyloid-β protein in the brain of Alzheimer's disease patients, *J Neuropathol Exp Neurol* **60** (2001), 94–104.

[71] E. Levy-Lahad, W. Wasco, P. Poorkaj, D.M. Romano, J. Oshima, W.H. Pettingell, C.E. Yu, P.D. Jondro, S.D. Schmidt, K. Wang, A.C. Crowley, Y.-H. Fu, S.Y. Guenette, D. Galas, E. Nemens, E.M. Wijsman, T.D. Bird, G.D. Schellenberg and R.E. Tanzi, Candidate gene for the chromosome 1 familial Alzheimer's disease locus, *Science* **269** (1995), 973–977.

[72] W. Luyendijk, G.T. Bots, M. Vegter-van der Vlis, L.N. Went and B. Frangione, Hereditary cerebral haemorrhage caused by cortical amyloid angiopathy, *J Neurol Sci* **85** (1988), 267–280.

[73] D.M. Mann, S.M. Pickering-Brown, A. Takeuchi and T. Iwatsubo, Amyloid angiopathy and variability in amyloid β deposition is determined by mutation position in presenilin-1-linked Alzheimer's disease, *Am J Pathol* **158** (2001), 2165–2175.

[74] K. Maruyama, S. Ikeda, T. Ishihara, D. Allsop and N. Yanagisawa, Immunohistochemical characterization of cerebrovascular amyloid in 46 autopsied cases using antibodies to β protein and cystatin C, *Stroke* **21** (1990), 397–403.

[75] K. Maruyama, M. Usami, W. Yamao-Harigaya, K. Tagawa and S. Ishiura, Mutation of Glu693 to Gln or Val717 to Ile has no effect on the processing of Alzheimer amyloid precursor protein expressed in COS-1 cells by cDNA transfection, *Neurosci Lett* **132** (1991), 97–100.

[76] C.L. Masters, G. Simms, N.A. Weinman, G. Multhaup, B.L. McDonald and K. Beyreuther, Amyloid plaque core protein in Alzheimer disease and Down syndrome, *Proc Natl Acad Sci USA* **82** (1985), 4245–4249.

[77] M.O. McCarron, J.A. Nicoll, J. Stewart, J.W. Ironside, D.M. Mann, S. Love, D.I. Graham and D. Dewar, The apolipoprotein E ε2 allele and the pathological features in cerebral amyloid angiopathy-related hemorrhage, *J Neuropathol Exp Neurol* **58** (1999), 711–718.

[78] P.L. McGeer, T. Kawamata and D.G. Walker, Distribution of clusterin in Alzheimer brain tissue, *Brain Res* **579** (1992), 337–341.

[79] E. McGowan, S. Sanders, T. Iwatsubo, A. Takeuchi, T. Saido, C. Zehr, X. Yu, S. Uljon, R. Wang, D. Mann, D. Dickson and K. Duff, Amyloid phenotype characterization of transgenic mice overexpressing both mutant amyloid precursor protein and mutant presenilin 1 transgenes, *Neurobiol Dis* **6** (1999), 231–244.

[80] J.P. Melchor, L. McVoy and W.E. Van Nostrand, Charge alterations of E22 enhance the pathogenic properties of the amyloid β-protein, *J Neurochem* **74** (2000), 2209–2212.

[81] L. Miravalle, T. Tokuda, R. Chiarle, G. Giaccone, O. Bugiani, F. Tagliavini, B. Frangione and J. Ghiso, Substitutions at codon 22 of Alzheimer's Aβ peptide induce diverse conformational changes and apoptotic effects in human cerebral endothelial cells, *J Biol Chem* **275** (2000), 27110–27116.

[82] O.R. Monro, J.B. Mackic, S. Yamada, M.B. Segal, J. Ghiso, C. Maurer, M. Calero, B. Frangione and B.V. Zlokovic, Substitution at codon 22 reduces clearance of Alzheimer's amyloid-β peptide from the cerebrospinal fluid and prevents its transport from the central nervous system into blood, *Neurobiol Aging* **23** (2002), 405–412.

[83] L. Morelli, R. Llovera, S. Ibendahl and E.M. Castano, The degradation of amyloid β as a therapeutic strategy in Alzheimer's disease and cerebrovascular amyloidoses, *Neurochem Res* **27** (2002), 1387–1399.

[84] L. Morelli, R.E. Llovera, I. Mathov, L.F. Lue, B. Frangione, J. Ghiso and E.M. Castano, Insulin-degrading enzyme in brain microvessels: proteolysis of amyloid β vasculotropic variants and reduced activity in cerebral amyloid angiopathy, *J Biol Chem* **279** (2004), 56004–56013.

[85] M. Mullan, F. Crawford, K. Axelman, H. Houlden, L. Lilius, B. Winblad and L. Lannfelt, A pathogenic mutation for probable Alzheimer's disease in the amyloid precursor protein gene at the N-terminus of β-amyloid, *Nature Genet* **1** (1992), 345–347.

[86] J. Murrell, M. Farlow, B. Ghetti and M.D. Benson, A mutation in the amyloid precursor protein associated with hereditary Alzheimer's disease, *Science* **254** (1991), 97–99.

[87] Y. Nakamura, M. Takeda, H. Suzuki, H. Hattori, K. Tada, S. Hariguchi, S. Hashimoto and T. Nishimura, Abnormal distribution of cathepsins in the brain of patients with Alzheimer's disease, *Neurosci Lett* **130** (1991), 195–198.

[88] Y. Namba, M. Tomonaga, H. Kawasaki, E. Otomo and K. Ikeda, Apolipoprotein E immunoreactivity in cerebral amyloid deposits and neurofibrillary tangles in Alzheimer's dis-

ease and kuru plaque amyloid in Creutzfeldt-Jakob disease, *Brain Res* **541** (1991), 163–166.

[89] S. Naruse, S. Igarashi, H. Kobayashi, K. Aoki, T. Inuzuka, K. Kaneko, T. Shimizu, K. Iihara, T. Kojima, T. Miyatake and S. Teuji, Mis-sense mutation Val–Ile in exon 17 of amyloid precursor protein gene in Japanese familial Alzheimer's disease, *Lancet* **337** (1991), 978–979.

[90] J.A. Nicoll, C. Burnett, S. Love, D.I. Graham, D. Dewar, J.W. Ironside, J. Stewart and H.V. Vinters, High frequency of apolipoprotein E ε2 allele in hemorrhage due to cerebral amyloid angiopathy, *Ann Neurol* **41** (1997), 716–721.

[91] C. Nilsberth, A. Westlind-Danielsson, C.B. Eckman, M.M. Condron, K. Axelman, C. Forsell, C. Stenh, J. Luthman, D.B. Teplow, S.G. Younkin, J. Naslund and L. Lannfelt, The 'Arctic' APP mutation (E693G) causes Alzheimer's disease by enhanced Aβ protofibril formation, *Nat Neurosci* **4** (2001), 887–893.

[92] R.A. Nixon, A.M. Cataldo, P.A. Paskevich, D.J. Hamilton, T.R. Wheelock and L. Kanaley-Andrews, The lysosomal system in neurons. Involvement at multiple stages of Alzheimer's disease pathogenesis, *Ann N Y Acad Sci* **674** (1992), 65–88.

[93] D. Nochlin, T.D. Bird, E.J. Nemens, M.J. Ball and S.M. Sumi, Amyloid angiopathy in a Volga German family with Alzheimer's disease and a presenilin-2 mutation (N141I), *Ann Neurol* **43** (1998), 131–135.

[94] J.M. Olson, K.A. Goddard and D.M. Dudek, A second locus for very-late-onset Alzheimer disease: a genome scan reveals linkage to 20p and epistasis between 20p and the amyloid precursor protein region, *Am J Hum Genet* **71** (2002), 154–161.

[95] F. Prelli, E. Castano, G.G. Glenner and B. Frangione, Differences between vascular and plaque core amyloid in Alzheimer's disease, *J Neurochem* **51** (1988), 648–651.

[96] F. Prelli, E. Levy, S.G. van Duinen, G.T. Bots, W. Luyendijk and B. Frangione, Expression of a normal and variant Alzheimer's β-protein gene in amyloid of hereditary cerebral hemorrhage, Dutch type: DNA and protein diagnostic assays, *Biochem Biophys Res Commun* **170** (1990), 301–307.

[97] D.L. Price and S.S. Sisodia, Mutant genes in familial Alzheimer's disease and transgenic models, *Annu Rev Neurosci* **21** (1998), 479–505.

[98] S.B. Prusiner, M.P. McKinley, K.A. Bowman, D.C. Bolton, P.E. Bendheim, D.F. Groth and G.G. Glenner, Scrapie prions aggregate to form amyloid-like birefringent rods, *Cell* **35** (1983), 349–358.

[99] G.W. Rebeck, S.D. Harr, D.K. Strickland and B.T. Hyman, Multiple, diverse senile plaque-associated proteins are ligands of an apolipoprotein E receptor, the ε2-macroglobulin receptor/low-density-lipoprotein receptor-related protein, *Ann Neurol* **37** (1995), 211–217.

[100] N.K. Robakis, N. Ramakrishna, G. Wolfe and H.M. Wisniewski, Molecular cloning and characterization of a cDNA encoding the cerebrovascular and the neuritic plaque amyloid peptides, *Proc Natl Acad Sci USA* **84** (1987), 4190–4194.

[101] G. Rossi, G. Giaccone, R. Maletta, M. Morbin, R. Capobianco, M. Mangieri, A.R. Giovagnoli, A. Bizzi, C. Tomaino, M. Perri, M. Di Natale, F. Tagliavini, O. Bugiani and A.C. Bruni, A family with Alzheimer disease and strokes associated with A713T mutation of the APP gene, *Neurology* **63** (2004), 910–912.

[102] A.M. Saunders, W.J. Strittmatter, D. Schmechel, P.H. George-Hyslop, M.A. Pericak-Vance, S.H. Joo, B.L. Rosi, J.F. Gusella, D.R. Crapper-MacLachlan, M.J. Alberts, C. Hulette, B. Crain, D. Goldgaber and A.D. Roses, Association of apolipoprotein E allele ε4 with late-onset familial and sporadic Alzheimer's Disease, *Neurology* **43** (1993), 1467–1472.

[103] G.D. Schellenberg, T.D. Bird, E.M. Wijsman, D.K. Moore, M. Boehnke, E.M. Bryant, T.H. Lampe, D. Nochlin, S.M. Sumi, S.S. Deeb, K. Beyreuther and G.M. Martin, Absence of linkage of chromosome 21q21 markers to familial Alzheimer's disease, *Science* **241** (1988), 1507–1510.

[104] P. Seubert, C. Vigo-Pelfrey, F. Esch, M. Lee, H. Dovey, D. Davis, S. Sinha, M. Schlossmacher, J. Whaley, C. Swindlehurst, R. McCormack, R. Wolfert, D.J. Selkoe, I. Lieberburg and D. Schenk, Isolation and quantification of soluble Alzheimer's β-peptide from biological fluids, *Nature* **359** (1992), 325–327.

[105] R. Sherrington, E.I. Rogaev, Y. Liang, E.A. Rogaeva, G. Levesque, M. Ikeda, H. Chi, C. Lin, G. Li, K. Holman, T. Tsuda, L. Mar, J.F. Foncin, A. Bruni, M. Montesi, S. Sorbi, I. Rainero, L. Pinessi, L. Nee, I. Chumakov, D. Pollen, A. Brookes, P. Sanseau, R.J. Polinsky, W. Wasco, H.A.R. Da Silva, J.L. Haines, M.A. Pericak-Vance, R.E. Tanzi, A.D. Roses, P.E. Fraser, J.M. Rommens and P. St George-Hyslop, Cloning of a gene bearing missense mutations in early-onset familial Alzheimer's disease, *Nature* **375** (1995), 754–760.

[106] T. Shimizu, H. Fukuda, S. Murayama, N. Izumiyama and T. Shirasawa, Isoaspartate formation at position 23 of amyloid β peptide enhanced fibril formation and deposited onto senile plaques and vascular amyloids in Alzheimer's disease, *J Neurosci Res* **70** (2002), 451–461.

[107] M. Shoji, T.E. Golde, J. Ghiso, T.T. Cheung, S. Estus, L.M. Shaffer, X.D. Cai, D.M. McKay, R. Tintner, B. Frangione and S.G. Younkin, Production of the Alzheimer amyloid β protein by normal proteolytic processing, *Science* **258** (1992), 126–129.

[108] A.D. Snow, J. Willmer and R. Kisilevsky, Sulfated glycosaminoglycans: a common constituent of all amyloids?, *Lab Invest* **56** (1987), 120–123.

[109] C. Soto, M.S. Kindy, M. Baumann and B. Frangione, Inhibition of Alzheimer's amyloidosis by peptides that prevent β-sheet conformation, *Biochem Biophys Res Commun* **226** (1996), 672–680.

[110] P.H. St George-Hyslop, R.E. Tanzi, R.J. Polinsky, J.L. Haines, L. Nee, P.C. Watkins, R.H. Myers, R.G. Feldman, D. Pollen, D. Drachman, J. Growdon, A. Bruni, J.-F. Foncin, D. Salmon, P. Frommelt, L. Amaducci, S. Sorbi, S. Piacentini, G.D. Stewart, W.J. Hobbs, P.M. Conneally, J.F. Gusella, The genetic defect causing familial Alzheimer's disease maps on chromosome 21, *Science* **235** (1987), 885–890.

[111] W.J. Strittmatter, A.M. Saunders, D. Schmechel, M. Pericak-Vance, J. Enghild, G.S. Salvesen and A.D. Roses, Apolipoprotein E: high-avidity binding to β-amyloid and increased frequency of type 4 allele in late-onset familial Alzheimer's Disease, *Proc Natl Acad Sci USA* **90** (1993), 1977–1981.

[112] C. Sturchler-Pierrat, D. Abramowski, M. Duke, K.H. Wiederhold, C. Mistl, S. Rothacher, B. Ledermann, K. Burki, P. Frey, P.A. Paganetti, C. Waridel, M.E. Calhoun, M. Jucker, A. Probst, M. Staufenbiel and B. Sommer, Two amyloid precursor protein transgenic mouse models with Alzheimer disease-like pathology, *Proc Natl Acad Sci USA* **94** (1997), 13287–13292.

[113] N. Suzuki, T.T. Cheung, X.D. Cai, A. Odaka, L. Otvos, Jr., C. Eckman, T.E. Golde and S.G. Younkin, An increased percentage of long amyloid β protein secreted by familial

amyloid β protein precursor (βAPP717) mutants, *Science* **264** (1994), 1336–1340.

[114] A. Tamaoka, A. Odaka, Y. Ishibashi, M. Usami, N. Sahara, N. Suzuki, N. Nukina, H. Mizusawa, S. Shoji, I. Kanazawa and H. Monin, APP717 missense mutation affects the ratio of amyloid β protein species (Aβ1-42/43 and Aβ1-40) in familial Alzheimer's disease brain, *J Biol Chem* **269** (1994), 32721–32724.

[115] R.E. Tanzi and L. Bertram, New frontiers in Alzheimer's disease genetics, *Neuron* **32** (2001), 181–184.

[116] R.E. Tanzi, J.F. Gusella, P.C. Watkins, G.A. Bruns, P. St George-Hyslop, M.L. Van Keuren, D. Patterson, S. Pagan, D.M. Kurnit and R.L. Neve, Amyloid β protein gene: cDNA, mRNA distribution, and genetic linkage near the Alzheimer locus, *Science* **235** (1987), 880–884.

[117] R.E. Tanzi, P.H. St George-Hyslop, J.L. Haines, R.J. Polinsky, L. Nee, J.F. Foncin, R.L. Neve, A.I. McClatchey, P.M. Conneally and J.F. Gusella, The genetic defect in familial Alzheimer's disease is not tightly linked to the amyloid β-protein gene, *Nature* **329** (1987), 156–157.

[118] R.E. Tanzi, G. Vaula, D.M. Romano, M. Mortilla, T.L. Huang, R.G. Tupler, W. Wasco, B.T. Hyman, J.L. Haines, B.J. Jenkins, M. Kalaitsidaki, A.C. Warren, M.C. McInnis, S.E. Antonarakis, H. Karlinsky, M.E. Percy, L. Connor, J. Growdon, D.R. Crapper-Mclachlan, J.F. Gusella and P.H. St George-Hyslop, Assessment of amyloid β-protein precursor gene mutations in a large set of familial and sporadic Alzheimer disease cases, *Am J Hum Gen* **51** (1992), 273–282.

[119] W.F. Timmers, F. Tagliavini, J. Haan and B. Frangione, Parenchymal preamyloid and amyloid deposits in the brains of patients with hereditary cerebral hemorrhage with amyloidosis–Dutch type, *Neurosci Lett* **118** (1990), 223–226.

[120] S. Tsubuki, Y. Takaki and T.C. Saido, Dutch, Flemish, Italian, and Arctic mutations of APP and resistance of Aβ to physiologically relevant proteolytic degradation, *Lancet* **361** (2003), 1957–1958.

[121] C. Van Broeckhoven, A.M. Genthe, A. Vandenberghe, B. Horsthemke, H. Backhovens, P. Raeymaekers, W. Van Hul, A. Wehnert, J. Gheuens, P. Cras, M. Bruyland, J.J. Martin, M. Salbaum, G. Multhaup, C.L. Masters, K. Beyreuther, H.M.D. Gurling, M.J. Mullan, A. Holland, A. Barton, N. Irving, R. Williamson, S.J. Richards and J.A. Hardy, Failure of familial Alzheimer's disease to segregate with the A4-amyloid gene in several European families, *Nature* **329** (1987), 153–155.

[122] C. Van Broeckhoven, J. Haan, E. Bakker, J.A. Hardy, W. Van Hul, A. Wehnert, M. Vegter-van der Vlis and R.A. Roos, Amyloid β protein precursor gene and hereditary cerebral hemorrhage with amyloidosis (Dutch), *Science* **248** (1990), 1120–1122.

[123] J. Van Dorpe, L. Smeijers, I. Dewachter, D. Nuyens, K. Spittaels, C. Van Den Haute, M. Mercken, D. Moechars, I. Laenen, C. Kuiperi, K. Bruynseels, I. Tesseur, R. Loos, H. Vanderstichele, F. Checler, R. Sciot and F. Van Leuven, Prominent cerebral amyloid angiopathy in transgenic mice overexpressing the london mutant of human APP in neurons, *Am J Pathol* **157** (2000), 1283–1298.

[124] S.G. van Duinen, E.M. Castano, F. Prelli, G.T. Bots, W. Luyendijk and B. Frangione, Hereditary cerebral hemorrhage with amyloidosis in patients of Dutch origin is related to Alzheimer disease, *Proc Natl Acad Sci USA* **84** (1987), 5991–5994.

[125] D. Van Gool, B. De Strooper, F. Van Leuven, E. Triau and R. Dom, ε2-Macroglobulin expression in neuritic-type plaques in patients with Alzheimer's disease, *Neurobiol Aging* **14** (1993), 233–237.

[126] W.E. Van Nostrand, J.P. Melchor, H.S. Cho, S.M. Greenberg and G.W. Rebeck, Pathogenic effects of D23N Iowa mutant amyloid β-protein, *J Biol Chem* **276** (2001), 32860–32866.

[127] W.E. Van Nostrand, J.P. Melchor and L. Ruffini, Pathologic amyloid β-protein cell surface fibril assembly on cultured human cerebrovascular smooth muscle cells, *J Neurochem* **70** (1998), 216–223.

[128] R.G. Vidal, I. Fernandez-Madrid, B. Frangione and E. Levy, Sequencing of the Alzheimer's APP gene Dutch variant (APP-D), *Human Mutation* **2** (1993), 496–497.

[129] H.V. Vinters, G.S. Nishimura, D.L. Secor and W.M. Pardridge, Immunoreactive A4 and γ-trace peptide colocalization in amyloidotic arteriolar lesions in brains of patients with Alzheimer's disease, *Am J Pathol* **137** (1990), 233–240.

[130] M.P. Vitek, C.G. Rasool, F. de Sauvage, S.M. Vitek, R.T. Bartus, B. Beer, R.A. Ashton, A.F. Macq, J.M. Maloteaux, A.J. Blume and J.-N. Octave, Absence of mutation in the β-amyloid cDNAs cloned from the brains of three patients with sporadic Alzheimer's disease, *Brain Res* **464** (1988), 121–131.

[131] L.C. Walker and R.A. Durham, Cerebrovascular amyloidosis: experimental analysis *in vitro* and *in vivo*, *Histol Histopathol* **14** (1999), 827–837.

[132] D.M. Walsh, D.M. Hartley, M.M. Condron, D.J. Selkoe and D.B. Teplow, *In vitro* studies of amyloid β-protein fibril assembly and toxicity provide clues to the aetiology of Flemish variant (Ala692→Gly) Alzheimer's disease, *Biochem J* **355** (2001), 869–877.

[133] Z. Wang, R. Natte, J.A. Berliner, S.G. van Duinen and H.V. Vinters, Toxicity of Dutch (E22Q) and Flemish (A21G) mutant amyloid β proteins to human cerebral microvessel and aortic smooth muscle cells, *Stroke* **31** (2000), 534–538.

[134] D.J. Watson, D.J. Selkoe and D.B. Teplow, Effects of the amyloid precursor protein Glu693→Gln 'Dutch' mutation on the production and stability of amyloid β-protein, *Biochem J* **340**(Pt 3) (1999), 703–709.

[135] A.R. Wattendorff, G.T. Bots, L.N. Went and L.J. Endtz, Familial cerebral amyloid angiopathy presenting as recurrent cerebral hemorrhage, *J Neurol Sci* **55** (1982), 121–135.

[136] P. Westermark, M.D. Benson, J.N. Buxbaum, A.S. Cohen, B. Frangione, S. Ikeda, C.L. Masters, G. Merlini, M.J. Saraiva and J.D. Sipe, Amyloid fibril protein nomenclature – 2002, *Amyloid* **9** (2002), 197–200.

[137] D.T. Winkler, L. Bondolfi, M.C. Herzig, L. Jann, M.E. Calhoun, K.H. Wiederhold, M. Tolnay, M. Staufenbiel and M. Jucker, Spontaneous hemorrhagic stroke in a mouse model of cerebral amyloid angiopathy, *J Neurosci* **21** (2001), 1619–1627.

[138] T. Wisniewski, J. Ghiso and B. Frangione, Peptides homologous to the amyloid protein of Alzheimer's disease containing a glutamine for glutamic acid substitution have accelerated amyloid fibril formation, *Biochem Biophys Res Commun* **179** (1991), 1247–1254.

[139] K. Yoshioka, T. Miki, T. Katsuya, T. Ogihara and Y. Sakaki, The 717Val – Ile substitution in amyloid precursor protein is associated with familial Alzheimer's disease regardless of ethnic groups, *Biochem Biophys Res Commun* **178** (1991), 1141–1146.

[140] S.G. Younkin, The amyloid β protein precursor mutations linked to familial Alzheimer's disease alter processing in a way that fosters amyloid deposition, *Tohoku J Exp Med* **174** (1994), 217–223.

Segregation of a missense mutation in the amyloid β-protein precursor gene with familial Alzheimer's disease

Alison Goate
Departments of Psychiatry, Neurology & Genetics, Washington University School of Medicine, 660 S. Euclid Avenue, St. Louis, MO 63110, USA
Tel.: +1 314 362 8691; Fax: +1 314 747 2983; E-mail: goate@icarus.wustl.edu

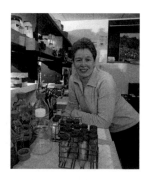

Abstract. In 1991 we described a missense mutation in the amyloid β-protein precursor (AβPP) gene in two familial Alzheimer's disease (FAD) kindreds. This gene encodes the amyloid β peptide deposited in senile plaques in AD. We made four predictions based upon these results: 1. Other FAD kindreds would be identified wth AβPP mutations; 2. FAD is genetically heterogeneous; 3. Aβ deposition is central to the pathogenesis of AD and 4, Regulatory variants in the AβPP gene lead to late onset AD. In the ensuing years substantial evidence has accrued in support of these predictions. Nineteen mutations in the AβPP gene have been reported. These mutations have all been shown to alter AβPP processing or Aβ fibrillogenesis, leading to early Aβ deposition. Furthermore, mutations in the genes encoding presenilin 1 and presenilin 2, that cause FAD, also lead to changes in AβPP processing and Aβ deposition. Together these observations strongly support the hypothesis that Aβ deposition is central to AD pathogenesis. Suprisingly, the fourth prediction, that variation in AβPP expression may predispose to late onset AD, has not been rigorously tested, despite the fact that overexpression of AβPP is sufficient to cause dementia and AD neuropathology in Down Syndrome.

Keywords: Familial Alzheimer's disease, Amyloid β-protein precursor, Amyloid β, gene, mutation, pathogenesis

1. Introduction

In 1991 little was known about the pathobiology of Alzheimer's disease. Earlier studies had demonstrated that plaques contain amyloid β (Aβ) and that neurofibrillary tangles were composed of paired-helical filaments of hyperphosphorylated tau [7,11,21]. However, it was unclear whether either of these inclusions was causative, largely because Aβ plaques were believed to be common in non-demented elderly and NFT were known to occur in many neurodegenerative diseases. Thus neither inclusion appeared to be specific for AD. Early studies suggested that NFT showed a better correlation with dementia than plaques and thus it was argued they were more likely to be the cause of disease. A major impediment to the molecular dissection of AD was the absence of cellular or animal models of disease.

2. Genetic linkage to chromosome 21 in Familial Alzheimer's disease

Although it had been known for more than 50 years that families existed in which AD had an early onset (< 60 yrs) (FAD), and was inherited as an autosomal dominant trait [20], the techniques of molecular genetics only began to make analysis of these families feasible in the late 1980s. The Human Genome Project led to major methodological advances including the development of genetic and physical maps of the human genome, methods for linkage analysis and PCR. Initial studies of FAD focused on chromosome 21 for two reasons, all individuals with Down syndrome (trisomy of chromosome 21) develop AD by middle age and Aβ had been shown to be derived from a larger precursor protein, the amyloid β protein precursor (AβPP) encoded by a gene on chromosome 21 [10,17,34,48]. Linkage was first reported between DNA markers on chromosome 21 and FAD in 1987 [43]. However, some groups failed to replicate these results in other family series [32,37]. When AβPP was shown to be encoded by a gene on chromosome 21 it was clearly a very strong candidate gene. However, the AβPP gene was quickly excluded because recombination events were observed between the AβPP gene and AD in several families [49,50]. At this time FAD was assumed to be a genetically homogeneous disorder and therefore the observation of recombinants in one family excluded the gene in all families. With the benefit of hindsight this appears to be a very naive viewpoint. Fifteen years on, non-allelic genetic heterogeneity in neurodegenerative diseases is common [41].

3. Familial Alzheimer's disease is genetically heterogeneous

A turning point in AD genetics was the multi-center investigation headed by Peter Hyslop and John Hardy [42]. This paper analyzed data from many families and came to the conclusion that FAD exhibited non-allelic genetic heterogeneity i.e. that some families were linked to a locus on chromosome 21 but that many families were not. Furthermore, there was more than one linkage signal on chromosome 21 raising the possibility of more than one gene on chromosome 21 leading to AD. This observation meant that a gene on chromosome 21 could only be excluded if the family showed evidence of linkage to chromosome 21 and that data from families should be analyzed individually, not pooled with other families, unless the families show linkage individually.

4. A Missense mutation in the AβPP gene causes FAD

After this paper, and two other papers describing linkage to the AβPP gene and a mutation in AβPP in a disorder called Hereditary cerebral hemorrhage with amyloidosis, Dutch type (HCHWA-D) [18,51] John Hardy and myself resolved to re-evaluate the AβPP gene in our own series of FAD kindreds. We had previously reported linkage to chromosome 21 in these families, and a large part of the linkage signal around AβPP in the multi-center study came from one of our families [9,42]. Segregation analysis of multiple markers along the entire length of chromosome 21 in this family demonstrated a common disease haplotype in all affected individuals. However, there were two unaffected individuals who provided important information. An unaffected cousin of the main sibship shared 10 Mb of chromosome 21 telomeric of D21S17. This individual was fifteen years over the mean age of onset in the family and remained unaffected. This ruled out the telomeric region as the site of the disease locus. The second unaffected individual was a sibling of the main sibship who shared 19 Mb centromeric of D21S1. This person, while unaffected, was only two years older than the mean age of onset, giving odds of two to one against this person developing AD. If the person remained healthy the disease locus must lie between D21S1 and D21S17, a region that includes the AβPP gene. Although the odds were not huge we decided to evaluate the AβPP gene because we could not exclude the gene genetically. Exons 16 and 17 were sequenced first because these exons encode the part of AβPP that gives rise to the Aβ peptide and because the mutation that causes HCHWA-D is in exon 17. This sequencing identified a single nucleotide substitution that results in a missense mutation, V717I [8]. This substitution was present in all of the affected individuals in the family but none of the unaffected individuals. Furthermore, it was absent from 100 unrelated normal individuals but present in one of sixteen early onset FAD kindreds screened. A polymorphism, in the 3' end of the AβPP gene, distinguished the two V717I families indicating that the mutation had arisen independently in these two families. The V717I substitution is conservative but its location, close to the C-terminus of the Aβ peptide suggested that it may influence production of Aβ.

We made several predictions based upon these results: 1. Other FAD kindreds would be identified that carry AβPP mutations; 2. FAD is genetically heterogeneous; 3. Aβ deposition is the central event in the pathogenesis of the disorder and 4, Regulatory variants in AβPP might lead to late onset AD.

5. Mutations in AβPP cause AD and stroke resulting from cerebral hemorrhage

Eight months after our original report, we reported a second mutation in AβPP that caused FAD [2]. This mutation was also at codon 717 but resulted in a V717G amino acid substitution. Based upon the two mutations we hypothesized that FAD mutations in AβPP alter AβPP processing to enhance Aβ production and thus Aβ deposition. At this time nothing was known about AβPP processing, indeed it was not even known that Aβ was produced in normal individuals. However, these observations clearly gave urgency to the need to understand more about the proteolytic processing of AβPP.

In the fourteen years since the publication of these papers 23 amino acid substitutions have been described in the *AβPP* gene (http//:www.alzforum.org/home.asp). The majority of these substitutions (19/23) have unambiguously been demonstrated to be pathogenic (Fig. 1). Many of the mutations have been shown to segregate with disease in an FAD kindred [2,8,22,23], and are not observed in unrelated controls. Some have also been shown to alter Aβ metabolism *in vitro* or cause age-dependent Aβ deposition *in vivo* (reviewed in [39]). Strikingly, all of these mutations occur in exons 16 and 17, the exons that code for the Aβ sequence and flanking regions (Fig. 1). The location of these mutations strongly supported our hypothesis that FAD mutations in AβPP result in altered Aβ processing.

The analysis of AβPP processing in neuronal and non-neuronal cells has subsequently demonstrated that AβPP can be proteolytically cleaved via two mutually exclusive pathways (Fig. 2). The first pathway, which is the most common in all cells except neurons, results in cleavage within the Aβ sequence by an activity termed α-secretase, to release a soluble N-terminal fragment called sAβPPα and a membrane associated C-terminal fragment called C83. In neurons an alternate pathway, called the β-secretase (BACE) pathway, cleaves at the N-terminus of Aβ generating sAβPPβ and a C-terminal fragment C99, which is subsequently cleaved by γ-secretase to generate Aβ and AβPP intracellular domain (AICD). C83 can also be cleaved by γ-secretase to generate P3 and AICD.

In vitro overexpression of AβPP FAD mutations has demonstrated that all mutations affect AβPP processing leading to changes in the amount of Aβ produced, changes in the ratios of the Aβ species produced and/or changes in the physico-chemical properties of the Aβ [3,12,47]. Some but not all of these mutations also alter the production of AICD [12]. The so-called Swedish mutation, located at the N-terminus of Aβ, results in an AβPP molecule that is a better substrate for BACE resulting in higher levels of Aβ [3]. In contrast FAD mutations located between AβPP714 and AβPP723 result in altered cleavage by γ-secretase [47]. The effect of these mutations is more complex in that the amount of Aβ and the ratios of the different Aβ species (Aβ37-Aβ43) vary with each mutation [12]. However, a common feature of all mutations seems to be an increase in Aβ42 relative to other Aβ species. Five mutations have been reported within the Aβ sequence at residues AβPP692-694. These mutations are often associated with cerebral hemorrhage rather than AD [13,18,27]. Although these mutations are located near the α-secretase cleavage site and thus could alter AβPP processing they are also within the Aβ peptide and thus alter the physico-chemical properties of the peptide leading to increase protofibril formation [27,44].

Several of these mutations have also been used to develop transgenic animals [6,16,46]. A consistent property of these animals is an age dependent Aβ deposition. However, unlike humans these mice do not develop overt neurodegeneration or neurofibrillary tangles. Another, striking observation coming from these mice is that overexpression of Aβ42 leads to parenchymal Aβ deposition, such as that seen in AD, while overexpression of Aβ40 leads to Aβ desposition primarily in the cerebral vessels [14]. Thus AβPPSwe, which results in higher levels of both Aβ40 and Aβ42 leads to both pathologies [5], while AβPP717 mutations lead to parenchymal Aβ deposition [6] and AβPP692 leads to Aβ deposition in the cerebral vessels [14].

6. Mutations in at least three genes can cause FAD

The second prediction was that FAD exhibited non-allelic genetic heterogeneity. This has also been demonstrated to be correct. In 1992, Schellenberg & colleagues reported linkage to chromosome 14 in early onset FAD and in 1995 St. George-Hyslop and colleagues identified mutations in a novel gene, later named *presenilin 1* [38,40]. A third FAD gene, *presenilin 2* was identified only a few months later because of its homology to *presenilin 1* [19,35]. *In vitro* and *in vivo* studies have demonstrated that FAD mutations in *PS1* and *PS2* also lead to changes in γ-secretase cleavage of AβPP, resulting in higher Aβ42/Aβ40 ratios and early Aβ deposition (reviewed in [39]). All known

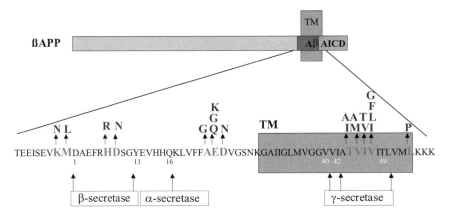

Fig. 1. Location of disease causing mutations in AβPP a type 1 transmembrane protein. FAD mutations in AβPP are located within and flanking the Aβ sequence and close to the proteolytic cleavage sites. FAD mutations are shown in grey above the normal sequence of the protein. Numbers indicate the amino acid position within the Aβ peptide. The location of the major proteolytic cleavage sites in AβPP are indicated by arrows below the sequence.

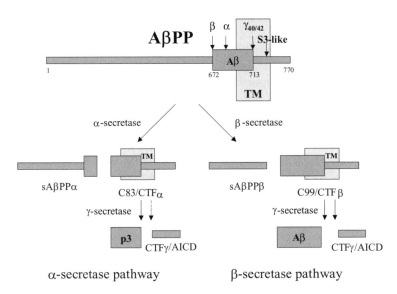

Fig. 2. AβPP is proteolytically cleaved via two pathways. In most cells AβPP is cleaved by α-secretase followed by γ-secretase. In neurons the predominant pathway involves sequential cleavage by β-secretase and γ-secretase.

FAD mutations appear to alter AβPP processing to produce more Aβ, increase the propensity of Aβ to form protofibrils or alter the ratio of the Aβ species. Most early onset FAD kindreds appear to carry a mutation in either the substrate or the enzyme that generates Aβ. It is unclear how many other FAD genes there may be because most large FAD kindreds carry a mutation in one of the three known genes.

A major focus of current genetic research is the identification of genetic risk factors for late onset AD (LOAD). Currently the only known genetic risk factor for LOAD is *APOE4* [4,45]. However, only 50% of AD cases carry one or more copies of the E4 allele suggesting that there must be other risk factors. Genetic linkage studies have implicated several chromosomal regions (e.g. chromosomes 9, 10, 12 and 21) but no consistent evidence has been reported for any single gene on these or any other chromosomes [1,24,25,31].

7. Is Aβ deposition central to the disease process?

The third prediction has proven to be the most controversial. While it is clear that FAD mutations in AβPP result in increased Aβ deposition, it is unclear whether the deposition is itself pathogenic. Several alternative hypotheses have been put forward. Rather than the deposited Aβ being neurotoxic some have suggested that the neurodegeneration observed in AD is caused by either soluble oligomers of Aβ, the build up of C-terminal fragments of AβPP or abnormal signaling by the intracellular domain of AβPP [26,52].

A key question for many years was whether late onset AD also involves an Aβ-centric mechanism. Elegant transgenic animal studies have demonstrated that APOE is required for Aβ fibrillogenesis (amyloid formation) and that APOE4 promotes Aβ deposition and amyloid formation when compared to the other *APOE* alleles, E3 and E2 [15]. A second intriguing observation in these mice is that the distribution of Aβ deposition is altered in mice lacking *APOE* and in mice carrying only human *APOE2*. These results suggest that in addition to being necessary for amyloid formation APOE is likely to be involved in the transport or clearance of Aβ. Indeed, we have shown that APOE genotype influences the age of onset of AD in individuals with FAD mutations suggesting an additive effect of PS mutations and the *APOE4* allele [30,53].

The fact that all four known AD genes implicate Aβ and that APOE implicates Aβ fibrillogenesis directly, provides support for the hypothesis that Aβ deposition is central to the disease.

8. Can overexpression of AβPP lead to AD?

The fourth prediction was that variants in AβPP that altered the level of AβPP expression might also result in AD. This is strongly supported by the observation that Down syndrome individuals with partial trisomy of chromosome 21, who are not trisomic for the *AβPP* gene, do not develop AD neuropathology, i.e. AD pathology in DS is associated with three copies of the *AβPP* gene [33]. Suprisingly, this hypothesis has not been rigorously tested with respect to late onset AD. Genetic linkage studies in late onset AD families have reported evidence for linkage on the long arm of chromosome 21, suggesting that a genetic risk factor is present on this chromosome [25]. Subsidiary analyses suggest that this linkage is associated with absence of an *APOE4* allele and later age of onset [28,29]. Despite these promising results genetic analyses of the *AβPP* gene in late onset AD have been very limited and inadequate to test the hypothesis. The *AβPP* gene is a large gene spanning more than 300 kb [36]. No published study has looked at more than a couple of SNPs within the gene, an inadequate number to rigorously exclude AβPP as a candidate gene. Thus more than fourteen years after the original report of a missense mutation in the AβPP gene causing early onset FAD, the AβPP gene remains a promising but untested candidate risk factor for late onset AD.

In summary, our report of a missense mutation in the AβPP gene that caused FAD provided an important turning point in AD research. This paper and subsequent papers provided information that has led to the development of cellular and animal models that recapitulate at least part of the AD phenotype. These models have greatly enhanced our understanding of the pathobiology of AD and have ultimately led to the identification of drug targets for AD and the development of drugs that are currently in clinical trials. Furthermore, the major predictions of this paper have withstood the test of time remarkably well.

On a more personal note this paper also had a large impact on the lives and careers of many of the paper's authors. The paper was the most cited scientific paper in 1991 and obviously received an immense amount of publicity in the media. John and I received both the Potamkin Award from the American Academy of Neurology and the MetlLife Award for Alzheimer's disease research for this work. We shared the Potamkin Award with Dr. Blas Frangione and Christine Van Broeckhoven because of the importance of the work on HCHWA-D in leading to the discovery of the AβPP mutations in AD. Although most of the authors on our paper were junior scientists (graduate students, postdoctoral fellows and research assistants), half of them continue to publish in the AD research field more than ten years later. As so often happens with success many members of the team were lured away from St. Mary's Hospital Medical School to other academic institutions. Within eighteen months of the publication of this paper John Hardy and several members of the laboratory moved to the University of South Florida in Tampa, while myself and several others moved to Washington University in St. Louis, where I took up a faculty position. Despite moving to different institutions within the USA, John and I have continued to collaborate on the genetics of dementia for the last fifteen years. This collaboration continues to be a stimulating and productive endeavor, but the fall of 1990 remains a high-water mark with regard to the special excitement felt by all who were involved in the project.

References

[1] D. Blacker, L. Bertram, A.J. Saunders, T.J. Moscarillo, M.S. Albert, H. Wiener, R.T. Perry, J.S. Collins, L.E. Harrell, R.C.

Go, A. Mahoney, T. Beaty, M.D. Fallin, D. Avramopoulos, G.A. Chase, M.F. Folstein, M.G. McInnis, S.S. Bassett, K.J. Doheny, E.W. Pugh and R.E. Tanzi, Results of a high-resolution genome screen of 437 Alzheimer's disease families, *Hum Mol Genet* **12** (2003), 23–32.

[2] M.C. Chartier-Harlin, F. Crawford, H. Houlden, A. Warren, D. Hughes, L. Fidani, A. Goate, M. Rossor, P. Roques, J. Hardy et al., Early-onset Alzheimer's disease caused by mutations at codon 717 of the beta-amyloid precursor protein gene, *Nature* **353** (1991), 844–846.

[3] M. Citron, T. Oltersdorf, C. Haass, L. McConlogue, A.Y. Hung, P. Seubert, C. Vigo-Pelfrey, I. Lieberburg and D.J. Selkoe, Mutation of the beta-amyloid precursor protein in familial Alzheimer's disease increases beta-protein production, *Nature* **360** (1992), 672–674.

[4] E.H. Corder, A.M. Saunders, W.J. Strittmatter, D.E. Schmechel, P.C. Gaskell, G.W. Small, A.D. Roses, J.L. Haines and M.A. Pericak-Vance, Gene dose of apolipoprotein E type 4 allele and the risk of Alzheimer's disease in late onset families, *Science* **261** (1993), 921–923.

[5] J.D. Fryer, K. Simmons, M. Parsadanian, K.R. Bales, S.M. Paul, P.M. Sullivan and D.M. Holtzman, Human apolipoprotein E4 alters the amyloid-beta 40:42 ratio and promotes the formation of cerebral amyloid angiopathy in an amyloid precursor protein transgenic model, *J Neurosci* **25** (2005), 2803–2810.

[6] D. Games, D. Adams, R. Alessandrini, R. Barbour, P. Berthelette, C. Blackwell, C. Carr, J. Clemens, T. Donaldson, F. Gillespie et al., Alzheimer-type neuropathology in transgenic mice overexpressing V717F beta-amyloid precursor protein, *Nature* **373** (1995), 523–527.

[7] G.G. Glenner and C.W. Wong, Alzheimer's disease: initial report of the purification and characterization of a novel cerebrovascular amyloid protein, *Biochem Biophys Res Commun* **120** (1984), 885–890.

[8] A. Goate, M.C. Chartier-Harlin, M. Mullan, J. Brown, F. Crawford, L. Fidani, L. Giuffra, A. Haynes, N. Irving, L. James et al., Segregation of a missense mutation in the amyloid precursor protein gene with familial Alzheimer's disease, *Nature* **349** (1991), 704–706.

[9] A.M. Goate, A.R. Haynes, M.J. Owen, M. Farrall, L.A. James, L.Y. Lai, M.J. Mullan, P. Roques, M.N. Rossor, R. Williamson et al., Predisposing locus for Alzheimer's disease on chromosome 21, *Lancet* **1** (1989), 352–355.

[10] D. Goldgaber, M.I. Lerman, W.O. McBride, U. Saffiotti and D.C. Gajdusek, Isolation, characterization, and chromosomal localization of human brain cDNA clones coding for the precursor of the amyloid of brain in Alzheimer's disease, Down's syndrome and aging, *J Neural Transm Suppl* **24** (1987), 23–28.

[11] I. Grundke-Iqbal, K. Iqbal, M. Quinlan, Y.C. Tung, M.S. Zaidi and H.M. Wisniewski, Microtubule-associated protein tau. A component of Alzheimer paired helical filaments, *J Biol Chem* **261** (1986), 6084–6089.

[12] S. Hecimovic, J. Wang, G. Dolios, M. Martinez, R. Wang and A.M. Goate, Mutations in APP have independent effects on Abeta and CTFgamma generation, *Neurobiol Dis* **17** (2004), 205–218.

[13] L. Hendriks, C.M. van Duijn, P. Cras, M. Cruts, W. Van Hul, F. van Harskamp, A. Warren, M.G. McInnis, S.E. Antonarakis, J.J. Martin et al., Presenile dementia and cerebral haemorrhage linked to a mutation at codon 692 of the beta-amyloid precursor protein gene, *Nat Genet* **1** (1992), 218–221.

[14] M.C. Herzig, D.T. Winkler, P. Burgermeister, M. Pfeifer, E. Kohler, S.D. Schmidt, S. Danner, D. Abramowski, C. Sturchler-Pierrat, K. Burki, S.G. van Duinen, M.L. Maat-Schieman, M. Staufenbiel, P.M. Mathews and M. Jucker, Abeta is targeted to the vasculature in a mouse model of hereditary cerebral hemorrhage with amyloidosis, *Nat Neurosci* **7** (2004), 954–960.

[15] D.M. Holtzman, K.R. Bales, T. Tenkova, A.M. Fagan, M. Parsadanian, L.J. Sartorius, B. Mackey, J. Olney, D. McKeel, D. Wozniak and S.M. Paul, Apolipoprotein E isoform-dependent amyloid deposition and neuritic degeneration in a mouse model of Alzheimer's disease, *Proc Natl Acad Sci USA* **97** (2000), 2892–2897.

[16] K. Hsiao, Transgenic mice expressing Alzheimer amyloid precursor proteins, *Exp Gerontol* **33** (1998), 883–889.

[17] J. Kang, H.G. Lemaire, A. Unterbeck, J.M. Salbaum, C.L. Masters, K.H. Grzeschik, G. Multhaup, K. Beyreuther and B. Muller-Hill, The precursor of Alzheimer's disease amyloid A4 protein resembles a cell-surface receptor, *Nature* **325** (1987), 733–736.

[18] E. Levy, M.D. Carman, I.J. Fernandez-Madrid, M.D. Power, I. Lieberburg, S.G. van Duinen, G.T. Bots, W. Luyendijk and B. Frangione, Mutation of the Alzheimer's disease amyloid gene in hereditary cerebral hemorrhage, Dutch type, *Science* **248** (1990), 1124–1126.

[19] E. Levy-Lahad, E.M. Wijsman, E. Nemens, L. Anderson, K.A. Goddard, J.L. Weber, T.D. Bird and G.D. Schellenberg, A familial Alzheimer's disease locus on chromosome 1, *Science* **269** (1995), 970–973.

[20] K. Lowenberg and R. Waggoner, Familial organic psychosis (Alzheimer's type), *Arch. Neurol. Psychiatr* **31** (1934), 737.

[21] C.L. Masters, G. Simms, N.A. Weinman, G. Multhaup, B.L. McDonald and K. Beyreuther, Amyloid plaque core protein in Alzheimer disease and Down syndrome, *Proc Natl Acad Sci USA* **82** (1985), 4245–4249.

[22] M. Mullan, H. Houlden, M. Windelspecht, L. Fidani, C. Lombardi, P. Diaz, M. Rossor, R. Crook, J. Hardy, K. Duff et al., A locus for familial early-onset Alzheimer's disease on the long arm of chromosome 14, proximal to the alpha 1-antichymotrypsin gene, *Nat Genet* **2** (1992), 340–342.

[23] J. Murrell, M. Farlow, B. Ghetti and M.D. Benson, A mutation in the amyloid precursor protein associated with hereditary Alzheimer's disease, *Science* **254** (1991), 97–99.

[24] A. Myers, P. Holmans, H. Marshall, J. Kwon, D. Meyer, D. Ramic, J. Shears, J. Booth, F.W. DeVrieze, R. Crook, M. Hamshere, R. Abraham, N. Tunstall, F. Rice, S. Carty, S. Lillystone, P. Kehoe, V. Rudrasingham, L. Jones, S. Lovestone, J. Perez-Tur, J. Williams, M.J. Owen, J. Hardy and A.M. Goate, Susceptibility locus for Alzheimer's disease on chromosome 10, *Science* **290** (2000), 2304–2305.

[25] A. Myers, F. Wavrant De-Vrieze, P. Holmans, M. Hamshere, R. Crook, D. Compton, H. Marshall, D. Meyer, S. Shears, J. Booth, D. Ramic, H. Knowles, J.C. Morris, N. Williams, N. Norton, R. Abraham, P. Kehoe, H. Williams, V. Rudrasingham, F. Rice, P. Giles, N. Tunstall, L. Jones, S. Lovestone, J. Williams, M.J. Owen, J. Hardy and A. Goate, Full genome screen for Alzheimer disease: stage II analysis, *Am J Med Genet* **114** (2002), 235–244.

[26] R.L. Neve and N.K. Robakis, Alzheimer's disease: a re-examination of the amyloid hypothesis, *Trends Neurosci* **21** (1998), 15–19.

[27] C. Nilsberth, A. Westlind-Danielsson, C.B. Eckman, M.M. Condron, K. Axelman, C. Forsell, C. Stenh, J. Luthman, D.B. Teplow, S.G. Younkin, J. Naslund and L. Lannfelt, The 'Arctic' APP mutation (E693G) causes Alzheimer's disease by en-

[28] J.M. Olson, K.A. Goddard and D.M. Dudek, The amyloid precursor protein locus and very-late-onset Alzheimer disease, *Am J Hum Genet* **69** (2001), 895–899.

[29] J.M. Olson, K.A. Goddard and D.M. Dudek, A second locus for very-late-onset Alzheimer disease: a genome scan reveals linkage to 20p and epistasis between 20p and the amyloid precursor protein region, *Am J Hum Genet* **71** (2002), 154–161.

[30] P. Pastor, C.M. Roe, A. Villegas, G. Bedoya, S. Chakraverty, G. Garcia, V. Tirado, J. Norton, S. Rios, M. Martinez, K.S. Kosik, F. Lopera and A.M. Goate, Apolipoprotein Eepsilon4 modifies Alzheimer's disease onset in an E280A PS1 kindred, *Ann Neurol* **54** (2003), 163–169.

[31] M.A. Pericak-Vance, M.L. Bass, L.H. Yamaoka, P.C. Gaskell, W.K. Scott, H.A. Terwedow, M.M. Menold, P.M. Conneally, G.W. Small, A.M. Saunders, A.D. Roses and J.L. Haines, Complete genomic screen in late-onset familial Alzheimer's disease, *Neurobiol Aging* **19** (1998), S39–S42.

[32] M.A. Pericak-Vance, L.H. Yamaoka, C.S. Haynes, M.C. Speer, J.L. Haines, P.C. Gaskell, W.Y. Hung, C.M. Clark, A.L. Heyman, J.A. Trofatter et al., Genetic linkage studies in Alzheimer's disease families, *Exp Neurol* **102** (1988), 271–279.

[33] V.P. Prasher, M.J. Farrer, A.M. Kessling, E.M. Fisher, R.J. West, P.C. Barber and A.C. Butler, Molecular mapping of Alzheimer-type dementia in Down's syndrome, *Ann Neurol* **43** (1998), 380–383.

[34] N.K. Robakis, H.M. Wisniewski, E.C. Jenkins, E.A. Devine-Gage, G.E. Houck, X.L. Yao, N. Ramakrishna, G. Wolfe, W.P. Silverman and W.T. Brown, Chromosome 21q21 sublocalisation of gene encoding beta-amyloid peptide in cerebral vessels and neuritic (senile) plaques of people with Alzheimer disease and Down syndrome, *Lancet* **1** (1987), 384–385.

[35] E.I. Rogaev, R. Sherrington, E.A. Rogaeva, G. Levesque, M. Ikeda, Y. Liang, H. Chi, C. Lin, K. Holman, T. Tsuda et al., Familial Alzheimer's disease in kindreds with missense mutations in a gene on chromosome 1 related to the Alzheimer's disease type 3 gene, *Nature* **376** (1995), 775–778.

[36] K. Rooke, C. Talbot, L. James, R. Anand, J.A. Hardy and A.M. Goate, A physical map of the human APP gene in YACs, *Mamm Genome* **4** (1993), 662–669.

[37] G.D. Schellenberg, T.D. Bird, E.M. Wijsman, D.K. Moore, M. Boehnke, E.M. Bryant, T.H. Lampe, D. Nochlin, S.M. Sumi, S.S. Deeb et al., Absence of linkage of chromosome 21q21 markers to familial Alzheimer's disease, *Science* **241** (1988), 1507–1510.

[38] G.D. Schellenberg, H. Payami, E.M. Wijsman, H.T. Orr, K.A. Goddard, L. Anderson, E. Nemens, J.A. White, M.E. Alonso, M.J. Ball et al., Chromosome 14 and late-onset familial Alzheimer disease (FAD), *Am J Hum Genet* **53** (1993), 619–628.

[39] D.J. Selkoe and M.B. Podlisny, Deciphering the genetic basis of Alzheimer's disease, *Annu Rev Genomics Hum Genet* **3** (2002), 67–99.

[40] R. Sherrington, E.I. Rogaev, Y. Liang, E.A. Rogaeva, G. Levesque, M. Ikeda, H. Chi, C. Lin, G. Li, K. Holman et al., Cloning of a gene bearing missense mutations in early-onset familial Alzheimer's disease, *Nature* **375** (1995), 754–760.

[41] A. Singleton, A. Myers and J. Hardy, The law of mass action applied to neurodegenerative disease: a hypothesis concerning the etiology and pathogenesis of complex diseases, *Hum Mol Genet* **13 Spec No 1** (2004), R123–R126.

[42] P.H. St George-Hyslop, J.L. Haines, L.A. Farrer, R. Polinsky, C. Van Broeckhoven, A. Goate, D.R. McLachlan, H. Orr, A.C. Bruni, S. Sorbi et al., Genetic linkage studies suggest that Alzheimer's disease is not a single homogeneous disorder. FAD Collaborative Study Group, *Nature* **347** (1990), 194–197.

[43] P.H. St George-Hyslop, R.E. Tanzi, R.J. Polinsky, J.L. Haines, L. Nee, P.C. Watkins, R.H. Myers, R.G. Feldman, D. Pollen, D. Drachman et al., The genetic defect causing familial Alzheimer's disease maps on chromosome 21, *Science* **235** (1987), 885–890.

[44] C. Stenh, C. Nilsberth, J. Hammarback, B. Engvall, J. Naslund and L. Lannfelt, The Arctic mutation interferes with processing of the amyloid precursor protein, *Neuroreport* **13** (2002), 1857–1860.

[45] W.J. Strittmatter, A.M. Saunders, D. Schmechel, M. Pericak-Vance, J. Enghild, G.S. Salvesen and A.D. Roses, Apolipoprotein E: high-avidity binding to beta-amyloid and increased frequency of type 4 allele in late-onset familial Alzheimer disease, *Proc Natl Acad Sci USA* **90** (1993), 1977–1981.

[46] C. Sturchler-Pierrat, D. Abramowski, M. Duke, K.H. Wiederhold, C. Mistl, S. Rothacher, B. Ledermann, K. Burki, P. Frey, P.A. Paganetti, C. Waridel, M.E. Calhoun, M. Jucker, A. Probst, M. Staufenbiel and B. Sommer, Two amyloid precursor protein transgenic mouse models with Alzheimer disease-like pathology, *Proc Natl Acad Sci USA* **94** (1997), 13287–13292.

[47] N. Suzuki, T.T. Cheung, X.D. Cai, A. Odaka, L. Otvos, Jr., C. Eckman, T.E. Golde and S.G. Younkin, An increased percentage of long amyloid beta protein secreted by familial amyloid beta protein precursor (beta APP717) mutants, *Science* **264** (1994), 1336–1340.

[48] R.E. Tanzi, J.F. Gusella, P.C. Watkins, G.A. Bruns, P. St George-Hyslop, M.L. Van Keuren, D. Patterson, S. Pagan, D.M. Kurnit and R.L. Neve, Amyloid beta protein gene: cDNA, mRNA distribution, and genetic linkage near the Alzheimer locus, *Science* **235** (1987), 880–884.

[49] R.E. Tanzi, P.H. St George-Hyslop, J.L. Haines, R.J. Polinsky, L. Nee, J.F. Foncin, R.L. Neve, A.I. McClatchey, P.M. Conneally and J.F. Gusella, The genetic defect in familial Alzheimer's disease is not tightly linked to the amyloid beta-protein gene, *Nature* **329** (1987), 156–157.

[50] C. Van Broeckhoven, A.M. Genthe, A. Vandenberghe, B. Horsthemke, H. Backhovens, P. Raeymaekers, W. Van Hul, A. Wehnert, J. Gheuens, P. Cras et al., Failure of familial Alzheimer's disease to segregate with the A4-amyloid gene in several European families, *Nature* **329** (1987), 153–155.

[51] C. Van Broeckhoven, J. Haan, E. Bakker, J.A. Hardy, W. Van Hul, A. Wehnert, M. Vegter-Van der Vlis and R.A. Roos, Amyloid beta protein precursor gene and hereditary cerebral hemorrhage with amyloidosis (Dutch), *Science* **248** (1990), 1120–1122.

[52] D.M. Walsh and D.J. Selkoe, Oligomers on the brain: the emerging role of soluble protein aggregates in neurodegeneration, *Protein Pept Lett* **11** (2004), 213–228.

[53] E.M. Wijsman, E.W. Daw, X. Yu, E.J. Steinbart, D. Nochlin, T.D. Bird and G.D. Schellenberg, APOE and other loci affect age-at-onset in Alzheimer's disease families with PS2 mutation, *Am J Med Genet B Neuropsychiatr Genet* **132** (2005), 14–20.

My story: The discovery and mapping to chromosome 21 of the Alzheimer amyloid gene

Dmitry Goldgaber
Department of Psychiatry and Behavioral Science, School of Medicine, State University of New York at Stony Brook, Stony Brook, New York 11794-8101, NY, USA
Tel.: +1 631 444 1369; Fax: +1 631 444 7534; E-mail: dmitry.goldgaber@sunysb.edu

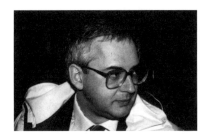

Abstract. When I decided to clone the amyloid gene I did not know that there were some twenty groups around the research world that desperately tried to do the same. If I knew that I would have never started the project. I was so ignorant about the disease that I did not know how to spell the name Alzheimer. I had to look at the papers of other researchers to make sure that my spelling was correct. After the cloning, I was invited to numerous national and international meetings on AD. These meetings became my University where I majored in AD.

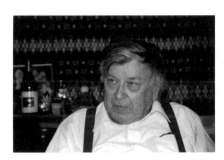

Fig. 1. Dr. Carleton Gajdusek at his home in Yonkers, New York, Christmas 1994.

To Carleton Gajdusek.

We wish we know more about the work that lead to the first paper describing Alzheimer's disease (AD) that was published 100 years ago. We wish we know more about the people who were involved in that work and the circumstances that lead Alois Alzheimer to the realization that the patient had indeed a novel disease. The aim of my story is to describe events that took place 20 years ago and that may be of interest to a few people later.

The following is the story of my work on the cloning of the amyloid gene. The facts are correct. At the very least they are as I remember them.

When I decided to clone the amyloid gene I did not know that there were some twenty groups around the research world that desperately tried to do the same. If I knew that I would have never started the project because I hate competitions. Competition in most projects in science means that the problem will be solved sooner or later. I, on the other hand, am always looking for novel ideas and new things to do, and always tried to open new doors instead of jumping on a band wagon.

I was so ignorant about the disease that I did not know how to spell the name Alzheimer. I had to look at the papers of other researchers to make sure that my spelling was correct.

After the cloning, I was invited to numerous national and international meetings on AD. I never refused and during the next several years I went to every one. These meeting provided me with a great education. The irony was that people at the meeting hoped to learn new things about AD from me, who knew nothing about the disease. I, on the other hand, was eager to learn from them who knew so much. I would come to a seasoned established scientist and ask- Could you tell me what you think about AD? What are you working on? And most people were very generous with me. They liked to talk about their work and about their ideas. These meetings became my University where I majored in AD.

And now back to the story.

1984 was my fourth year in America and I happily studied hantaviruses in Carleton Gajdusek's lab at NIH. It was my fourteenth year in the field of virology and I became a bit restless. I wanted to go back to my roots – molecular biology, in which I majored at the Leningrad Polytechnic Institute (LPI) in the Department of Semion Bresler, the father of molecular biology in the Soviet Union. In fact, I had two majors – physics and molecular biology. However, since graduation I worked in the area of virology using biochemical and molecular biological techniques.

Luckily, there, at the National Cancer Institute (NCI) was Michael (Misha) Lerman, a molecular biologist from Moscow. Michael was a well known scientist in the Soviet Union and he had publications in international journals. He was very knowledgeable with a hands-on experience in molecular biology. In our conversations he praised working with DNA and urged me to forget about my viruses and come to work for him. Misha came to America while he was in his early 50's. In the US he had to start, as many immigrants do, at a lower position. He had to work once more as a bench scientist. He did and he did it well. He was hunting oncogenes. By the time we met he already had several publications in peer-reviewed journals. Misha was working at Fort Detrick in Frederick, MD, in the NCI building located next to Carleton's building. He worked in the laboratory of Dr. Saffiotti and had a single technician.

It looked like that we would both benefit if I could spend some time with him and pick up techniques. I asked Carleton if I could spend a few months working at NCI with Michael Lerman. I told him that I wanted to pick up some modern molecular biological techniques and then use them in projects that were central in Carleton's lab – the Laboratory of Central Nervous System Studies (LCNSS). At that time there were no molecular biologists in his lab and Carleton agreed.

I understood that Misha's primary motivation was to get some additional help that he could not get from the NCI. That was fine with me. I told him that I would be coming as an apprentice. I didn't need any "pay" in the form of papers. I told him that I always work hard and that the knowledge I gain will be my pay.

Early 1985.

I plunged into Misha's projects spending most of my waking hours in the lab of Dr. Saffiotti. Dr. Saffiotti was very supportive and a real gentleman. We worked on chemical cancerogenesis trying to find oncogenes that were responsible for the transformation of keratinocytes treated with cancer inducing chemicals. I enjoyed working with Misha very much and I learned a lot. I learned many new methods including making various cDNA and genomic libraries and gene cloning. I know that he too was very happy with me because I was a quick learner, worked hard, generated a lot of data, and had great respect for Misha.

The idea

Time passed very quickly and in the fall of 1985 I finally felt that I have to begin working on a project that Carleton would be interested in. Carleton at that time, as well as now, was very interested in brain amyloid. He saw a lot of similarities between amyloid found in scrapie, Kuru, Creutzfeldt-Jakob disease on one hand and AD on the other hand.

Colin Masters, who spent many years in Carleton's lab, and his colleagues in Germany in Konrad Beyreuter's lab just published a paper in PNAS with a sequence of the A4 peptide that was almost identical to the sequence of amyloid beta protein (Aβ) that was published 1984 by George G. Glenner and his associate C.W. Wong. The Americans purified the peptide from leptomeninges of AD and Down's syndrome (DS) brain [1,2]. Colin and company purified the peptide from the plaques of AD and DS brains [3]. The sequence of a peptide called A4 by a German group was almost identical to the sequence of the Aβ peptide of George Glenner, except for minor differences and the fact that the sequence of A4 was longer. In fact, Colin and colleagues would not have been able to understand the protein sequencing results if not for the published peptide sequence of Glenner. Plaque amyloid is composed of a mixture of peptides of identical sequence but of different length because of the ragged N- and C-termini. Therefore, it was practically impossible to decipher the sequencing signals of peptide mixture without knowing the Aβ peptide sequence of Glenner.

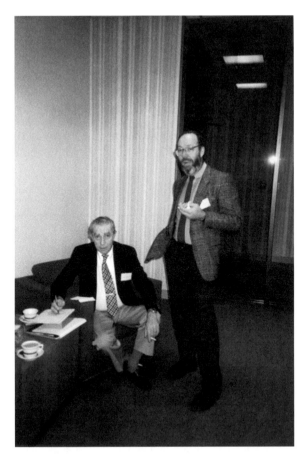

Fig. 2. George G. Glenner (left) and Colin L. Masters at the First International Conference on Alzheimer's Disease and Related Disorders, Las Vegas, 1988.

In the fall of 1985 I went to Carleton and proposed to clone the Alzheimer's amyloid gene – the gene that encodes the Aβ protein that Glenner and Wong purified from the AD brain and published in 1984. Carleton supported me. The paper of Masters and his colleagues in Germany was just published in PNAS and Carleton was very excited by it [3]. He later told me that at that time he did not believe that I would succeed. But, as it happened before me to others, Carleton never prohibited people in his lab from doing what they thought was important. He might have discouraged them if he did not believe in their ideas, but he never stopped them from trying.

First attempts

It was known that amyloid was detected in extracellular plaques and in intraneuronal neurofibrillary tangles (NFTs). I discussed the project with Carleton and we decided that there was a good chance that Aβ could be a fragment of one of the neurofilament proteins (NF). At that time only the sequence of the NF small was known and it did not contain Aβ. The sequence of NF medium was known only partially and therefore it could have had Aβ. The sequence of NF large was not known. I thought that at first I will try to clone NF large by screening of brain cDNA expression libraries with antibodies generated against NF large.

I found that Virginia Lee from the University of Pennsylvania published a number of papers using anti NF antibodies that she generated. I contacted Virginia and she sent me some antibodies. However, screening of cDNA expression libraries did not produce a single positive clone and I abandoned this direction.

Soon afterwards I learned that Ivan Lieberburg from the Rockefeller University was planning to present the sequence of NF large at a cell biology meeting (American Society for Cell Biology). I went to the meeting to see the sequence, but Ivan did not show up at his poster. After the meeting I contacted him and learned that he had only partial sequence of NF large and it did not contain an Aβ region. Later, I sequenced Ivan's NF large clone during the sequencing course that I took at University of North Carolina in the spring of 1986. I found that the sequence of NF large did not contain an Aβ sequence and therefore Aβ was not a fragment of any of the three NF proteins.

Conception

In parallel I was developing an alternative strategy – screening of brain cDNA libraries with an oligonucleotide probe that was based on Glenner's and Colin Masters' sequences of Aβ [1–3]. The sequence of the probe could not be precisely known because of the degeneracy of the code. At that time researchers were using a mixture of partially correct probes. Usually it was done either by mixing different oligos (with variable nucleotides at every ambiguous position), or by synthesis of a mixture of oligonucleoltides using a mixture of nucleotides at every step that corresponded to an ambiguous position. None of these approaches produced really good probes and successes in cloning were far fewer than failures.

Luckily, in 1985 a group from Japan published a paper in PNAS [4]. In this paper they proposed a very clever approach of generating probes for gene cloning. They also proved that this approach worked by cloning several known genes. The main idea was to use deoxyinosine in ambiguous positions. Because deoxyinosine is a small molecule it does not interfere during hybridization with sequences of genes containing any of the four nucleotides at the position opposite to deoxyinosine.

Another problem in cloning was the existence of sequences in many proteins that were similar to the sequence of the peptide or to one of it regions. I understood that it was important to find a unique region in the sequence of Aβ. At that time very few researchers knew how to compare sequences and BLAST was not at their fingertips as it is now.

Nina Goldgaber, who was my wife at that time, was working for a computer firm that serviced NIH scientists at Fort Detrick. One of her duties was analysis of protein and DNA sequences. I asked Nina to compare the sequence of Aβ with the database of known proteins and protein sequences predicted from the cloned genes in the GeneBank. The purpose was to identify regions of Aβ that had the least similarities to known sequences. I wanted to use the sequence of the unique region of Aβ for generating a probe with deoxyinosine in every ambiguous position. Nina compared the sequences and I saw that there was indeed a region of Aβ that was similar to regions found in many proteins. However, there was another region of Aβ that had no significant homology to known sequences in the GeneBank. These two steps – the use of deoxyinosine and the identification of a unique region of Aβ (plus a bit of luck) – were crucial in the successful cloning of the amyloid gene.

I told Misha about Nina's results, showed him the unique region of Aβ and the sequence of the probe with deoxyinosine. Misha had no objections and I ordered the probe in the fall of 1985. There were only two companies in the United States that made deoxyinosine at that time. I send the request to one of these companies. Surprisingly, I did not receive my probe for several months. When I called to find why the probe was not made, I was told that there was an explosion in the room next to the one where they were making deoxyinosine and the hallway and all adjacent rooms were sealed for investigation. But they told me that the investigation was almost over. After my call they opened the room, made deoxyinosine, and synthesized my probe.

I continued to work with Misha on his projects in Saffiotti's lab. It was an exiting time. I spent days and sometimes nights in the lab. I remember that one day in 1986 I came out of the lab during the daytime and was surprised to see it was already spring. I was working

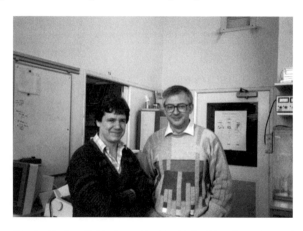

Fig. 3. Dmitry Goldgaber with Alan T. Bankier, Sanger's MRC Laboratory of Molecular Biology, Cambridge, 1987.

so hard and spent so much time in the lab that I actually missed the passing of winter!

Around that time I learned from Bob Rohwer, who spent many years in Carleton's lab and who had moved to UNC, that there was a sequencing course that was being given by Alan T. Bankier from Sanger's lab (MRC Laboratory of Molecular Biology, Cambridge). The very same Sanger who received two Nobel prizes – one was for sequencing proteins, and the second for sequencing DNA. Alan learned sequencing directly from Sanger! I was very excited about a possibility to learn sequencing from Alan, in a way making me a student of a student of Sanger.

Bob sent me the application form and I applied for the course. I was however late – they already had enough students. Bob knew the director of the course who promised to notify me if some of the participants will not be able to come. G-d was on my side again and I received a call that one place became available and I could come. I decided to drive to North Carolina. However, after a few hours I began loosing oil. I bought a lot of cans of oil and kept adding oil every time I saw that the level of oil became too low. Finally, I made it to UNC, but the gasket of the engine was blown and the engine suffered irreparable damage. I had to buy a new engine. It did not stop me. I was happy that I could be learning sequencing from the student of Sanger.

The two weeks of the course passed very quickly. I stayed at Bob's place and every day he drove me to the course. My first sequencing gel was the worst of all students. But I kept making and running gels and in the end I generated many more sequences than anyone else. I was very happy, because I became a master of sequencing.

Among the genes that I brought with me for sequencing, as I mentioned earlier, was a clone of NF large

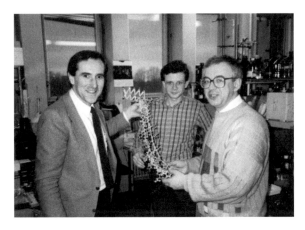

Fig. 4. Dmitry Goldgaber with Konrad Beyreuther (left) and Gerd Multhaup at the University of Cologne, 1987.

from Ivan Lieberburg. I sequenced it but it did not contain the Aβ region. I also had several clones from Misha's projects and sequenced all of them. During the course at UNC I learned from Misha that my probe with deoxyinosine has finally arrived.

Birth

It was already June of 1986. Misha's project on chemical cancerogenesis was finished. Unfortunately, we did not find the oncogene. Misha was leaving the NCI. He had a good offer from the Dental Institute in Bethesda – he would get his own lab with several positions and a good research budget. Finally, I had time to work on my own project on the amyloid gene.

I had several cDNA and genomic libraries to screen with my deoxyinosine containing probe. Some of these libraries were purchased and some I made myself. At first I screened my best libraries. Each time, after the first round of screening I had some weak positive signals. I picked the clones from the positive areas and re-screened them. No signals. They were false positives. Finally, in the second half of the summer, only one library was left unscreened. It was a library from a commercial source with very poor characteristics and short inserts. After so many failed attempts I did not believe that screening of this library would bring anything different. But I had nothing else to do. And I hate to miss chances. Even if I had only one chance in a million, I would rather try it than later feel that I had this chance, however small it was, and did not take it.

So, I screened the last library with my deoxyinosine containing probe and, as before, I got several weak signals. Without much hope I re-screened the picked colonies and WOW – there was a HUGE signal!

When Misha showed up in the lab (at that time he spent most of his time in Bethesda) I showed him the X-ray film with the signals. For the first time in this project Misha seemed to be interested. I finished screening and isolated several clones. Three clones contained cDNA inserts of similar size and I picked one for sequencing. I cut the insert with several restriction enzymes and did a Southern with my probe to determine which fragment might contain the Aβ. I sequenced the fragment using the Sanger method that I learned from Alan Bankier at UNC just a couple of months ago. The first sequencing reaction brought me terrific news: the clone contained the Aβ sequence!!!

I remember it as if it was yesterday ... I finished sequencing Friday night and put an X-ray film for overnight exposure. Next morning I developed the film and read the sequence. It was around 11 am on Saturday, and there it was – the sequence of the Aβ peptide! I was very, very lucky! The size of the cDNA fragment that I cloned was 1000 bp. The sequence that was recognized by my deoxyinosine containing probe was located at the 5' end of the clone and was only 53 bp long. If this clone was just 50 bp shorter, I would not have had the gene.

I was so excited that I could not work. Misha came to the lab to collect some of his stuff. I showed him the sequence and said "Look, I will not work today. I am going to a liquor store to buy the best bottle of cognac they have. And then I will go to Carleton's house on Prospect Hill and will have a drink with Carleton. Let's go and celebrate!" Misha was somewhat reluctant, but I insisted and we went to the liquor store. I bought XO cognac, the best they had, and we went to Prospect Hill, Carleton's house.

Carleton was home, upstairs. There were several foreign guests in the house, as usual. I asked to find glasses for everyone, and call Carleton. He came down asking what the occasion was. I poured XO cognac into glasses and told Carleton that we have the amyloid gene. I said that I have a toast: "Carleton," I said with a chock in my throat, "Thank you Carleton for giving me a chance!"

I felt very emotional at that moment. I did not how to express my feelings. I was thinking about the years in the Soviet Union and threats, the immigration I faced and the uncertainties of an immigrant life and the years in Carleton's lab. What else was there to say? I was so grateful to him for inviting me, an unknown Russian Jewish immigrant, to work in his lab. So many people from all over the world were dreaming of working in his lab and he invited me. I will never forget his kindness and his support. He changed my life by giving me a chance to work in his laboratory.

Carleton did not meet me personally during his trips to Russia. I saw him at one of his lectures at my Institute in 1977. I wrote him a letter during my journey from Russia to the United States (November, 1979 – March, 1980). It was my very first letter in English. I did not know how to write letters in English. As an example of how to write letters, I used a book from a hotel in Vienna. It was a book for hotel managers with examples of business correspondence in five major European languages.

I remember that I wrote him that I had left the Soviet Union, that I am in Vienna, and on my way to the United States. That I am ready to do any work in the United States, be it a parking attendant, to pump gas, or to sweep floors. But, I said in the letter, I prefer to do science, because this it what I was trained to do, this is what I am good at, and this is where I can contribute. I did not ask for a job. I asked him to guide me in my search for a job.

It is hard to imagine how stunned I was when, while still in Italy, I received his letter inviting me to work on a project in his lab, if I find it interesting! "Interesting"?!!! It was a dream. No. It was more than a dream, because I did not dream of having THIS opportunity. And this is why I said the toast – "Thank you Carleton for giving me a chance!"

Soon after that Saturday Misha talked to Wesley McBride, a senior scientist at NCI, about mapping of the amyloid gene. Wesley had hybrid human-mouse cell lines each containing various sets of human chromosomes. By hybridizing the gene of interest to DNA from these cell lines one can find the chromosomal location of the gene. One week after he received the amyloid clone, Wesley called and told us with amusement that the gene was on chromosome 21!!!

This was really exciting! The location of the amyloid gene on chromosome 21 meant that the long-standing puzzle – why there was such a similarity between brain pathology in DS and AD – was solved!

Postpartum

Carleton told me that we should quickly find a place where we can present this discovery. Carleton attended a FESN meeting in the Pierre Hotel in New York in the fall of 1986 and already talked about this work to a number of people, including Henry Wisniewski, the director of the Institute for Basic Research on Staten Island and Floyd Bloom from the Scripps Clinic Research Institute [5].

I began looking for meetings to present our work. Luckily, in 1986 the Society for Neuroscience had a meeting on November 9–14 in Washington, DC, in our backyard so to speak. I looked at the schedule and found one session with an appropriate title. The chair of the session was John Morrison. He was from Floyd Bloom's place in California. A few weeks ago Floyd Bloom attended the FESN meeting in New York when Carleton announced that we cloned the amyloid gene. Carleton called Floyd and he talked to John Morrison. John called me and said that he can't allow me to present my work at his session because only those who submitted abstracts before the deadline were allowed to present their data. However, he said that he will announce there will be my presentation on cloning and chromosomal localization of the Alzheimer amyloid gene AFTER his session is over. The word spread around and by the end of the session, the room was full.

Bob Rohwer, who came from North Carolina for the meeting, helped me with my presentation, correcting my English. In the afternoon, I think it was November 12th, I went to the Convention Center and paced in the hallway near the room where I would present my talk.

There were several people in the hallway. I did not know any of them. I learned later that one was Ken Kosik, a "Tau man" from Harvard. The other one was his friend from Harvard-Huntington Potter. A third was Rudy Tanzi, a graduate student of Jim Guzella and Rachel Neve. One of them realized that I was the guy who will make the presentation after the session and asked me what chromosome the gene was on. I said that I would reveal it during my talk. I was somewhat nervous before the talk, but not too much. Finally, my time came.

John Morrison was announcing my presentation after each of the talks and ended the session saying that now those who are interested will hear my presentation. Then he left the podium.

I climbed up and saw that this huge room was full of people. They were even sitting in the walkways and more people were coming in. I gave my talk. At the end I said: And the gene was mapped to chromosome 21. There was silence. I waited – no questions. I was somewhat confused because questions were a norm. But there was this silence. I will never forget it. So, I said, if there were no questions, I thank you for your attention. I was ready to leave the podium.

At that moment some one in the third row stood up, scratched his head and loudly said – what do you mean there are no questions, of course we have questions, lots of questions. It was Peter Davies, one of the leading researchers in Alzheimer's field who just made the discovery of NFT specific antibody Alz50. I did not know him as I did not know anybody in the field of AD research.

There were a lot of questions. Finally, I stepped down from the podium and went to the hall. People were congratulating me, asking more questions, asking for my clone, patted my shoulder. And then there was a press conference and more questions. Reporters at the press conference wrote about our discovery and newspapers and magazines published the story on the discovery of the Alzheimer amyloid gene and the location of the gene on chromosome 21 [6,7].

After the press conference Dennis Selkoe, whom I also did not know, wanted to talk to me. He brought me to a room in a hotel next to the meeting, introduced me to a lot of people, and asked if I would be interested in working for a newly formed company specializing in AD research. The name of the company was Athena Neuroscience. I said, thank you, no. I wanted to stay in academia.

We moved to a lobby and Dennis introduced me to some of the people in his lab. I remember one, Carmela Abraham. Carmela told me that she also tried to clone the amyloid gene, but did not get it. She used antibody generated against amyloid preps from brains of patients with AD for screening of expression libraries. She cloned an inhibitor of proteases and was very upset that it was not the amyloid gene. I told her not to despair. I explained that her work was very valuable because the sequence of the amyloid gene predicted a large protein that has to be cleaved in order to make $A\beta$. Therefore, the next step was to find proteases that will do the job and inhibitors of proteases to control the processing of $A\beta PP$. I said that she is already two steps ahead of the game and therefore should finish her work and be happy.

The other person who came to talk to me was Rudy Tanzi. Rudy asked if I was interested in genetic studies of AD. I said that I am interested but that I am not a geneticist and that we don't have AD families. He offered collaboration and asked if I can give him my clone. I agreed under the conditions that Carleton and Misha Lerman will be coauthors of the collaborative paper and said that I will give him the clone. Rudy agreed to my conditions. He mentioned that he also tried to clone the gene but he did not sequence the candidate clones and did not know if any of them actually had the $A\beta$ sequence. And of course he did not know the chromosomal localization of the gene. He told me that during my presentation he and Rachel Neve decided to write down the sequence of my clone. He wrote from one end and Rachel wrote the sequence from the other so they had as much sequence as they could get. So did, apparently many others in the room.

Rudy was very interested in seeing actual Southern blots because he wanted to see polymorphisms of the gene. I suggested that we go to NIH by Metro and he would see the blots and pick up the clone. I called Wesley McBride. He was in his lab and agreed to show the blots. So we went. Wesley showed Rudy the blots and the EcoR1 polymorphism that he found. I gave Rudy my clone and Rudy left a very happy fellow.

During the next several months Rudy called many times. He told me that he was under a lot of pressure from his bosses to write a paper. At one point he offered me a co-authorship on a paper without Carleton and Misha Lerman. I refused. He managed to publish his paper without our names in the same issue of Science that had my paper. But all of this happened later.

My priority after the November 1986 Neuroscience meeting was to write the paper. This was the time when I had to look at other papers in order to make sure that I spell correctly the name Alzheimer. Not only did I write this paper describing our work. I understood that overexpression of $A\beta$ was the basis of AD and wrote about this in the discussion part of the paper.

For a long period of time researchers knew about the similarity between AD and DS. But nobody could understand why there was such a similarity between these two different diseases: a simple genetic disease of the young (DS) and a very complex and complicated (from the point of view of etiology) disease of the aged (AD).

Involvement of chromosome 21 in AD was suspected, but was never understood. Now, the puzzle was solved. Because the amyloid gene was located on chromosome 21 there were three copies of the gene in patients with DS. The gene was overexpressed in patients with DS and this overexpression led to the increase in the amount of $A\beta$ and consequently to the pathological changes that were so similar to AD. That was obvious.

However, I went further. I understood, that the increased quantity of $A\beta$ was the key not only to the pathology of DS. It should explain the pathology of AD!!! However, numerous cytogenetic studies found no trisomy 21 in AD. Therefore, the increased quantity of $A\beta$ in AD must have been achieved by other means.

I speculated that overexpression of the $A\beta$ peptide at the level of transcription, translation and/or posttranslational modifications or processing would result in overexpression of $A\beta$? Such over-expression could be a result of mutations in the gene or a gene dosage effect. Because $A\beta$ turned out to be only a part of much larger precursor molecule, the proteolytic processing of this molecule was essential. Therefore, mutations in other genes that were involved in the processing of the precursor protein could also lead to the increase amount of $A\beta$. It was also possible that the level of the precursor and/or $A\beta$ could increase in response to changes in the environment. I speculated that these and other possible mechanisms could lead to the over-production of $A\beta$, its subsequent aggregation, formation of amyloid, and other neuropathological changes observed in AD.

Thus, the mapping of the gene to chromosome 21 not only explained why brain pathology in DS was similar to AD, but it gave me a clue to the origin of the brain pathology in AD.

Subsequent work in many laboratories showed that almost all of these predictions were correct. Mutations were found in the amyloid gene and these mutations led to the increased generation of $A\beta$. Other genes (presenilin 1 and 2) that are involved in the processing of the $A\beta PP$ gene were discovered. Mutations in these genes led to overproduction of $A\beta$. We found that the level of the $A\beta PP$ gene expression was increased by cytokine IL-1β, an inflammation marker, and by a growth factor bFGF, thus showing that $A\beta PP$ overexpression might be a result of environmental influence. In fact, inflammation was shown to be a major feature in AD with the increased prominent expression of IL-1β in the brain.

I wrote the paper in a few short weeks. It was an easy task. I did all the key experiments and Wesley McBride mapped the gene to chromosome 21. We named the gene Alzheimer's Disease Amyloid Precursor (ADAP). It was later renamed the amyloid β protein precursor (APP or $A\beta PP$). The discussion was short and contained my speculation on the over-expression of $A\beta$ as the key event in the pathology of the disease. Carleton went over the paper and corrected it. Misha read it and left it without corrections.

When I was finishing the paper, Carleton told me that Konrad Beyreuther called him and said that they (Colin and Konrad) too have the gene. They had not mapped the gene but learned about its localization to chromosome 21 from Carleton and from my presentation. Konrad asked Carleton to wait and to publish their paper back to back with our paper in PNAS. He asked to give them 3 or 4 weeks to finish writing the paper. Carleton agreed. Konrad and his people quickly found a group in Germany to do the mapping of the gene. The results confirmed that we were correct – the gene was indeed on chromosome 21.

Two weeks later we learned from Colin that their paper was sent to Nature and they are waiting for the decision. He said that Benno Muller-Hill did not want to send their paper to PNAS and insisted on sending it to Nature. Benno was a well-known molecular biologist and a co-author of their paper. In fact, it was his student J. Kang who finally succeeded in the cloning of the full length cDNA of the gene using a cDNA library made by Axel Unterbeck who was a student of Konrad. So they decided that if Nature would turn them down, then they would send the paper to Carleton for PNAS. However, they did not tell this to Carleton. When he later learned the news from Colin, he was shocked and asked me what should we do? Wait or not wait for Konrad. I said that because he promised Konrad to wait, we have to wait. But, I said we should send our paper to Science right after the four weeks period that Carleton promised to Konrad was over. Carleton agreed. He waited till four weeks have passed and made a call to Science. The associate Editor sounded very enthusiastic and asked to send her the paper. I told Carleton that I would personally deliver the paper to Science. So I took a Metro to downtown Washington, DC and handed my paper to the Associate Editor.

We began waiting for the reviewers' response. Very soon we learned that the reviewers liked the paper and that it will be published in Science. The editors liked that paper so much that they put on the cover the picture showing the expression of our gene in the prefrontal cortex of the brain.

Meanwhile Bob Rohwer told us that he reviewed for Nature Colin and Konrad's paper from Germany. Bob was very enthusiastic about the paper. He was present at my talk at the Neuroscience meeting in Washington and saw the reaction of the people, the press conference, and the enthusiasm. He understood the significance of this work. However, he learned that their paper was rejected by Nature despite his enthusiasm. Bob knew that our paper was already accepted to Science. So he wrote a passionate letter to the editors of Nature and told them about our work, the reaction to my presentation at the Neuroscience meeting, and the fact that the paper just now was accepted to Science. Nature editors reversed their decision and accepted the paper from Germany.

Someone from Nature later called me and asked if my paper was indeed accepted to Science. I naively said yes. She asked the second question – when it will

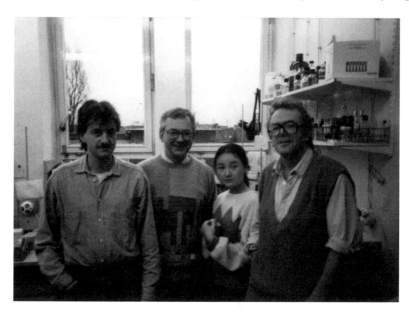

Fig. 5. Dmitry Goldgaber with Benno Müller-Hill (right) and J. Kang (next to Benno) at the University of Cologne, 1987.

it be published. I said February 20. Thank you very much said the voice with the perfect English accent and hung up the phone. Thank you very much indeed. What a fool I was.

Apparently Nature, after accepting the paper, planned to publish it in March. After the "lovely" talk with me they changed the date of publication and published the paper in February 19 issue of Nature [8]. Science published my paper in the February 20 issue. Thus, Nature beat Americans by one day, which is apparently so important in journalism. I, of course, was a bloody fool, using their expression.

During my work on the galley proofs of our paper we exchanged the galley proofs with Colin. When I compared the sequences I found few minor discrepancies. I checked my sequencing X-ray films and found that they were right. I had misread a few nucleotides. I made corrections in our galley proofs and acknowledged the German group in my paper.

Meanwhile, the editors of Science decided to make an Alzheimer's issue of Science. They called Dennis Selkoe and invited him to resubmit his paper describing amyloid depositions in several different mammals including the polar bear.

They also waited for two papers from Jim Gusella. One was Rudy's paper on the cloning of the amyloid gene and the other was the genetic paper from Peter St George-Hyslop. Using several families with AD Peter showed a positive linkage to a region of chromosome 21 [9]. That paper had a major impact on the thinking about AD by showing that in some familial cases AD is indeed a genetic disease.

Mapping the amyloid gene to chromosome 21 made a big impression on everybody in the field, including Peter. He thought, as many others at that time, that our gene was the gene that caused AD. Peter later told me that they tried to use my clone that I gave to Rudy, but that it was not informative. Then they found a marker located near the amyloid gene and succeeded in the linkage analysis.

It turned out that none of Peter's families was linked to chromosome 21 because they had mutations in the gene located on a different chromosome. I believe that at least some of them had mutations in the presenilin 1 gene located on chromosome 14. In any case, Peter's was the first paper that brought the genetic aspects of AD into the center of research. Mutations later were found in the amyloid gene in other families.

As a result of all these actions, the publication of our paper was delayed and everybody except for us gained from it. Our paper was supposed to be first to be published. But now it became only one of several papers published simultaneously.

At present, 20 years later, a few days, a few months, or even a year does not seem to make much difference. But at that time it was so important and publications of these other papers in Science and Nature had a major affect on lives and careers of a large number of people.

The stories of publications in Science and Nature in February 1987 do not cover the whole story of this

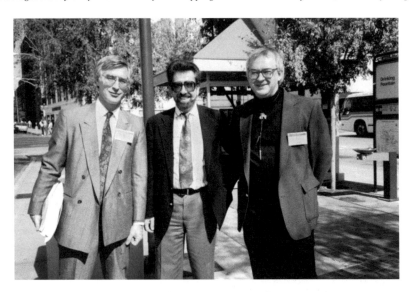

Fig. 6. Dmitry Goldgaber with Allen D. Roses (center) and Don E. Schmechel (undated).

discovery. Peter Davies who was present at my talk at the Neurosciences in November 1986, called me several days later and invited me to attend a Banbury meeting in Cold Spring Harbor Laboratories at the end of the month.

At that meeting I met several remarkable people including George Glenner who had sequenced $A\beta$, Allen D. Roses from Duke who later discovered the role of apolipoprotein E4 as a risk factor for AD, Peter Davies from the Albert Einstein, Tuck Finch from the University of Southern California, an old Alzheimer hand, Nick Robakis from the Henry Wisniewski's Institute on Staten Island, and Jim Gusella from Harvard famous for his pioneering work on Huntington disease.

During my presentation I emphasized the contribution of Glenner. In fact, I said that without his sequence of the $A\beta$ none of what I was going to present would have been done. George appreciated it because there were people who tried to diminish or undermine his contribution.

Nick had also tried to clone the gene. At the time of Banbury meeting he presented sequences of several genomic clones. However, none of his clones contained the correct sequence of $A\beta$. Some of his clones had partial sequences of $A\beta$ but they were followed by unrelated sequences. Nick of course heard about our work from Henry and he tried to verify that the gene was on chromosome 21. But at the time of the meeting he told us that he had no information about the mapping of the gene. However, a few weeks later Nick had the correct information and his paper on the chromosomal location of the amyloid gene appeared in Lancet as a letter to the editor in February 1987 [10]. His full paper with the correct sequence was published later in PNAS.

While my presentation at the Neuroscience meeting was covered only by newspapers and magazines including New Scientist and Science News [6,7], my presentation at the November 1986 Banbury meeting was published in the middle of 1987 in Banbury Report 27 [11]. It became the third official publication of our work. Our paper in the February issue of Science was the second publication [12]. The first scientific publication of our results was in the proceedings of a meeting that was organized by MIT and held in Zurich in January 1987. The proceedings of the meeting were published before the meeting and were given to the participants at the meeting. Thus it became the first scientific publication of our results [13].

I also remember that Carleton made several presentations in 1986 and 1987 but I don't have information about the dates and places of his presentations. Once the paper was published I sent the $A\beta PP$ clones to every researcher who requested it. One request came from Dr. Chamer Wei, vice president RD, Transgenic Sciences Inc. (TSI), who wanted to create a transgenic mouse model of AD. I sent him a full length $A\beta PP$ clone and Dr. Montoya, who worked for TSI at that time, created the very first transgenic mouse with amyloid depositions. Later this transgenic mouse line was purchased by Athena Neuroscience Inc. and became known as the Athena mouse.

Next step

For a long period of time, $A\beta$ was believed to be a pathological product of processing of $A\beta PP$. However, in the early 90s, it was shown that $A\beta$ was present in serum and in CSF of people who did not have AD. These results changed the prevailing view because they showed that $A\beta$ was a normal product of $A\beta PP$ processing. By that time it was known that $A\beta$ is cytotoxic and self-aggregates easily forming oligomers and amyloid. Because $A\beta$ was a product of normal cellular events the organism must have had a mechanism of neutralizing and disposing of this toxic self-aggregating product. So, I switched from thinking about the processes of generation of $A\beta$ to the ideas of its disposal and neutralization. I reasoned that this mechanism must work well in healthy individuals, otherwise we would all have AD pathology, and that the pathological changes observed in AD might develop because of the failure of this mechanism. At the molecular level this mechanism must involve an interaction of $A\beta$ with other molecules. Such interaction may neutralize cytotoxicity of $A\beta$ and prevent amyloid formation. My sequestration hypothesis was published in 1993 and we began the search for $A\beta$ sequestering molecules. We found that indeed there was a major protein in CSF that formed complex with $A\beta$. Surprisingly, it was a well known transporter protein transthyretin (TTR). TTR transports thyroid hormone T4 as well as retinol A. TTR is produced primarily in liver and choroids plexus. TTR is a well known nutritional marker and a negative response protein. It is down regulated by inflammation. We found TTR- $A\beta$ complexes in human CSF and showed that interaction of TTR with $A\beta$ prevented formation of amyloid. In addition, TTR neutralized $A\beta$ toxicity. A number of studies directly or indirectly supported the sequestration hypothesis. For example, the levels of TTR is low in CSF of patients with AD. The levels of TTR in CSF inversely correlated with amount of neuritic plaques in hippocampus. Recently, a dramatic increase of TTR was detected in transgenic mice that overproduced $A\beta$ but did not develop massive amyloid depositions. Infusion of anti TTR antibody into the brains of these mice resulted in an increase of amyloid, phosphorylation of tau, and caused neuronal cell loss. It seems that TTR protects these transgenic mice from the detrimental effects of $A\beta$. Reversely, conditions that lead to a decrease of amyloid burden in model systems were accompanied by an increase in the amounts of TTR and TTR- $A\beta$ complexes. Epidemiological data pointed to the role of non-steroidal anti-inflammatory drugs (NSAIDs) in protection from AD. The mechanism of protection is not known. We found that a number of NSAIDs increased the levels of TTR in TTR producing cultured human HepG2 cells. These results suggest that the protection by NSAIDs might work by the increase in TTR, the protein that sequesters and neutralize $A\beta$. Thus, neutralization and removal of $A\beta$ by TTR is an important mechanism impairment of which may lead to AD. Therefore, agents that increase levels of TTR might not only protect from AD, but might help patients with AD.

References

[1] G.G. Glenner and C.W. Wong, Alzheimer's disease. Initial report of the purification and characterization of a novel cerebrovascular amyloid protein, *Biochem. Biophys. Res. Commun.* **120** (1984), 885–890.

[2] G.G. Glenner and C.W. Wong, Alzheimer's disease and Down's syndrome – Sharing of a unique cerebrovascular amyloid fibril protein, *Biochem. Biophy Res Commun.* **122** (1984), 1131–1135.

[3] C.L. Masters, G. Simms, N.A. Weinman, G. Multhaup, B.L. McDonald and K. Beyreuther, Amyloid plaque core protein in Alzheimer disease and Down syndrome, *Proc. Nat. Acad. Sci. USA* **82** (1985), 4245–4249.

[4] Y. Takahashi, K. Kato, Y. Hayashizaki, T. Wakabayashi, E. Ohtsula, S. Matsuki, M. Ikehara and K. Matsubara, Molecular cloning of the human cholecystokinin gene by use of a synthetic probe containing deoxyinosine, *Proc. Nat. Acad. Sci. USA* **82** (1985), 1931–1935.

[5] D. Goldgaber, M.I. Lerman, W.O. McBride, U. Saffiotti and D.C. Gajdusek, Isolation and characterization of human brain cDNA clones coding for the precursor of the amyloid of brain in Alzheimer's disease, Downs syndrome and aging, *J. Neural Transmission* **28** (1987), Suppl. 24.

[6] G. Ferry, Journey to the centre of Dementia, *New Scientist* (November 20, 1986), 20.

[7] I. Amato, Alzheimer's Disease: Scientists report advances, *Science News* (November 22, 1986), 327.

[8] J. Kang, H.G. Lemaire, A. Unterbeck, J.M. Salbaum, C.L. Masters, K.H. Grzeschik, G. Multhaup, K. Beyreuther and B. Muller-Hill, The precursor of Alzheimer's disease amyloid A4 protein resembles a cell surface receptor, *Nature* **325** (1987), 733–736.

[9] P.H. St.George-Hyslop, R.E. Tanzi, R.J. Polinsky, J.L. Haines, L. Nee, P.C. Watkins, R.H. Myers, R.G. Feldman, D. Pollen, D. Drachman, J. Crowdon, A. Bruni, J.F. Foncini, D. Salmon, P. Frommelt, L. Amaducci, S. Sorbi, S. Piacentinni, G.D. Stewart, W.J. Hobbs, P.M. Conneally and J.F. Gusella, The genetic defect causing familial Alzheimer's disease maps to chromosome 21, *Science* **235** (1987), 885–890.

[10] N.K. Robakis, H.M. Wisniewski, E.C. Jenkins, E.A. Devinegage, G.E. Houck, X.L. Yao, N. Ramakrishna, G. Wolfe, W.P. Silverman and W.T. Brown, Chromosome 21q21 sublocalization of gene encoding beta-amyloid peptide in cerebral vessels and neuritic (senile) plaques of people with Alzheimer's disease and Down syndrome, *Lancet* **1-8529** (1987), 384–385.

[11] D. Goldgaber, M.I. Lereman, W.O. McBride, U. Saffiotti and D.C. Gajdusek, Isolation and characterization of human brain cDNA clones coding for the precursor of the amyloid of brain in Alzheimer's disease, Downs syndrome and aging, in: *Molecular Neuropathology of Aging. Banbury Reports 27,* P. Davies and C.E. Finch, eds, CSHL Press, New York, 1988.

[12] D. Goldgaber, M.I. Lerman, W.O. McBride, U. Saffiotti and D.C. Gajdusek, Isolation and characterization of human brain cDNA clones coding for the precursor of theamyloid of brain in Alzheimer's disease, Downs syndrome and aging, *Science* **235** (1987), 877–880.

[13] D. Goldgaber, M.I. Lerman, W.O. McBride, U. Saffiotti and D.C. Gajdusek, Isolation and characterization of human brain cDNA clones coding for the precursor of the amyloid of brain in Alzheimer's disease, Downs syndrome and aging, in: *Alzheimer's Disease: Advances in Basic Research and Therapies, Proceedings of the Fourth Meeting of the International Study Group on the Pharmacology of Memory Disorders Associated with Aging, Zurich, January 16–18,* R.J. Wurtman, S.H. Corkin and J.H. Growdon, eds, Center for Brain Sciences and Metabolism Charitable Trust, Cambridge, Mass., pp. 209–217.

On the discovery of the genetic association of Apolipoprotein E genotypes and common late-onset Alzheimer disease

Allen D. Roses
Genetic Research, GlaxoSmithKline Research and Development, Five Moore Drive, 5.5616, Research Triangle Park, NC 27709, USA
Tel.: +1 919 483 3771; E-mail: allen.d.roses@gsk.com

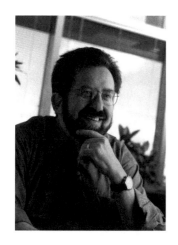

Abstract. The association of Apolipoprotein E-4 with the age of onset of common late-onset Alzheimer's disease (AD) was originally reported in three 1993 papers from the Duke ADRC (Alzheimer's Disease Research Center) group [1–3]. The Center was investigating two diverse experimental streams that led to this discovery. The first being a genetic linkage study performed in multiplex familial late-onset AD in which a linkage was discovered at chromosome 19q13 [4,5]. The 1991 multilocus analysis of linkage had been considered very controversial [6]. The second stream came from a series of amyloid-β binding studies in which a consistent protein "impurity" was present on gel separation analyses [1]. After sequencing this "impurity" band, several tryptic peptide sequences were found to be identical for apoE which, at that time, had no known association with Alzheimer's disease.

The flash of recognition was the knowledge that APOE was one of the first genes localized to chromosome 19 in the mid-1980's. Within a three week period in late 1992, a highly significant association was identified in clinical patients from multiplex families, in sporadic clinical patients, and in autopsy diagnosed series [1,2]. Within the first two months of 1993, it was possible to clearly demonstrate that the APOE isoforms were associated with differing ages of onset, but the course of illness following diagnosis was related more to age than APOE genotype [3]. The earliest submitted paper reported the familial association and amyloid-β binding [1]. The second reported the association with common sporadic late-onset, [not-known to be familial] AD patients [2]. The third reported that APOE4 carriers had earlier rates of onset of clinical disease than APOE2 or APOE3 carriers [3]. Subsequently, over more than a decade, the biological expression of apoE in human neurons was confirmed as distinct from rodent brain [7,8] Proteomic experiments and positron emission tomography data have led to a series of clinical trials with agents selected to increase glucose utilization. These agents also regulate inflammatory responses of neural cells. Rosiglitazone, a PPARγ agonist which also leads to mitochondrial proliferation shown efficacy as a monotherapy in a Phase IIB clinical trial of 511 patients in an APOE allele-specific analysis.

1. Introduction

At the time of the APOE/AD discovery in 1992, the Joseph and Kathleen Bryan Alzheimer's Disease Research Center group had been involved in testing a genetic susceptibility theory for AD for more than a dozen years. In the late 1970's, Dr. Albert Heyman initiated clinical studies of AD patients, each of whom

ISSN 1387-2877/06/$17.00 © 2006 – IOS Press and the authors. All rights reserved

had more than one family member with AD which suggested a familial contribution to the disease [4] In 1979, our group at Duke University initiated a Brain Bank and a DNA Bank for neurological diseases [9]. In the early 1980's, before the initiation of the NIA ADRC program, the Duke group began collecting multiplex AD families and storing the clinical phenotypes in early computer databases [4].

When the NIA issued a call for Research Center applications in 1983, Dr. Albert Heyman was contacted. Dr. Heyman was a former Chief of Neurology at Duke who had published in the field of Alzheimer's Disease. Dr. Heyman, the then-Head of the NIA Duke Aging Center and the Chancellor of Duke Medical School called me for a meeting to tell me that they would like me to be the principal investigator for an ADRC application. My colleagues and I followed the guidelines and submitted an application based on a genetic strategy for AD including susceptibility locus identification and use of subtraction cDNA hybridization of rapidly autopsied brain from patients and age-matched normal controls to identify genes. After a flurry of three months to prepare the application, we simply went back to our funded research in muscular dystrophies and inherited neuropathies.

One afternoon about eight months later I received a call from Dr. Zavin Khachaturian. He identified himself as the Head of the AD Section of the NIA and asked me if I wanted the "good news or the bad news." I took the good news first: the application came out #6 of 21 applications – the bad news was that only five would be funded. Instead of ending it there, he told me that our application was quite distinct from the others, but that none of the reviewers felt that we could get rapid-autopsied brain from AD patients and controls with intact "preserved RNA" in less than one hour after death. He suggested that we re-apply because the second round would have a site visit.

I met Dr. Khachaturian for the first time, face to face, months later during our site visit. We presented our application before the lunch break, allowed the Visitors to dine and commune, at which time they continued to show their concern that we could not get autopsied material from AD patients and controls fast enough to confirm our "preserved RNA" theory. We presented the results of our first two "rapid autopsies," one at 23 minutes and the other at 41 minutes [delayed by a coal train crossing between the hospital and the autopsy suite!] [9]. We demonstrated the quality of the mRNA which was not degraded – a heavily quoted paper at the time actually blamed AD on the degradation of RNA seen in late autopsies [10]. After this surprising demonstration, the application was approved and later funded.

2. The linkage

In 1988, after the ADRC was founded, my first non-ADRC research funding in AD [and my last!] was an NIA LEAD [Leadership and Excellenxe in Alzheimer's Disease] Award for seven years. Shortly after, we had increased the rate of ascertainment, examination, and DNA sampling of patients in our Clinical Core and their families, our statistical geneticist reported significant linkage in late-onset AD multiplex families on chromosome 19q13 by a newly applied method of "multipoint analysis" [6,11]. It is now hard to believe the level of skepticism in 1991 when barely a decade later we can perform genome wide screening based on variants in the sequenced Human Genome. We also had identified a large single family with 12 siblings, several of whom were diagnosed with early-onset autosomal dominant AD, and several more family members who were at risk. We determined chromosome 21 linkage, then gave the information and DNA samples to a collaborating St. Mary's Hospital group [12]. In addition, we generated a relatively huge family resource with early onset autosomal dominant AD that we transferred to Dr. Gerry Schellenberg's laboratory where they were searching for loci other than chromosome 21 [13]. Both families were included on the first reports of AβPP717 mutations (of the two families [12]) and what turned out to be chromosome 14-linked presenilin mutations (the largest family of the four [13]). The fractious nature of the AD genetic field was illustrated early when the initial submission of the AβPP717 paper eliminated any mention of the collaboration and had to be corrected "in proof". The second paper never acknowledged the very large familiy and collaboration.

We were actively participants in the early chromosome 19 Gene Mapping Consortium by concentrating on the then-laborious task of discovering, sequencing and testing candidate genes at or near 19q13. It also helped that our major research had been in myotonic muscular dystrophy which had also mapped to chromosome 19. The first gene localized to chromosome 19 had been apolipoprotein E – which everyone knew had nothing to do with either myotonic dystrophy or AD.

3. The intercept of data

In 1990, Dr. Warren Strittmatter joined our ADRC. He was an "amyloidologist" which made him, by definition, an AD researcher. He generated CSF binding data for amyloid peptide that was repeatedly contaminated by another protein band of different molecular size [1]. In trying to figure out the identity of this protein, I charged Dr. Strittmatter to extract the protein from gels, make tryptic peptides and sequence the peptide fragments. Two of the tryptic peptides were identical to sequences of apoE.

It was still crystal clear that apoE was not related to AD. Dr. Strittmater had spent four months on the peptide analysis and was quite agitated with his results. He walked into my office with two large volumes – Hurst's "Cardiology" and Stanbury et al.'s "Metabolic Basis of Inherited Diseases" – slammed them on my desk and stated that the #7*@$** peptides were apoE and they have nothing to do with AD.

My own laboratory, with seven post-doctoral scientists, was devoted to looking for candidate genes on chromosome 19q13. I felt like another lightening bolt hit me – similar, but less painful, than the myocardial infarction of two years earlier. I knew the location of APOE was on chromosome 19q13! Using the references provided in the textbooks, I found that there were three known alleles that could be accurately measured by PCR. I was a laboratory director and had no ability to set up a PCR assay – but my seven post-docs did – however none would – the Chief was off on one of his crazy ideas. Each had their own genes to work on.

It was the first week of December 1991, and Duke had defeated Harvard in the first basketball game of the season. My new daughter was two days old and had attended her first Duke game. My wife, Dr. Ann Saunders, was home on maternity leave. She was a scientist, known in gene mapping circles as the "mouse lady," because of her work in mapping genes in syntenic mice, but she knew how PCR reactions were done [14]. We cut a deal: she would go to my lab and set up the PCR for APOE and I would stay home with our new daughter.

Before Christmas the PCR was working, validated, and producing markedly different results on gels of fifty AD patients versus fifty controls. By the end of January, the strong associations of APOE4 with familial AD, sporadic AD and brain pathology were identified. By April, we had mapped genotypes against age of onset and determined that APOE4 alleles were associated with earlier age of onset compared to APOE3 – and that APOE2/3 individuals had very late age-of-onset perhaps indicating that APOE2 was a longevity gene. Dr. Saunders never went back to the syntenic mouse laboratory and has been committed and productive. She was the lead author on the initial genetic association with sporadic AD and continued the subsequent experiments and later headed the "APOE Team" in GSK that led to the clinical trial problem for glucose metabolism and apoptosis research [34].

4. The follow-up

The first presentation of the familial APOE data was in November 1992 at the Society for Neurosciences ADRC meeting [15]. Three papers were prepared. The first described the amyloid experiments leading to the association of APOE4 to familial AD and was published in the Proc Nat Acad Sci USA in 1993 [1]. The third paper prepared was published a month later by Science [3]. The critical paper describing the sporadic AD association was published eleven months after submission to Neurology [2]. (No press releases accompanied the first three papers, and the data were duly ignored by the AD community.)

At the Academy of Neurology meeting in New York City in April 1993, a ten minute presentation on the sporadic AD data [at the time in press] was followed by a seriously heated attack on the data during the discussion [16]. A reporter for the Wall Street Journal, Michael Waldholz, was in attendance. Every good reporter likes controversy – so he followed the presentation up by calling folks in the AD research world during May 1993. He did not call me but others told me of the calls.

My life changed on June 7, 1993, when I awoke on a Monday morning to a telephone call from a post-doc that my picture was on the front page of the Wall Street Journal [17]. Subsequent public meetings went from vicious to nasty, with prominent colleagues explicitly stating that they could not replicate the association [but later quietly retracted due to lab errors!]. However, a series of published letters in Lancet and other medical journals in which multiple investigators in Europe and Japan confirmed the APOE4 association with relatively small series of AD patients using their hospital laboratory APOE genotyping.

5. Towards a treatment

Space and decorum does not permit my view of academic science from 1993–1997. When my seven year NIA grant ended, so did my academic career. Only grant applications that implicated amyloid as a causative factor were fundable at the NIA study sections. Our work in apoE expression differences in neurons from mice and humans went unnoticed [7, 8,18–24]. Moving to a leadership position in GlaxoWellcome provided me the opportunity to apply genomics, proteomics and genetics in ways which were unimaginable in academia. This work continued into GSK [merger of GW and SmithKlineBeecham] and has led to one of several AD programs active within the company – some novel, some based on amyloid involvement, and one based on the differences found in protein expression between brain tissue expressing neuronal human apoE4 and tissue expressing neuronal apoE3 [25,26].

Positron emission tomography data developed first by Dr. Eric Reiman in Arizona, and confirmed by Dr. Gary Small at UCLA, clearly demonstrated that patients who carry the APOE4 allele – either homozygous or heterozygous – metabolize glucose [FDG] at a lower rate than patients with APOE3 and APOE2 alleles [27, 28].

A series of proteomic experiments in which brain from APOE knock-out mice and APOE knock-out mice transfected with human genomic APOE isoform-specific genes [with human-like neuronal apoE expression] identified a small number of genes with decreased or increased protein expression [25,26]. In additional these experiments are supported by a wealth of physiological supporting data, such as the use of thermography as a heat surrogate for measuring the rate of glucose metabolism in synaptosomes. A group of these genes clearly identified by proteomic screening supported decreased glucose utilization associated with apoE4, and these data were supported by thermography data.

In a series of *in vitro* thermography, glucose utilization and glucose utilization experiments with compounds known to affect glucose utilization through several mechanisms, we generated data with several lead compounds that increased glucose utilization in APOE4 animals to the level found in APOE3 animals. These compounds are at various stages in the pipeline [26].

The compounds were Perioxisome Proliferator-activated Receptor γ Activators. The GW experiments concentrated on PPAR γ agonists, including one under development for type 2 diabetes mellitus, called 570. At the merger, however, GSK already had an approved drug for type 2 diabetes, rosiglitizone. A Phase IIA clinical trial performed by Dr. Suzanne Craft at the University of Washington with rosiglitizone provided promising efficacy data [29–31]. Despite the fact that rosiglitizone was originally selected to have low blood-brain-barrier penetrance, because it was so far ahead of other compounds in the pipeline GSK initiated a Phase IIB proof of concept clinical trial of rosiglitizone as primary therapy which completed in August 06 [34]. There were as expected, no serious adverse events with a marketed product that has been proven to be quite safe in hundreds of thousands of patients. A parallel clinical trial in patients accompanied by PET is also ongoing in Phoenix [Reiman] and UCLA [Small]. The low brain penetrance may limit maximum clinical effectiveness for AD – but other GSK compounds are moving forward in the queue. One possibility is that the inflammation associated with AD will enhance access of rosiglitizone, which also has direct effects on neuronal cell inflammation responses.

The efficiency of a well organized pharmaceutical company has led to a wealth of experimental data that may lead to new classes of drugs based on the glucose utilization, inflammation and also apoptotic responses associated in an APOE isoform-specific manner in brain. Much of this work has remained under the academic radar screen which has focused on pathological manifestations of late disease. The association of APOE4 to the earlier age of onset of AD [now known to occur in early-onset autosomal dominant AD diseases as well] will soon lead to symptomatic and preventive therapies. The complex "causes" and "effects" of AD will soon be clarified.

Our current speculation is that neither amyloid-β nor APOE4 causes AD. In its simplest form, our hypothesis is that apoE isoforms affect glucose metabolism over many years and the APOE4 form binds tighter to amyloid-β [32]. Over years of decreased glucose metabolism protein aggregations occur differentially so that the onset of late symptoms relates to the kinetics of amyloid and tau aggregation. Once the aggregation begins and reaches a similar state in patients with, or without an APOE allele, the cascade of disease progression relates to the similar rates of protein aggregation. A prototype may be observed in the prion literature, when protein aggregations also cause neuronal pathologies [33]. In the case of AD, the critical rate – or incubation period – relates to the APOE4/amyloid-β aggregations in the presence of chronic, low level degrees of decreased glucose utilization and oxygen metabolism. The practical significance separates out symptomatic therapy programs from those that can confer prevention.

Rosiglitazone, a PPARγ agonist used in the treatment of type 2 diabetes mellitus has been tested as a monotherapy in a Phase IIB clinical trial of 511 patients and demonstrated clinical efficacy in an APOE allele-specific analysis. Patients who did not carry an APOE4 allele responded to all three doses of rosiglitazone, while the response in patients who carried an APOE4 allele was not significant in this trial, but a higher dose effect was suggested [34]. PET studies had previously demonstrated decreased glucose utilisation in subjects with an APOE4 allele compared to APOE4 non-carriers [25,26]. Rosiglitazone is a mitochondrial proliferator which results in stimulation of gulcose utilization in neuronal cells. The C-terminal degradation product of apoE4 protein binds to the outer mitochondrial membrane and disrupts mitochondrial dynamics. Providing newly proliferated mitochondrial enhances neuronal metabolism [35–37].

References

[1] W. Strittmatter, A. Saunders, D. Schmechel, M. Pericak-Vance, J. Enghild, G. Salvesen and A. Roses, Apolipoprotein E: high-avidity binding to beta-amyloid and increased frequency of type 4 allele in late-onset familial Alzheimer disease, *Proceedings of the National Academy of Sciences of the United States of America* **90** (2004), 1977–1981.

[2] A. Saunders, W. Strittmatter, D. Schmechel, P. George-Hyslop, M. Pericak-Vance, S. Joo, B. Rosi, J. Gusella, D. Crapper-MacLachlan, M. Alberts, C. Hulette, B. Crain, D. Goldgaber and A. Roses, Association of apolipoprotein E allele epsilon 4 with late-onset familial and sporadic Alzheimer's disease, *Neurology* **43** (1993), 1467–1472.

[3] E. Corder, A. Saunders, W. Strittmatter, D. Schmechel, P. Gaskell, G. Small, A. Roses, J. Haines and M. Pericak-Vance, Gene dose of apolipoprotein E type 4 allele and the risk of Alzheimer's disease in late onset families, *Science* **261** (1993), 921–923.

[4] Heyman, W. Wilkinson, B. Hurwitz, D. Schmechel, A. Sigmon, T. Weinberg, M. Helms and M. Swift, Alzheimer's disease: genetic aspects and associated clinical disorders, *Annals of Neurology* **14** (1983), 507–515.

[5] A. Roses, M. Pericak-Vance, L. Yamaoka, C. Haynes, M. Speer, P. Gaskell, W. Hung, C. Clark, A. Heyman, J. Trofatter, N. Earl, J. Gilbert, J. Lee, M. Alberts, D. Dawson, R. Bartlett, T. Siddique, J. Vance and P. Conneally, Linkage studies in familial Alzheimer's disease, *Progress in Clinical & Biological Research* **317** (1989), 201–215.

[6] C. Hulette, K. Welsh-Bohmer, B. Crain, M. Szymanski, N. Sinclaire and A. Roses, Rapid brain autopsy. The Joseph and Kathleen Bryan Alzheimer's Disease Research Center experience, *Archives of Pathology & Laboratory Medicine* **121** (1997), 615–618.

[7] E. Sajdel-Sulkowska and C. Marotta, Alzheimer's disease brain: alterations in RNA levels and in a ribonuclease-inhibitor complex, *Science* **225** (1984), 947–949.

[8] M. Pericak-Vance, J. Bebout, P. Gaskell, L. Yamaoka, W. Hung, M. Alberts, A. Walker, R. Bartlett, C. Haynes, K. Welsh, N. Earl, A. Heyman, C. Clark and A. Roses, Linkage studies in familial Alzheimer disease: evidence for chromosome 19 linkage, *American Journal of Human Genetics* **48** (1991), 1034–1050.

[9] M. Pericak-Vance, P. St George-Hyslop, P. Gaskell, J. Growdon, B. Crain, C. Hulette, J. Gusella, L. Yamaoka, R. Tanzi, A. Roses and J. Haines, Linkage analysis in familial Alzheimer disease: description of the Duke and Boston data sets, *Genetic Epidemiology* **10** (1993), 361–364.

[10] A. Goate, M. Chartier-Harlin, M. Mullan, J. Brown, F. Crawford, L. Fidani, L. Giuffra, A. Haynes, N. Irving, L. James, R. Mant, P. Newton, K. Rooke, P. Roques, C. Talbot, M. Pericak-Vance, A. Roses, R. Williamson, M. Rossor, M. Owen and J. Hardy, Segregation of a missense mutation in the amyloid precursor protein gene with familial Alzheimer's disease, *Nature* **349** (1991), 704–706.

[11] G. Schellenberg, T. Bird, E. Wijsman, H. Orr, L. Anderson, E. Nemens, J. White, L. Bonnycastle, J. Weber, M. Alonso, H. Potter, L. Heston and G. Martin, Genetic linkage evidence for a familial Alzheimer's disease locus on chromosome 14, *Science* **258** (1992), 668–671.

[12] A. Saunders and M. Seldin, The syntenic relationship of proximal mouse chromosome 7 and the myotonic dystrophy gene region on human chromosome 19q, *Genomics* **6** (1990), 324–332.

[13] Editorial, Society for Neuroscience Annual Meeting Report: Roses supposes that APOE predisposes to amyloidosis, *Journal of NIH Research* (December 1992).

[14] A. Roses, A. Saunders, W. Strittmatter, M. Pericak-Vance and D. Schmechel, Apolipoprotein E-E4 isoform is associated with susceptibility to Alzheimer's disease, *Neurology* **43** (1993), 192A.

[15] M. Waldholz, One of the main enigmas of the Alzhiemer's disease is said to be untangled, *Wall Street Journal* (Nov. 1993).

[16] S. Han, G. Einstein, K. Weisgraber, W. Strittmatter, A. Saunders, M. Pericak-Vance, A. Roses and D. Schmechel, Apolipoprotein E is localized to the cytoplasm of human cortical neurons: a light and electron microscopic study, *Journal of Neuropathology & Experimental Neurology* **53** (1994), 535–544.

[17] B. Teter, P. Xu, J. Gilbert, A. Roses, D. Galasko and G. Cole, Human apolipoprotein E isoform-specific differences in neuronal sprouting in organotypic hippocampal culture, *Journal of Neurochemistry* **73** (1999), 2613–2616.

[18] S. Chapman, T. Sabo, A. Roses and D. Michaelson, Reversal of presynaptic deficits of apolipoprotein E-deficient mice in human apolipoprotein E transgenic mice, *Neuroscience* **97** (2000), 419–424.

[19] G. Einstein, V. Patel, P. Bautista, M. Kenna, L. Melone, R. Fader, K. Karson, S. Mann, A. Saunders, C. Hulette, D. Mash, A. Roses and D. Schmechel, Intraneuronal ApoE in human visual cortical areas reflects the staging of Alzheimer disease pathology, *Journal of Neuropathology & Experimental Neurology* **57** (1998), 1190–1201.

[20] P. Xu, J. Gilbert, H. Qiu, T. Rothrock-Christian, D. Settles, A. Roses and D. Schmechel, Regionally specific neuronal expression of human APOE gene in transgenic mice, *Neuroscience Letters* **246** (1998), 65–68.

[21] Roses, J. Gilbert, P. Xu, P. Sullivan, B. Popko, D. Burkhart, T. Christian-Rothrock, A. Saunders, N. Maeda and D. Schmechel, Cis-acting human ApoE tissue expression element is associated with human pattern of intraneuronal ApoE in transgenic mice, *Neurobiology of Aging* **19** (1998), S53–S58.

[22] K. Williams, V. Pye, A. Saunders, A. Roses and P. Armati, Apolipoprotein E uptake and low-density lipoprotein receptor-related protein expression by the NTera2/D1 cell line: a cell culture model of relevance for late-onset Alzheimer's disease, *Neurobiology of Disease* **4** (1997), 58–67.

[23] D. Huang, M. Goedert, R. Jakes, K. Weisgraber, C. Garner, A. Saunders, M. Pericak-Vance, D. Schmechel, A. Roses and W. Strittmatter, Isoform-specific interactions of apolipoprotein E with the microtubule-associated protein MAP2c: implications for Alzheimer's disease, *Neuroscience Letters* **182** (1994), 55–58.

[24] W. Strittmatter, A. Saunders, M. Goedert, K. Weisgraber, L. Dong, R. Jakes, D. Huang, M. Pericak-Vance, D. Schmechel and A. Roses, Isoform-specific interactions of apolipoprotein E with microtubule-associated protein tau: implications for Alzheimer disease, *Proceedings of the National Academy of Sciences of the United States of America* **91** (1994), 11183–11186.

[25] E. Reiman, R. Caselli, L. Yun, K. Chen, D. Bandy, S. Minoshima, S. Thibodeau and D. Osborne, Preclinical evidence of Alzheimer's disease in persons homozygous for the epsilon 4 allele for apolipoprotein E, *New England Journal of Medicine* **334** (1996), 752–758.

[26] G. Small, L. Ercoli, D. Silverman, S. Huang, S. Komo, S. Bookheimer, H. Lavretsky, K. Miller, P. Siddarth, N. Rasgon, J. Mazziotta, S. Saxena, H. Wu, M. Mega, J. Cummings, A. Saunders, M. Pericak-Vance, A. Roses, J. Barrio and M. Phelps, Cerebral metabolic and cognitive decline in persons at genetic risk for Alzheimer's disease, *Proceedings of the National Academy of Sciences of the United States of America* **97** (2000), 6037–6042.

[27] A. Saunders, M. Trowers, R. Shimkets, S. Blakemore, D. Crowther, T. Mansfield, D. Wallace, W. Strittmatter and A. Roses, The role of apolipoprotein E in Alzheimer's disease: pharmacogenomic target selection, *Biochimica et Biophysica Acta* **1502** (2000), 85–94.

[28] A. Roses and M. Pangalos, Drug development and Alzheimer disease, *American Journal of Geriatric Psychiatry* **11** (2003), 123–130.

[29] G. Watson and S. Craft, The role of insulin resistance in the pathogenesis of Alzheimer's disease: implications for treatment, *CNS Drugs* **17** (2003), 27–45.

[30] S. Craft and G. Watson, Insulin and neurodegenerative disease: shared and specific mechanisms, *Lancet Neurology* **3** (2004), 169–178.

[31] G. Watson and S. Craft, Modulation of memory by insulin and glucose: neuropsychological observations in Alzheimer's disease, *European Journal of Pharmacology* **490** (2004), 97–113.

[32] A. Roses, Causes or consequences of inflammation and pathological signs of Alzheimer disease, *Neurobiology of Aging* **21** (2000), 423–425.

[33] J. Shorter and S. Lindquist, Prions as asaptive conduits of memory and inheritance, *Nature Reviews Genetics* **6** (2005), 435–450.

[34] M.E. Risner, A.M. Saunders, J.F.B. Altman, G.C. Ormandy, S. Craft, I.M. Foley, M. Zyartau-Hind, D.A. Hosford and A.D. Roses, Efficacy of rosiglitazone in a genetically defined population with mild-to-moderate Alzheimer's Disease, *The Pharmacogenetics Journal*, advance online publication 31 January 2006; doi:10.1038/sj.tpj.6500369.

[35] Y. Huang, X.Q. Liu, T. Wyss-Coray, W.J. Brecht, D.A. Sanan and R.W. Mahley, Apolipoprotein E fragments present in Alzheimer's disease brains induce neurofibrillary tangle-like intracellular inclusions in neurons, *Proc Natl Acad Sci USA* **98** (2001), 8838–8843.

[36] S. Chang, T.R. Ma, R.D. Miranda, M.E. Balestra, R.W. Mahley and Y. Huang, Lipid- and receptor-binding regions of apolipoprotein E4 fragments act in concert to cause mitochondrial dysfunction and neurotoxicity, *Proc Natl Acad Sci USA* **102** (2005), 18694–18699.

[37] A.D. Roses, A.M. Saunders, Y. Huang, J. Strum, K.H. Weisgraber and R.W. Mahley, Complex disease-associated pharmacogenetics: drug efficacy, drug safety, and confirmation of a pathogenetic hypothesis (Alzheimer's disease), *The Pharmacogenomics Journal* (2006), in press.

Early Alzheimer's disease genetics

Gerard D. Schellenberg
E-mail: Zachdad@u.washington.edu

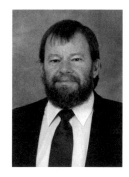

Abstract. The genetics community working on Alzheimer's disease and related dementias has made remarkable progress in the past 20 years. The cumulative efforts by multiple groups have lead to the identification of three autosomal dominant genes for early onset AD. These are the amyloid-β protein precursor gene (APP), and the genes encoding presenilin1 and 2. The knowledge derived from this work has firmly established Aβ as a critical disease molecule and lead to candidate drugs currently in treatment trials. Work on a related disease, frontotemporal dementia with parkinsonism – chromosome 17 type has also added to our understanding of pathogenesis by revealing that tau, the protein component of neurofibrillary tangles, is also a critical molecule in neurodegeneration. Lessons learned that still influence work on human genetics include the need to recognize and deal with genetic heterogeneity, a feature common to many genetic disorders. Genetic heterogeneity, if recognized, can be source of information. Another critical lesson is that clinical, molecular, and statistical scientists need to work closely on disease projects to succeed in solving the complex problems of common genetic disorders.

Keywords: Alzheimer disease, APP, genetics, mutation, tau

My entry into Alzheimer's disease genetics and really into human genetics began with a casual hallway conversation with Tom Bird, a colleague in Neurology at the University of Washington. He showed me some dementia pedigrees, both large and small, and wondered if I was interested in working on a linkage study of Alzheimer's disease. The year was 1984, an exciting time in human genetics. James Gusella had just used linkage analysis and newly developed DNA markers to map Huntington's disease to the short arm of chromosome 4 [9]. Even though at this time, only 20–30% of human chromosomes had been mapped, DNA sequencing was a tedious manual process, PCR had not been invented, and the word "genome" was rarely used in the same phrase with "human", the optimistic view was that the Huntington's disease gene would be identified in 2–3 years, no problem. So why not do the same for thing with Alzheimer's disease?

I was trained as a biochemist, and recognized the power of genetics to find molecules responsible for biologic function. However, even though I had used genetic tools throughout my career, just like using antibodies does not make you an immunologist, I was not a geneticist. My real interest in Tom's proposition was not out of an interest in genetics, but rather I figured that if I helped map and clone the Alzheimer's disease gene, I would have a leg-up on working on the protein. After all, this was only going to take a few years, so I started to work with Tom. We were both highly enthusiastic about the project for different reasons. I was enthusiastic out of complete ignorance about how difficult the work was going to be. Tom's enthusiasm, on the other hand, came from an earlier success. He and Jurg Ott in 1980 had used non-DNA blood markers to map a Charcot-Marie-Tooth locus to the Duffy locus, a polymorphic antigen mapped to chromosome 1 [3]. At the time when this work was done, genetic markers covered only a few percent of the genome, and there were no off-the-shelf analysis packages. The Charcot-Marie-Tooth locus was the first autosomal neurologic disease to be mapped, and was used as an example in Jurg Ott's classic book, "Analysis of human genetic linkage" [16]. I figured I couldn't go wrong, working with Tom, an astute clinical neurogeneticist who also had been so well prepared for an early moment of good luck.

We started in 1984 with three large families and several smaller kindreds, each with multiple cases of early-onset Alzheimer's disease, or at least some form of dementia, and a disease pattern that looked autosomal dominant. Each of these kindreds were to play a prominent part in our work but not always for the reason we initially thought. We had hoped that these large families could be pooled and linkage analysis could be used to find an Alzheimer's disease gene. However, as autopsies were accumulated, and antibodies for different amyloid proteins became available, it was clear that not all of these families had the same disease. In 1984, we also had to complete our research team and recruit a statistical geneticist, since the University of Washington had not been able to retain Jurg Ott. We first tried to recruit Mike Boehnke from the University of Michigan, but could not, but are still trying to get him to come to this day. We did succeed in getting Ellen Wijsman to come, which not only completed our group for the early work, but also, because of her efforts to develop new statistical methodologies, she brought novel quantitative trait analysis methods to Alzheimer's disease genetics.

One family, the BK or Seattle A family, was particularly perplexing. I call this the blind men and the elephant family. When psychiatrists saw family members early in the disease course, the diagnosis was mid-life onset psychosis similar to schizophrenia. When the subjects got to neurologists, late in the course of disease, the diagnosis was severe dementia like or related to Alzheimer's disease. The neuropathologists, Mark Sumi and David Nochlin, presumably with eyes wide open, really could do no better in assigning this family to a known disease. The brains had abundant neurofibrillary tangles throughout the cortex, with the hippocampus relatively spared, but no amyloid plaques [23]. This neuopathologic picture was consistently observed in multiple autopsies. Michelle Goedert and Maria Spillantini [21] later showed that the tangles in this family were composed of tau and the isoform and phosphor-epitope pattern was indistinguishable from Alzheimer's disease. The combined clinical and neuropathologic pattern did not match any other families in the literature, and to this day is unique. It would be another 13 years before we could make any sense of this family.

Another family added shortly after we started, the GCSA family, had large diffuse non-neuritic plaques that were eventually shown to be $A\beta$-negative but PRP-positive. In collaboration with Karen Hsaio, a mutation in the PRP gene (alanine to valine change at amino acid 117) was identified in 1991 [10]. This was one of the first Gerstmann-Straussler-Scheinker syndrome families where a causative PRP mutation was identified.

The remaining families did fortunately have Alzheimer's disease. These included 2 large families, the L and SNW kindreds, the latter had been described earlier by Lowell Weitkamp [25], and several smaller families, the H and V pedigrees. Tom continued to expand our families focusing initially on early-onset onset families but subsequently he began collecting late-onset kindreds. Through this continual evaluation of Alzheimer's disease families, Tom made two remarkable discoveries. First, in interviewing family members from some of the early-onset group, he heard the same phrase from two different people in two different families. Both mentioned their families were from Russia, but were actually Germans. The people turned out to be descendants from Germans who had emigrated in the 17th century to Russia and subsequently to the US at the end of the 19th and beginning of the 20th century. With a little more detective work, Tom found we had a total of five families with the same history and what is more remarkable, all had come from one of two towns, Frank and Walter, that were no more than 5 km apart near the Volga river in Russia [2]. Clearly a common ancestor, within Germany, or one of the original migrants to Russia had carried an Alzheimer's disease mutation and had been the founder of these families.

The second finding from these studies was really a prediction. Tom noted that based on age-of-onset, our families fell into three classes. First were the very early onset pedigrees with first symptoms occurring in the late 30's and early 40's (e.g., the L and SNW families). Second, were the Volga German families, with an intermediate onset age ranging from early 50's to 60's and even into the 70's. And finally, there were families where all cases had late-onset disease. The conclusion was that the genetics of Alzheimer's disease was going to involve at least 3 different genes and that onset-age was useful in classifying the different types of families [1] (Fig. 1). This prediction that Alzheimer's disease was genetically heterogeneous was not particularly popular at the time, because this meant that not all the families could be pooled and finding Alzheimer's disease genes was going to be more difficult than initially thought. To this day, age-of-onset is still the best quan-

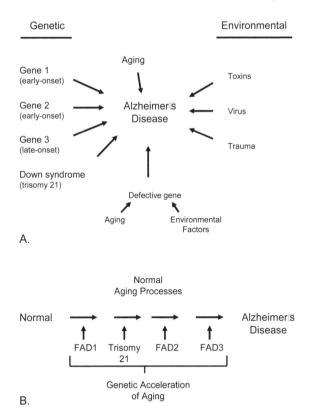

Fig. 1. (A) Potential genetic and environmental factors producing etiologic heterogeneity in AD. Possible gene/environment interactions are noted in the bottom. (B) AD may represent a common end result of the normal aging process. Several different genetic factors could accelerate this process and produce AD at younger ages. Note that in contrast to (A) above we show here that different mutations and trisomy 21 could affect different steps in a single pathway, all eventually leading to the AD phenotype. Reprinted from Neurobiology of Aging, Volume 10, Bird TD, Schellenberg GD, Wijsman EM, Martin GM, Evidence for etiologic heterogeneity in Alzheimer's disease, pp. 432–434, 1989, with permission from Elsevier.

titative phenotype for genetic analysis of Alzheimer's disease, though other traits such as Aβ levels may at some point get us closer to the disease.

The molecular genetics and biology really started in 1987 when the gene that encodes the Aβ peptide in Alzheimer's disease amyloid was cloned [13]. The gene/protein is called the amyloid-β protein precursor (APP). The gene, its location, and deduced protein sequence lead immediately to several interesting conclusions. First, the gene location on chromosome 21 was intriguing because an extra copy of this chromosome leads to Down syndrome, a genetic condition where Alzheimer's disease -like amyloid plaques accumulate. Second, the Aβ peptide that ended up in plaques was a proteolytic fragment of a larger protein, APP, and the mature Aβ peptide was the result of at least 2 proteolytic cleavage events. However, what the sequence could not tell us was whether Aβ was at the heart of the disease, or just a by-product of neurodegeneration. However, as George Glenner reminded me at a meeting in Niigata, Japan in 1988, in every amyloid he had studied, causative mutations had been found in the gene that encoded the amyloid protein.

In the same year, 1987, genetic linkage studies suggest that the APP gene accounted for Alzheimer's disease in early-onset Alzheimer's disease families. This was a frustrating time for our group because not only could we not find a mutation in the APP gene, despite sequencing over 500 subjects, but our linkage studies of the APP region using our early-onset families were also negative. When we published this in 1988 [18], one of our conclusions was that more than one gene was responsible for Alzheimer's disease genetics.

The first mutation found in APP in 1990 was not in Alzheimer's disease but rather in a familial cerebral disorder where Aβ was deposited in the cerebral vascular system [14,24]. Finally in 1991, Alison Goate and John Hardy found an APP mutation in two Alzheimer's disease kindreds, firmly establishing that at least for some families, Aβ caused Alzheimer's disease. During this early phase of Alzheimer's disease genetics, the closest we came to finding an APP mutation was a Glu to Gly change at amino acid 693 of the APP gene [12]. This was at the same position as the Glu to Gln mutation described for the hereditary cerebral hemorrhage with amyloidosis – Dutch type kindred [14]. However, the subject with the mutation (onset 63 years) had a sibling with Alzheimer's disease (onset 65 years) who did not have the mutation, so we could not demonstrate co-segregation and we could not find the same mutation in any other family. We published this mutation as an ambiguous result and had to wait 9 years before Lars Lannfelt and colleagues found the same mutation in a very large Swedish pedigree where he could show the change, dubbed the Artic mutation, was clearly pathogenic [15]. Remarkable, our US family was a distant branch of the Swedish kindred. This mutation is particularly interesting as Lars showed that the mutation does not affect Aβ production but only accelerates Aβ aggregation rates. This finding points to Aβ aggregates as the pathogenic molecule rather than the naked Aβ peptide.

Because we could not find APP mutations in any of our early-onset families, and could find no evidence for any other gene on chromosome 21, in 1988 we set off looking for genes on other chromosomes. We were using early-onset, Volga German, and late-onset families, but keeping them separate because we were convinced that genetic heterogeneity was important. This was still a risky project since there were substantial segments of the genome not covered by genetic markers. When we finally did get a positive linkage signal in 1992 [19], the results were breathtaking. I guess it should not have been surprising that given the right families, appropriate analysis, and good genetic markers the project would pay off. However, the fact that the approach really worked after years of preparation, was still startling. There were several important conclusions that immediately jumped out of the results. First, we had statistically unambiguous evidence from our early-onset families for a new Alzheimer's disease gene on chromosome 14. The results were so strong that the L family, one of our original kindreds, gave a significant signal by itself. A second gratifying result was that the Volga German families did not show a chromosome 14 signal, confirming our suspicions of genetic heterogeneity. Finally, early the next year, we also showed that the chromosome 14 gene was not responsible for late-onset Alzheimer's disease [20]. Not only did this start the race to identify the actual chromosome 14 gene, but also justified searching for genes for the Volga German and late-onset Alzheimer's disease. Work on the latter continues to this day.

The early-onset families where Alzheimer's disease was caused by the chromosome 14 gene were relatively straight-forward. Disease inheritance was clearly autosomal dominant, and the age-of-onset and disease duration were fairly tightly clustered in a given family. The Volga German kindreds, on the other hand, were significantly more complex. Onset ages ranged from 40 to 82 years with one obligate carrier dying apparently cognitively intact at age 89. Also the disease duration was not as short as in the chromosome 14 families and ranged in the Volga Germans from 8 to over 20 years. Because of the late-onset of Alzheimer's disease in the Volga German families, some kindreds had a fairly low density of cases, presumably with some family members dying of other causes prior to Alzheimer's disease onset. Thus the possibility existed that the etiology of cases in these families could be mixed, with some having an autosomal dominant disease and others simply having late-onset Alzheimer's disease. Another problem with these families was that not only were most of the parents of the affected subjects missing, there were also inbreeding loops in several of the families, making analysis particularly cumbersome. Because of these difficulties, once we did get an initial signal in 1994 to a marker on chromosome 1, it took Ellen Wijsman a full year of intensive analysis before we felt comfortable in publishing the results. While Ellen worked on the analysis, a bright young post-doctoral fellow, Ephrat Levy-Lahad, who was focusing on the Volga German project, had narrowed the region of interest down to a single yeast artificial chromosome clone that was a mere 300 kb. After the manuscript was submitted, Peter St George-Hyslop's group identified the chromosome 14 gene called presenilin 1, and also a homologue on chromosome 1. Once we determined that the presenilin 1 homolog was on our target YAC, we were sure that this homologue was the gene responsible for Alzheimer's disease in the Volga German kindreds.

Thus by 1995, after over a decade of work, we had been able to solve the genetics of most of the larger families that we had started with. However, the neurofibrillary tangle-only BK family remained unsolved. This kindred was clearly autosomal dominant with a high density of cases in the family. Unfortunately, most of the affected subjects had died before we could obtain a DNA sample. Thus we did not have enough sampled cases to be able to do linkage analysis just on this family. Usually in genetics, if no single large family is available for linkage analysis, data from other kindreds with the same disease are pooled in hopes all have the same underlying genetic cause. In this case, the reverse occurred with linkage analysis really identifying families that should be pooled. Kirk Wilhelmsen and colleagues had used linkage analysis to identify a region of chromosome 17 responsible for a disorder in a single large family where affected subjects had a complex spectrum of symptoms that included behavioral features such as disinhibition, and neurologic signs including parkinsonism and amyotrophy in a single large family [26]. When we examined the same region of chromosome 17, we also observed a positive linkage signal indicating these two rather dissimilar families possible had the same disease. By 1997, 13 families, all with substantially varied phenotypes all had been mapped to the same region of chromosome 17 [7]. Though the genome had not been fully sequenced, and thus the genes present in the target region not fully described, it was clear that the gene that encoded tau, called MAPT, was in the linkage region. Tau of course is the protein component in neurofibrillary tangles and our BK family had abundant tangle pathology. Existing genetic data also pointed to MAPT. Chris Conrad, a graduate student in the late Tsunao Saitoh's laboratory had reported that a specific allele of MAPT increased risk for supranuclear palsy (PSP) [5]. Even though this was a genetic association study, a method notorious for producing false-positive results, remarkably, this result was confirmed by multiple groups. However, extensive sequence analysis has not yielded a PSP-specific mutation, and the evidence suggested that there is a susceptibility rather than causative allele that contributes to PSP.

The first gene sequenced in my laboratory was MAPT. Parvoneh Poorkaj, a post-doctoral fellow in my group, almost immediately found a mutation in this family, a valine 337 site change to a methionine [17]. However, the interpretation of this mutation was not straight-forward. MAPT had already been sequenced in one chromosome 17 family and no mutation found [8]. Also the conventional wisdom being discussed at meetings was that MAPT was not the chromosome 17 gene because it had been sequenced in several families and no mutations found. Was the V337M a rare private change unrelated to disease only to be found in one family? Since at least some of the chromosome 17 families did not appear to have frank neurofibrillary tangles, was there more than one neurodegenerative gene in this region of chromosome 17? Had others simply missed mutations in this gene? It was not until Mike Hutton and an international consortium assembled a large panel of chromosome 17 families and found MAPT mutations in most of their [11], and Michelle Goedert and Maria Spillantini [22] had found a tau mutation in a multiple system atrophy family, that became clear that the V337M mutation mutation was responsible for disease in the BK family.

The chromosome 17 story is not finished. While most families where disease maps to chromosome 17 have mutations in or near the MAPT coding regions, there are several families that do not have mutations. These are large autosomal dominant kindreds where rare pathogenic mutations should be easily recognized, yet none have been found in MAPT. Are there mutations in MAPT non-coding regulatory sequences within or flanking MAPT tau responsible for disease in these families? Though improbable, is there another gene in the region that causes a neurodegenerative disease? Since these families do not have obvious tau pathology, perhaps another gene is responsible. Hopefully in the next year or so, one of the groups working on this problem will find the answer. Whatever the answer, the result will almost certainly tell us much about the neurodegenerative process.

In retrospect, our work in Seattle has been driven in part by what families Tom Bird and collaborators were able to identify. By solving the genetics of these families, we and others have firmly established the role of Aβ as a pathogenic molecule, identified the presenilins as part of the Aβ metabolism, and established tau as a contributor to pathogenesis rather than neurofibrillary tangles being simply an end-product of neurodegeneration. Lessons we have learned along the way that influence our current work include the importance of addressing genetic heterogeneity. While heterogeneity is usually considered a stumbling block in disease genetics, if dealt with, heterogeneity can be a rich source of information concerning disease pathogenesis. Another lesson learned is that scientists studying the clinical and neuropathology of families need to interact closely and continually with scientists with molecular and statistical expertise.

The genetic problems in Alzheimer's disease and dementia genetic that remain to be solved include finding the genetic risk factors for late-onset Alzheimer's disease. Ellen Wijsman's analysis of late-onset families suggests that there are 4–5 more genes with effect sizes comparable to ApoE that remain to be identified [6]. Other out standing genetic problems in Alzheimer's disease and dementia genetics include identifying the causative gene in the chromosome 17 families that do not have MAPT mutations. Also the risk allele presumably in a regulatory component of MAPT that elevates PSP risk also needs to be identified. This may require a more detailed understanding of how MAPT expression and alternative splicing is regulated. New methods are being applied to these problems including novel statistical methods for dealing with quantitative trait data in families, and methods for genome-wide association studies. Hopefully the lessons learned including an appreciation for heterogeneity and the need for detailed phenotype information, both from clinical data and autopsy results that comes from close collaborations scientists of different expertise.

References

[1] T.D. Bird, J.P. Hughes, S.M. Sumi, D. Nochlin, G.D. Schellenberg, T.H. Lampe et al., A proposed classification of familial Alzheimer's disease based on analysis of 32 multigeneration pedigrees. Alzheimer's Disease, in: *Epidemiology, Neuropathology, Neurochemistry, and Clinics, Key Topics in Brain Research*, K. Maurer, P. Riederer and H. Beckman, eds, 1990, pp. 51–57.

[2] T.D. Bird, T.H. Lampe, E.J. Nemens, G.W. Miner, S.M. Sumi and G.D. Schellenberg, Familial Alzheimer's disease in American Descendents of the Volga Germans: Probable genetic founder effect, *Ann. Neurol.* **23** (1988), 25–31.

[3] T.D. Bird, J. Ott and E.R. Giblett, Evidence for linkage of Charcot-Marie-Tooth neuropathy to the Duffy locus on chromosome 1, *Am. J. Hum. Genet.* **34** (1982), 388–394.

[4] T.D. Bird, G.D. Schellenberg, E.M. Wijsman and G.M. Martin, Evidence for etiologic heterogeneity in Alzheimer's disease, *Neurobiol Aging* **10** (1989), 432–434.

[5] C. Conrad, A. Andreadis, J. Trojanowski, D. Dickson, D. Kang, X. Chen et al., Genetic evidence for the involvement of Tau in progressive supranuclear palsy, *Ann. Neurol.* **47** (1997), 277–281.

[6] E.W. Daw, H. Payami, E.J. Nemens, D. Nochlin, T.D. Bird, G.D. Schellenberg et al., The number of trait loci in late-onset Alzheimer Disease, *Am. J. Hum. Genet.* **66** (2000), 196–204.

[7] N.L. Foster, K. Wilhelmsen, A.A.F. Sima, M.Z. Jones, C.J. D'Amato, S. Gilman et al., Frontotemporal dementia and parkinsonsim linked to chromosome 17: A consensus conference, *Ann. Neurol.* **41** (1997), 706–715.

[8] S. Froelich, H. Basun, C. Forsell, L. Lilius, K. Axelman, A. Andreadis et al., Mapping of a disease locus for familial rapidly progressive frontotemporal dementia to chromosome 17q12–21, *Am. J. Med. Genet.* **74** (1997), 380–385.

[9] J.F. Gusella, N.S. Wexler, P.M. Conneally, S.L. Naylor, M.A. Anderson, R.E. Tanzi et al., A polymorphic DNA marker genetically linked to Huntington's disease, *Nature* **306** (1983), 234–238.

[10] K.K. Hsiao, C.S.G.D. Cass, T.D. Bird, E. Devine-Gage, H. Wisniewski and S.B. Prusiner, A prion protein variant in a family with the telencephalic form of Gerstmann-Straussler-Scheinker syndrome, *Neurology* **41** (1991), 681–684.

[11] M. Hutton, C.L. Lendon, P. Rizzu, M. Baker, S. Froelich, H. Houlden et al., Association of missense and 5'-splice-site mutations in tau with the inherited dementia FTDP-17, *Nature* **393** (1998), 702–705.

[12] K. Kamino, H.T. Orr, H. Payami, E.M. Wijsamn, M.E. Alonso, S.M. Pulst et al., Linkage and mutational analysis of familial Alzheimer disease kindreds for the APP gene region, *Am. J. Hum. Genet.* **51** (1992), 998–1014.

[13] J. Kang, H.-G. Lemaire, A. Unterbeck, J.M. Salbaum, C.L. Masters, H.-H. Grzeschik et al., The precursor of Alzheimer's disease amyloid A4 protein resembles a cell-surface receptor, *Nature* **325** (1987), 733–736.

[14] E. Levy, M.D. Carman, I.J. Fernandez-Madrid, M.D. Power, I. Lieberburg, S.G. van Duinen et al., Mutation of the Alzheimer's disease amyloid gene in hereditary cerebral hemorrhage, Dutch type, *Science* **248** (1990), 1124–1126.

[15] C. Nilsberth, A. Westlinddanielsson, C.B. Eckman, M.M. Condron, K. Axelman, C. Forsell et al., The 'Arctic' APP mutation (E693G) causes Alzheimer's disease by enhanced A beta protofibril formation, *Nat. Neurosci.* **4** (2001), 887–893.

[16] J. Ott, *Analysis of human genetic linkage*, The Johns Hopkins University Press, Baltimore 1991.

[17] P. Poorkaj, T.D. Bird, E. Wijsman, E. Nemens, R.M. Garruto, L. Anderson et al., Tau is a candidate gene for chromosome 17 frontotemporal dementia, *Ann. Neurol.* **43** (1998), 815–825.

[18] G.D. Schellenberg, T.D. Bird, E.M. Wijsman, D.K. Moore, M. Boehnke, E.M. Bryant et al., Absence of linkage of chromosome 21q21 markers to familial Alzheimer's disease, *Science* **241** (1988), 1507–1510.

[19] G.D. Schellenberg, T.D. Bird, E.M. Wijsman, H.T. Orr, L. Anderson, E. Nemens et al., Genetic linkage evidence for a familial Alzheimer's disease locus on chromosome 14, *Science* **258** (1992), 668–671.

[20] G.D. Schellenberg, H. Payami, E.M. Wijsman, H.T. Orr, K.A.B. Goddard, L. Anderson et al., Chromosome-14 and Late-Onset Familial Alzheimer Disease (FAD), *Am. J. Hum. Genet.* **53** (1993), 619–628.

[21] M.G. Spillantini, R.A. Crowther and M. Goedert, Comparison of the neurofibrillary pathology in Alzheimer's disease and familial presenile dementia with tangles, *Acta Neuropathol* **92** (1996), 42–48.

[22] M.G. Spillantini, J.R. Murrell, M. Goedert, M.R. Farlow, A. Klug and B. Ghetti, Mutation in the tau gene in familial multiple system tauopathy with presenile dementia, *Proc. Natl. Acad. Sci. USA.* **95** (1998), 7737–7741.

[23] S.M. Sumi, T.D. Bird, D. Nochlin and M.A. Raskind, Familial presenile dementia with psychosis associated with cortical neurofibrillary tangles and neurodegeneration of the amygdala, *Neurology* **42** (1992), 120–127.

[24] C. Van Broeckhoven, J. Haan, E. Bakker, J.A. Hardy, W. Van Hul, A. Wehnert et al., Amyloid beta protein precursor gene and hereditary cerebral hemorrhage with amyloidosis (Dutch), *Science* **248** (1990), 1120–1122.

[25] L.R. Weitkamp, L. Nee, B. Keats, R.J. Polinskky and S. Guttormsen, Alzheimer disease: evidence for susceptibility loci on chromosomes 6 and 14, *Am. J. Hum. Genet.* **35** (1983), 443–453.

[26] K.C. Wilhelmsen, T. Lynch, E. Pavlou, M. Higgens and T.G. Nygaard, Localization of disinhibition-dementia-Parkinsonism-Amyotropy complex to 17q21–22, *Am. J. Hum. Genet.* **55** (1994), 1159–1165.

Mutations in the tau gene (MAPT) in FTDP-17: The family with Multiple System Tauopathy with Presenile Dementia (MSTD)

Maria Grazia Spillantini[a,*], Jill R. Murrell[b], Michel Goedert[c], Martin Farlow[b], Aaron Klug[c] and Bernardino Ghetti[b]

[a]*Centre for Brain Repair, Department of Clinical Neurosciences, University of Cambridge, Robinson Way, Cambridge CB2 2PY, UK*
[b]*Departments of Pathology and Laboratory Medicine (Division of Neuropathology) and Neurology, Indiana University School of Medicine, Indianapolis, IN 47202, USA*
[c]*MRC Laboratory of Molecular Biology, Hills Road, Cambridge CB2 2QH, UK*

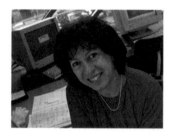

Abstract. Work in 1980s and early 1990s established that the microtubule-associated protein tau is the major component of the paired helical filament of Alzheimer's disease. Similar filamentous deposits are also present in a number of other diseases, including progressive supranuclear palsy, corticobasal degeneration and Pick's disease. In 1998, the relevance of tau dysfunction for the neurodegenerative process became clear, when mutations in the tau gene were found to cause the inherited "frontotemporal dementia and parkinsonism linked to chromosome 17 (FTDP-17)." The paper highlighted here [Spillantini M.G., Murrell J.R., Goedert M., Farlow M., Klug A. and Ghetti B. (1998) Mutation in the tau gene in familial multiple system tauopathy with presenile dementia. Proc. Natl. Acad. Sci. USA 95, 7737–7741] reported a mutation at position +3 in the intron following alternatively spliced exon 10 of the tau gene in a family with abundant filamentous deposits made exclusively of four-repeat tau. Levels of soluble four-repeat tau were increased in individuals with this mutation. It was proposed that the +3 mutation destabilises a stem-loop structure located at the end of exon 10 and the beginning of the intron, thus resulting in an abnormal ratio of three-repeat to four-repeat tau isoforms.

Keywords: Mutation, tau, tauopathy

1. Tau protein and the paired helical filament of Alzheimer's disease

On 3 November 1906, at the 37th meeting of the Society of Southwest German Psychiatrists in Tübingen, Alois Alzheimer presented the clinical and neuropathological characteristics of the disease that was subsequently named after him. The work in question was published in the short paper of 1907 [1] and the more extensive article of 1911 [2]. To this day, abundant neuritic plaques and neurofibrillary lesions constitute the defining neuropathological characteristics of Alzheimer's disease (AD). Although Kidd had described the paired helical filament (PHF) as the major structural component of the neurofibrillary lesions in 1963 [21], the molecular nature of the PHF was only

*Corresponding author. Tel.: +44 1223 331145; Fax: +44 1223 331174; E-mail: mgs11@cam.ac.uk.

uncovered in the late 1980s. By the early 1990s, it was clear that tau was the major component of the PHF and that the latter was composed of the six brain tau isoforms, each full-length and hyperphosphorylated [13, 24]. By that time, tau protein-like immunoreactivity had also been described in the pathological deposits of Pick's disease (PiD), progressive supranuclear palsy (PSP) and corticobasal degeneration (CBD). In contrast to AD and PiD, the abnormal deposits of PSP and CBD were present in neurons and glia. Subsequently, filamentous tau deposits were described in a number of additional neurodegenerative diseases.

The molecular dissection of the PHF of AD gave quite a complete description of the composition of the filament. It also provided important clues regarding the mechanisms of filament formation. However, it did not provide any direct information as to the relevance of filament formation for the disease process. As a result, tau-positive inclusions were frequently considered to be nothing more than epiphenomena of little or no consequence. What was missing was genetic evidence linking the formation of tau filaments to neurodegeneration and dementia. This was provided by studies of an inherited dementia.

2. Frontotemporal dementia and parkinsonism linked to chromosome 17 (FTDP-17)

In 1994, Kirk Wilhelmsen, Tim Lynch and colleagues described a family with frontotemporal dementia, parkinsonism and amyotrophy [Disinhibition-Dementia-Parkinsonism-Amyotrophy Complex (DDPAC)] and mapped the genetic defect to chromosome 17q21–22 [26,43]. These reports attracted the attention of those working on tau in AD, because the gene encoding tau (*MAPT*) is located in this region of the long arm of chromosome 17 [30]. A subsequent neuropathological examination of three cases of DDPAC described the presence of abundant argyrophilic, filamentous inclusions in neurons and glia, in conjunction with ballooned neurons, circumscribed nerve cell loss, gliosis and spongiosis [33]. The neuronal inclusions were reported to stain for phosphorylated neurofilaments and ubiquitin, but not for tau protein. The oligodendroglial inclusions, by contrast, were tau-immunoreactive, as were ballooned neurons and some spheroids. In 1995, a familial form of progressive subcortical gliosis was linked to chromosome 17q21–22 [23,31], and in 1996 pallido-ponto-nigral degeneration (PPND) [42,44] and the frontotemporal dementia in Duke family 1684 [46]

were also mapped to 17q21–22. Neuropathological examination of PPND revealed the presence of extensive nerve cell loss and gliosis in the substantia nigra and amygdala, in the apparent absence of Lewy bodies, neurofibrillary tangles and amyloid plaques, but in the presence of tau-immunoreactive neuropil threads and oligodendroglial microtubular masses. In Duke family 1684, senile plaques, neurofibrillary tangles, Pick bodies and Lewy bodies were not observed. In early 1997, hereditary forms of frontotemporal dementia in three Dutch families were linked to chromosome 17q21–22, with the apparent absence of tau deposits [17].

Having worked on filamentous tau inclusions for a number of years, we were naturally very interested in the existence of inherited neurodegenerative diseases characterized by the presence of abundant tau inclusions, in the absence of extracellular Aβ or prion protein deposits. The condition reported by Sumi et al. in 1992 [39] provided a striking illustration of this novel concept. This disease is inherited in an autosomal-dominant manner and is characterized clinically by presenile dementia and psychosis. Neuropathologically, tau-positive neurofibrillary tangles and PHFs are present in a number of brain regions, chiefly neocortex, amygdala and parahippocampal gyrus. In 1994, Michel Goedert obtained brain tissue from an affected individual of what is now known as Seattle family A from Mark Sumi and Tom Bird, which Maria Grazia Spillantini, Tony Crowther and Goedert used to characterize the tau deposits [34]. By using phosphorylation-dependent anti-tau antibodies, they showed that these deposits had the same staining characteristics as the neurofibrillary lesions of AD. Glial deposits were not observed. By electron microscopy, PHFs and straight filaments (SFs) were present in the same proportions as in AD. By immunoblotting, the sarkosyl-insoluble tau bands from Seattle family A and AD were identical, indicating the presence of all six human brain tau isoforms. In 1997, Bird and colleagues linked the genetic defect in Seattle family A to chromosome 17q21–22 [3].

In 1994, Bernardino Ghetti contacted Spillantini and Goedert and proposed to join forces in the characterization of the tau pathology in an autosomal-dominantly inherited form of presenile dementia that he and Martin Farlow had identified. Tau deposits were extremely abundant and widespread and were present in neurons and glia (Fig. 1). In view of this severe phenotype, the disease was named "Multiple System Tauopathy with Presenile Dementia" (MSTD), the first use of the term "tauopathy" [35]. Tau-positive lesions were stained

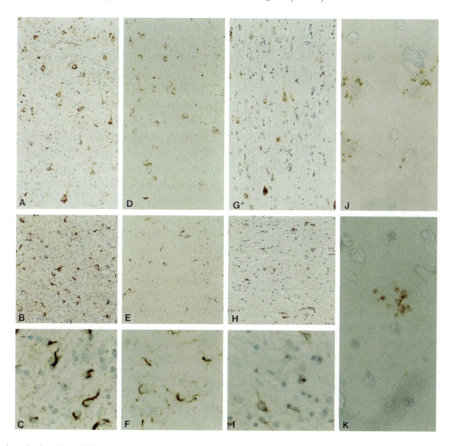

Fig. 1. Tau inclusions in familial MSTD brain. Temporal cortex from a patient with familial MSTD showing neurons and glia stained with phosphorylation-dependent anti-tau antibodies. Neurons and glia in grey matter stained with antibodies AT8 (A), AT180 (D) and PHF1 (G). In white matter AT8 (B and C), AT180 (E and F) and PHF1 (H and I) stained numerous glial cells with cytoplasmic inclusions (C, F and I). Antibody 12E8 stained granular deposits in neurons and glia in both grey (J) and white matter (K). Magnifications: A, B, D, E, G and H, ×140; C,F and I, ×448; J, ×760 and K, ×112. Taken from Spillantini et al. [35] Copyright (1997) National Academy of Sciences, USA.

by a large number of phosphorylation-independent and phosphorylation-dependent anti-tau antibodies. By immunoelectron microscopy, Crowther showed that the anti-tau antibodies decorated isolated filaments, which had a twisted ribbon morphology and differed markedly from PHFs and SFs (Fig. 2). By immunoblotting, tau protein extracted from filament preparations ran as two major bands of 64 and 68 kDa and a minor band of 72 kDa (Fig. 3). This pattern of sarkosyl-insoluble tau bands differed from that of AD, but was similar to that previously described in PSP and CBD [5,22], two diseases with neuronal and glial tau pathology. It raised the question of the isoform composition of the sarkosyl-insoluble tau in MSTD. Dephosphorylation was used to show the presence of four repeat-containing isoforms, in the absence of three-repeat tau [35]. In parallel, Jill Murrell performed linkage analyses to show that the genetic defect in MSTD mapped to chromosome 17q21–22 [27]. This work made *MAPT* a strong candidate gene for MSTD. The open reading frame of *MAPT* was therefore sequenced, but no pathogenic mutation was found.

The work on Seattle family A and familial MSTD established the presence of abundant tau pathology in two families linked to chromosome 17q21–22. Affected individuals from both families suffered from presenile dementia, but the clinical pictures were otherwise quite different. Similarly, the tau deposits had some characteristics in common, such as the sites of hyperphosphorylation, but also showed significant differences. In particular, tau filaments had different morphologies and were made of all six brain isoforms in Seattle family A, but comprised only four-repeat tau in MSTD. Furthermore, tau deposits were present in nerve cells in Seattle family A and in both neurons and glia in familial MSTD.

In October 1996, Ghetti, Murrell and Spillantini attended the consensus conference on chromosome 17-

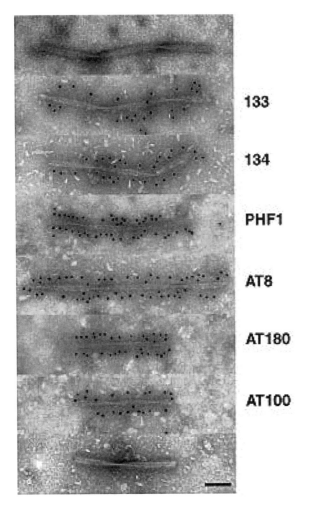

Fig. 2. Tau filaments from familial MSTD brain. Immunoelectron microscopy of isolated twisted ribbon-like filaments. The top and bottom panels are unlabelled, and the others are immunogold decorated with phosphorylation-dependent (PHF1, AT8, AT180 and AT100) and phosphorylation-independent (133 and 134) anti-tau antibodies. Scale bar, 100 nm. Taken from Spillantini et al. [35] Copyright (1997) National Academy of Sciences, USA.

linked dementias organized by Norman Foster at the University of Michigan, which brought together many of those working in this emerging field. At the time, 13 kindreds were considered to have sufficient evidence of linkage to be included in what was named "Frontotemporal Dementia and Parkinsonism linked to chromosome 17" (FTDP-17) [6]. At the conference, it became clear that a variety of techniques, some suboptimal, had been used to look for tau pathology and that Seattle family A and familial MSTD were the only pedigrees where a systematic analysis had been carried out. Spillantini therefore began to collaborate with a number of groups, to look for the presence of tau pathology in

their families. These included DDPAC [26,43], Dutch families I-III [17], Duke family 1684 [46], the Swedish FTDP-17 family [7] and hereditary dysphasic disinhibition dementia (HDDD2) [25]. When using state of the art techniques, abundant tau deposits were detected in DDPAC, Dutch families I and II and Duke family 1684. In HDDD2, tau deposits were also present, but their abundance varied between cases. Some of this work was later published [19,36,38]. These findings, together with our earlier work, left little doubt that tau deposits were an important feature of FTDP-17.

3. Mutation in MAPT in familial MSTD

The exclusive presence of four-repeat tau in the MSTD filaments led us to examine the isoform composition of soluble tau. One possibility (among several) was that certain tau isoforms might be abnormally expressed in MSTD brain [35]. It was well established that upon dephosphorylation soluble tau from normal human cerebral cortex runs as four strong and two weak bands on SDS-PAGE, which align with the six recombinantly expressed human brain isoforms [8, 9]. In normal adult human cerebral cortex, the ratio of three-repeat to four-repeat tau isoforms is approximately 1:1. Over the years, many experiments on both control and diseased human brains had failed to reveal a significant departure from this 1:1 ratio. Therefore, the striking pattern of alternating stronger and weaker bands that we observed upon immunoblotting of dephosphorylated soluble tau from MSTD brain was unprecedented (Fig. 3). It showed a marked increase in the level of four-repeat tau isoforms and a corresponding reduction in tau isoforms with three repeats, with no apparent change in total tau levels. This finding provided a straightforward explanation for the exclusive presence of four-repeat tau in MSTD filaments and suggested, rather unexpectedly, that increased splicing of exon 10 of *MAPT* might be the cause of familial MSTD.

In early 1998, Spillantini, Bird and Ghetti wrote a review article on FTDP-17 for "Brain Pathology" (it was published on-line in early March that year) [36]. In it they summarized what was known about the presence of tau deposits in FTDP-17 and mentioned the increase in soluble four-repeat tau in familial MSTD. They also mentioned the V337M change in exon 12 of *MAPT* that Parvoneh Poorkaj, Gerard Schellenberg and Bird had identified in Seattle family A. However, it was unclear then whether this amino acid change in the

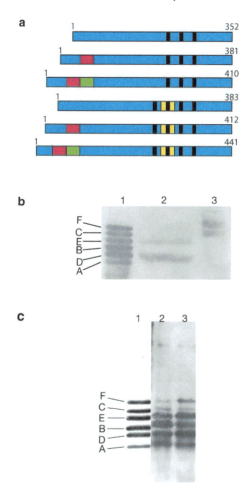

Fig. 3. Abnormal filaments from familial MSTD brain consist of tau isoforms with four repeats and the level of soluble four-repeat tau is increased in MSTD brain. (a), Schematic representation of the six human brain tau isoforms. (b), Immunoblots of sarkosyl-insoluble tau from familial MSTD brain before (lane 3) and after (lane 2) alkaline phosphatase treatment using antibody 133. Note that before alkaline phosphatase treatment, two major tau bands of 64 and 68 kDa and a minor band of 72 kDa are present. After alkaline phosphatase treatment, two major bands are visible that align with four repeat-containing recombinant tau isoforms (lane 1) of 383 and 412 amino acids (isoforms D and E in schematic diagram). (c), Immunoblots of dephosphorylated soluble tau protein from the frontal cortex of a control subject (lane 2) and a patient with familial MSTD (lane 3) using antibody 133. Six tau isoforms are present in lanes 2 and 3. They align with the six recombinant human brain tau isoforms (lane 1). In the frontal cortex from the familial MSTD patient, tau isoforms with four repeats (isoforms D-F) are more abundant and tau isoforms with three repeats (isoforms A-C) are less abundant than in frontal cortex from the control. Taken from Spillantini et al. [35,37] Copyright (1997, 1998) National Academy of Sciences, USA.

microtubule-binding repeat region of tau represented a benign polymorphism, or was in some way involved in the pathogenesis of the disease in this family.

In familial MSTD, sequencing of the intronic regions flanking exon 10 had revealed a guanine (G) to adenine (A) transition at position +3 in the intron following exon 10. It segregated with the disease and was not found in control samples. Furthermore, no change was found in MAPT cDNA isolated from familial MSTD brain, indicating that the MAPT exons were spliced correctly. This raised the question of how this nucleotide change might lead to increased splicing of exon 10. Following examination of the nucleotide sequence of exon 10 and the 5' intron junction by Aaron Klug, and discussions with Gabriele Varani and Kiyoshi Nagai of the MRC Laboratory of Molecular Biology, it became apparent that the G to A transition at position +3 destabilized a putative stem-loop structure encompassing the last 6 nucleotides of exon 10 and 19 nucleotides of the intron, including the GT splice-donor site. Varani then set out to determine the three-dimensional structure of the stem-loop, disruption of which was predicted to result in increased splicing of exon 10. A role for premRNA structure in the regulation of alternative splicing had been well documented in other systems. Moreover, experimental studies had shown that the formation of stem-loop structures at the 5' splice sites leads to inefficient splicing. We also noticed that the G to A transition at position +3 could increase binding of the U1 snRNA to the 5' splice site of exon 10, resulting in increased splicing of exon 10.

4. Mutations in MAPT in FTDP-17

Towards the end of April 1998, Michael Hutton and Spillantini presented their respective discoveries of MAPT mutations in FTDP-17 at a closed meeting of the US Alzheimer Center Directors in Minneapolis, which was held ahead of the annual meeting of the American Academy of Neurology. The news spilled over into the main meeting and was discussed at the Potamkin Prize Symposium.

In June 1998, the papers by Poorkaj et al. [32], Hutton et al. [20] and Spillantini et al. [37] were published. Poorkaj et al. reported two exonic mutations in MAPT (V337M in Seattle family A and P301L in Seattle family D). Hutton et al. reported six different mutations in ten FTDP-17 families. Three of these mutations (G272V, P301L and R406W) were in exons. The other three were located in the intron following exon 10 (at positions +13, +14 and +16), where they disrupted a predicted stem-loop. By exon trapping, the intronic mutations caused an increase in the transcripts encoding four-repeat tau. Spillantini et al. reported the +3

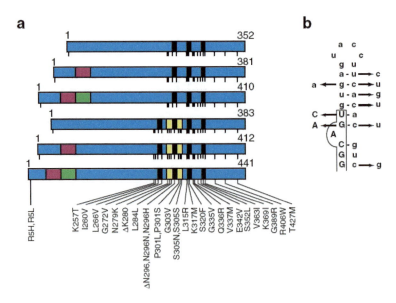

Fig. 4. Mutations in the tau gene (*MAPT*) in FTDP-17. (a), Schematic diagram of the six tau isoforms (352 to 441 amino acids) that are expressed in the adult human brain, with mutations in the coding region indicated using the numbering of the 441 amino acid isoform. Twenty-five missense mutations, two deletion mutations and three silent mutations are shown. The six tau isoforms are produced by alternative mRNA splicing from a single gene. They differ by the presence or absence of three inserts, shown in red (encoded by exon 2), green (encoded by exon 3) and yellow (encoded by exon 10), respectively. The migotubule binding repects are indicated by black bars. (b), Stem-loop structure in the pre-mRNA at the boundary between exon 10 and the intron following exon 10. Nine mutations are shown, two of which (S305N and S305S) are located in exon 10. Exon sequences are boxed and shown in capitals, with intron sequences shown in lowercase letters. The two-dimensional representation of the *MAPT* exon splicing regulatory element RNA is based on the three-dimensional structure determined in [41].

intronic mutation in familial MSTD and its effect on the predicted stem-loop, as well as the increase in soluble four-repeat tau in MSTD brain. Later that year, the reported missense mutations were shown to reduce the ability of tau to promote microtubule assembly [15, 18]. Some mutations also promote tau filament assembly [11,28].

Varani determined the three-dimensional structure of a 25 nucleotide-long synthetic RNA (extending from position −5 to +19) from the exon 10-intron junction by nuclear magnetic resonance (NMR) spectroscopy. This work, which was eventually published in 1999 [41], established that the synthetic RNA does form a stable stem loop with a structure similar to that originally proposed [37]. The stem consists of a single stable guanine-cytosine (G-C) base pair, which is separated from a double helix of 6 base pairs by an unpaired adenine. The apical loop consists of 6 nucleotides that adopt multiple conformations in rapid exchange. Functional experiments showed that the +3 mutation caused a marked reduction in the thermodynamic stability of the stem-loop. The same was also true of the +13, +14 and +16 mutations.

In 1999, coding region mutations in exon 10 itself were identified which increase splicing by affecting RNA regulatory elements [4,16]. By that time, mutations in *MAPT* had been identified in most of the FTDP-17 families mentioned in this article. Besides Seattle family A (mutation V337M [32]) and familial MSTD (+3 intronic mutation [37]), mutations were identified in DDPAC (+14 intronic mutation [20]), familial progressive subcortical gliosis (+16 intronic mutation [12]), Duke family 1684 (+16 intronic mutation [19]), PPND (mutation N279K [4]), Dutch family I (mutation P301L [20]) and Dutch family II (mutation G272V [20]).

Since 1999, the number of known mutations in *MAPT* has grown steadily. At the time of writing, 37 different mutations, mostly affecting the sequence or splicing of the repeat region, have been reported in over 100 families with FTDP-17 (Fig. 4). About half of these mutations influence the alternative splicing of *MAPT* pre-mRNA, whereas the other half have their primary effect at the protein level. Besides MSTD, two additional families with the +3 intronic mutation have been described [29,40]. Overall, the existence of mutations in *MAPT* in FTDP-17 established that dysfunction of tau is sufficient to cause neurodegeneration and dementia.

References

[1] A. Alzheimer, Über eine eigenartige Erkrankung der Hirnrinde, *Allg Z Psychiat Psych Gerichtl Med* **64** (1907), 146–148.

[2] A. Alzheimer, Über eigenartige Krankheitsfälle des späteren Alters, *Z Ges Neurol Psychiat* **4** (1911), 356–385.

[3] T.D. Bird, E.M. Wijsman, D. Nochlin, M. Leehey, S.M. Sumi, H. Payami, P. Poorkaj, E. Nemens, M.A. Raskind and G.D. Schellenberg, Chromosome 17 and hereditary dementia: linkage studies in three non-Alzheimer families and kindreds with late-onset FAD, *Neurology* **48** (1997), 949–954.

[4] I. D'Souza, P. Poorkaj, M. Hong, D. Nochlin, V.M.-Y. Lee, T.D. Bird and G.D. Schellenberg, Missense and silent tau gene mutations cause frontotemporal dementia with parkinsonism-chromosome 17 type, by affecting multiple alternative RNA splicing regulatory elements, *Proc Natl Acad Sci USA* **96** (1999), 5598–5603.

[5] S. Flament, A. Delacourte, M. Verny, J.J. Hauw and F. Javoy-Agid, Abnormal tau proteins in progressive supranuclear palsy. Similarities and differences with the neurofibrillary degeneration of the Alzheimer type, *Acta Neuropathol* **81** (1991), 591–596.

[6] N.L. Foster, K. Wilhelmsen, A.A.F. Sima, M.Z. Jones, C.J. D'Amato, S. Gilman, M.G. Spillantini, T. Lynch, R.P. Mayeux, P.C. Gaskell, C. Hulette, M.A. Pericak-Vance, K.A. Welsh-Bohmer, D.W. Dickson, P. Heutink, J. Kros, J.C. van Swieten, F. Arwert, B. Ghetti, J. Murrell, L. Lannfelt, M. Hutton, C.H. Phelps, D.S. Snyder, E. Oliver, M.J. Ball, J.L. Cummings, B.L. Miller, R. Katzman, L. Reed, R.L. Schelper, D.J. Lanska, A. Brun, J.K. Fink, D.E. Khul, D.S. Knopman, Z. Wszolek, C.L. Miller, T.D. Bird, C. Lendon and C. Elechi, Frontotemporal dementia and parkinsonism linked to chromosome 17: a consensus conference, *Ann Neurol* **41** (1997), 706–715.

[7] S. Froelich, H. Basun, C. Forsell, L. Lilius, K. Axelman, A. Andreadis and L. Lannfelt, Mapping of a disease locus for familial rapidly progressive frontotemporal dementia to chromosome 17q12–21, *Am J Med Genet* **74** (1997), 380–385.

[8] M. Goedert, M.G. Spillantini, R. Jakes, D. Rutherford and R.A. Crowther, Multiple isoforms of human microtubule-associated protein tau: Sequences and localization in neurofibrillary tangles of Alzheimer's disease, *Neuron* **3** (1989), 519–526.

[9] M. Goedert and R. Jakes, Expression of separate isoforms of human tau protein: Correlation with the tau pattern in brain and effects on tubulin polymerization, *EMBO J* **9** (1990), 4225–4230.

[10] M. Goedert, M.G. Spillantini, N.J. Cairns and R.A. Crowther, Tau proteins of Alzheimer paired helical filaments: Abnormal phosphorylation of all six brain isoforms, *Neuron* **8** (1992), 159–168.

[11] M. Goedert, R. Jakes and R.A. Crowther, Effects of frontotemporal dementia FTDP-17 mutations on heparin-induced assembly of tau filaments, *FEBS Lett* **450** (1999), 306–311.

[12] M. Goedert, M.G. Spillantini, R.A. Crowther, S.G. Chen, P. Parchi, M. Tabaton, D.J. Lanska, W.R. Markesbery, K.C. Wilhelmsen, D.W. Dickson, R.B. Petersen and P. Gambetti, Tau gene mutation in familial progressive subcortical gliosis, *Nature Med* **5** (1999), 454–457.

[13] M. Goedert, A. Klug and R.A. Crowther, Tau protein, the paired helical filament and Alzheimer's disease, *J Alz Dis* (in press).

[14] S. Greenberg and P. Davies, A preparation of Alzheimer paired helical filaments that displays distinct tau proteins by polyacrylamide gel electrophoresis, *Proc Natl Acad Sci USA* **87** (1990), 5827–5831.

[15] M. Hasegawa, M.J. Smith and M. Goedert, Tau proteins with FTDP-17 mutations have a reduced ability to promote microtubule assembly, *FEBS Lett* **437** (1998), 207–210.

[16] M. Hasegawa, M.J. Smith, M. Iijima, T. Tabira and M. Goedert, FTDP-17 mutations N279K and S305N in tau produce increased splicing of exon 10, *FEBS Lett* **443** (1999), 93–96.

[17] P. Heutink, M. Stevens, P. Rizzu, E. Bakker, J.M. Kros, A. Tibben, M.F. Niermeijer, M. van Duin, B.A. Oostra and J.C. van Swieten, Hereditary frontotemporal dementia is linked to chromosome 17q21–22: a genetic and clinicopathological study of three Dutch families, *Ann Neurol* **41** (1997), 150–159.

[18] M. Hong, V. Zhukareva, V. Vogelsberg-Ragaglia, Z. Wszolek, L. Reed, B.I. Miller, D.H. Geschwind, T.D. Bird, D. McKeel, A. Goate, J.C. Morris, K.C. Wilhelmsen, G.D. Schellenberg, J.Q. Trojanowski and V.M.-Y. Lee, Mutation-specific functional impairments in distinct tau isoforms of hereditary FTDP-17, *Science* **282** (1998), 1914–1917.

[19] C.M. Hulette, M.A. Pericak-Vance, A.D. Roses, D.E. Schmechel, L.H. Yamaoka, P.C. Gaskell, K.A. Welsh-Bohmer, R.A. Crowther and M.G. Spillantini, Neuropathological features of frontotemporal dementia and parkinsonism linked to chromosome 17q21–22 (FTDP-17): Duke family 1684, *J Neuropathol Exp Neurol* **58** (1999), 859–866.

[20] M. Hutton, C.L. Lendon, P. Rizzu, M. Baker, S. Froelich, H. Houlden, S. Pickering-Brown, S. Chakraverty, A. Isaacs, A. Grover, J. Hackett, J. Adamson, S. Lincoln, D. Dickson, P. Davies, R.C. Petersen, M. Stevens, E. de Graaff, E. Wauters, J. van Baren, M. Hillebrand, M. Joosse, J.M. Kwon, P. Nowotny, L.K. Che, J. Norton, J.C. Morris, L.A. Reed, J. Trojanowski, H. Basun, L. Lannfelt, M. Neystat, S. Fahn, F. Dark, T. Tannenberg, P.R. Dodd, N. Hayward, J.B.J. Kwok, P.R. Schofield, A. Andreadis, J. Snowden, D. Craufurd, D. Neary, F. Owen, B.A. Oostra, J. Hardy, A. Goate, J. van Swieten, D. Mann, T. Lynch and P. Heutink, Association of missense and 5'-splice-site mutations in tau with the inherited dementia FTDP-17, *Nature* **393** (1998), 702–705.

[21] M. Kidd, Paired helical filaments in electron microscopy of Alzheimer's disease, *Nature* **197** (1963), 192–193.

[22] H. Ksiezak-Reding, K. Morgan, L.A. Mattiace, P. Davies, W.K. Liu, S.-H. Yen, K. Weidenheim and D.W. Dickson, Ultrastructure and biochemical composition of paired helical filaments in corticobasal degeneration, *Am J Pathol* **145** (1994), 1496–1508.

[23] D.J. Lanska, R.D. Currier, M. Cohen, P. Gambetti, E.E. Smith, J. Bebin, J.F. Jackson, P.J. Whitehouse and W.R. Markesbery, Familial progressive subcortical gliosis, *Neurology* **44** (1994), 1633–1643.

[24] V.M.-Y. Lee, M. Goedert and J.Q. Trojanowski, Neurodegenerative Tauopathies, *Annu Rev Neurosci* **24** (2001), 1121–1159.

[25] C.L. Lendon, T. Lynch, J. Norton, D.W. McKeel, F. Busfield, N. Craddock, S. Chakraverty, G. Gopalakrishnan, S.D. Shears, W. Grimmett, K.C. Wilhelmsen, L. Hansen, J.C. Morris and A.M. Goate, Hereditary dysphasic disinhibition dementia: a frontotemporal dementia linked to 17q21–22, *Neurology* **50** (1998), 1546–1555.

[26] T. Lynch, M. Sano, K.S. Marder, K.L. Bell, N.L. Foster, R.F. Defendini, A.A.F. Sima, C. Keohane, T.G. Nygaard, S. Fahn, R. Mayeux, L.P. Rowland and K.C. Wilhelmsen, Clinical characteristics of a family with chromosome

17-linked disinhibition-dementia-parkinsonism-amyotrophy complex, *Neurology* **44** (1994), 1878–1884.

[27] J.R. Murrell, D. Koller, T. Foroud, M. Goedert, M.G. Spillantini, H.J. Edenberg, M.R. Farlow and B. Ghetti, Familial multiple system tauopathy with presenile dementia is localized to chromosome 17, *Am J Hum Genet* **61** (1997), 1131–1138.

[28] P. Nacharaju, J. Lewis, C. Easson, S. Yen, J. Hackett, M. Hutton and S.-H. Yen, Accelerated filament formation from tau protein with specific FTDP-17 mutations, *FEBS Lett* **447** (1999), 195–199.

[29] M. Neumann, M. Mittelbronn, P. Simon, B. Vanmassenhove, R. de Silva, A. Lees, J. Klapp, R. Meyermann and H.A. Kretzschmar, A new family with frontotemporal dementia with intronic 10 + 3 splice site mutation in the tau gene: neuropathology and molecular effects, *Neuropathol Appl Neurobiol* **31** (2005), 362–373.

[30] R.L. Neve, P. Harris, K.S. Kosik, D.M. Kurnit and T.A. Donlon, Identification of cDNA clones for the human microtubule-associated protein tau and chromosomal localization of the genes for tau and microtubule-associated protein 2, *Mol Brain Res* **1** (1986), 271–280.

[31] R.B. Petersen, M. Tabaton, S.G. Chen, L. Monari, S.L. Richardson, T. Lynch, V. Manetto, D.J. Lanska, W.R. Markesbery, R.D. Currier, L. Autilio-Gambetti, K.C. Wilhelmsen and P. Gambetti, Familial progressive subcortical gliosis: Presence of prions and linkage to chromosome 17, *Neurology* **45** (1995), 1062–1067.

[32] P. Poorkaj, T.D. Bird, E. Wijsman, E. Nemens, R.M. Garruto, L. Anderson, A. Andreadis, W.C. Wiederholt, M. Raskind and G.D. Schellenberg, Tau is a candidate gene for chromosome 17 frontotemporal dementia, *Ann Neurol* **43** (1998), 815–825.

[33] A.A.F. Sima, R. Defendini, C. Keohane, C. D'Amato, N.L. Foster, P. Parchi, P. Gambetti, T. Lynch and K.C. Wilhelmsen, The neuropathology of chromosome 17-linked dementia, *Neurology* **39** (1996), 734–743.

[34] M.G. Spillantini, R.A. Crowther and M. Goedert, Comparison of the neurofibrillary pathology in Alzheimer's disease and familial presenile dementia with tangles, *Acta Neuropathol* **92** (1996), 42–48.

[35] M.G. Spillantini, M. Goedert, R.A. Crowther, J.R. Murrell, M.J. Farlow and B. Ghetti, Familial multiple system tauopathy with presenile dementia: a disease with abundant neuronal and glial tau filaments, *Proc Natl Acad Sci USA* **94** (1997), 4113–4118.

[36] M.G. Spillantini, T.D. Bird and B. Ghetti, Frontotemporal dementia and parkinsonism linked to chromosome 17: a new group of tauopathies, *Brain Pathol* **8** (1998), 387–402.

[37] M.G. Spillantini, J.R. Murrell, M. Goedert, M.R. Farlow, A. Klug and B. Ghetti, Mutation in the tau gene in familial multiple system tauopathy with presenile dementia, *Proc Natl Acad Sci USA* **95** (1998), 7737–7741.

[38] M.G. Spillantini, R.A. Crowther, W. Kamphorst, P. Heutink and J.C. van Swieten, Tau pathology in two Dutch families with mutations in the microtubule-binding region of tau, *Am J Pathol* **153** (1998), 1359–1363.

[39] S.M. Sumi, T.D. Bird, D. Nochlin and M.A. Raskind, Familial presenile dementia with psychosis associated with cortical neurofibrillary tangles and degeneration of the amygdala, *Neurology* **42** (1992), 120–127.

[40] M. Tolnay, M.G. Spillantini, C. Rizzini, D. Eccles, J. Lowe and D. Ellison, A new case of frontotemporal dementia and parkinsonism resulting from an intron 10 + 3-splice site mutation in the tau gene: clinical and pathological features, *Neuropathol Appl Neurobiol* **26** (2000), 368–378.

[41] L. Varani, M. Hasegawa, M.G. Spillantini, M.J. Smith, J.R. Murrell, B. Ghetti, A. Klug, M. Goedert and G. Varani, Structure of tau exon 10 splicing regulatory element RNA and destabilization by mutations of frontotemporal dementia and parkinsonism linked to chromosome 17, *Proc Natl Acad Sci USA* **96** (1999), 8229–8234.

[42] M. Wijker, Z.K. Wszolek, E.C.H. Wolters, M.A. Rooimans, G. Pals, R.F. Pfeiffer, T. Lynch, R.L. Rodnitzky, K.C. Wilhelmsen and F. Awert, Localization of the gene for rapidly progressive autosomal dominant parkinsonism and dementia with pallido-ponto-nigral degeneration to chromosome 17q21, *Hum Mol Genet* **5** (1996), 151–154.

[43] K.C. Wilhelmsen, T. Lynch, E. Pavlou, M. Higgins and T.G. Nygaard, Localization of disinhibition-dementia-parkinsonism-amyotrophy complex to 17q21–22, *Am J Hum Genet* **55** (1994), 1159–1165.

[44] Z.K. Wszolek, R.F. Pfeiffer, M.H. Bhatt, R.L. Schelper, M. Cordes, B.J. Snow, R.L. Rodnitzky, E.C. Wolters, F. Arwert and D.B. Calne, Rapidly progressive autosomal dominant parkinsonism and dementia with pallido-ponto-nigral degeneration, *Ann Neurol* **32** (1992), 312–320.

[45] T. Yamada, E.G. McGeer, R.L. Schelper, Z.K. Wszolek, P.L. McGeer, R.F. Pfeiffer and R.L. Rodnitzky, Histological and biochemical pathology in a family with autosomal dominant Parkinsonism and dementia, *Neurol Psychiat Brain Res* **2** (1993), 26–35.

[46] L.H. Yamaoka, K.A. Welsh-Bohmer, C.M. Hulette, P.C. Gaskell, M. Murray, J.L. Rimmler, B.R. Helms, M. Guerra, A.D. Roses, D.E. Schmechel and M.A. Pericak-Vance, Linkage of frontotemporal dementia to chromosome 17: clinical and neuropathological characterization of phenotype, *Am J Hum Genet* **59** (1996), 1306–1312.

Genetic complexity of Alzheimer's disease: Successes and challenges

Ekaterina Rogaeva[a,b], Toshitaka Kawarai[a] and Peter St George-Hyslop[a,b,c,*]
[a]Centre for Research in Neurodegenerative Diseases, Department of Medicine, University of Toronto, 6 Queen's Park Crescent West, Toronto, ON, Canada M5S 3H2
[b]Department of Medicine, Division of Neurology, University of Toronto, Toronto, ON, Canada
[c]Toronto Western Hospital Research Institute, Toronto Western Hospital, University of Toronto, Toronto, ON, Canada

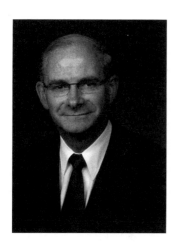

Abstract. About 1% of Alzheimer's Disease (AD) cases have an early-onset autosomal dominant familial form of the disease, genetic analyses of which have found three causal genes: amyloid β-protein precursor (AβPP), presenilin 1 (PS1) and presenilin 2 (PS2). The APOE gene is the only robustly replicated risk factor for the common form of AD with onset after 65 years of age. In at least half of the AD cases, there is no known cause of the disease. Here we provide an overview on known AD-linked genes and discuss the strategies of searching for novel AD genetic risk factors.

Keywords: Alzheimer's disease, presenilin, gene, AβPP, APOE

Abbreviations used in text: AD – Alzheimer's disease; AβPP – amyloid β-protein precursor; PS1 – presenilin 1; PS2 – presenilin 2; APOE – apolipoprotein E.

1. Introduction

Alzheimer's Disease (AD) is progressive dementia accompanied by neuronal loss, neurofibrillary tangles (formed of hyper-phosphorylated tau microtubule associated protein) and amyloid plaques, consisting mainly of A$\beta_{40/42}$ peptides generated by cleavage of the amyloid β-protein precursor (AβPP). Multiple studies suggest a complex etiology for AD, with both environmental and genetic factors influencing disease pathogenesis. Twin-studies found the concordance rate for AD among monozygotic twins to be 78%, indicating a strong genetic influence [2]. More than 95% of AD cases are sporadic with onset after 65 years of age.

The earliest sign of AD brain pathology is the deposition of extracellular amyloid plaques. The longer and more neurotoxic isoform (Aβ_{42}) appears to be elevated in the brains of individuals affected with AD. Numerous genetic and biochemical data support the amyloid cascade hypothesis, which suggests that Aβ

---

*Corresponding author: Peter St George-Hyslop, Centre for Neurodegenerative Diseases, Department of Medicine, University of Toronto, 6 Queen's Park Crescent West, Toronto, OO, Canada, M5S 3H2. Tel.: +1 416 946 7927; Fax: +1 416 978 1878; E-mail: p.hyslop@utoronto.ca.

deposition is the primary event in disease pathogenesis [12,15,33]. The link between Aβ production and tau protein is not currently established, although it is clear that abnormal formation of neurofibrillary tangles has neurotoxic consequences itself; because mutations in the tau gene cause frontotemporal dementia [16]. Nevertheless, currently there is no convincing data that tau is genetically involved in AD.

To date four AD genes have been identified: AβPP [13], presenilin 1 (PS1) [35], presenilin 2 (PS2) [19,26] and Apolipoprotein E (APOE) [30,31]. The disease in AβPP-, PS1- and PS2-linked families is transmitted as an autosomal dominant trait. In contrast, the APOE ε4-allele acts as an AD risk factor and age-at-onset modifier for the late-onset and early-onset forms of AD. Importantly, the common pathological effect of all these genetic factors is to alter AβPP processing and promote Aβ deposition (reviewed in [27,36]).

AβPP: The AβPP gene is located on chromosome 21q21 and encodes a protein that can be cleaved by at least two separate pathways. One involves α-secretase cleavage within the Aβ peptide sequence. The other pathway requires proteolysis by β- and γ-secretases to generate the Aβ_{40-42} peptides (reviewed in [36]). All known pathological AβPP mutations have a direct effect on its processing and are clustered near the α-, β-, or γ-secretase cleavage sites [14]. The majority of them lead to either an elevation of the Aβ_{42} peptide, to a more amyloidogenic peptide, or to an increase of both the short and long forms of Aβ. To date 25 different AD-associated mutations in the AβPP gene have been published (including the duplications of the AβPP locus), which affect more than 71 families with the age-at-onset ranging between 30 and 65 years (http://www.molgen.ua.ac.be/ADMutations/). The most frequent pathological mutation is the Val717Ile substitution, which is found in $\sim$ 50% of AβPP-linked families. In addition, some of the AβPP mutations are related to hereditary cerebral hemorrhage with amyloid (congophilic) angiopathy [20,37].

PS1 and PS2: Mutations in the PS1 gene, located on chromosome 14q24.3, account for 18%–50% of all early-onset AD cases and are responsible for the most severe form of the disease with the age-at-onset ranging between 16 and 65 years [9,35]. To date 155 different PS1 mutations (mainly missense substitutions) have been found in more than 315 AD families (http://molgen-www.uia.ac.be/ADMutations/). The Gly206Ala is the most frequent PS1 mutation observed in 18 unrelated Caribbean Hispanic families [1]. In contrast with AβPP mutations, PS1 mutations are not clustered in any particular region, but rather broadly distributed throughout the gene and cumulatively affect $\sim$ 25% of the coding region.

In 15 families with different PS1 mutations the disease (in addition to dementia) is associated with spastic paraplegia characterized by progressive weakness of the lower limbs (reviewed in [27]). The brain pathology of these cases differs from the typical picture for AD. Mature plaques are scarce. Instead, there are diffuse, Aβ-positive cotton wool plaques without a congophilic core and with only minor neuritic pathology and markers of inflammation [8]. The fact that, an identical PS1 mutation has been found in a family with variant AD, as well as in a family with typical AD argues in favor of the existence of genetic or environmental modifier(s) in the variant AD families.

PS1 shares amino acid and structural similarities with PS2 mapped to chromosome 1q31-q42. In contrast to PS1, mutations in PS2 gene are rare, variably penetrant and associated with a much later age-at-onset [26,34]. To date only 10 different PS2 mutations have been reported in 18 families with age-at-onset ranging between 40 and 85 years (http://molgen-www.uia.ac.be/ADMutations/).

Mutations in the PS1 and PS2 genes cause the overproduction of Aβ_{42}, which further supports the concept that changes in AβPP processing are central to AD pathology [6]. The PS1 and PS2 proteins have a very complex functional profile as integrators of several signaling pathways. In addition to AβPP processing, PS1 and PS2 are essential for the proteolytic cleavage of several other proteins including Notch [10]. Currently, it is not clear whether a dysfunction of these other pathways could in part contribute to the neurodegeneration process in mutation carriers.

APOE: The three common isoforms of the APOE gene on chromosome 19q13.2 are encoded by alleles ε2, ε3 and ε4. The link between the ε4-allele and AD has been confirmed in numerous studies across multiple ethnic groups (reviewed in [36]). The APOE ε4-allele is considerably over-represented in AD subjects ($\sim$ 40% versus $\sim$ 15% in the general population). On the other hand, the frequency of the protective ε2-allele is reduced from 10% in the normal population to 2% in AD cases [7,31]. Many studies suggest that AβPP processing is affected by the APOE polymorphisms. For instance, the absence or presence of one or two ε4-alleles was found to correlate in a dose-dependent manner with the relative density of amyloid plaques [32].

While the presence of the APOE ε4-allele may not be sufficient to cause AD, it acts both as an AD risk factor

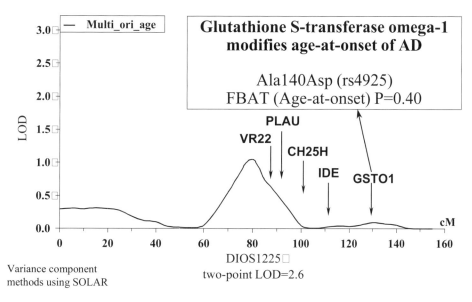

Fig. 1. Linkage of age-at-onset to chr10 with AD as a co-variate. Variance component methods using SOLAR were applied to study linkage/association between chromosome 10 markers and age-at-onset of AD.

and modifier of disease onset (the mean age-at-onset of AD is less than 70 years among the $\varepsilon 4/\varepsilon 4$ population, but over 90 years for the $\varepsilon 2/\varepsilon 3$ population) [30]. Unlike the AβPP, PS1 and PS2 genes, the APOE gene itself is not suitable for pre-symptomatic testing since not all ε4-carriers will develop AD and ε4-association is not entirely specific to AD. In the future however APOE may be used in combination with other yet to be discovered AD risk factors. Indeed, more than half of AD cases do not have an APOE ε4-allele indicating that additional factors are involved in the late-onset form of AD.

Search for novel AD genes: Genome-wide linkage surveys on late-onset AD datasets have identified more than 20 different AD loci as the site of potential susceptibility genes, with the strongest support for linkage being on chromosomes 10 and 12 [4,17,25]. A subsequent follow-up study confirmed the presence of an AD susceptibility loci on chromosome 12 [23,29] and on chromosome 10 [3,11,18,24]. As is typical for disorders with complex inheritance, these initial map-intervals have been very broad (> 30 Mb), and not infrequently do not point to exactly the same regions on the chromosome, but depict intervals that may be several million base pairs apart. Although not the most parsimonious explanation, some have suggested that these broad, weakly or non-overlapping genetic mapping results may in fact represent the presence of several distinct AD genes on the same chromosomal arm.

In our dataset (133 North American AD families) the overall evidence for an AD-susceptibility locus on chromosome 10 is weak: linkage analysis of 39 microsatellite markers generated only a marginally significant result at position 133 cM (NPL = 1.14; $p = 0.06$). However, we have obtained suggestive evidence for an age-of-onset modifying locus near position 80 cM on chromosome 10 (Fig. 1). In addition, we genotyped several case-control and familial datasets with > 140 single nucleotide polymorphisms (SNPs) in the region 90–119 cM that is within 1-LOD score of the of the peak locations identified in the previsouly published linkage reports [3,11,24]. Our data do not support the notion that any of the previously proposed candidate genes on chromosome 10 are sites of prevalent and high effect alleles causing AD. Thus, analysis of SNPs in insulin-degrading enzyme (IDE), cholesterol 25-hydroxylase (CH25H), plasminogen activator, urokinase (PLAU) have not generated evidence for linkage or association ($p > 0.05$). We have also tested allelic associations using a non-synonymous SNP (rs4925) in Glutathione S-Transferase Omega 1 gene (GSTO1), which has previously been implicated to modify age-at-onset of AD [22] (Fig. 1). Contrary to the prior report, our results show no evidence to support a role for GSTO1 as an age-at-onset modifying locus. However, we identified 15 SNPs in a cluster of 10 different genes, which generate significant results in our case-control or familial datasets. The investigation of addition SNPs in these genes is currently on the way.

In our North American familial dataset there is much better evidence for an AD locus on chromosome 12: 34

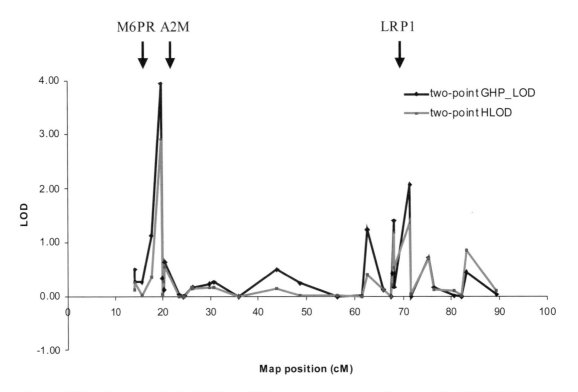

Fig. 2. Linkage of AD to Chromosome 12. The HLODs and GHP_lods were generated using Genehunter Plus (GHP). HLODs are parametric LODscores under heterogeneity, where alpha (fraction of pedigrees linked) was allowed to vary until the HLOD is maximized.

microsatellite markers generated a peak overall LOD score of 3.57 and a peak overall NPL score of 2.57 ($p = 0.0025$) in a ~ 5 Mb interval near position 20 cM (Fig. 2). Furthermore, a second chromosome 12 AD-linkage peak in our dataset exists in a ~ 4 Mb interval near position 70 cM (NPL = 1.94).

The identity of the chromosome 12 AD-susceptibility gene remains to be identified. Currently we are examining > 200 polymorphisms (45% of which are coding SNPs) in the regions with the highest support for linkage. Both case-control methods and family-based association studies are being used to investigate the genotype data from the North European sporadic dataset and two familial AD datasets of North American and Caribbean Hispanic origin. These analyses generated several nominally significant results in the North European sporadic case-control set for 22 SNPs ($p = 0.05 - 0.005$). Three of these SNPs were positive in at least one of the familial datasets, including a SNP in the glyceraldehyde-3-phosphate dehydrogenase (GAPD) gene. GAPD has recently been assosciated with late-onset AD in an independent case-control dataset [21]. Haplotype analysis of our datasets with additional SNPs gave modest support for association of the GAPD gene with AD in the Caribbean Hispanic familial AD dataset [unpublished data]. However, the specific alleles and haplotypes associated with AD in this datset were not the same as those in the prior report. Furthermore, we have also observed positive association with SNPs in four other nearby genes, including pregnancy zone protein (a homologue of α2-macroglobulin (A2M)). A2M, which binds Aβ and has previously been proposed as a site of AD-associated polymorphism [5], maps to the telomeric end of this interval. In agreement with our previous results [28], none of the SNPs in A2M itself were associated with AD. Consequently, the most likely interpretation of the recent association reports with GAPD and other genes in this region is that there is an AD susceptibility in this region, but it is probably not any of the genetic variant assessed to date.

Another way to identify AD risk factors is to select a gene by function (regardless of its chromosomal location) and then to test if SNPs within the gene are associated with AD. Since the common pathological effect imparted by all known AD-linked genes is to alter AβPP processing and promote Aβ deposition, the genes that encode the proteins involved in excessive production or reduced degradation of the Aβ peptides represent strong functional candidate genes. In recent years, many genes have been reported to be associated with AD (http://www.alzforum.org/res/com/gen/alzgene/chromo.asp?c=1); however, none of these findings have received the same robust replication as the association between AD and the APOE ε4-allele (reviewed in [27,36]). A possible explanation for the contradictory results in different datasets is that several genes (with different population allele frequencies) could impart susceptibility to late-onset AD. In addition, it is likely that the effect of these genes could be modulated by gene-gene interactions, which may explain the genetic, clinical and neuropathological heterogeneity of AD.

2. Conclusion

The identification of genes bearing polymorphisms or mutations that cause familial AD has already provided otherwise unattainable starting points from which to explore the pathogenesis of this disease. Mutations in the four known AD genes all cause the accumulation of Aβ peptides as a central and initiating event in the pathogenesis of disease. Cumulatively the four known AD genes account for about half of the genetic risk factors and recent studies have further confirmed the genetic heterogeneity of AD. However, the conflicting genetic data generated for numerous gene candidates and late-onset AD loci in the recent past, reflects the difficulty of genetic approaches to complex traits in general, and is not a specific difficulty of AD genetics. Various strategies have been proposed including the use of surrogate, simpler endophenotypes (e.g. psychosis, myoclonus, rapid decline, etc.) [38]. There are several caveats about these strategies, and currently the most robust strategy is still the incorporation of biologically reasonable candidate genes, assessment in large cohorts of well characterized cases and controls, and replication in independent datasets. An additional important emerging target for future research in AD is the increasing focus on the genetic epidemiology of AD with the objective of investigating gene/environment interactions, which are in fact likely to be a significant cause of the current difficulty as environmental factors can modify the effects of genetic factors and also introduce purely non-genetic phenocopies, which confound the genetic analysis unless their occurrence is incorporated into the genetic statistical model.

References

[1] E.S. Athan, J. Williamson, A. Ciappa, V. Santana, S.N. Romas, J.H. Lee, H. Rondon, R.A. Lantigua, M. Medrano, M. Torres, S. Arawaka, E. Rogaeva, Y.Q. Song, C. Sato, T. Kawarai, K.C. Fafel, M.A. Boss, W.K. Seltzer, Y. Stern, P. St George-Hyslop, B. Tycko and R. Mayeux, A founder mutation in presenilin 1 causing early-onset Alzheimer disease in unrelated Caribbean Hispanic families, JAMA **286**(18) (14 Nov 2001), 2257–2263.

[2] A.L. Bergem, K. Engedal and E. Kringlen, The role of heredity in late-onset Alzheimer disease and vascular dementia. A twin study, Arch Gen Psychiatry **54**(3) (March 1997), 264–270.

[3] L. Bertram, D. Blacker, K. Mullin, D. Keeney, J. Jones, S. Basu, S. Yhu, M.G. McInnis, R.C. Go, K. Vekrellis, D.J. Selkoe, A.J. Saunders and R.E. Tanzi, Evidence for genetic linkage of Alzheimer's disease to chromosome 10q, Science **290**(5500) (22 Dec 2000), 2302–2303.

[4] D. Blacker, L. Bertram, A.J. Saunders, T.J. Moscarillo, M.S. Albert, H. Wiener, R.T. Perry, J.S. Collins, L.E. Harrell, R.C. Go, A. Mahoney, T. Beaty, M.D. Fallin, D. Avramopoulos, G.A. Chase, M.F. Folstein, M.G. McInnis, S.S. Bassett, K.J. Doheny, E.W. Pugh and R.E. Tanzi, NIMH Genetics Initiative Alzheimer's Disease Study Group. Results of a high-resolution genome screen of 437 Alzheimer's disease families, Hum Mol Genet **12**(1) (1 Jan 2003), 23–32.

[5] D. Blacker, M.A. Wilcox, N.M. Laird, L. Rodes, S.M. Horvath, R.C. Go, R. Perry, B. Watson Jr, S.S. Bassett, M.G. McInnis, M.S. Albert, B.T. Hyman and R.E. Tanzi, Alpha-2 macroglobulin is genetically associated with Alzheimer disease, Nat Genet **19**(4) (Aug 1998), 357–360.

[6] M. Citron, D. Westaway, W. Xia, G. Carlson, T. Diehl, G. Levesque, K. Johnson-Wood, M. Lee, P. Seubert, A. Davis, D. Kholodenko, R. Motter, R. Sherrington, B. Perry, H. Yao, R. Strome, I. Lieberburg, J. Rommens, S. Kim, D. Schenk, P. Fraser, H.P. St George and D.J. Selkoe, Mutant presenilins of Alzheimer's disease increase production of 42- residue amyloid beta-protein in both transfected cells and transgenic mice, Nat Med **3** (1997), 67–72.

[7] E.H. Corder, A.M. Saunders, N.J. Risch, W.J. Strittmatter, D.E. Schmechel, P.C. Gaskell Jr., J.B. Rimmler, P.A. Locke, P.M. Conneally and K.E. Schmader, Protective effect of apolipoprotein E type 2 allele for late onset Alzheimer disease, Nat Genet **7** (1994), 180–184.

[8] R. Crook, A. Verkkoniemi, J. Perez-Tur, N. Mehta, M. Baker, H. Houlden, M. Farrer, M. Hutton, S. Lincoln, J. Hardy, K. Gwinn, M. Somer, A. Paetau, H. Kalimo, R. Ylikoski, M. Poyhonen, S. Kucera and M. Haltia, A variant of Alzheimer's disease with spastic paraparesis and unusual plaques due to deletion of exon 9 of presenilin 1, Nat Med **4**(4) (April 1998), 452–455.

[9] M. Cruts, C.M. van Duijn, H. Backhovens, B.M. Van den, A. Wehnert, S. Serneels, R. Sherrington, M. Hutton, J. Hardy, P.H. George-Hyslop, A. Hofman and C. Van Broeckhoven, Estimation of the genetic contribution of presenilin-1 and -2 mutations in a population-based study of presenile Alzheimer disease, Hum Mol Genet **7** (1998), 43–51.

[10] B. De Strooper, W. Annaert, P. Cupers, P. Saftig, K. Craessaerts, J.S. Mumm, E.H. Schroeter, V. Schrijvers, M.S. Wolfe, W.J. Ray, A. Goate and R. Kopan, A presenilin-1-dependent gamma-secretase-like protease mediates release of Notch intracellular domain, Nature **398** (1999), 518–522.

[11] N. Ertekin-Taner, N. Graff-Radford, L.H. Younkin, C. Eckman, M. Baker, J. Adamson, J. Ronald, J. Blangero, M. Hutton and S.G. Younkin, Linkage of plasma Abeta42 to a quantita-

tive locus on chromosome 10 in late-onset Alzheimer's disease pedigrees, *Science* **290**(5500) (22 Dec 2000), 2303–2304.

[12] G.G. Glenner and C.W. Wong, Alzheimer's disease: initial report of the purification and characterization of a novel cerebrovascular amyloid protein, *Biochem Biophys Res Commun* **120**(3) (16 May 1984), 885–890.

[13] A.M. Goate, M.C. Chartier-Harlin, M.C. Mullan, J. Brown, F. Crawford, L. Fidani, L. Giuffra, A. Haynes, N. Irving, L. James, R. Mant, P. Newton, K. Rooke, P. Roques, C. Talbot, M. Pericak-Vance, A. Roses, R. Williamson, M.N. Rossor, M. Owen and J. Hardy, Segregation of a missense mutation in the amyloid precursor protein gene with familial Alzheimer's disease, *Nature* **349** (1991), 704–706.

[14] J. Hardy, Amyloid, the presenilins and Alzheimer's disease, *Trends Neurosci* **20**(4) (April 1997), 154–159.

[15] J.A. Hardy and G.A. Higgins, Alzheimer's disease: the amyloid cascade hypothesis, *Science* **286** (1992), 184–185.

[16] M. Hutton, C.L. Lendon, P. Rizzu, M. Baker, S. Froelich, H. Houlden, S. Pickering-Brown, S. Chakraverty, A. Isaacs, A. Grover, J. Hackett, J. Adamson, S. Lincoln, D. Dickson, P. Davies, R.C. Petersen, M. Stevens, E. de Graaff, E. Wauters, J. van Baren, M. Hillebrand, M. Joosse, J.M. Kwon, P. Nowotny, L.K. Che, J. Norton, J.C. Morris, L.A. Reed, J. Trojanowski, H. Basun, L. Lannfelt, M. Neystat, S. Fahn, F. Dark, T. Tannenberg, P.R. Dodd, N. Hayward, J.B.J. Kwok, P.R. Scho. eld, A. Andreadis, J. Snowden, D. Craufurd, D. Neary, F. Owen, B.A. Oostra, J. Hardy, A. Goate, J. van Swieten, D. Mann, T. Lynch and P. Heutink, Association of missense and 5'-splice-site mutations in tau with the inherited dementia FTDP-17, *Nature* **393** (1998), 702–705.

[17] P. Kehoe, F. Wavrant-De Vrieze, R. Crook, W.S. Wu, P. Holmans, I. Fenton, G. Spurlock, N. Norton, H. Williams, N. Williams, S. Lovestone, J. Perez-tur, M. Hutton, M.C. Chartier-Harlin, S. Shears, K. Roehl, J. Booth, W. Van Voorst, D. Ramic, J. Williams, A. Goate, J. Hardy and M.J. Owen, A full genome scan for late onset Alzheimer's disease, *Hum Mol Genet* **8** (1999), 237–245.

[18] J.H. Lee, R. Mayeux, D. Mayo, J. Mo, V. Santana, J. Williamson, A. Flaquer, A. Ciappa, H. Rondon, P. Estevez, R. Lantigua, T. Kawarai, A. Toulina, M. Medrano, M. Torres, Y. Stern, B. Tycko, E. Rogaeva, P. St George-Hyslop and J.A. Knowles, Fine mapping of 10q and 18q for familial Alzheimer's disease in Caribbean Hispanics, *Mol Psychiatry* **9**(11) (Nov 2004), 1042–1051.

[19] E. Levy-Lahad, W. Wasco, P. Poorkaj, D.M. Romano, J. Oshima, W.H. Pettingell, C.E. Yu, P.D. Jondro, S.D. Schmidt, K. Wang et al., Candidate gene for the chromosome 1 familial Alzheimer's disease locus, *Science* **269**(5226) (18 Aug 1995), 973–977.

[20] E. Levy, M.D. Carman, I.J. Fernandez-Madrid, M.D. Power, I. Lieberburg, S.G. van Duinen, G.T. Bots, W. Luyendijk and B. Frangione, Mutation of the Alzheimer's disease amyloid gene in hereditary cerebral hemorrhage, Dutch type, *Science* **248**(4959) (1 June 1990), 1124–1126.

[21] Y. Li, P. Nowotny, P. Holmans, S. Smemo, J.S. Kauwe, A.L. Hinrichs, K. Tacey, L. Doil, R. van Luchene, V. Garcia, C. Rowland, S. Schrodi, D. Leong, G. Gogic, J. Chan, A. Cravchik, D. Ross, K. Lau, S. Kwok, S.Y. Chang, J. Catanese, J. Sninsky, T.J. White, J. Hardy, J. Powell, S. Lovestone, J.C. Morris, L. Thal, M. Owen, J. Williams, A. Goate and A. Grupe, Association of late-onset Alzheimer's disease with genetic variation in multiple members of the GAPD gene family, *Proc Natl Acad Sci USA* **101**(44) (2 Nov 2004), 15688–15693.

[22] Y.J. Li, S.A. Oliveira, P. Xu, E.R. Martin, J.E. Stenger, C.R. Scherzer, M.A. Hauser, W.K. Scott, G.W. Small, M.A. Nance, R.L. Watts, J.P. Hubble, W.C. Koller, R. Pahwa, M.B. Stern, B.C. Hiner, J. Jankovic, C.G. Goetz, F. Mastaglia, L.T. Middleton, A.D. Roses, A.M. Saunders, D.E. Schmechel, S.R. Gullans, J.L. Haines, J.R. Gilbert, J.M. Vance, M.A. Pericak-Vance, C. Hulette and K.A. Welsh-Bohmer, Glutathione S-transferase omega-1 modifies age-at-onset of Alzheimer disease and Parkinson disease, *Hum Mol Genet* **12**(24) (15 Dec 2003), 3259–3267.

[23] R. Mayeux, J.H. Lee, S.N. Romas, D. Mayo, V. Santana, J. Williamson, A. Ciappa, H.Z. Rondon, P. Estevez, R. Lantigua, M. Medrano, M. Torres, Y. Stern, B. Tycko and J.A. Knowles, Chromosome-12 mapping of late-onset Alzheimer disease among Caribbean Hispanics, *Am J Hum Genet* **70**(1) (Jan 2002), 237–243. Epub 2001 Nov 19.

[24] A. Myers, P. Holmans, H. Marshall, J. Kwon, D. Meyer, D. Ramic, S. Shears, J. Booth, F.W. DeVrieze, R. Crook, M. Hamshere, R. Abraham, N. Tunstall, F. Rice, S. Carty, S. Lillystone, P. Kehoe, V. Rudrasingham, L. Jones, S. Lovestone, J. Perez-Tur, J. Williams, M.J. Owen, J. Hardy and A.M. Goate, Susceptibility locus for Alzheimer's disease on chromosome 10, *Science* **290**(5500) (22 Dec 2000), 2304–2305.

[25] M.A. Pericak-Vance, M.P. Bass, L.H. Yamaoka, P.C. Gaskell, W.K. Scott, H.A. Terwedow, M.M. Menold, P.M. Conneally, G.W. Small, J.M. Vance, A.M. Saunders, A.D. Roses and J.L. Haines, Complete genomic screen in late-onset familial Alzheimer disease. Evidence for a new locus on chromosome 12, *JAMA* **278**(15) (15 Oct 1997), 1237–1241.

[26] E.I. Rogaev, R. Sherrington, E.A. Rogaeva, G. Levesque, M. Ikeda, Y. Liang, H. Chi, C. Lin, K. Holman and T. Tsuda, Familial Alzheimer's disease in kindreds with missense mutations in a gene on chromosome 1 related to the Alzheimer's disease type 3 gene, *Nature* **376** (1995), 775–778.

[27] E. Rogaeva, The solved and unsolved mysteries of the genetics of early-onset Alzheimer's disease, *Neuromolecular Med* **2**(1) (2002), 1–10.

[28] E.A. Rogaeva, S. Premkumar, J. Grubber, L. Serneels, W.K. Scott, T. Kawarai, Y. Song, D.L. Hill, S.M. Abou-Donia, E.R. Martin, J.J. Vance, G. Yu, A. Orlacchio, Y. Pei, M. Nishimura, A. Supala, B. Roberge, A.M. Saunders, A.D. Roses, D. Schmechel, A. Crane-Gatherum, S. Sorbi, A. Bruni, G.W. Small, P.M. Conneally, J.L. Haines, F. Van Leuven, P.H. St George-Hyslop, L.A. Farrer and M.A. Pericak-Vance, An alpha-2-macroglobulin insertion-deletion polymorphism in Alzheimer disease, *Nat Genet* **22**(1) (May 1999), 19–22.

[29] E. Rogaeva, S. Premkumar, Y. Song, S. Sorbi, N. Brindle, A. Paterson, R. Duara, G. Levesque, G. Yu, M. Nishimura, M. Ikeda, C. O'Toole, T. Kawarai, R. Jorge, D. Vilarino, A.C. Bruni, L.A. Farrer and P.H. George-Hyslop, Evidence for an Alzheimer disease susceptibility locus on chromosome 12 and for further locus heterogeneity, *JAMA* **280** (1998), 614–618.

[30] A.D. Roses, Apolipoprotein E and Alzheimer's disease. The tip of the susceptibility iceberg, *Ann N Y Acad Sci* **855** (1998), 738–743.

[31] A.M. Saunders, W.J. Strittmatter, D. Schmechel, P.H. George-Hyslop, M.A. Pericak-Vance, S.H. Joo, B.L. Rosi, J.F. Gusella, D.R. Crapper-MacLachlan and M.J. Alberts, Association of apolipoprotein E allele epsilon 4 with late-onset familial and sporadic Alzheimer's disease, *Neurology* **43** (1993), 1467–1472.

[32] D.E. Schmechel, A.M. Saunders, W.J. Strittmatter, B.J. Crain, C.M. Hulette, S.H. Joo, M.A. Pericak-Vance, D. Goldgaber and A.D. Roses, Increased amyloid beta-peptide deposition in

cerebral cortex as a consequence of apolipoprotein E genotype in late-onset Alzheimer disease, *Proc Natl Acad Sci USA* **90** (1993), 9649–9653.

[33] D.J. Selkoe, The molecular pathology of Alzheimer's disease, *Neuron* **6**(4) (April 1991), 487–498.

[34] R. Sherrington, S. Froelich, S. Sorbi, D. Campion, H. Chi, E.A. Rogaeva, G. Levesque, E.I. Rogaev, C. Lin, Y. Liang, M. Ikeda, L. Mar, A. Brice, Y. Agid, M.E. Percy, F. Clerget-Darpoux, S. Piacentini, G. Marcon, B. Nacmias, L. Amaducci, T. Frebourg, L. Lannfelt, J.M. Rommens and P.H. George-Hyslop, Alzheimer's disease associated with mutations in presenilin 2 is rare and variably penetrant, *Hum Mol Genet* **5** (1996), 985–988.

[35] R. Sherrington, E.I. Rogaev, Y. Liang, E.A. Rogaeva, G. Levesque, M. Ikeda, H. Chi, C. Lin, G. Li and K. Holman, Cloning of a gene bearing missense mutations in early-onset familial Alzheimer's disease, *Nature* **375** (1995), 754–760.

[36] A. Tandon, E.A. Rogaeva, M. Mullan and P. St George-Hyslop, Molecular genetics of Alzheimer's disease: the role of beta-amyloid and the presenilins, *Current Opinion in Neurology* **13** (2000), 377–384.

[37] C. Van Broeckhoven, J. Haan, E. Bakker, J.A. Hardy, W. Van Hul, A. Wehnert, M. Vegter-Van der Vlis and R.A. Roos, Amyloid beta protein precursor gene and hereditary cerebral hemorrhage with amyloidosis (Dutch), *Science* **248**(4959) (1 June 1990), 1120–1122.

[38] J.L. Kennedy, L.A. Farrer, N.C. Andreasen, R. Mayeux and P. St George-Hyslop, The genetics of adult-onset neuropsychiatric disease: Complexities and conundra? *Science* **302**(5646) (31 Oct. 2003), 822–826.

Genetics and pathology of alpha-secretase site AβPP mutations in the understanding of Alzheimer's disease

Christine Van Broeckhoven* and Samir Kumar-Singh
Department of Molecular Genetics, Neurodegenerative Brain Diseases Research Group, Flanders Interuniversity Institute for Biotechnology, Institute Born-Bunge and University of Antwerp, Antwerpen, Belgium

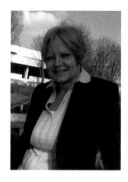

Abstract. Development of therapeutics begins with delineating the precise disease pathology along with a reasonable understanding of the sequence of events responsible for the development of disease, or disease pathogenesis. For Alzheimer's disease (AD), the classical pathology is now known for quite some time; however, the disease pathogenesis has eluded our understanding for a complete century. This review, in addition to providing a brief overview of all primary events, will highlight those aspects of AD genetics and novel pathological descriptions linked to unique mutations within AβPP that have led to our better understanding of the pathogenesis of AD. Specifically, we will discuss how pathologies linked to the Dutch (E693Q) and Flemish AβPP (A692G) mutations have helped in understanding the role of CAA in dementia and in the development of dense-core plaques. In addition, this review will also point directions that warrant additional studies.

Keywords: Dementia, Alzheimer's disease, Cerebral Amyloid Angiopathy (CAA), cerebral hemorrhages, AβPP mutations, Flemish APP692 disease, HCHWAD

1. Amyloid is the culprit protein in Alzheimer's Disease (AD)

Ever since Alois Alzheimer provided his first clinical and neuropathological description of presenile dementia in a 51-year old woman with senile plaques (*Herdchen*) and neurofibrillary tangles ("*Knäueln*") in 1906 [1], started the controversies some of which continue to mystify AD research today. The first confusion was in the use of the term presenile Alzheimer dementia because similar neuropathological features were soon identified in senile dementia patients. However, we now well accept that AD is not strictly a presenile disorder and arbitrarily set a cut-off of 65 years to differentiate *early*-onset AD from the late-onset. As we shall see later, it is important to differentiate these two subsets of disease populations as the genetic alterations in the causation of early and late-onset AD have been shown to be different. Consecutive findings demonstrated the presence of amyloid in the senile plaque core by Paul Divry [17] and in blood vessels by Scholtz [72]. The atherosclerotic vascular lesions were already well recognized since 1911, when Simchowicz differentiated senile dementia into 'proper' senile dementia characterized by neurofibrillary tangles (NFT) and amyloid

---

*Corresponding author: Prof. Dr. Christine Van Broeckhoven PhD DSc, VIB8 Department of Molecular Genetics, University of Antwerp – Campus CDE, Universiteitsplein 1, B-2610 Antwerpen, Belgium. Tel.: +32 3 265 1001; Fax: +32 3 265 1012; E-mail: christine.vanbroeckhoven@ua.ac.be.

plaques, and arteriosclerotic senile dementia characterized by vascular degeneration; the latter entity is still recognized today as vascular dementia. However, the recognition of *congophilic (cerebral) amyloid angiopathy* (CAA) as another hallmark of AD led into yet another controversy that continues even today: is there an overlap between AD and vascular dementia? This controversy is most important to this review, as we shall discuss AβPP mutations that are linked to strokes and present recent findings that development of senile plaques could be related to cerebral vessels.

A better structural characterization of the aggregate lesions was obtained by electron microscopy showing that tangles contained 10–20 nm paired helical filaments (PHF) and that the amyloid within vessels contained 10 nm thick filaments similar to the amyloid observed in the senile plaques. The subsequent use of x-ray diffraction and infrared spectroscopy demonstrated a characteristic cross-β conformation and suggested that the common features of amyloid protein in different diseases might be the cross-β conformation.

Purification and biochemical characterization of AD aggregates launched another era of AD research. Ironically, the first amyloid characterized to be ≈4 kDa amyloid-β (Aβ) peptides were amyloid isolated from CAA from AD and Down's syndrome (DS) patients and not from senile plaques [23,24]. Soon after, the amyloid protein of senile plaques was shown to be identical to the Aβ peptide [60]. Studies on neurofibrillary tangles (NFT) and PHF were a bit more intricate due to their difficult solubilization, but the breakthrough came from histochemistry. Initially, however, microtubules were implicated because microtubule-associated proteins (MAP) like MAP-2 and tau inadvertently contaminated the purification process of microtubules [31, 100], but soon this controversy was closed with phosphorylated tau being recognized as the major, if not the only, component of PHF [26,30,48,68].

2. The amyloid gene is central to AD genetics

Though increasingly better descriptions of the clinical symptoms and pathological hallmarks became available, the biochemical nature of the disease remained largely unknown. One way to approach this problem was by using molecular genetic techniques that allowed identification of a disease gene and its respective protein using "positional cloning" techniques, i.e., segregation studies using genetic markers in extended pedigrees to map the genetic defect to a chromosomal region from which the actual gene could be identified using recombinant DNA technologies. The mapping approach had been successful for several monogenic diseases like Duchenne muscular dystrophy and cystic fibrosis. However, it was the successful mapping of Huntington's disease, another neurodegenerative brain disease, to chromosome 4p that stimulated molecular genetic studies in AD [32]. Rare families with presenile AD had been documented in which the disease was apparently inherited according to an autosomal dominant trait. In our research group, we had access to two large Belgian families, nicknamed AD/A and AD/B, with presenile AD and onset age around 35 years that had been followed for many years at the Institute Born-Bunge, and of which very detailed clinical and pathological descriptions were available [59,83].

While we did not have the access to the current dense genetic maps for genome-wide scanning, alternative strategies had to be used that would allow rapid mapping of the disease genes. Initial genetic studies were targeted at chromosome 21 because almost all middle-aged DS patients develop AD pathology [97]. It was hypothesized that in DS, AD is caused by over-representation of a gene on chromosome 21 as a result of the trisomy 21, while in AD a mutation in that same gene leads to the production of an abnormal protein or to the overproduction of a normal protein. While segregation studies identified chromosome 21 linked presenile AD families [80], a major breakthrough came from the mapping of the amyloid-β protein precursor gene (AβPP) to chromosome 21 in the region linked to the disease [47]. Proteolytic cleavage of the 677–770 amino acid, type 1 integral membrane protein AβPP produces Aβ, the culprit protein in senile plaques and blood vessels in AD, making it the candidate gene for AD. However, what some of us do not like to remember is that we first excluded AβPP as an AD gene, and Aβ as a key protein in AD pathogenesis [82,85]. The AβPP did not cosegregate with the disease in families that later were shown to be linked to chromosome 14 [79,84], and segregated mutations in the *presenilin 1 (PSEN1)* gene [8,73]. It took up to 3 years to revive the interest in AβPP and Aβ, and ultimately restore its central position in the amyloid cascade, a working hypothesis underlying the important role of amyloid plaques in AD [35,36].

2.1. AβPP mutations linked to CAA and AD

While basically most geneticists had turned their backs on AβPP and Aβ, and were searching in other areas of chromosome 21 or the human genome for the ultimate AD gene(s), we started analyzing AβPP in an AD related disorder namely hereditary cerebral hemorrhages with amyloidosis – Dutch type (HCHWAD). HCHWAD is an autosomal dominant form of CAA characterized by recurrent hemorrhages due to extensive amyloid Aβ deposition in cerebral blood vessel walls in the absence of senile plaques and NFT [33,88]. We showed that HCHWAD co-segregated with AβPP in 3 families [2,86] and published the data side by side with that of Levy and colleagues who identified a mutation in exon 17 of AβPP in two Dutch HCHWAD patients [55]. The mutation predicted an amino acid substitution at codon 693 (AβPP 770 isoform) replacing a glutamate (Glu, A) by a glutamine (Gln, G), and is since then known by its nickname Dutch APP693 mutation. Subsequently, a mutation, dubbed London AβPP mutation, was identified in a chromosome 21 linked presenile AD family [25], and so far 16 missense mutations in AβPP have been identified causing autosomal dominant forms of early-onset AD (EOAD) [9]; www.molgen.ua.ac.be/ADMutations/ (Fig. 1). Support for the genetic evidence of the role of AβPP in AD was provided by the finding that AβPP and PSEN mutations linked to familial early-onset forms of AD altered AβPP processing to lead to increased Aβ42 production [3,71], the more fibrillogenic Aβ species compared to the physiological and more abundantly secreted Aβ40 [45].

The following year, we reported a second AβPP mutation near the α-secretase site, the Flemish APP692 mutation replacing a glycine (Gly, G) by an alanine (Ala, A) [39]. Patients carrying the Flemish APP692 mutation suffer from presenile dementia and cerebral hemorrhage inherited in an autosomal dominant pattern. In a recent follow-up of this family, we have confirmed these data and shown that indeed the clinical phenotypes overlap, i.e., cerebral hemorrhages are reported in offsprings of demented patients and vice versa [70]. Neuropathological studies performed on brains from Flemish APP692 patients supported the clinical diagnosis of AD [7,49]. Numerous senile plaques with the largest central dense-cores ever noted in AD – accompanied by a very severe degree of leptomeningeal and parenchymal CAA – characterize these brains. Also, in contrast to HCHWAD and consistent with a clinical diagnosis of probable AD, Flemish APP692 patients deposit abundant tau-PHF in pyramidal neurons and dystrophic neurites [7,49,56]. The uniqueness of Dutch APP693 and Flemish APP692 mutations from the other AβPP mutation linked to the classical AD was in their location near the α-secretase cleavage site. While the full-length Aβ (Aβ1–40 or Aβ1–42) is generated by sequential activity of α-secretase [77,90] and α-secretase/presenilin complex [12], α-secretase activity prevents the generation of full-length Aβ [78] (Fig. 1). Because of the altered AβPP cleavage and because these mutations would also change the primary Aβ sequence and therefore the fibrillogenic potential of the resulting mutant Aβ peptide, these genetic forms of vascular amyloidosis linked to α-secretase site were again a strong support of AβPP in the disease mechanism and provided one of the strongest rationales for studies of factors that influence abnormal metabolism and aggregation of Aβ in the causation of CAA with or without AD. With subsequent identification of a series of AβPP mutations in the proximity of α-secretase site -'Arctic' (E693G), 'Italian' (E693K), and 'Iowa' (D694N) [27,46,63,66]- the Dutch and Flemish AβPP pathology became the prototypes of pure cerebral hemorrhage at one end and mixed AD/cerebral hemorrhage at the other, respectively, and the clinicopathological descriptions of most of these mutations fitted into this spectrum. For instance, the Italian AβPP mutation had clinical manifestations similar to HCHWAD patients [63], the Arctic [46,66] and Iowa AβPP [27] mutations showed features of probable EOAD along with vascular features, subsequently confirmed on neuropathology at least for the Iowa pedigree (Table 1).

3. AβPP mutations near the α-secretase site cause disease by different mechanisms

One of the primary reasons to study the α-secretase site mutations was how did mutations on the same or adjacent codons although causing distinct diseases, invariably lead to a severe degree of CAA. Ever since the first description of CAA in AD brain by Scholtz [72], there was a strong interest in understanding, firstly, how CAA develops, secondly, by what all mechanism(s) does the vascular amyloidosis cause dementia, and thirdly, what precise role does CAA play in the development of AD?

Two lines of investigation were immediately apparent with studying α-secretase site mutations: one, whether the mutations altered the aggregation property as they also altered the primary sequence of Aβ, and two, whether the mutations affect the AβPP processing as they might affect α-secretase processing. The altered aggregation property gained popularity as it was

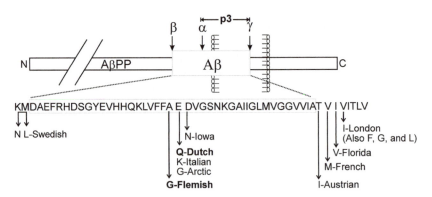

Fig. 1. The AβPP mutations within the region encoding for Aβ at the α-secretase site associate with CAA, and some associate with AD changes as well. This location contrasts with AβPP mutations associated primarily with AD that flank the Aβ region (i.e., Swedish and London AβPP mutations).

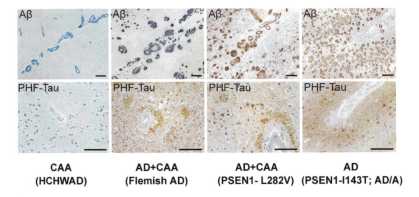

Fig. 2. Spectrum of diseases from primarily hereditary amyloidosis to pure familial forms of Alzheimer's disease. The upper panel depicts Aβ staining with 4G8 in an HCHWAD (E693Q) patient with CAA, Flemish AD patient with both CAA and plaques, PSEN1 (L282V) AD with prominent CAA, and classical AD patient with PSEN1 (I143T) from our AD/A pedigree. The lower panel is AT8-phosphorylated tau staining in temporal cortical region of the same patients. Note HCHWAD brain does not show tau staining and both Flemish AD and PSEN1 L282V show phosphorylated tau (AT8) staining around CAA as observed for the neuritic plaques. Bars represent 10 μm.

soon recognized that cerebrovascular amyloid deposits are chiefly composed of Aβ40, the less fibrillogenic Aβ form. It turned out that most of the α-secretase site mutations use both mechanisms in causing disease. For instance, the Dutch APP693 substitution alters AβPP processing by increasing Aβ in vitro beginning at D1, V18 and Y19 [95] with an overall decrease in Aβ42 in plasma of HCHWAD patients. However, more importantly, Dutch peptide has accelerated fibrillogenic kinetics [5,6,19,52,64,75,98] and stability [21], and leads to an increased in situ aggregation on cultured cell surfaces, and enhances neurotoxicity to both smooth muscle and endothelial cells [10,63,89,94]. It was thus reasonable to presume that HCHWAD is a result of increased propensity of the Dutch peptide to aggregate in association with vascular smooth muscle and endothelial cells and also the aggregates were more stable to degradation.

The search for the pathogenic mechanism by which Flemish APP692 mutation caused its pathology was more intriguing. Early studies showed that Flemish APP692 leads to an increased production of Aβ beginning at D1, R5, and E11 [34] proposed to be mediated by a β-secretase homologue, BACE 2 [20]. This results in an increase in both Aβ40 and Aβ42 [11]. In addition, Flemish Aβ peptide fibrilizing slower than wild-type Aβ, forms larger aggregates [5,6,64,92]. While the large aggregates were characteristic of Flemish AD pathology, the fibrillogenic property of these two mutant Aβ peptides led to an apparent paradox where the most fibrillogenic Dutch Aβ peptide neither caused AD clinically nor pathologically, while the least fibrillogenic Aβ in the Flemish APP692 patients caused a clinical and pathological AD. This contrasted with the 'amyloid cascade of AD' where increased fibrillogenic propensity of Aβ42 was thought to be responsible for the disease.

Table 1
Clinical and biochemical characteristics of mutations near the α-secretase site of AβPP

AβPP Codon*	Substitution	Position within Aβ	Nick name	Clinics	References
692	Ala–>Gly	A21G	Flemish	EOAD/Cerebral hemorrhage	[39,49]
693	Glu–>Gln	E22Q	Dutch	Cerebral hemorrhage	[55,86]
	Glu–>Gly	E22G	Arctic	EOAD/Vascular symptomatology	[46,66]
	Glu–>Lys	E22K	Italian	Cerebral hemorrhage	[63]
694	Asp–>Asn	D23N	Iowa	EOAD	[27]

*Numbered according to the largest AβPP transcript AβPP 770.

4. Flemish APP692 pathology sheds light on one of the mechanisms of dense-core plaque formation

In our laboratory, we studied this apparent paradox of how Flemish APP692 patients, but not HCHWAD, present with PHF-tau aggregates, dense-core plaques and a clinical AD [7,56]. We first inferred on differentiated SH-SY5Y cells that the observed differences were not due to a direct interaction between mutant Aβ and/or AβPP and tau phosphorylation by studying a few epitopes commonly phosphorylated in AD [52]. Next, we showed that exogenous synthetic Flemish, Dutch, and wild-type Aβ although increased phosphorylation of AD-specific tau epitopes but not differently from each other [52]. It was the in vitro aggregation properties, however, that pinpointed the likely cause. Confirming earlier studies, we showed that Flemish Aβ although was the least fibrillogenic peptide [5,6,52,64, 92], but was most toxic to differentiated SH-SY5Y cells in the early stages of aggregation (compared to wild type and Dutch Aβ) [52]. In the late stages of aggregation, the Dutch peptide was the most species, suggesting that Aβ, at least in in vitro conditions, might be neurotoxic in an initial phase due to its soluble oligomeric or other early toxic Aβ intermediate(s), which was distinct from the late neurotoxicity incurred by aggregated larger assemblies of Aβ [52]. This fitted well with recent data showing that in addition to a direct toxicity caused by Aβ fibril formation [69], non-aggregated oligomeric, diffusible, and/or protofibrillar forms are neurotoxic both in vitro and in vivo [37,54,93]. Moreover, it has been suggested that cytotoxic potential of Aβ might lie in their ability to form extensive fibrils directly on the cell surface, as preaggregation of Aβ abolishes its neurotoxic effect as in smooth muscle cells [10]. Thus, Dutch Aβ once released from the sites of generation, aggregate almost instantaneously in the parenchymal matrix as diffuse plaques. With this it also loses its neurotoxic potential and therefore diffuse plaques with a few exceptions [50] are commonly non-neuritic [52,56]. The observed increased in vitro toxicity potential of Dutch Aβ thus might be relevant only for vessels and not for parenchyma as the enormous aggregates observed in vitro never occur in close proximity to neuronal cells in HCHWAD patients. Conversely, slowly fibrilizing Flemish Aβ diffuse more readily in a relatively soluble or low-fibrillar toxic form to the nidi of plaque formation. The same year, we also showed that dense-core plaques in Flemish APP692 patients were centered on vascular walls [49], which might be one of the major pathways of Aβ brain clearance for Flemish Aβ as suggested for wild type Aβ [4,14,15, 61,74,87,96,101]. This not only brought the 2 major types of amyloid deposits as spectrum of the same disease mechanism, but also connected parenchymal and vascular dementia.

The remaining α-secretase site-related AβPP mutations neatly fit into the spectrum of HCHWAD and Flemish AD clinical and pathological descriptions (where available). For the Italian peptide, increased propensity to make fibrils and peptide-mediated pathogenic effects was similar to the Dutch peptide and not surprisingly, resembled clinicopathology of HCHWAD (CAA and hemorrhagic strokes) [62, 64]. The Arctic mutation is also most likely due to increased propensity of protofibril formation without necessarily increasing the rate of fibril formation or the amounts of Aβ [66]. Iowa mutation resembling both Flemish APP692 and HCHWAD pathologically (a severe degree of CAA and predominantly diffuse plaques with some dense-core plaques [27]), shows cytotoxicity and aggregation properties that lie between those caused by the Flemish and Dutch Aβ peptides [64]. None of these pathological descriptions, however, recapitulate the large and abundant dense-cores characteristic of Flemish AD pathology as none of the mutant Aβ parallel the low fibrillogenic potential of Flemish Aβ.

5. Transgenic mice studies deciphering CAA and dense-core plaque pathology: potential for therapeutics

Essential clues in Aβ catabolism, trafficking, and formation of CAA and dense-core plaques have also come from transgenic mouse studies. Although Dutch and Flemish AβPP mice do not deposit Aβ in brain [42, 51] or deposit only at a very late stage [40], clues have come from transgenesis with AD mutations exhibiting progressive age-related development of dense-core and diffuse plaques as well as of CAA [22,41,43,81]. Formation of CAA in these mouse AD models, where only neurons are designed to secrete Aβ, was proposed to be due to Aβ entrapment in the periarterial ISF drainage, one of the principal routes of Aβ elimination from brain in these models [4,87,96]. Utilizing some of these mouse models in the study of development of dense-core plaques, we have recently shown that a great majority of dense-core plaques are also centered on vessel walls or in the immediate perivascular regions [53]. In addition, we also identified ultrastructural microvascular abnormalities occurring in association with dense-core plaques, similar to those described in AD [53]. Aβ is normally cleared through vessels by either periarterial ISF drainage pathway or by an active transport across the blood brain barrier [14,15,61,74,101]. Thus, in mouse models that secrete supraphysiological amounts of Aβ, the majority of the Aβ (that cannot be catabolized in brain) traffics towards blood vessels by an undefined mechanism, and precipitates to form dense-core plaques. This is similar to Flemish AD pathology where the less fibrillogenic Flemish Aβ is upregulated ≈2 fold. As yet, we do not know if this could be a mechanism of dense-core plaque formation in general AD. If indeed this were a major site and a mechanism of dense-core plaque formation, increasing Aβ brain clearance by peripheral sequestering as those tried recently by immune [15] or non-immune [13,61] mechanisms will decrease the burden of 'neuritic' dense-core plaques, so far the best pathological substrate of AD. Moreover, there should also be a concurrent search for molecules like select gangliosides [38] that might help seed plaque deposition in close proximity to vascular walls and in turn could also serve as a therapeutic target.

6. CAA causes progressive dementia in AD

Firstly, cerebral hemorrhage is not limited to Dutch and Flemish AβPP pathology. While the majority of cases of symptomatic CAA are sporadic, CAA leading to strokes has also been described in Down's syndrome cases [18]. Some PSEN linked AD mutations have abundant amyloid angiopathy, including those described by us [16,44,57,76,99]. Some correlations have also been made to the PSEN topology where a severe degree of CAA has been linked to PSEN1 mutation occurring after codon 200 [58]. Some of the PSEN mutations also appear capable of causing hemorrhagic strokes as those described for some of the members of the Volga-German AD family [67].

Secondly, cerebral hemorrhage is also not the only manifestation of CAA. Although the most common clinical manifestation of CAA is indeed vessel rupture and lobar hemorrhagic stroke, other clinical syndromes also occur, including a progressive dementing illness [28,29]. In a recent study on 19 HCHWAD patients, extensive CAA was found to be sufficient to cause progressive dementia in these patients [65]. As yet, it is unknown how CAA per se can contribute to the gradual progressive neurodegeneration seen in AD. One of the mechanisms could be that Aβ depositing within CAA can trigger a perivascular neurodegenerative response, similar to that caused by dense-core plaques. A similar explanation was recently suggested in a neuropathological study of 2 cases with senile dementia presenting with CAA and perivascular tau pathology in the absence of neuritic dense-core plaques [91]. Secondly, severe degree of CAA might also cause restricted blood flow. For instance, in HCHWAD patients that have almost no PHF-tau pathology, the observed progressive dementia [65] is most likely due to restricted blood flow through the amyloid-laden blood vessels. In Flemish AD patients, where dense-core plaques occur in association with blood vessels, the role of vascular insufficiency as a cofactor in neuronal toxicity is also strongly implicated.

7. Conclusions

With a brief historical recount of all major events in AD research, we focused in this review on the genotype-proteotype-phenotype studies related to AβPP α-secretase site mutations and show how research in this direction has facilitated in pinpointing the role of CAA and other vascular abnormalities in the clinics and in the pathology of AD. Especially, we suggested that CAA should be considered an important contributing factor in the progressive cognitive decline observed in AD. We also discussed how multi-level investigations on Flemish AD have helped identify the mechanism of dense-core plaque formation, which has also been extended to some of the mouse AD models. While future studies will address the generality of some of the observations, detailed clinical, neuropathological, and biochemical descriptions of families or individual patients with unusually severe CAA are likely to contribute to our understanding of the role of CAA in dementia.

References

[1] Alzheimer A. über eine eigenartige erkrankung der Hinrinde, *Zentralblatt für Nervenheilkunde und Psychiatrie* **18** (1907), 177–179.

[2] E. Bakker, C. Van Broeckhoven, J. Haan et al., DNA diagnosis for hereditary cerebral hemorrhage with amyloidosis (Dutch type), *Am J Hum Genet* **49** (1991), 518–521.

[3] D.R. Borchelt, G. Thinakaran, C.B. Eckman et al., Familial Alzheimer's disease-linked presenilin 1 variants elevate Abeta1-42/1-40 ratio *in vitro* and *in vivo*, *Neuron* **17** (1996), 1005–1013.

[4] M.E. Calhoun, P. Burgermeister, A.L. Phinney et al., Neuronal overexpression of mutant amyloid precursor protein results in prominent deposition of cerebrovascular amyloid, *Proc Natl Acad Sci USA* **96** (1999), 14088–14093.

[5] A. Clements, D. Allsop, D.M. Walsh and C.H. Williams, Aggregation and metal-binding properties of mutant forms of the amyloid A beta peptide of Alzheimer's disease, *J Neurochem* **66** (1996), 740–747.

[6] A. Clements, D.M. Walsh, C.H. Williams and D. Allsop, Effects of the mutations Glu22 to Gln and Ala21 to Gly on the aggregation of a synthetic fragment of the Alzheimer's amyloid beta/A4 peptide, *Neurosci Lett* **161** (1993), 17–20.

[7] P. Cras, F. van Harskamp, L. Hendriks et al., Presenile Alzheimer dementia characterized by amyloid angiopathy and large amyloid core type senile plaques in the APP 692Ala->Gly mutation, *Acta Neuropathol* **96** (1998), 253–260.

[8] M. Cruts, H. Backhovens, S.Y. Wang et al., Molecular genetic analysis of familial early-onset Alzheimer's disease linked to chromosome 14q24.3, *Hum Mol Genet* **4** (1995), 2363–2371.

[9] M. Cruts and C. Van Broeckhoven, Presenilin mutations in Alzheimer's disease, *Human Mutation* **11** (1998), 183–190.

[10] J. Davis-Salinas and W.E. Van Nostrand, Amyloid beta-protein aggregation nullifies its pathologic properties in cultured cerebrovascular smooth muscle cells, *J Biol Chem* **270** (1995), 20887–20890.

[11] C. De Jonghe, C. Zehr, D. Yager et al., Flemish and Dutch mutations in amyloid beta precursor protein have different effects on amyloid beta secretion, *Neurobiol Dis* **5** (1998), 281–286.

[12] B. De Strooper, P. Saftig, K. Craessaerts et al., Deficiency of presenilin-1 inhibits the normal cleavage of amyloid precursor protein, *Nature* **391** (1998), 387–390.

[13] R. Deane, Y.S. Du, R.K. Submamaryan et al., RAGE mediates amyloid-beta peptide transport across the blood-brain barrier and accumulation in brain, *Nat Med* **9** (2003), 907–913.

[14] R. Deane, Z.H. Wu, A. Sagare et al., LRP/amyloid beta-peptide interaction mediates differential brain efflux of A beta isoforms, *Neuron* **43** (2004), 333–344.

[15] R.B. DeMattos, K.R. Bales, D.J. Cummins, S.M. Paul and D.M. Holtzman, Brain to plasma amyloid-beta efflux: a measure of brain amyloid burden in a mouse model of Alzheimer's disease, *Science* **295** (2002), 2264–2267.

[16] B. Dermaut, S. Kumar-Singh, C. De Jonghe et al., Cerebral amyloid angiopathy is a pathogenic lesion in Alzheimer's disease due to a novel presenilin 1 mutation, *Brain* **124** (2001), 2383–2392.

[17] P. Divry, Etude histochimique des plaques séniles, *J Neurol Psychiat* **27** (1934), 643–657.

[18] J.E. Donahue, J.S. Khurana and L.S. Adelman, Intracerebral hemorrhage in two patients with Down's syndrome and cerebral amyloid angiopathy, *Acta Neuropathol (Berl)* **95** (1998), 213–216.

[19] H. Fabian, G.I. Szendrei, H.H. Mantsch and L. Otvos Jr., Comparative analysis of human and Dutch-type Alzheimer beta-amyloid peptides by infrared spectroscopy and circular dichroism, *Biochem Biophys Res Commun* **191** (1993), 232–239.

[20] M. Farzan, C.E. Schnitzler, N. Vasilieva, D. Leung and H. Choe, BACE2, a beta-secretase homolog, cleaves at the beta site and within the amyloid-beta region of the amyloid-beta precursor protein, *Proc Natl Acad Sci USA* **97** (2000), 9712–9717.

[21] P.E. Fraser, J.T. Nguyen, H. Inouye et al., Fibril formation by primate, rodent and Dutch-hemorrhagic analogues of Alzheimer amyloid b-protein, *Biochem* **31** (1992), 10716–10723.

[22] D. Games, D. Adams, R. Alessandrini et al., Alzheimer-type neuropathology in transgenic mice overexpressing V717F beta-amyloid precursor protein, *Nature* **373** (1995), 523–527.

[23] G.G. Glenner and C.W. Wong, Alzheimer's disease and Down's syndrome: Sharing of a unique cerebrovascular amyloid fibril protein, *Biochem Biophys Res Commun* **122** (1984), 1131–1135.

[24] G.G. Glenner and C.W. Wong, Alzheimer's disease: Initial report of the purification and characterization of a novel cerebrovascular amyloid protein, *Biochem Biophys Res Commun* **122** (1984), 885–890.

[25] A. Goate, H.M. Chartier, M. Mullan et al., Segregation of a missense mutation in the amyloid precursor protein gene with familial Alzheimer's disease, *Nature* **349** (1991), 704–706.

[26] M. Goedert, C.M. Wischik, R.A. Crowther, J.E. Walker and A. Klug, Cloning and sequencing of the cDNA encoding a core protein of the paired helical filament of Alzheimer disease: identification as the microtubule-associated protein tau, *Proc Natl Acad Sci USA* **85** (1988), 4051–4055.

[27] T.J. Grabowski, H.S. Cho, J.P. Vonsattel, G.W. Rebeck and S.M. Greenberg, Novel Amyloid Precursor Protein Mutation in an Iowa Family with Dementia and Severe Cerebral Amyloid Angiopathy, *Ann Neurol* **49** (2001), 697–705.

[28] F. Gray, F. Dubas, E. Roullet and R. Escourolle, Leukoencephalopathy in diffuse hemorrhagic cerebral amyloid angiopathy, *Ann Neurol* **18** (1985), 54–59.

[29] S.M. Greenberg, J.P. Vonsattel, J.W. Stakes, M. Gruber and S.P. Finklestein, The clinical spectrum of cerebral amyloid angiopathy: presentations without lobar hemorrhage, *Neurology* **43** (1993), 2073–2079.

[30] I. Grundke-Iqbal, K. Iqbal, Y.C. Tung, M. Quinlan, H.M. Wisniewski and L.I. Binder, Abnormal phosphorylation of the microtubule-associated protein tau (tau) in Alzheimer cytoskeletal pathology, *Proc Natl Acad Sci USA* **83** (1986), 4913–4917.

[31] I. Grundke-Iqbal, A.B. Johnson, H.M. Wisniewski, R.D. Terry and K. Iqbal, Evidence that Alzheimer neurofibrillary tangles originate from neurotubules, *Lancet* **1** (1979), 578–580.

[32] J.F. Gusella, N.S. Wexler, P.M. Conneally et al., A polymorphic DNA marker genetically linked to Huntington's disease, *Nature* **306** (1983), 234–238.

[33] J. Haan, J.A. Hardy and R.A.C. Roos, Hereditary cerebral hemorrhage with amyloidosis-Dutch type: its importance for Alzheimer research, **14** (TINS), 231–234.

[34] C. Haass, A.Y. Hung, D.J. Selkoe and D.B. Teplow, Mutations associated with a locus for familial Alzheimer's disease result in alternative processing of amyloid beta-protein precursor, *J Biol Chem* **269** (1994), 17741–17748.

[35] J. Hardy and D.J. Selkoe, The amyloid hypothesis of Alzheimer's disease: progress and problems on the road to therapeutics, *Science* **297** (2002), 353–356.

[36] J.A. Hardy and G.A. Higgins, Alzheimer's disease: The amyloid cascade hypothesis, *Science* **256** (1992), 184–185.

[37] D.M. Hartley, D.M. Walsh, C.P. Ye et al., Protofibrillar intermediates of amyloid beta-protein induce acute electrophysiological changes and progressive neurotoxicity in cortical neurons, *J Neurosci* **19** (1999), 8876–8884.

[38] H. Hayashi, N. Kimura, H. Yamaguchi et al., A seed for Alzheimer amyloid in the brain, *J Neurosci* **24** (2004), 4894–4902.

[39] L. Hendriks, C.M. van Duijn, P. Cras et al., Presenile dementia and cerebral haemorrhage linked to a mutation at condon 692 of the b-amyloid precursor protein gene, *Nat Genet* **1** (1992), 218–221.

[40] M.C. Herzig, D.T. Winkler, P. Burgermeister et al., A beta is targeted to the vasculature in a mouse model of hereditary cerebral hemorrhage with amyloidosis, *Nature Neuroscience* **7** (2004), 954–960.

[41] L. Holcomb, M.N. Gordon, E. McGowan et al., Accelerated Alzheimer-type phenotype in transgenic mice carrying both mutant amyloid precursor protein and presenilin 1 transgenes, *Nat Med* **4** (1998), 97–100.

[42] D.S. Howland, M.J. Savage, F.A. Huntress et al., Mutant and native human beta-amyloid precursor proteins in transgenic mouse brain, *Neurobiol Aging* **16** (1995), 685–699.

[43] K. Hsiao, P. Chapman, S. Nilsen et al., Correlative memory deficits, Abeta elevation, and amyloid plaques in transgenic mice, *Science* **274** (1996), 99–102.

[44] M. Ikeda, V. Sharma, S.M. Sumi et al., The clinical phenotype of two missense mutations in the presenilin I gene in Japanese patients, *Ann Neurol* **40** (1996), 912–917.

[45] J.T. Jarrett, E.P. Berger and P.T. Lansbury Jr., The carboxy terminus of the -amyloid protein is critical for the seeding of amyloid formation: Implications for the pathogenesis of Alzheimer's disease, *Biochemistry* **32** (1993), 4693–4697.

[46] K. Kamino, H.T. Orr, H. Payami et al., Linkage and mutational analysis of familial Alzheimer disease kindreds for the APP gene region, *Am J Hum Genet* **51** (1992), 998–1014.

[47] J. Kang, H-G. Lemaire, A. Unterbeck et al., The precursor of Alzheimer's disease amyloid A4 protein resembles a cell-surface receptor, *Nature* **325** (1987), 733–736.

[48] K.S. Kosik, L.D. Orecchio, L. Binder, J.Q. Trojanowski, V.M. Lee and G. Lee, Epitopes that span the tau molecule are shared with paired helical filaments, *Neuron* **1** (1988), 817–825.

[49] S. Kumar-Singh, P. Cras, R. Wang et al., Dense-core senile plaques in the Flemish variant of Alzheimer's disease are vasocentric, *Am J Pathol* **161** (2002), 507–520.

[50] S. Kumar-Singh, C. De Jonghe, M. Cruts et al., Nonfibrillar diffuse amyloid deposition due to a gamma(42)-secretase site mutation points to an essential role for N-truncated abeta(42) in Alzheimer's disease, *Hum Mol Genet* **9** (2000), 2589–2598.

[51] S. Kumar-Singh, I. Dewachter, D. Moechars et al., Behavioral disturbances without amyloid deposits in mice overexpressing human amyloid precursor protein with Flemish (A692G) or Dutch (E693Q) mutation, *Neurobiol Dis* **7** (2000), 9–22.

[52] S. Kumar-Singh, A. Julliams, D. Nuyens et al., In vitro studies of Flemish, Dutch, and wild type Amyloid β (Aβ) provide evidence for a two-stage Aβ neurotoxicity, *Neurobiol Dis* **11** (2002), 300–310.

[53] S. Kumar-Singh, D. Pirici, E. McGowan et al., Dense core plaques in Tg2576 and PSAPP mouse models of Alzheimer's disease are centered on vessel walls, *Am J Pathol* **167** (2005), 527–543.

[54] M.P. Lambert, A.K. Barlow, B.A. Chromy et al., Diffusible, nonfibrillar ligands derived from Abeta1–42 are potent central nervous system neurotoxins, *Proc Natl Acad Sci USA* **95** (1998), 6448–6453.

[55] E. Levy, M.D. Carman, I.J. Fernandez-Madrid et al., Mutation of the Alzheimer's disease amyloid gene in hereditary cerebral hemorrhage, Dutch type, *Science* **248** (1990), 1124–1126.

[56] M.L. Maat-Schieman, S.G. van Duinen, M. Bornebroek, J. Haan and R.A. Roos, Hereditary cerebral hemorrhage with amyloidosis-Dutch type (HCHWA-D): II–A review of histopathological aspects, *Brain Pathol* **6** (1996), 115–120.

[57] D.M. Mann, T. Iwatsubo, N.J. Cairns et al., Amyloid beta protein (Abeta) deposition in chromosome 14-linked Alzheimer's disease: predominance of Abeta42(43), *Ann Neurol* **40** (1996), 149–156.

[58] D.M. Mann, S.M. Pickering-Brown, A. Takeuchi and T. Iwatsubo, Amyloid Angiopathy and Variability in Amyloid beta Deposition Is Determined by Mutation Position in Presenilin-1-Linked Alzheimer's Disease, *Am J Pathol* **158** (2001), 2165–2175.

[59] J.-J. Martin, J. Gheuens, M. Bruyland et al., Early-onset Alzheimer's disease in 2 large Belgian families, *Neurology* **41** (1991), 62–68.

[60] C.L. Masters, G. Simms, N.A. Weinman, G. Multhaup, B.L. McDonals and K. Beyreuther, Amyloid plaque core protein in Alzheimer disease and Down syndrome, *Proc Natl Acad Sci USA* **82** (1985), 4245–4249.

[61] Y. Matsuoka, M. Saito, J. LaFrancois et al., Novel therapeutic approach for the treatment of Alzheimer's disease by peripheral administration of agents with an affinity to beta-amyloid, *J Neurosci* **23** (2003), 29–33.

[62] J.P. Melchor, L. McVoy and W.E. Van Nostrand, Charge alterations of E22 enhance the pathogenic properties of the amyloid beta-protein, *J Neurochem* **74** (2000), 2209–2212.

[63] L. Miravalle, T. Tokuda, R. Chiarle et al., Substitutions at codon 22 of Alzheimer's A{beta} peptide induce conformational changes and diverse apoptotic effects in human cerebral endothelial cells, *J Biol Chem* **275** (2000), 27110–27116.

[64] K. Murakami, K. Irie, A. Morimoto et al., Synthesis, aggregation, neurotoxicity, and secondary structure of various A beta 1–42 mutants of familial Alzheimer's disease at positions 21–23, *Biochem Biophys Res Commun* **294** (2002), 5–10.

[65] R. Natte, M.L. Maat-Schieman, J. Haan, M. Bornebroek, R.A. Roos and S.G. van Duinen, Dementia in hereditary cerebral hemorrhage with amyloidosis-Dutch type is associated with cerebral amyloid angiopathy but is independent of plaques and neurofibrillary tangles, *Ann Neurol* **50** (2001), 765–772.

[66] C. Nilsberth, A. Westlind-Danielsson, C. Eckman et al., The Arctic APP mutation (E693G) causes Alzheimer's disease by enhanced Abeta protofibril formation, *Nat Neurosci* **4** (2001), 887–893.

[67] D. Nochlin, T.D. Bird, E.J. Nemens, M.J. Ball and S.M. Sumi, Amyloid angiopathy in a Volga German family with Alzheimer's disease and a presenilin-2 mutation (N141I), *Ann Neurol* **43** (1998), 131–135.

[68] G. Perry, N. Rizzuto, L. Autilio-Gambetti and P. Gambetti, Paired helical filaments from Alzheimer disease patients contain cytoskeletal components, *Proc Natl Acad Sci USA* **82** (1985), 3916–3920.

[69] C.J. Pike, A.J. Walencewicz, C.G. Glabe and C.W. Cotman, Aggregation-related toxicity of synthetic beta-amyloid protein in hippocampal cultures, *Eur J Pharmacol* **207** (1991), 367–368.

[70] G. Roks, F. van Harskamp, K.I. De et al., Presentation of amyloidosis in carriers of the codon 692 mutation in the amyloid precursor protein gene (APP692), *Brain* **123** (2000), 2130–2140.

[71] D. Scheuner, C. Eckman, M. Jensen et al., Secreted amyloid beta-protein similar to that in the senile plaques of Alzheimer's disease is increased *in vivo* by the presenilin 1 and 2 and APP mutations linked to familial Alzheimer's disease [see comments], *Nat Med* **2** (1996), 864–870.

[72] W. Scholtz, Studien zur Pathologie der Hirngefässe. II. Die drüsige Entartung der Hirnarterien und -capillären, *Z Gesamte Neurol Psychiat* **162** (1938), 694–715.

[73] R. Sherrington, E.I. Rogaev, Y. Liang et al., Cloning of a gene bearing mis-sense mutations in early-onset familial Alzheimer's disease, *Nature* **375** (1995), 754–760.

[74] M. Shibata, S. Yamada, S.R. Kumar et al., Clearance of Alzheimer's amyloid-ss(1–40) peptide from brain by LDL receptor-related protein-1 at the blood-brain barrier, *J Clin Invest* **106** (2000), 1489–1499.

[75] A.K. Sian, E.R. Frears, O.M. El Agnaf et al., Oligomerization of beta-amyloid of the Alzheimer's and the Dutch-cerebral-haemorrhage types, *Biochem J* **349** (2000), 299–308.

[76] A.B. Singleton, R. Hall, C.G. Ballard et al., Pathology of early-onset Alzheimer's disease cases bearing the Thr113-114ins presenilin-1 mutation, *Brain* **123**(12) (2000), 2467–2474.

[77] S. Sinha, J.P. Anderson, R. Barbour et al., Purification and cloning of amyloid precursor protein beta-secretase from human brain [see comments], *Nature* **402** (1999), 537–540.

[78] S.S. Sisodia, E.H. Koo, K. Beyreuther, A. Unterbeck and D.L. Price, Evidence that b-amyloid protein in Alzheimer's disease is not derived by normal processing, *Science* **248** (1990), 492–495.

[79] P. St George-Hyslop, J. Haines, E. Rogaev et al., Genetic evidence for a novel familial Alzheimer's disease locus on chromosome 14, *Nature Genet* **2** (1992), 330–334.

[80] P. St George-Hyslop, R.E. Tanzi, P.J. Polinsky et al., The genetic defect causing familial Alzheimer's disease maps on chromosome 21, *Science* **235** (1987), 885–890.

[81] C. Sturchler-Pierrat, D. Abramowski, M. Duke et al., Two amyloid precursor protein transgenic mouse models with Alzheimer disease-like pathology, *Proc Natl Acad Sci USA* **94** (1997), 13287–13292.

[82] R.E. Tanzi, P. St George-Hyslop, J.L. Haines et al., The genetic defect in familial Alzheimer's disease is not tightly linked to the amyloid b-protein gene, *Nature* **329** (1987), 156–157.

[83] L. van Bogaert, M. Maere and E. de Smedt, Sur les formes familiales précoces de la maladie d'Alzheimer, *Mschr Psychiat Neurol* **102** (1940), 249–301.

[84] C. Van Broeckhoven, H. Backhovens, M. Cruts et al., Mapping of a gene predisposing to early-onset Alzheimer's disease to chromosome 14q24.3, *Nat Genet* **2** (1992), 335–339.

[85] C. Van Broeckhoven, A.M. Genthe, A. Vandenberghe et al., Failure of familial Alzheimer's disease to segregate with the A4-amyloid gene in several European families, *Nature* **329** (1987), 153–155.

[86] C. Van Broeckhoven, J. Haan, E. Bakker et al., Amyloid beta protein precursor gene and hereditary cerebral hemorrhage with amyloidosis (Dutch), *Science* **248** (1990), 1120–1122.

[87] J. Van Dorpe, L. Smeijers, I. Dewachter et al., Prominent cerebral amyloid angiopathy in transgenic mice overexpressing the london mutant of human APP in neurons [In Process Citation], *Am J Pathol* **157** (2000), 1283–1298.

[88] S.G. van Duinen, E.M. Castaño, F. Prelli, G.T.A.B. Bots, W. Luyendijk and B. Frangione, Hereditary cerebral hemorrhage with amyloidosis in patients of Dutch origin is related to Alzheimer disease, *Proc Natl Acad Sci USA* **84** (1987), 5991–5994.

[89] W.E. Van Nostrand, J. Davis-Salinas and S.M. Saporito-Irwin, Amyloid beta-protein induces the cerebrovascular cellular pathology of Alzheimer's disease and related disorders, *Ann N Y Acad Sci* **777** (1996), 297–302.

[90] R. Vassar, B.D. Bennett, S. Babu-Khan et al., Beta-secretase cleavage of Alzheimer's amyloid precursor protein by the transmembrane aspartic protease BACE [see comments], *Science* **286** (1999), 735–741.

[91] R. Vidal, M. Calero, P. Piccardo et al., Senile dementia associated with amyloid beta protein angiopathy and tau perivascular pathology but not neuritic plaques in patients homozygous for the APOE-epsilon4 allele, *Acta Neuropathol (Berl)* **100** (2000), 1–12.

[92] D.M. Walsh, D.M. Hartley, M.M. Condron, D.J. Selkoe and D.B. Teplow, In vitro studies of amyloid beta-protein fibril assembly and toxicity provide clues to the aetiology of Flemish variant (Ala692->Gly) Alzheimer's disease, *Biochem J* **355** (2001), 869–877.

[93] D.M. Walsh, I. Klyubin, J.V. Fadeeva et al., Naturally secreted oligomers of amyloid beta protein potently inhibit hippocampal long-term potentiation *in vivo*, *Nature* **416** (2002), 535–539.

[94] Z. Wang, R. Natte, J.A. Berliner, S.G. van Duinen, H.V. Vinters and W.I. Rosenblum, Toxicity of Dutch (E22Q) and Flemish (A21G) mutant amyloid beta proteins to human cerebral microvessel and aortic smooth muscle cells, *Stroke* **31** (2000), 534–538.

[95] D.J. Watson, D.J. Selkoe and D.B. Teplow, Effects of the amyloid precursor protein Glu693->Gln Dutch mutation on the production and stability of amyloid beta-protein, *Biochem J* **340** (1999), 703–709.

[96] R.O. Weller, A. Massey, T.A. Newman, M. Hutchings, Y.M. Kuo and A.E. Roher, Cerebral amyloid angiopathy: amyloid beta accumulates in putative interstitial fluid drainage pathways in Alzheimer's disease, *Am J Pathol* **153** (1998), 725–733.

[97] K.E. Wisniewski, A.J. Dalton, D.R. Crapper-McLachlan, G.Y. Wen and H.M. Wisniewski, Alzheimer's disease in Down's syndrome: Clinicopathologic studies, *Neurology* **35** (1985), 957–961.

[98] T. Wisniewski, J. Ghiso and B. Frangione, Peptides homologous to the amyloid protein of Alzheimer's disease contain-

ing a glutamine for glutamic acid substitution have accelerated amyloid fibril formation, *Biochem Biophys Res Commun* **179** (1991), 1247–1254.

[99] M. Yasuda, K. Maeda, Y. Ikejiri, T. Kawamata, S. Kuroda and C. Tanaka, A novel missense mutation in the presenilin-1 gene in a familial Alzheimer's disease pedigree with abundant amyloid angiopathy, *Neurosci Lett* **232** (1997), 29–32.

[100] S.H. Yen, F. Gaskin and R.D. Terry, Immunocytochemical studies of neurofibrillary tangles, *Am J Pathol* **104** (1981), 77–89.

[101] B.V. Zlokovic, Clearing amyloid through the blood-brain barrier, *J Neurochem* **89** (2004), 807–811.

Diagnosis and Treatment

Preclinical characterization of amyloid imaging probes with multiphoton microscopy

Jesse Skoch, Bradley T. Hyman and Brian J. Bacskai*
MassGeneral Institute for Neurodegenerative Disease, Department of Neurology/Alzheimer's Disease Research Laboratory, Massachusetts General Hospital, 114 16th Street, Charlestown, MA 02129, USA

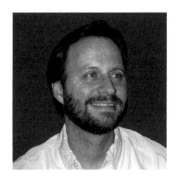

Abstract. Multiphoton microscopy is an optical imaging technique that allows high resolution detection of fluorescence in thick, scattering tissues. The technique has been used for trans-cranial imaging of the brains of living transgenic mouse models of Alzheimer's disease. Direct detection of senile plaques in these mice has allowed the characterization of the natural history of individual senile plaques, the evaluation of plaque clearance during immunotherapy, and the characterization of the kinetics and biodistribution of the PET ligand, PIB. With the expanding repertoire of structural and functional fluorescent probes, and the preclinical characterization of new contrast agents for complementary imaging modalities like MRI, PET, SPECT, and NIRS, multiphoton microscopy will continue to be a powerful tool in understanding and combating Alzheimer's disease.

1. Introduction

Despite the advances of the last century, the most significant hurdle to the development of effective therapeutics for Alzheimer's disease is, perhaps, a sensitive, specific biomarker of disease progression. It is hard to argue with the elegance of an imaging technique that would allow early diagnosis and anatomically specific monitoring of the disease. Diseases like cancer and stroke have benefited from diagnostic imaging that allows direct assessment of therapeutic interventions. No such technique has existed for AD until recently. There have been several advances in indirect imaging of the disease with FDG-PET and high resolution MRI, that while lacking specificity, have been used with success to help diagnose and monitor disease progression [5, 14,15,17]. Although the role of senile plaques in AD is still debated, the accumulation of amyloid deposits with progression is accepted. Therefore, the detection of amyloid deposits in the brain, and efforts to prevent or remove them have received considerable attention. Recent advances using PET [21,22,31] and MRI [16, 29,35] to image plaques in mice show great promise. This review, however, will focus on the efforts to image senile plaques *in vivo* using multiphoton microscopy in transgenic mouse models. While these efforts added to our understanding of the natural progression of plaque deposition, they were also instrumental in both evaluating anti-amyloid-β therapeutics and the preclinical characterization of an *in vivo* amyloid ligand that is currently in clinical trials as a PET imaging agent [22].

Multiphoton microscopy has an advantage over other *in vivo* imaging approaches since the high spatial resolution inherent to the technique allows direct immuno- or histochemical confirmation of the imaged structures. Multiphoton microscopy, therefore, allows direct eval-

---

*Corresponding author: Brian J. Bacskai, PhD, Department of Neurology/Alzheimer's Disease Research Laboratory, Massachusetts General Hospital, 114 16th Street, #2850, Charlestown, MA 02129, USA. Tel.: +1 617 724 5306; Fax: +1 617 724 1480; E-mail: bbacskai@partners.org.

uation of the binding specificity and kinetics of novel amyloid targeting reagents. It can be anticipated that the screening of new clinical imaging agents for PET, SPECT, MRI, NIRS, or any other *in vivo* technique will be facilitated by testing with multiphoton microscopy in animal models of AD.

2. Multiphoton microscopy

Multiphoton microscopy is an optical imaging technique similar to confocal microscopy that allows diffraction-limited spatial resolution of cellular and sub-cellular structures using a scanning laser for excitation of fluorescence. Both techniques result in 3-dimensional images with optical sectioning achieved in different ways. Multiphoton microscopy is advantageous when imaging thick scattering tissue like intact brain, live cells, and fluorophores that require UV excitation. The photophysical phenomenon of multi-photon excitation of fluorescence is simply described as the simultaneous acceptance of two low energy photons (in the near infrared) that would normally match the single photon acceptance of a higher energy photon (in the UV or blue region.) This is achieved by means of a pulsed near infrared laser with low average power, but very high peak power, and concomitant focusing of the light to further increase the local photon flux. This increases the probability that a fluorophore will accept two low-energy photons nearly simultaneously. The end result is that near infrared excitation, possessing the advantage of deeper penetration through scattering tissue with minimal phototoxicity, excites a broad range of fluorophores only at the plane of focus, allowing a narrow depth of field with confocal-like optical sectioning without photodamage above or below the plane of focus or the need for a signal-reducing pinhole [9]. The end result is sub-micron spatial resolution in three dimensions deep within living tissue. Figure 1 shows an example of simultaneous 2-color fluorescence detection in the brain of a living transgenic mouse using multiphoton microscopy.

While the technique can exploit extrinsic signals, they are inherently weak. Alzheimer's disease research, however, has been endowed with a selection of amyloid binding fluorophores that have been used and characterized for decades. Our initial studies exploited the fluorescence of thioflavin S as an amyloid binding reagent. Thioflavin S is a small, diffusible, nontoxic fluorophore that binds specifically to the beta-sheet structure of dense-core plaques in the brain. It ab-

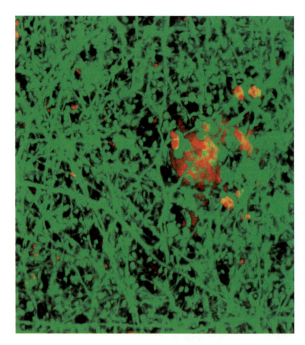

Fig. 1. Simultaneous 2 channel *in vivo* multi-photon micrograph of an amyloid plaque (red pseudocolor) amongst cortical YFP-expressing neurites (green pseudocolor). The blood-brain barrier permeant methoxy-X04 labeling agent was administered systemically to label dense-core deposits in a PDAPP transgenic mouse. A maximum intensity projection of 55 μm depth is displayed here.

sorbs UV light and emits fluorescence in the blue/green spectrum. It is a bright, sensitive fluorophore amenable to multiphoton excitation. Our first studies applied this compound directly to the surface of the brain of living transgenic mice to label amyloid deposits. Thioflavin S allowed sensitive, chronic imaging of both plaques and cerebrovascular amyloid angiopathy (CAA) up to 400 μm deep into the cortex, and enabled the characterization of the natural history of dense core plaques in the Tg2576 mouse model [8]. This report demonstrated that senile plaques form quickly, and are then stable in size. Very little growth or shrinking was detected in the chronic imaging experiments.

The establishment of a reliable *in vivo* imaging approach then permitted the evaluation of the efficacy of anti-Aβ immunotherapy [3,4]. These studies used topical application of anti-Aβ antibodies to the surface of the brain to monitor directly the clearance of Aβ deposits *in vivo*. Multiphoton imaging allowed detection of individual deposits before and after treatment. The imaging approach was further exploited to characterize the effects of therapies on structural and functional fluorescent readouts in the living mouse brain [6,23]. These assays used fluorescent outcomes as indicators of oxidative stress or neuritic morphology *in vivo*, and illustrate one of the major advantages of the fluorescence imaging approach; the availability and selection of fluorescent probes is extremely large, and ever expanding. This allows multi-dimensional imaging of structure and function at the cellular or subcellular level *in vivo*. For example, genetically encoded fluorescent reporters based on GFP for calcium, pH, kinase activity, oxidative metabolism, and proteases have been developed [13,26,37]. Furthermore, small molecule fluorescent probes have recently been introduced into mature brain *in vivo* and monitored with multiphoton microscopy [27]. Together, these tools permit application of a broad range of structural and functional fluorophores that were previously limited to *in vitro* preparations.

3. 4-D imaging of PIB

William E. Klunk, Chester A. Mathis, and their team at the University of Pittsburgh have been developing rationally designed derivatives of known amyloid binding agents for the ultimate goal of clinical diagnostic imaging of amyloid pathology in humans using PET. Their synthetic approach started with known binding agents like thioflavin T, which, although relatively specific for amyloid deposits in brain tissue, is too polar to cross blood-brain barrier, and therefore not suitable as a PET ligand. After several generations of derivatives, Pittsburgh compound B (PIB), appeared to satisfy the requirements for a suitable ligand. The compound is small, somewhat lipophilic, crosses the blood-brain barrier, and still retains high affinity for Aβ fibrils (Kd $\sim$ 20 nM). *In vitro* assays have shown high specificity, and *in vivo* radio tracer studies demonstrated promising brain entry and clearance [20,36]. The compound is radiolabeled with C^{11} which has a half-life of $\sim$ 20 min, dictating the need for rapid brain entry, and rapid efflux of unbound probe. As a derivative of the compound thioflavin T, however, PIB retained the fluorescent properties of its parent, and was readily detected using multiphoton microscopy in the AβPP mouse models. Because PIB is fluorescent even when not bound to amyloid deposits, the appearance and clearance from the brain was easily monitored. Time-lapse imaging of the biodistribution of PIB after IV injection in the mouse models allowed direct examination of the appearance in circulation, entry into the brain, labeling of amyloid pathology, and egress of unbound agent from the parenchyma [2]. A 4-dimensional im-

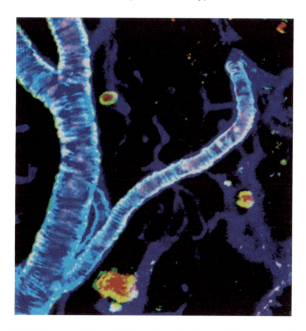

Fig. 2. Representation of 4-dimensional *in vivo* multiphoton recording of the fluorescent biomarker PIB in the brain of a Tg2576 mouse. Three discreet time points are shown here simultaneously as two-dimensional projections (maximum intensity) of their respective 3D volumes. Blue pseudocolor corresponds to the dye visible in the volume immediately after i.v. injection, green 5 min later, and red at $t = 20$ min. PIB enters the brain, is rapidly cleared from circulation, and targets vascular and parenchymal amyloid deposits with high specificity, making it a suitable *in vivo* biomarker.

age, showing the time-course of PIB distribution in an imaged volume of mouse brain is shown in Figure 2. These imaging results, not possible with PET or SPECT imaging, demonstrated directly that PIB met the criteria of a PET amyloid imaging agent. While the animal experiments cannot replace experience with human imaging, they do lend a considerable amount of confidence that the agent is binding to the appropriate pathological target, particularly since the amyloid plaques are too small to be imaged individually with PET, due to the lower spatial resolution of the technique.

PIB has been evaluated for imaging in humans, and is currently under more widespread evaluation in several imaging centers [19]. This radiolabel is now considered the "gold standard" for amyloid imaging, partially due to the overwhelming pre-clinical characterization of the compound. While multiphoton microscopy played only a small part in its development, it allowed direct detection of binding in animal models with immunohistochemical confirmation. It is no surprise, therefore, that other compounds are being evaluated using this technique. Indeed, relatively low resolution imaging modalities like MRI, SPECT, or NIRS would benefit from the characterization of *in vivo* binding using multiphoton microscopy.

4. New probes for imaging with NIRS

An alternative non-invasive approach for diagnostic imaging in humans is based on near infrared spectroscopy (NIRS). This technique capitalizes on the deep transmission of near infrared light through scattering tissue. It is commonly used to take advantage of the unique absorption spectra of oxy- and deoxy- hemoglobin to detect changes in cerebral blood flow and local oxygen utilization [7,10,24,34]. In this sense, NIRS has been applied for functional imaging in animals and humans, allowing regional detection of metabolic changes in the brain associated with physiological stimuli [30]. The spatial resolution of this technique varies with depth, but can surpass 1 mm at up to several centimeters into the brain [12]. Using multiple source and detector arrays and sophisticated image reconstruction algorithms, 3D optical tomography can be performed, leading to PET or SPECT like images of the brain, non-invasively, and without radioligands [32]. The functional imaging of hemoglobin relies on an intrinsic absorption spectra, however, targeted fluorescent probes could be detected even more sensitively, particularly if the excitation and emission spectra lie within the range of 650–850 nm, between the strong absorption bands of hemoglobin and water. It is the development of novel molecular imaging probes with spectra in this region that will accelerate varied applications of non-invasive optical imaging in the brain and periphery. Indeed, a number of studies have been performed with applications to peripheral imaging using existing near infrared fluorophores targeted with antibodies or peptide recognition sequences [1,11,18,25,28].

In the case of Alzheimer's disease, diagnostic imaging of amyloid-β deposits in the brain could be accomplished with a near infrared fluorophore that enters the brain and targets amyloid plaques specifically. To this end, a small fluorescent molecule like PIB could be used as long as the fluorescent spectrum was shifted from the UV/blue to the near infrared region. This will require some clever chemistry, as maintaining the necessary qualities possessed by PIB is not trivial. However, we have begun to develop molecular amyloid binding reagents small enough to cross the blood-brain barrier that are near infrared fluorescent [33]. Figure 3 demonstrates our early proof-in-principle approaches towards non-invasive detection of fluorescence deep in the brain. Because the detection hardware and imaging software is already established, the development of a chemical ligand is the last step for non-invasive optical detection of amyloid in the brain. Successful development of such a probe would have significant advantages over PET or SPECT imaging for several reasons. First, no radioactivity is required. Besides minimizing the exposure to radioactivity (which is extremely low-dose for PET or SPECT), ligands with short half-life isotopes need to be synthesized on site, or delivered with great speed and expense. Second, the technology, maintenance, training, and staffing required for optical imaging is much less expensive than for a PET or even SPECT scanner. Together these factors will contribute to easier accessibility for a massive and growing population of potential patients. Lastly, optical biomarkers can be exploited for greater sensitivity and increased contrast because a probe can be designed such that the optical properties can be sensitive to the local environment. For instance, the intensity, wavelength, or lifetime of the dye can change whether bound to the amyloid target or not. By capitalizing on these physical changes in the dye, it is no longer necessary to clear unbound dye from the brain, since bound vs unbound probe can be discriminated based on the differences in spectroscopic properties. This permits background subtraction, and therefore substantially improved contrast.

As with the characterization of PIB in mouse models, multiphoton microscopy is useful for characterizing other novel molecular imaging probes. New amyloid targeting reagents can be evaluated in tissue sections and *in vivo* in mouse models with subcellular resolution to confirm non-invasive imaging results. Like PET or SPECT, NIRS will not permit imaging of individual senile plaques, but rather a collective amyloid burden representing binding to plaque-containing regions in the brain. Therefore, imaging results will need to be compared with immunostaining of post-mortem brains. Chronic studies, however, can be performed in parallel with multiphoton imaging of plaques in the cortex. Multiphoton microscopy uses a near-infrared laser source for excitation that can also be used as a tunable single-photon source for near infrared fluorophores.

Lastly, while the mouse models have been exceptionally valuable for the preclinical development of amyloid imaging agents, the utility of these agents for amyloid imaging in mice has been underappreciated. Screening of anti-amyloid therapeutics depends on reliable biomarkers to evaluate efficacy, and quantitative

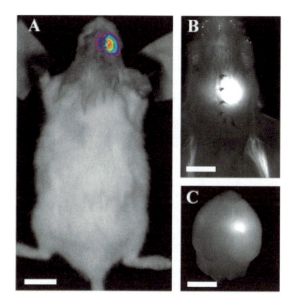

Fig. 3. Non-invasive detection of NIR fluorescence *in vivo* in the brain of an intact mouse. A bolus intracerebral injection of Alexafluor 750 labeled BAM10 antibody (8 μL) was made in an anesthetized mouse in the right hemisphere several millimeters deep from the cortical surface. The skin was restored and sutured closed along the midline. Shortly thereafter, the anesthetized mouse was imaged using a commercial, laser scanning, small animal imaging platform (eXplore Optix prototype, ART, Quebec) (A), and again on a flatbed NIR laser scanner (LiCor Odyssey) (B). Imaging was performed through the skin and skull of the intact, live animal with the focal plane set at eye level in the eXplore Optix imager and at 4 mm from the scanner surface of the Odyssey plate reader. The fluorescent signal was readily detected with both instruments, and was confined to the injected hemisphere. 24 hrs after injection, the mouse was sacrificed, and the post-mortem brain was isolated and fixed in 4% paraformaldehyde. The isolated brain was imaged using the LiCor Odyssey with a 3 mm focus offset from the scanner surface (C). The eXplore Optix image was captured at 0.5 mm resolution (pseudocolor from purple to red) and superimposed on a white light CCD image (A), *in vivo* Licor Odyssey image at 42 μm resolution (B), and *ex vivo* brain image at 21 μm (C). Scale bars A = 1.8 cm B = 1 cm C = 5.5 mm. Reprinted with permission from Skoch et al. [33]. Copyright SPIE, 2005.

imaging of amyloid burden is the most direct approach. Thus, the combination of transgenic mouse models and a reliable non-invasive imaging technique should lead to rapid screening of anti-amyloid drugs without the need for large cohorts of animals sacrificed at individual time-points. To date, the attempts to use radiolabeled PIB and micro-PET imaging in transgenic mice have proven unsuccessful. While not completely understood, this failure may result from low contrast in the mouse brain due to non-specific binding that is not observed with fluorescence imaging, or a lack of sensitivity in the micro-PET devices. Future studies should be able to overcome this obstacle, although an all optical approach based on NIRS may well represent the best alternative for low-cost non-invasive imaging in the mouse brain, pending development of a suitable molecular imaging probe.

5. Conclusions

This review describes the current and future impact of multiphoton microscopy for increasing our understanding of AD as well as for developing diagnostic tools suitable for use in mouse models and humans. Multiphoton microscopy provides a bridge between histo- and immunohisto-logical examination of tissue and live animal imaging of Aβ pathology. This is due to the very high spatial resolution afforded by the technique. This spatial resolution also limits the applications of multiphoton imaging to small regions of cortex in animal models. As a tool for preclinical characterization of amyloid binding agents, however, multiphoton has been successfully used to characterize the PET ligand PIB, which is now in use for clinical imaging in humans. Development of other probes for PET, SPECT, MRI, or NIRS will also benefit from characterization with direct imaging in animal models with multiphoton microscopy. There is much to be learned about the etiology of AD and the effects of therapeutics upon pathology in the mouse models from direct, *in vivo* imaging with multiphoton microscopy. Indeed, because of the extremely large collection of existing fluorescent probes for structural and functional imaging, and because the molecular imaging probe library is constantly expanding, multiphoton microscopy is positioned for many years of fruitful studies. At this moment, multiphoton microscopy is the best-characterized *in vivo* amyloid imaging approach in the transgenic mouse models, and is therefore, the method of choice to evaluate new anti-Aβ therapeutics *in vivo*. We believe that better, faster, and cheaper imaging approaches will be developed for amyloid imaging in mice and humans, and we predict that multiphoton microscopy will be an operative, if not essential reference for the characterization of these new probes and modalities.

Acknowledgements

This work was supported by NIH AG020570, EB00768 (BJB), AG08487, and a Pioneer Award from the Alzheimer Association (BTH).

References

[1] S. Achilefu, R.B. Dorshow, J.E. Bugaj and R. Rajagopalan, Novel receptor-targeted fluorescent contrast agents for in vivo tumor imaging, *Invest Radiol.* **35** (2000), 479–485.

[2] B.J. Bacskai, G.A. Hickey, J. Skoch, S.T. Kajdasz, Y. Wang, G.F. Huang, C.A. Mathis, W.E. Klunk and B.T. Hyman, Four-dimensional multiphoton imaging of brain entry, amyloid binding, and clearance of an amyloid-beta ligand in transgenic mice, *Proc Natl Acad Sci USA* **100** (2003), 12462–12467.

[3] B.J. Bacskai, S.T. Kajdasz, R.H. Christie, C. Carter, D. Games, P. Seubert, D. Schenk and B.T. Hyman, Imaging of amyloid-beta deposits in brains of living mice permits direct observation of clearance of plaques with immunotherapy, *Nat Med* **7** (2001), 369–372.

[4] B.J. Bacskai, S.T. Kajdasz, M.E. McLellan, D. Games, P. Seubert, D. Schenk and B.T. Hyman, Non-Fc-mediated mechanisms are involved in clearance of amyloid-beta in vivo by immunotherapy, *J Neurosci* **22** (2002), 7873–7878.

[5] J. Barnes, R.I. Scahill, R.G. Boyes, C. Frost, E.B. Lewis, C.L. Rossor, M.N. Rossor and N.C. Fox, Differentiating AD from aging using semiautomated measurement of hippocampal atrophy rates, *Neuroimage* **23** (2004), 574–581.

[6] R.P. Brendza, B.J. Bacskai, J.R. Cirrito, K.A. Simmons, J.M. Skoch, W.E. Klunk, C.A. Mathis, K.R. Bales, S.M. Paul, B.T. Hyman and D.M. Holtzman, Anti-Abeta antibody treatment promotes the rapid recovery of amyloid-associated neuritic dystrophy in PDAPP transgenic mice, *J Clin Invest* **115** (2005), 428–433.

[7] A.F. Cannestra, I. Wartenburger, H. Obrig, A. Villringer and A.W. Toga, Functional assessment of Broca's area using near infrared spectroscopy in humans, *Neuroreport* **14** (2003), 1961–1965.

[8] R.H. Christie, B.J. Bacskai, W.R. Zipfel, R.M. Williams, S.T. Kajdasz, W.W. Webb and B.T. Hyman, Growth arrest of individual senile plaques in a model of Alzheimer's disease observed by in vivo multiphoton microscopy, *J Neurosci* **21** (2001), 858–864.

[9] W. Denk, J.H. Strickler and W.W. Webb, Two-photon laser scanning fluorescence microscopy, *Science* **248** (1990), 73–76.

[10] A.K. Dunn, A. Devor, H. Bolay, M.L. Andermann, M.A. Moskowitz, A.M. Dale and D.A. Boas, Simultaneous imaging of total cerebral hemoglobin concentration, oxygenation, and blood flow during functional activation, *Optics Letters* **28** (2003), 28–30.

[11] J.V. Frangioni, In vivo near-infrared fluorescence imaging, *Curr Opin Chem Biol* **7** (2003), 626–634.

[12] E.E. Graves, J. Ripoll, R. Weissleder and V. Ntziachristos, A submillimeter resolution fluorescence molecular imaging system for small animal imaging, *Med Phys* **30** (2003), 901–911.

[13] O. Griesbeck, Fluorescent proteins as sensors for cellular functions, *Curr Opin Neurobiol* **14** (2004), 636–641.

[14] J.A. Helpern, J. Jensen, S.P. Lee and M.F. Falangola, Quantitative MRI assessment of Alzheimer's disease, *J Mol Neurosci* **24** (2004), 45–48.

[15] K. Herholz, E. Salmon, D. Perani, J.C. Baron, V. Holthoff, L. Frolich, P. Schonknecht, K. Ito, R. Mielke, E. Kalbe, G. Zundorf, X. Delbeuck, O. Pelati, D. Anchisi, F. Fazio, N. Kerrouche, B. Desgranges, F. Eustache, B. Beuthien-Baumann, C. Menzel, J. Schroder, T. Kato, Y. Arahata, M. Henze and W.D. Heiss, Discrimination between Alzheimer dementia and controls by automated analysis of multicenter FDG PET, *Neuroimage* **17** (2002), 302–316.

[16] C.R. Jack, Jr., M. Garwood, T.M. Wengenack, B. Borowski, G.L. Curran, J. Lin, G. Adriany, O.H. Grohn, R. Grimm and J.F. Poduslo, In vivo visualization of Alzheimer's amyloid plaques by magnetic resonance imaging in transgenic mice without a contrast agent, *Magn Reson Med* **52** (2004), 1263–1271.

[17] C.R. Jack, Jr., M.M. Shiung, J.L. Gunter, P.C. O'Brien, S.D. Weigand, D.S. Knopman, B.F. Boeve, R.J. Ivnik, G.E. Smith, R.H. Cha, E.G. Tangalos and R.C. Petersen, Comparison of different MRI brain atrophy rate measures with clinical disease progression in AD, *Neurology* **62** (2004), 591–600.

[18] S. Ke, X. Wen, M. Gurfinkel, C. Charnsangavej, S. Wallace, E.M. Sevick-Muraca and C. Li, Near-infrared optical imaging of epidermal growth factor receptor in breast cancer xenografts, *Cancer Res* **63** (2003), 7870–7875.

[19] W.E. Klunk, H. Engler, A. Nordberg, Y. Wang, G. Blomqvist, D.P. Holt, M. Bergstrom, I. Savitcheva, G.F. Huang, S. Estrada, B. Ausen, M.L. Debnath, J. Barletta, J.C. Price, J. Sandell, B.J. Lopresti, A. Wall, P. Koivisto, G. Antoni, C.A. Mathis and B. Langstrom, Imaging brain amyloid in Alzheimer's disease with Pittsburgh Compound-B, *Ann Neurol* **55** (2004), 306–319.

[20] W.E. Klunk, Y. Wang, G.F. Huang, M.L. Debnath, D.P. Holt and C.A. Mathis, Uncharged thioflavin-T derivatives bind to amyloid-beta protein with high affinity and readily enter the brain, *Life Sci* **69** (2001), 1471–1484.

[21] M.P. Kung, D.M. Skovronsky, C. Hou, Z.P. Zhuang, T.L. Gur, B. Zhang, J.Q. Trojanowski, V.M. Lee and H.F. Kung, Detection of amyloid plaques by radioligands for Abeta40 and Abeta42: potential imaging agents in Alzheimer's patients, *J Mol Neurosci* **20** (2003), 15–24.

[22] C.A. Mathis, B.J. Bacskai, S.T. Kajdasz, M.E. McLellan, M.P. Frosch, B.T. Hyman, D.P. Holt, Y. Wang, G.F. Huang, M.L. Debnath and W.E. Klunk, A lipophilic thioflavin-T derivative for positron emission tomography (PET) imaging of amyloid in brain, *Bioorg Med Chem Lett* **12** (2002), 295–298.

[23] M.E. McLellan, S.T. Kajdasz, B.T. Hyman and B.J. Bacskai, In vivo imaging of reactive oxygen species specifically associated with thioflavine S-positive amyloid plaques by multiphoton microscopy, *J Neurosci* **23** (2003), 2212–2217.

[24] J. Menke, H. Stocker and W. Sibrowski, Cerebral oxygenation and hemodynamics during blood donation studied by near-infrared spectroscopy, *Transfusion* **44** (2004), 414–421.

[25] S.M. Messerli, S. Prabhakar, Y. Tang, K. Shah, M.L. Cortes, V. Murthy, R. Weissleder, X.O. Breakefield and C.H. Tung, A novel method for imaging apoptosis using a caspase-1 near-infrared fluorescent probe, *Neoplasia* **6** (2004), 95–105.

[26] A. Miyawaki, Fluorescence imaging of physiological activity in complex systems using GFP-based probes, *Curr Opin Neurobiol* **13** (2003), 591–596.

[27] K. Ohki, S. Chung, Y.H. Ch'ng, P. Kara and R.C. Reid, Functional imaging with cellular resolution reveals precise microarchitecture in visual cortex, *Nature* **433** (2005), 597–603.

[28] A. Petrovsky, E. Schellenberger, L. Josephson, R. Weissleder and A. Bogdanov, Jr., Near-infrared fluorescent imaging of tumor apoptosis, *Cancer Res* **63** , (2003), 1936–1942.

[29] J.F. Poduslo, T.M. Wengenack, G.L. Curran, T. Wisniewski, E.M. Sigurdsson, S.I. Macura, B.J. Borowski and C.R. Jack, Jr., Molecular targeting of Alzheimer's amyloid plaques for contrast-enhanced magnetic resonance imaging, *Neurobiol Dis* **11** (2002), 315–329.

[30] K. Sakatani, Y. Xie, W. Lichty, S. Li and H. Zuo, Language-activated cerebral blood oxygenation and hemodynamic changes of the left prefrontal cortex in poststroke aphasic patients: a near-infrared spectroscopy study, *Stroke* **29** (1998), 1299–1304.

[31] K. Shoghi-Jadid, G.W. Small, E.D. Agdeppa, V. Kepe, L.M. Ercoli, P. Siddarth, S. Read, N. Satyamurthy, A. Petric, S.C. Huang and J.R. Barrio, Localization of neurofibrillary tangles and beta-amyloid plaques in the brains of living patients with Alzheimer disease, *Am J Geriatr Psychiatry* **10** (2002), 24–35.

[32] A.M. Siegel, J.P. Culver, J.B. Mandeville and D.A. Boas, Temporal comparison of functional brain imaging with diffuse optical tomography and fMRI during rat forepaw stimulation, *Phys Med Biol* **48** (2003), 1391–1403.

[33] J. Skoch, A. Dunn, B.T. Hyman and B.J. Bacskai, Development of an optical approach for non-invasive imaging of Alzheimer's disease pathology, *J Biomed Opt* **10** (2005), 011007.

[34] G. Strangman, J.P. Culver, J.H. Thompson and D.A. Boas, A quantitative comparison of simultaneous BOLD fMRI and NIRS recordings during functional brain activation, *Neuroimage* **17** (2002), 719–731.

[35] Y.Z. Wadghiri, E.M. Sigurdsson, M. Sadowski, J.I. Elliott, Y. Li, H. Scholtzova, C.Y. Tang, G. Aguinaldo, M. Pap polla, K. Duff, T. Wisniewski and D.H. Turnbull, Detection of Alzheimer's amyloid in transgenic mice using magnetic resonance microimaging, *Magn Reson Med* **50** (2003), 293–302.

[36] Y. Wang, W.E. Klunk, G.F. Huang, M.L. Debnath, D.P. Holt and C.A. Mathis, Synthesis and evaluation of 2-(3'-iodo-4'-aminophenyl)-6-hydroxybenzothiazole for *in vivo* quantitation of amyloid deposits in Alzheimer's disease, *J Mol Neurosci* **19** (2002), 11–16.

[37] F.S. Wouters, P.J. Verveer and P.I. Bastiaens, Imaging biochemistry inside cells, *Trends Cell Biol* **11** (2001), 203–211.

Diagnosis of Alzheimer's disease: Two-decades of progress

Zaven S. Khachaturian
Potomac, Maryland, USA
E-mail: zaven_khachaturian@kra.net

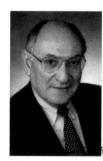

Abstract. A retrospective view of the critical events and advances in the development of criteria, instruments and algorithms in the diagnosis of Alzheimer's disease. The review is from the vantage point of the National Institute on Aging and its role in the development of the national infrastructure, in the US, for clinical research on dementia. The paper discusses future research needs and challenges for developing new diagnostic armamentarium for early and accurate detection of neurodegenerative processes of dementia in the early prodromal stages or during early mild cognitive impairments.

Keywords: Diagnosis, dementia, Alzheimer's disease, mild cognitive impairments, MCI, diagnostic criteria, biomarkers, diagnostic instruments, neuroimaging, National Institute on Aging, NIA, NIH

1. Introduction

The 1985 article in the Archives of Neurology, "*Diagnosis of Alzheimer's Disease*" [1] represents a small chapter in the prolonged efforts to characterize the distinct clinical-pathological features of Alzheimer's disease (AD). Although the study of dementia has a one hundred-year history, the attempt to address systematically the array of scientific and clinical issues related to differential diagnosis is a relatively recent phenomenon. This paper is an account of the early history of the struggles to define the disease and the more recent efforts at the National Institute on Aging (NIA)/National Institutes of Health (NIH) to establish: diagnostic criteria, standardized clinical assessment algorithms, and validated screening instruments and/or biological markers.

2. Early history

Although various forms of dementia have always been part of the human experience, the efforts for systematic description of the clinical-pathological characteristics of phenomenon gained traction in the late 1890s roughly paralleling advances in histology (chemistry of tissue stains), light microscopy, neuroanatomy and other areas of biology [2,3]. The early pioneers of the field were able to make some groundbreaking observations about dementia because of access to a wealth of new technologies for studying the brain and the emergence of vibrant academic environments that fostered interactions and cross-fertilization among psychiatrist, neurologist and neuropathologist. Reports by Blocq and Marinesco [1892] and later by Redlich [1898] began to describe the relationships between neocortical senile plaques and senile dementia. Oskar Fisher [1907] was one of the first to suggest that severity of dementia and memory loss might be associated with senile plaques. Alois Alzheimer, a psychiatrist with an abiding interest to "help psychiatry through the microscope," was among the first to exploit the newly emerging tools for histological study of the human brain. The 1907 paper by Alois Alzheimer became the index case for "Alzheimer's Disease", however the term did not receive broad endorsement until the eighth edition of Emil Kraepelin's "Textbook of Psychiatry" published in 1910.

Nearly a century later, Alzheimer's original report remains a crucial milestone in the annals of dementia research. The study approach, by Alzheimer, of combining meticulous clinical observations with systematic neuropathological analysis of brain lesions become the template for NIA's: a) strategy to develop its extramural program of research support for Alzheimer's disease and, b) program priority for promoting further interdisciplinary research on the causal relationships between the clinical-pathological phenotypes of dementia.

In the era between Alzheimer's initial report and the 1960s, the primary focus of the scholarship on dementia was the epistemology of the disease and the struggle for consensus on the clinical definitions. Progress in understanding the relationships between the behavioral expression and pathological phenotypes of dementia was relatively slow in this stage due to two impediments: first, the lack of validated standardized objective clinical assessment tools, and second, uncertainty in the definition of the clinical phenomenon.

During the two decades following WWII, arguably the start of the modern era of Alzheimer's disease (AD) research, the question of whether AD changes were simply an accentuation of normal senescence, gradually began to emerge as a central research question. The important clinical controversy revolved around the issue of whether "*presenile*" and "*senile*" dementias were the same disorder. Newton in 1948 and later Neuman and Cohn in 1953 suggested that these two forms of the disease were identical. The challenge of distinguishing brain changes due to pathology from those alterations due to healthy aging were started in a number of landmark investigations by the Blessed, Tomlinson and Roth in the mid-1960s [4]. However, the dispute could not be settled without comparisons of the clinical/biological/neuropathological phenotypes of the disease. Such comparisons became possible in the early 1960s with, the introduction of the electron microscope (EM) as a research tool, and the development of quantitative measures of dementia.

In 1963, Terry (in the US) and Kidd (in the UK) independently reported the findings of EM studies showing the ultrastructure of a single neurofibrillary tangle to contain masses of microscopic fibers with periodic structure: paired helical filaments (PHF). These landmark studies enabled the field to: 1) develop quantitative assessments of the hallmark lesions, 2) clearly delineate the ultrastructure of the amyloid core (neuritic plaque), 3) develop methods of isolating plaques, neurofibrillary tangles and preparation of enriched PHFs, and 4) set the stage for the discovery of more sophisticated molecular and immunological probes to further characterize the abnormal proteins associated with the disease. Thus, these early ultrastructural studies by Terry, Kidd and colleagues opened the door for more detailed molecular characterization of the two fibrous proteins and set the stage for the remarkable advances of the last few years in understanding the molecular neurobiology of AD.

The need for functional measures of severity and objective/quantitative tools to assess mental status was the crucial hurdles for progress in clinical/behavioral studies of this period. This problem was surmounted in 1968, with the publication of the Blessed, Tomlinson and Roth *Dementia Scale (Information-Memory-Concentration Test)*. This was an informant-based scale of memory function, orientation, information, concentration, activities of daily living, etc. The landmark prospective studies of this group for the first time correlated *quantitative measures of dementia* (cognitive and functional impairments) with estimates of the *number of the lesions* (plaques), and the volume of brain destroyed by infarcts. These efforts to quantify the relationships between the clinical and biological indices of the disease established the foundation for subsequent program initiatives and several collaborative multi-site longitudinal studies launched by NIA. In the mid-1960 to mid-1980 period, four categories of objective clinical measurement tools were developed and validated, some in longitudinal studies with autopsy confirmations. These include: *Mental Status Exams* (e.g., Dementia Scale or ICM Test-1968, Mini-Mental Status Exam -1975 [5], Short Blessed Test -1983), *Global Measures of Dementia Severity* (e.g., Clinical Dementia Rating – 1993, Global Deterioration Scale – 1982, CAMDEX -1986), Behavioral Scales (Geriatric Depression Scale – 1988, Agitation Inventory – 1986, CERAD Behavioral Rating Scale for Dementia – 1995, Clinical Impression of Global Change or CIBIC) and *Cognitive Assessment Batteries* (e.g., Alzheimer Disease Assessment Scale or ADAS-cog) [6]. The efforts to construct quantitative measures of cognition and the validation of instruments for objective evaluation of symptoms were critical to the refinements in the characterization of the disease. These advances in assessment of the severity of the disease became the foundation for much of the current "routine clinical-workup" and set the "standard" for clinical staging methods an essential element of clinical research.

While many investigators were laboring to develop objective measures for assessing the severity of symptoms, the uncertainty about the clinical "identity" of Alzheimer's diseases lingered until the 1976 editorial by Katzman [7]. This landmark paper for the first time framed Alzheimer's disease as an important public health/medical issue. The Katzman editorial was an important step towards: a) the recognition of a need for specific *diagnostic criteria* and b) reviving the argument for a common cause for late-onset and pre-senile dementia, an earlier thesis suggested by Newton [1948] and by Neuman and Cohn [1953].

Recent history: NIA initiatives on "diagnosis of Alzheimer's disease"

The recent history of efforts to improve the diagnostic armamentarium, particularly the impact of the 1985 article on *"Diagnosis of Alzheimer's Disease"*, becomes meaningful only in the context of the overall struggles to establish the neurobiology of disease program at the NIA.

The Institute was established in 1974 with an amorphous congressional authorization to address the *"problems and diseases of the aged."* But, the NIA's implicit directive was to develop and support *interdisciplinary* research on *healthy (normal) aging* as well as *disorders of aging*. In 1977, this author was recruited to translate the Institute's broad legislative directive into a specific a plan for organizing and developing a national program of research on the neurobiology of aging and AD. In the late-1970s the task of building the *"Neuroscience of Aging Program"* had to overcome a number of daunting challenges. Among these the most problematic hurdles were the: 1) lack of funds specifically targeted funds for program development, 2) rudimentary state of knowledge on diagnosis of AD, the neurobiology of aging and/or dementia, 3) low credibility of "aging research" and prevailing negative attitudes of the scientific community towards this field of study, and 4) difficulty in attracting competent new investigators into "aging" or "AD" research. Meanwhile, the efforts to develop a national program of clinical research on dementia faced additional special impediments and a more grueling uphill struggle to gain traction due to the lack of:

- consensus on diagnostic criteria
- standardized assessment instruments
- infrastructure to support longitudinal clinical studies
- expertise in clinical trials
- well characterized postmortem brain tissue for molecular studies

The strategy for addressing these challenges required NIA to adopt a different model, for developing, organizing and managing the Institutes extramural program, than those used by other well established institutes at NIH e.g., NINCDS or NIMH. The complexities of the multi-facetted problem, such as contrasting normal "aging" from "diseases of aging", required that the program structure be based on the replica of a *systems research*. This approach to program development de-emphasized disciplinary "silos" and focused on building linkages for the integration of knowledge, skills and points of views across a wide rang of disciplines. The NIA's program development efforts stressed: a) vertically integration of basic research with clinical studies, b) funding mechanisms to promote collaborative research, e.g., program projects, centers, research consortiums, c) building-up resources and infrastructure for conducting longitudinal clinical research and/or clinical trials, e.g., ADCS, and d) developing the "capabilities" of the field for clinical research, including development of diagnostic criteria, standardization of assessment tools and the methodologies of clinical trials. Thus the NIA plan to develop the nascent fields of AD and brain aging stressed the importance of not only on mechanisms of support for investigator initiated projects but also initiatives that encouraged: *coordination, organization, and infrastructure building*.

The series of *"Research Planning Workshops"*, organized by NIA since 1978, were primarily designed to solicit advice from extramural scientific community. These planning workshops were an essential tool for identifying gaps in knowledge and formulating strategies concerning new program directions. Also they served as a critical vehicle for establishing collaborating network of clinical investigator and creating the infrastructure necessary to developing standardized diagnostic procedures. The 1985 Archives of Neurology paper, which was based on the proceeding of one such *"Research Planning Workshop on Diagnosis of Alzheimer's Disease,"* was organized in December 1983. The recommendations of this workshop lead to several NIA initiatives in subsequent years and set the stage for some of today's 'hot topics'. The Neuropathology Panel of this Workshop took the first step toward defining the minimum microscopic criteria necessary for histological diagnosis of AD. The Neurology Panel suggested that the term 'Alzheimer Disease' be reserved for patients who show a compatible clinical course along with the histopathological and neurochemical changes associated with the disease. The panel also considered the problem of distinguishing

AD from benign senescent forgetfulness [MCI] and non-Alzheimer type dementia. Other topics and recommendations of this workshop included: neuroimaging, biomarkers, molecular genetics, longitudinal studies, brain banks, establishment of family registries and pedigree studies, animal models and the need for research on normal brain aging.

Prior to 1984, in the absence of specific diagnostic criteria for Alzheimer, the DSM-III (DSM-IV) criteria for diagnosis of dementia had fulfilled the requirements of clinical research [8]. Finally this need was address with the publications of the: a) "*Diagnosis of Alzheimer's Disease*" [1] and b) NINCDS-ADRDA Diagnostic Criteria [9], which specified inclusion-exclusion factors and three levels of confidence: probable, possible and definite [requiring histopathological confirmation]. Since the publication of these papers, substantial progress has been made in the accuracy, reliability, sensitivity and sophistication of diagnostic assessment instruments and algorithms. Some of the most significant contributions to current clinical knowledge on diagnosis stemmed from the early efforts to: a) refine the clinical description of the phenomenon/symptoms, b) establish clinical – pathological correlations, c) develop objective measures of behavior – psychometric assessment instrument, d) establish diagnostic criteria and standardize diagnostic procedures, e) establish infrastructure for longitudinal clinical-pathological studies and, the remarkable advances in understanding the neurobiology of dementia during the last three decades.

One of the earliest NIA initiatives to expand research on diagnosis and treatments focused on promoting the construction and validation of assessment tools specifically designed for cognitive changes in several domains. The best know example of this was the proposal funded in 1978 which resulted in the development of the Alzheimer's disease Assessment Scale (ADAS) published in 1984 [6]. Other strategies were required to address issues in the development of diagnostic criteria, standardization of assessment tools and the methodologies of clinical trials. Thus the mid-1980s were a watershed period for Alzheimer's research in general but in particular for improvements in the technologies for diagnosis. In 1984 several concurrent developments enabled multi-site collaborative clinical studies, these included: a) Alzheimer's Disease Centers provided necessary research infrastructure, b) Standardized cognitive assessment instruments and global measured of dementia severity were introduced [ADAS, CDR, CIBIC], c) NINCDS-ADRDA criteria provided a systematic clinical diagnostic system supporting comparisons across centers, d) Glenner and Wong identified amyloid, e) Consortium to Establish Registries for Alzheimer's disease (CERAD) (1987), and f) Alzheimer's Disease Cooperative Study (ADCS) (1991).

Once the challenges of developing diagnostic criteria and objective assessment instruments were overcome, the next major impediment for clinical research was the effort to 1) *validate* the diagnostic criteria with histopathological confirmations; thus the need for neuropathologic criteria, 2) *standardize* (reliability, sensitivity, specificity) various clinical assessment instruments, and 3) *construct* new measurements for changes in behaviors, symptoms of various domains of cognition. The availability of standardized, well-validated quantitative assessment instruments were indispensable prerequisites for NIA's subsequent initiatives [e.g., Centers Program; CERAD; ADCS; ADNI etc].

To address the long-term strategic goal of developing treatments, it was necessary for NIA to build a) mechanisms for promoting collaborative research, b) the capability of the field to conduct longitudinal clinical research and clinical trials and c) infrastructure for clinical research. The NIA began to create the necessary national research infrastructure. The Alzheimer's Disease Research Centers (ADRCs), established in 1984 and the Alzheimer's Disease Core Centers (ADCCs), established in 1990, were central components of the research and capability infrastructure. These programs referred to as the Alzheimer's Disease Centers or ADCs provide the infrastructure for integrating clinical and basic science research and allowed the augmentation of a wide range of studies on the etiology and pathogenesis of AD. In 1991 the 'Satellite Clinics' program was established to fund outreach to underserved or rural patient groups now Satellites are an integral part of many ADCs.

The 'Alzheimer's Disease Patient Registry' Program (ADPR) was launched in 1986 to address the goal of developing standardized diagnostic assessments. This program included the Consortium to Establish a Registry for AD (CERAD) led by Al Heyman and Gerda Fillenbarum, the Mayo Clinic Registry led by Len Kurland and Ron Peterson, the Seattle site led by Eric Larson, the Mon valley project with Lewis Kuller and Mary Ganguli, and Denis Evans's group in East Boston. The CERAD project was successful in establishing uniform methods for the diagnosis and assessment of AD because of the dedicated and effective leadership provided by Al Heyman and the cooperation of clinicians and investigators nation and worldwide. The ADPR program overall was instrumental in the development of assessment instruments and procedures but also in filling gaps the epidemiology of AD [10,11].

During the following two decades the improvements in the accuracy of the clinical diagnosis were remarkable. The procedures for clinical assessment steadily advanced towards well-validated algorithms for identification of positive clinical phenotypes of the diseases. Early diagnosis has become one of the most important clinical accomplishments with profound implications for: 1) research, 2) establishing the prevalence of AD, 3) initiating treatment when it may have optimal benefit, and 4) understanding the pathobiology of the disease. For example, the original cholinergic hypothesis was based on neuropathologic material from end-stage AD patients. Now that AD is diagnosed earlier, some investigators [e.g., Ken Davis and Steve DeKosky] have suggested that simple cholinergic hypofunction may not be a feature of the initial stages.

The introduction of the construct of "*mild cognitive impairment (MCI)*" as a potential precursor or prodrome of the disease was another significant milepost [11]. Several groups (e.g., Barry Reisberg, Steve Ferris and the NYU group, Thomas Crook at NIMH, Ron Petersen and the Mayo Clinic group, Marilyn Albert and the MGH group, and John Morris and the Washington University group) contributed to efforts to improve the definitions and algorithms for distinguishing the early stages, MCI, from non-demented aging and in characterizing border zone conditions.

The notion of prodromal stages of the disease energized the current explorations for early biomarkers. Advances in molecular neurobiology and emerging imaging technologies promise to provide much needed surrogate markers to detect and/or monitor progression during the early clinically asymptomatic stages. The classification of degenerative dementias is moving rapidly, not just toward diagnostic and prognostic biomarkers, but toward antecedent biomarkers; a system of categorization based on combined behavioral and protein abnormalities (e.g., amyloidopathy, tauopathies, synuceinopathies and prion protein disorders). The potential value of an amyloid imaging compound [Pittsburgh Compound] for early diagnosis was recently demonstrated by Bill Klunk and Chet Mathis (Pittsburgh), Henry Engler (Stockholm) and collaborators from Uppsala and Boston with their success in imagining $A\beta$-containing lesions in the living human brain.

The prospects that validated molecular and biochemical markers may soon complement clinical approaches in making early and valid diagnoses are very good [12]. However, any potential biomarker must detect a fundamental biological feature of the disease and be validated in neuropathologic confirmed cases prior to routine clinical use. Presently none of the many [proposed] putative bio-markers have been validated in adequately powered investigations. Recent advances in neuroimaging technologies [e.g., Pittsburgh Compound with PET] offer the potential to detect and follow longitudinally the clinical course of the disease. In the future, it might be possible for neuroimaging technologies, perhaps MRI, to allow more direct monitoring of some biological phenotypes of the disease (e.g., brain metabolic changes, $A\beta$, Tau, synapse loss or cell death via PET and other structural changes). In contrast to neuropsychological measurements, imaging measurements, when validated, will allow the more proximal brain changes associated with disease progression to be followed over time.

There is a general consensus that many of the advances in diagnosis, treatment(s), care and understanding the cause(s) would not have been possible without the creation of instruments, criteria, infrastructure and programs that support interdisciplinary research. Some of the spectacular clinical and research strides attributable in some measure to the NIA initiatives include:

– improvements in antimortem and postmortem diagnosis
– access to samples of blood, DNA, CSF and postmortem tissues from well-characterized patients for basic and clinical research
– advances in understanding the neurobiology of the normal aging brain, as well as the mechanisms of AD and related neurodegenerative diseases
– capacity to pool data on large cohorts of research participants through the NACC, for example, the landmark cooperative study assessing the diagnostic impact of the *APOE ε4* allele in the evaluation of dementia patients
– insights into the role of immune mechanisms, the complement cascade, proteases, glia, head trauma, etc. in the pathogenesis of dementing disorders
– benefits of NIA's "team science" are reflected in the sharing of data and samples fostered by the Alzheimer's Disease Centers network, Alzheimer Disease Cooperative Study and the National Alzheimer Disease Coordinating Center and the productivity of these groups.

3. Prospects for the future

- Only *thirty years* ago AD was regarded as a hopelessly untreatable condition. Except for a handful of investigators, the area attracted little interest and virtually no support for research.
- *Twenty five* years ago, the essential clinical infrastructures for longitudinal studies of well-characterized patients did not exist.
- *Twenty* years ago, ideas about "cure" and "prevention" were unconceivable; such things as diagnostic criteria, standardized assessment instruments, cadres of specialized professionals, memory disorder clinics, family support groups or outreach programs, all taken for granted now, were not fully developed.
- *Fifteen years* ago, the knowledge on biological underpinnings and the genes associated with the disease had not been identified.
- *Ten years* ago, animal models of the disease were not available.
- *Five years* ago, persons risk for the disease could not be identified and the concept of clinical trials to delay the symptoms was unconceivable.
- Until 2004, the $A\beta$ protein, hallmark lesions of the disease, could not be directly visualized in patients.

Today, the field is on the brink of major breakthroughs that may lead to more effective treatments and, ultimately, to prevention. A great deal has been learned about the pathogenesis of neurodegeneration, after less than three decades. Novel intervention strategies are being developed to ameliorate the neuro-toxicity caused by abnormal metabolic products and prevent processes that lead to cell death. A large number of clinical trials are underway, both industry and government (NIA-ADCS) sponsored studies, with widely-used drugs (e.g., antioxidants, anti-inflammatory agents, statins, vitamins and folate) that might reduce the risk of AD. Intensive studies are underway on multiple fronts, from basic science to genetics to drug therapy to care giving. Recent public policy initiatives on disease prevention and the gradual shift of emphasis in drug discovery research, toward disease modification, have underscored the need for validated surrogate markers of AD. However, the major impediment to prevention or interventions to slow disease progression remains to be the lack of a positive and validated marker or the technology for early and accurate detection of the prodromal neurodegenerative processes. The recently launched NIA "Alzheimer's Disease Neuroimaging Initiative" (ADNI) is the much needed strategy to address this critical need.

The remarkable progress towards understanding AD and the improved prospect of discovering disease modifying therapies would not have been possible without the: 1) worldwide network of investigators working closely and collaboratively, 2) research infrastructure established by NIA and, 3) the successful partnership between the NIA Alzheimer's Association. Now these partnerships need to be expanded to include industry, foundations and individual philanthropists. The goal for such public-private working partnership is to mobilize all the necessary international resource for a new initiative to discovery [and/or develop] of interventions to prevent the disease. Time is running out; the epidemic of AD will completely overwhelm the health care system due to the substantial growth in the numbers of people with AD. The demographic changes, resulting from the continuing increases in the life expectancy of the oldest-old, are going to have their full impact in 20 to 30 years from now. The projected costs in human suffering and lost opportunities will be incalculable and unthinkable.

References

[1] Z.S. Khachaturian, Diagnosis of Alzheimer's disease, *Arch Neurol* **42**(11) (1985), 1097–1105.
[2] N.C. Berchtold and C.W. Cotman, Evolution in the conceptualization of dementia and Alzheimer's disease: Greco-Roman period to the 1960s, *Neurobiol Aging* **19**(3) (1998), 173–189.
[3] T.G. Beach, The history of Alzheimer's disease: three debates, *J Hist Med Allied Sci* **42**(3) (1987), 327–349.
[4] G. Blessed, B.E. Tomlinson and M. Roth, The association between quantitative measures of dementia and of senile change in the cerebral grey matter of elderly subjects, *British Journal of Psychiatry* **114** (1968), 797–811.
[5] M.F. Folstein, S.E. Folstein and P.R. McHugh, Mini-Mental state. A practical method for grading the cognitive state of patients for the clinician, *Journal of Psychiatric Research* **12** (1975), 189–198.
[6] W.G. Rosen, R.C. Mohs and K.L. Davis, A new rating scale for Alzheimer's disease, *Am J Psychiatry* **141**(11) (1984), 1356–1364.
[7] R. Katzman, Editorial: The prevalence and malignancy of Alzheimer disease. A major killer, *Arch Neurol* **33**(4) (1976), 217–218.
[8] Diagnostic and Statistical Manual of Mental Disorders. 1987. Third Edition-Revised. 3 ed. Washington, D.C.: American Psychiatric Association
[9] G. McKhann, D. Drachman, M. Folstein, R. Katzman, D. Price and E.M. Stadlan, Clinical diagnosis of Alzheimer's disease: report of the NINCDS-ADRDA Work Group under the auspices of Department of Health and Human Services Task Force on Alzheimer's Disease, *Neurology* **34**(7) (1984), 939–944.

[10] S. Mirra, A. Heyman, D. McKeel, S.M. Sumi, B.J. Crain, L.M. Brownlee et al., The Consortium to Establish a Registry for Alzheimer's Disease (CERAD). Part II. Standardization of the neuropathologic assessment of Alzheimer's disease, *Neurology* **41**(4) (1991), 479–486.

[11] R.C. Petersen, Mild cognitive impairment: transition between aging and Alzheimer's disease, *Neurologia* **15**(3) (2000), 93–101.

[12] Consensus Report of the Work Group, Molecular and Biochemical Markers of Alzheimer's Disease, The Ronald and Nancy Reagan Research Institute of the Alzheimer's Association and the National Institute on Aging Work Group, *Neurobiol Aging* **19** (1998), 109–116.

Consensus guidelines for the clinical and pathologic diagnosis of dementia with Lewy bodies (DLB): Report of the Consortium on DLB International Workshop

Ian G. McKeith
Wolfson Research Centre, Institute for Ageing and Health, Newcastle General Hospital, Newcastle upon Tyne, NE4 6BE, UK
E-mail: i.g.mckeith@ncl.ac.uk

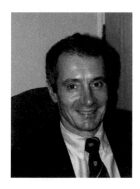

Abstract. Dementia with Lewy bodies (DLB) was considered to be an uncommon cause of dementia until improved neuropathological staining methods for ubiquitin were developed in the late 1980's. Subsequent recognition that 10–15% of dementia cases in older people were associated with Lewy body pathology led to the publication in 1996 of Consensus clinical and pathological diagnostic criteria for the disorder. These have greatly raised global awareness of DLB and helped to generate a body of knowledge which informs modern clinical management of this pharmacologically sensitive group of patients. They have also enabled important issues surrounding the relationships of DLB with Alzheimer's disease and Parkinson's disease to be addressed and partially resolved. A recent re-evaluation of the Consensus criteria has confirmed many aspects of the original recommendations, supplementing these with suggestions for improved pathological characterisation, clinical detection and management. Virtu-ally unrecognised 20 years ago, DLB could within this decade be one of the best characterised and potentially treatable neurodegenerative disorders of late life.

Keywords: Dementia with Lewy bodies, diagnosis

1. Background

This ambitiously titled paper [1] appeared in Neurology in November 1996 as an account of the "First International Workshop on Dementia with Lewy Bodies (DLB)" which Elaine and Robert Perry and I had organised in Newcastle upon Tyne in October 1995. We took this initiative for several reasons. Research into Lewy body (LB) related dementia had started to gain momentum during the previous 4 or 5 years with the publication of several articles about small series of patients who had a clinical history of dementia and neuropathological findings of cortical and sub-cortical LBs [2–9]. Similar case reports had been appearing in the literature since the 1960s [10] and some would argue even earlier [11–13]. Kosaka's group in Japan had been developing a spectrum model of Lewy body disease since the late 1970s [14,15] but it was generally considered to be an uncommon, if not rare, cause of dementia in old age. Clinical details of these early cases were often fairly limited.

A sudden upsurge of interest in LBs and dementia was triggered by the realisation that the combination might be more common than previously supposed. This coincided with the introduction of anti-ubiquitin immunocytochemistry as a sensitive way to visualise cortical LB [16]. In the early 1990s, the various groups most interested in the disorder (in Yokohama, San Diego, New York, Nottingham and Newcastle) were starting to diverge in developing concepts and terminology about what were in all probability the same group of patients. This was a potentially damaging trend. For LB dementia research to advance rapidly it needed a collaborative approach and a common brand. This was the prime mover behind "DLB1" as the First International Workshop is now known.

The outputs of DLB1 were the Consensus Guidelines paper and a edited book comprising chapters from 94 contributors who attended the meeting [17]. Looking back at the reports it is clear that the clinicians in the group were motivated to generate diagnostic criteria in the hope that the majority LB pathology cases might be detected by purely clinical methods. The pathologists by contrast wanted to agree a framework of methods for assessing and reporting LB and Lewy related pathologies without committing themselves to defining diagnostic categories. They succeeded in describing three patterns of LB disease (brainstem predominant, limbic [transitional] and neocortical) based upon semi-quantitative LB counts and they dealt with the ever troublesome issue of concomitant Alzheimer pathology (predominantly amyloid plaques, less frequently tangles) by saying that its presence should be documented and its significance was unclear. Brain areas to be examined were specified in detail, but staining methods for LB were left optional (H&E or anti-ubiquitin). The term DLB was agreed by all parties because it was agnostic as to the causative role of LB in symptom formation and because the term had not been used previously so "belonged" to the group rather than to any one of the participating players. Coalescing the various terms in use at the time under the one umbrella DLB, was probably the single most important step to secure acceptance of the disorder. Despite being a little unwieldy and containing the word "dementia" which is disliked by many, DLB has been adopted globally and the abbreviation seems useable by clinicians, carers and patients alike. It has made it possible to use standard criteria to recruit patients into clinical and neuroimaging trials and other investigative studies with a 30 fold expansion of published literature over the last ten years.

2. Immediate reaction

The 1996 paper was written within six months of the DLB1 meeting and published six months after that. Reaction was mixed. DLB appeared on the scene as a new "type" of dementia just at the time when clinicians and researchers had finally become comfortable with the idea that Alzheimer's disease (AD) and multi-infarct dementia (MID) as it was then called, were the two common causes of dementia and that other types were relatively uncommon or rare. DSM III and ICD 9 confirmed this view as did the major textbooks. It was bad enough to rock the boat by suggesting that a third common cause of dementia might exist (we suggested 10–15% of all elderly cases) and that even in expert hands relatively large numbers of people with DLB were probably being (mis)diagnosed as having AD or MID [18]. But even worse was the implication that our understanding of those two disorders was also imperfect. DLB was therefore an unwelcome newcomer. Clinicians dealing only or predominantly with dementia seemed to have less difficulty with the concept and quickly recognised patients in their own clinics who showed fluctuating cognition and consciousness, recurrent visual hallucinations and spontaneous motor parkinsonism. The associated features of syncope, falls and neuroleptic sensitivity reactions were also often familiar to them. The strongest rejections of DLB as a discrete entity came from two sources. The first was the research community itself. Several clinico-pathological "validation" studies were published shortly after the Consensus paper showing that although the clinical criteria had high specificity for predicting LB pathology at autopsy, their sensitivity to detect cases was very low, as low as 0% in some reports [19,20]. The interpretation was either that the clinical criteria were inadequate or that cortical LB were poor predictors of a dementia syndrome. A second source of rejection was from some Parkinson's disease (PD) clinicians who felt that DLB was simply a variant or late manifestation of that condition. The publication of the 1996 Consensus paper was designed to consolidate knowledge and advance the position of DLB. With hindsight it also had the effect of crystallising scientific and dogma-based rebuttals and it was in response to these that the real advances have followed.

3. Why did the DLB concept prosper?

Before moving to a quick review of the new information that has accumulated since DLB1, it is also important to acknowledge some other factors bearing on the "DLB or not-DLB" debate. The observation that DLB patients were susceptible to severe neuroleptic sensitivity reactions [21] and that these carried a

2–3 fold mortality risk was a powerful argument for taking DLB seriously. Unsurprisingly this observation has never been formally tested in a randomised clinical trial, although it has been reproduced [22–24]. The suggestion was also made, based upon post-mortem neurochemical pathological findings, that DLB patients might be particularly responsive to cholinesterase inhibitors (CHEIs) [25]. This soon found empirical support in case reports of patients enrolled in early trials of CHEI in AD who responded well to treatment and who turned out at autopsy to have DLB pathology [26, 27]. These reports combined two compelling pieces of evidence; a) that DLB cases were out there and being misdiagnosed as AD even when rigorous trial criteria were being applied and b) that they were capable of being good CHEI responders. An early open-label treatment of PDD patients with the CHEI tacrine reported spectacular cognitive and psychiatric improvements [28] that generated a brief *déja-vu* of the movie "Awakenings" and the race was on to set up the first trials of CHEIs in DLB patients. All of this was happening upon the background of a dementia field that was advancing very rapidly, producing a climate in which new ideas were more likely to be accepted than previously. New discoveries in molecular genetics were for example revolutionising our understanding of AD and the early cholinesterase inhibitor treatment trials were beginning to report some success.

4. Major advances following the publication of the 1996 paper

A systematic review of the DLB literature in 2005 is outside the scope of this article (and I suspect now beyond the scope of this author!) An attempt at such, published last year [29] was Lancet Neurology's most downloaded article of the year with 4420 requests, a good 1000 more than the second most requested. This suggests that we have not yet managed to keep up with the demand for information about DLB from clinical and non-clinical scientists and the general public. Advances in the last ten years that were identified in that review include a better understanding of the role of AD- type pathology. While some cases of DLB have little or none, it is a common feature in most. The 1996 paper suggested that the precise terminology used to describe AD-type pathology should be considered less important than the need to establish a common protocol for assessing and evaluating it. This approach, appropriate at the time, has probably exaggerated concerns about the diagnostic specificity and sensitivity of the clinical diagnostic criteria for DLB in predicting pathology because of uncertainty about the significance of the co-existing AD-type pathology that is so often seen.

A more productive view is that the likelihood that a patient has the DLB clinical syndrome is directly related to the severity of Lewy-related pathology, and is inversely related to the severity of concurrent AD-type pathology. This is consistent with the observations that "pure" DLB cases without any significant Alzheimer pathology are highly likely to have DLB core symptoms whereas those with high Braak stage AD changes are not [30]. Neocortical neurofibrillary tangles in particular alter the clinical profile to look more like AD with prominent amnestic symptoms, reducing the probability of fluctuation, visual hallucinations and parkinsonism [30–32]. The collollary of this is that a significant number of LB pathology cases will lack these core features and be extremely difficult to recognise clinically. This explains at least in part the apparently poor results of the early clinico-pathological validation studies referred to above and one reason why many clinicians still feel that they are poor at diagnosing DLB. It is not they who are lacking in their powers of observation, nor are the clinical diagnostic criteria incorrect. It is simply that not all DLB patients present with one typical picture.

5. Improved case detection

To detect these less typical cases additional pieces of clinical evidence are required, e.g. a history of REM sleep behaviour disorder (RBD) [33] or of severe neuroleptic sensitivity. Even so, not all DLB cases are going to be identifiable by clinical history and examination and biomarkers are needed to improve diagnostic sensitivity . The most promising of these so far are neuro-imaging methods, particularly those labelling the dopamine transporter site in the basal ganglia [34, 35]. Scintigraphy with [I-123]metaiodobenzyl guanidine ([I-123] (MIBG) which enables the quantification of postganglionic sympathetic cardiac innervation, is reduced in DLB has also been suggested to have high sensitivity and specificity in the differential diagnosis from AD [36,37]. Other imaging investigations can also be helpful including preservation of hippocampal and medial temporal lobe volume on MRI [38,39], atrophy of the putamen [40] and occipital hypoperfusion (SPECT) and hypometabolism (PET) [41–45] without occipital atrophy on MRI [46]. Other features such as the degree of generalised atrophy, rate of progressive brain atrophy and severity of white matter lesions do not aid in differential diagnosis from other dementia subtypes [47,48]. There are as yet no clinically applicable genotypic or CSF markers to support a diagnosis of DLB [29].

Identifying cortical LBs with traditional staining methods such as hematoxylin and eosin (H&E) is rather like looking for needles in a haystack. The development of ubiquitin immunohistochemistry, which unequivocally stains LBs and Lewy neurites (LNs) undoubtedly contributed to the "discovery" of DLB as common in the late1990s and was then recommended as the staining method of choice. However in cases with concurrent AD-type pathology, ubiquitin is also present in NFTs, which can be easily confused with LBs. Immunohistochemical staining for alpha-synuclein has therefore emerged as the most sensitive and specific method currently available for detecting LBs and Lewy-related pathology. Using such sensitive methods Lewy-related pathology has also been reported as frequently present in the amygdala and periamygdaloid cortex in AD [49] calling into question yet again the significance of LB in determining clinical phenotype. In these cases the amygdala is the only brain region so affected and the alpha-synuclein may simply represent a late-stage secondary change in neurones already metabolically overwhelmed by tau deposition and tangle formation [50]. Determining the presence of alpha-synuclein pathology in the amygdala in other dementias is a research priority.

6. Lewy body disease as a spectrum disorder

Most parties now accept that DLB represents one part of a spectrum of neurodegenerative disorders that share dysregulation and aggregation of alpha-synuclein. The clinical manifestations of LB disease include DLB, PD, and autonomic failure. Multiple system atrophy (MSA) is a related alpha-synucleinopathy in which LB formation is not seen. Drawing a distinction between these clinical syndromes is helpful in the clinic but less logical to laboratory researchers interested in understanding mechanisms of disease. The 1996 paper partially addressed the DLB/PD relationship in a straightforward way by suggesting that the temporal sequence of appearance of symptoms should determine diagnostic category. It was recommended that DLB should be diagnosed when dementia occurred before or concurrently with parkinsonism and PDD should be used to describe dementia that occurred in the context of PD which had already been present for twelve months or more. This now infamous "12 month rule" was acknowledged as being an arbitrary convenience and remains that to this day. Adoption of other (longer) time periods has been suggested but would simply serve to confound attempts at data pooling or comparison between research samples or studies. It has to be admitted that the classification of LB disorders/alpha-synucleinopathies remains unresolved and we should accept that different approaches work in different situations. A unitary approach may be preferable for molecular and genetic studies and for developing therapeutics whereas descriptive labels that include consideration of the temporal course (DLB, PDD) are preferred for clinical, operational definitions. The best term depends upon the clinical situation and generic terms such as LB disease are often helpful.

7. Genetics

It is clear from several case studies that familial cases of DLB occur [51,52] and that LBs are commonly seen in familial cases of AD [53]. There are recent reports that triplication of the alpha-synuclein gene (SNCA) can cause DLB, PD and PDD whereas gene duplication is associated only with motor PD suggesting a gene dose effect [54]. However, SCNA multiplication is not found in most LB disease patients [55]. Continued clinical, pathological and genetic evaluation of familial cases of DLB and AD is therefore an important and potential highly informative area for continued research.

8. Clinical advances

Probably one of the most important consequences of the paper was that publication of operationalised clinical diagnostic criteria meant that DLB patients could be recruited into clinical studies, in particular imaging studies and treatment trials. The imaging studies have shown possibilities to improve case detection and open label studies have demonstrated the effectiveness of all three generally available CHEIs in DLB and PDD. Placebo controlled trial data is only available to date for rivastigmine [56,57]. The reported reduction in symptom frequency and intensity of VH appears to be mediated at least in part by improved attentional function and the presence of VH is associated with greater cognitive improvement [58]. Side effects of hypersalivation, lacrimation, and urinary frequency may occur, in addition to the usual gastro-intestinal symptoms and a dose dependent exacerbation of extrapyramidal motor features may occur in a minority [59] The number of patients entered into trials has however been modest and neither DLB nor PDD are yet recognised indications for CHEIs. As a result prescribing remains off-licence and in some localities is actively discouraged by funding restrictions, formulary committees or other guidelines.

9. Patients, families and carers

For families dealing with DLB the recognition that the clinical picture and burden of care is different for them compared with AD sufferers is a major step forward. But it carries with it many frustrations, not least that they often are more aware of DLB than their professional carers. The Alzheimer and Parkinson's Associations and Societies, nationally and internationally provide rapid access via the internet to a growing range of fact-sheets and other sources of information about DLB. More recently a carer -based organisation specifically for Lewy body dementia has been established offering on-line communication with other families and providing more detailed and up to date information. The range of topics about which DLB sufferers and their carers need to know is extensive. In addition to the fluctuating cognitive impairments which predominantly affect attention and visuo-perceptual abilities, there may also be psychiatric and behavioural abnormalities, motor deficits, autonomic dysfunction and sleep disorders. How to impart such a diverse range of facts without instilling pessimistic anticipation of the worst is truly a challenge. The reality is that many of these symptoms of DLB are amenable to treatment, often but not always pharmacological. As treatment guidelines for DLB emerge, clinicians should become more confident about prescribing not only single therapies but combing them to target all symptoms identified by patient and carer as troublesome enough to warrant intervention.

10. The future of DLB

If so much progress has been made in the last decade, what can be hoped for in the next? The ideal would be a drug which significantly interrupted the pathological processing of alpha-synuclein and other proteins, arresting the neurodegenerative process. A useful clinical objective would be for our clinical diagnostic methods to have improved to such a point that patients with DLB were reliably identifiable in the earliest stages of disease when application of such a treatment would be of most benefit. If one makes analogy with the current status of amnestic mild cognitive impairment (MCI) as a predictor for AD, it is clear that defining the MCI equivalent of LB disease is likely to be a difficult task. Research effort needs to be directed towards early detection of LB disease, likely using biological markers such as dopamine transporter imaging in patients showing evidence of possible early symptoms. For those with established DLB we need better symptomatic treatments. This may involve new drug discovery but there is huge scope for improvement in the management of individual patients using tailored regimes of currently available medications. Specialist clinics for DLB patients may be one way to deliver these, and they could be embedded within existing provision for people with dementia or movement disorders.

One of the most important aspects of the 1996 paper was that it had impact on several fronts – clinical practice, clinical and laboratory research, dementia and movement disorder communities. A second report was published in 1999 [60] which reviewed the accumulating literature and made a few minor modifications to the clinical criteria. It performed a useful holding function while the exciting developments briefly outlined above were taking place. In October 2003 the Consortium on DLB met for the third time and significant amendments to the clinical and pathological guidelines were agreed and treatment recommendations offered for the first time [61]. These have been framed in response to critical reviews of "DLB1" with the aims of improving diagnostic reliability and sensitivity, clarifying the nature of relationships with AD and PD and recognising the broader concepts of LB disease/alpha-synucleinopathy. The hope is to maintain the pace of advance that followed the 1996 paper. Virtually unrecognised 20 years ago, DLB could within this decade be one of the best characterised and potentially treatable neurodegenerative disorders of late life.

References

[1] I.G. McKeith, D. Galasko, K. Kosaka et al., Consensus guidelines for the clinical and pathologic diagnosis of dementia with Lewy bodies (DLB): Report of the consortium on DLB international workshop, *Neurology* **47** (1996), 1113–1124.

[2] G. Lennox, J. Lowe, E.J. Byrne, M. Landon, R.J. Mayer and R.B. Godwin-Austen, Diffuse Lewy body disease, *Lancet* **11** (February 1989), 323–324.

[3] W.R.G. Gibb, M.M. Esiri and A.J. Lees, Clinical and pathological features of diffuse cortical Lewy body disease (Lewy body dementia), *Brain* **110** (1987), 1131–1153.

[4] C.R. Burkhardt, C.M. Filley, B.K. Kleinschmidt-DeMasters, S. de la Monte, M.D. Norenberg and S.A. Schneck, Diffuse Lewy body disease and progressive dementia, *Neurology* **38** (1988), 1520–1528.

[5] E.J. Byrne, G. Lennox, J. Lowe and R.B. Godwin-Austen, Diffuse Lewy body disease: clinical features in 15 cases, *Journal of Neurology, Neurosurgery and Psychiatry* **52** (1989), 709–717.

[6] R.H. Perry, D. Irving, G. Blessed, E.K. Perry and A.F. Fairbairn, Clinically and neuropathologically distinct form of dementia in the elderly, *Lancet* **21** (January 1989), 166.

[7] H.A. Crystal, D.W. Dickson, J.E. Lizardi, P. Davies and L.I. Wolfson, Antemortem diagnosis of diffuse Lewy body disease, *Neurology* **40** (1990), 1523–1528.

[8] L. Hansen, D. Salmon, D. Galasko et al., The Lewy body variant of Alzheimer's disease: A clinical and pathologic entity, *Neurology* **40** (1990), 1–8.

[9] I.G. McKeith, R.H. Perry, A.F. Fairbairn, S. Jabeen and E.K. Perry, Operational criteria for senile dementia of Lewy body type (SDLT), *Psychological Medicine* **22** (1992), 911–922.

[10] H. Okazaki, L.E. Lipkin and S.M. Aronson, Diffuse intracytoplasmic ganglionic inclusions (Lewy type) associated with progressive dementia and quadriparesis in flexion, *Journal of Neuropathology and Experimental Neurology* **20** (1961), 237–244.

[11] I. McKeith, Dementia with Lewy bodies: a clinical overview, in: *Dementia*, A. Burns, O.B. JT and D A, eds, London: Arnold, 2005.

[12] J.S. Woodard, Concentric hyaline inclusion body formation in mental disease: analysis of twenty-seven cases, *Journal of Neuropathology and Experimental Neurology* **21** (1962), 442–449.

[13] R. Hassler, Zur pathologie der paralysis agitans und des postenzephalitischen Parkinsonismus, *Journal f.Psychologie und Neurologie* **48** (1938), 387–476.

[14] K. Kosaka, M. Yoshimura, K. Ikeda and H. Budka, Diffuse type of Lewy body disease: progressive dementia with abundant cortical Lewy bodies and senile changes of varying degree – A new disease? *Clinical Neuropathology* **3**(5) (1984), 185–192.

[15] K. Kosaka, Lewy bodies in cerebral cortex. Report of three cases, *Acta Neuropathologica* **42** (1978), 127–134.

[16] G. Lennox, J. Lowe, M. Landon, E.J. Byrne, R.J. Mayer and R.B. Godwin-Austen, Diffuse Lewy body disease: correlative neuropathology using anti-ubiquitin immunocytochemistry, *Journal of Neurology, Neurosurgery and Psychiatry* **52** (1989), 1236–1247.

[17] R. Perry, I. McKeith and E. Perry, *Dementia with Lewy Bodies*, New York: Cambridge University Press, 1996.

[18] I.G. McKeith, A.F. Fairbairn, R.H. Perry and P. Thompson, The clinical diagnosis and misdiagnosis of senile dementia of Lewy body type (SDLT), *British Journal of Psychiatry* **165** (1994), 324–332.

[19] O.L. Lopez, I. Litvan, K.E. Catt et al., Accuracy of four clinical diagnostic criteria for the diagnosis of neurodegenerative dementias, *Neurology* **53** (1999), 1292–1299.

[20] I. Litvan, A. MacIntyre, C.G. Goetz et al., Accuracy of the clinical diagnoses of Lewy body disease, Parkinson's disease, and dementia with Lewy bodies, *Archives of Neurology* **55** (1998), 969–978.

[21] I. McKeith, A. Fairbairn, R. Perry, P. Thompson and E. Perry, Neuroleptic sensitivity in patients with senile dementia of Lewy body type, *British Medical Journal* **305** (1992), 673–678.

[22] D. Aarsland, C. Ballard, J.P. Larsen, I. McKeith, J. O'Brien and R. Perry, Marked neuroleptic sensitivity in dementia with Lewy bodies and Parkinson's disease, *J Clin Psychiatry* **66**(5) (2005), 633–637.

[23] C. Ballard, J. Grace, I. McKeith and C. Holmes, Neuroleptic sensitivity in dementia with Lewy bodies and Alzheimer's disease, *Lancet* **351** (1998), 1032–1033.

[24] J. Grace, C. Ballard and I.G. McKeith, Neuroleptic sensitivity in dementia with Lewy bodies (DLB) and Alzheimer's disease (AD), *Fifth International Geneva/Springfield Symposium on Advances in Alzheimer Therapy* (1998) 144.

[25] E.K. Perry, I. McKeith, P. Thompson et al., Topography, extent, and clinical relevance of neurochemical deficits in dementia of Lewy body type, Parkinson's disease and Alzheimer's disease, *Annals of the New York Academy of Sciences* **640** (1991), 197–202.

[26] G.K. Wilcock and M.I. Scott, Tacrine for senile dementia of Alzheimer's or Lewy body type, *Lancet* **344** (1994), 544.

[27] R. Levy, S. Eagger, M. Griffiths et al., Lewy bodies and response to tacrine in Alzheimer's disease, *Lancet* **343** (1994), 176.

[28] M. Hutchinson and E. Fazzini, Cholinesterase inhibitors in Parkinson's disease, *Journal of Neurology, Neurosurgery and Psychiatry* **61** (1996), 324–325.

[29] I. McKeith, J. Mintzer, D. Aarsland et al., Dementia with Lewy bodies, *Lancet Neurology* **3** (2004), 19–28.

[30] A.R. Merdes, L.A. Hansen, D.V. Jeste et al., Influence of Alzheimer pathology on clinical diagnostic accuracy in dementia with Lewy bodies, *Neurology* **60**(10) (2003), 1586–1590.

[31] T. Del Ser, V. Hachinski, H. Merskey and D.G. Munoz, Clinical and pathologic features of two groups of patients with dementia with Lewy bodies: Effect of coexisting Alzheimer-type lesion load, *Alzheimer Disease & Associated Disorders* **15**(1) (2001), 31–44.

[32] C.G. Ballard, R. Jacoby, T. Del Ser et al., Neuropathological substrates of psychiatric symptoms in prospectively studied patients with autopsy-confirmed dementia with Lewy bodies, *American Journal of Psychiatry* **161**(5) (2004), 843–849.

[33] B.F. Boeve, M.H. Silber and T.J. Ferman, REM sleep behavior disorder in Parkinson's disease and dementia with Lewy bodies, *Journal of Geriatric Psychiatry and Neurology* **17**(3) (2004), 146–157.

[34] Z. Walker, D.C. Costa, R.W.H. Walker et al., Striatal dopamine transporter in dementia with Lewy bodies and Parkinson disease – A comparison, *Neurology* **62**(9) (2004), 1568–1572.

[35] J.T. O'Brien, S.J. Colloby, J. Fenwick et al., Dopamine transporter loss visualised with FP-CIT SPECT in Dementia with Lewy bodies, *Archives of Neurology* **61**(6) (2004), 919–925.

[36] M. Yoshita, J. Taki and M. Yamada, A clinical role for I-123 MIBG myocardial scintigraphy in the distinction between dementia of the Alzheimer's-type and dementia with Lewy bodies, *Journal of Neurology Neurosurgery and Psychiatry* **71**(5) (2001), 583–588.

[37] J. Taki, M. Yoshita, M. Yamada and N. Tonami, Significance of I-123-MIBG scintigraphy as a pathophysiological indicator in the assessment of Parkinson's disease and related disorders:

It can be a specific marker for Lewy body disease, *Annals of Nuclear Medicine* **18**(6) (2004), 453–461.

[38] R. Barber, C. Ballard, I.G. McKeith, A. Gholkar and J.T. O'Brien, MRI volumetric study of dementia with Lewy bodies. A comparison with AD and vascular dementia, *Neurology* **54** (2000), 1304–1309.

[39] R. Barber, A. Gholkar, P. Scheltens, C. Ballard, I.G. McKeith and J.T. O'Brien, Medial temporal lobe atrophy on MRI in dementia with Lewy bodies, *Neurology* **52** (1999), 1153–1158.

[40] D.A. Cousins, E.J. Burton, D. Burn, A. Gholkar, I.G. McKeith and J.T. O'Brien, Atrophy of the putamen in dementia with Lewy bodies but not Alzheimer's disease: An MRI study, *Neurology* **61**(9) (2003), 1191–1195.

[41] K. Lobotesis, J.D. Fenwick, A. Phipps et al., Occipital hypoperfusion on SPECT in dementia with Lewy bodies but not AD, *Neurology* **56** (2001), 643–649.

[42] S.J. Colloby, J.D. Fenwick, E.D. Williams et al., A comparison of 99mTc-HMPAO SPECT changes in dementia with Lewy bodies and Alzheimer's disease using statistical parametric mapping, *European Journal of Nuclear Medicine* **29**(5) (2002), 615–622.

[43] K. Ishii, K. Hosaka, T. Mori and E. Mori, Comparison of FDG-PET and IMP-SPECT in patients with dementia with Lewy bodies, *Annals of Nuclear Medicine* **18**(5) (2004), 447–451.

[44] R.L. Albin, S. Minoshima, C.J. Damato, K.A. Frey, D.A. Kuhl and A.A.F. Sima, Fluoro-deoxyglucose positron emission tomography in diffuse Lewy body disease, *Neurology* **47**(2) (1996), 462–466.

[45] S. Minoshima, N.L. Foster, A.A.F. Sima, K.A. Frey, R.L. Albin and D.E. Kuhl, Alzheimer's disease versus dementia with Lewy bodies: Cerebral metabolic distinction with autopsy confirmation, *Annals of Neurology* **50**(3) (2001), 358–365.

[46] H.A.M. Middelkoop, W.M. van der Flier, E.J. Burton et al., Dementia with Lewy bodies and AD are not associated with occipital lobe atrophy on MRI, *Neurology* **57**(11) (2001), 2117–2120.

[47] R. Barber, A. Gholkar, P. Scheltens, C. Ballard, I.G. McKeith and J.T. O'Brien, MRI volumetric correlates of white matter lesions in dementia with Lewy bodies and Alzheimer's disease, *International Journal of Geriatric Psychiatry* **15** (2000), 911–916.

[48] J.T. O'Brien, S. Paling, R. Barber et al., Progressive brain atrophy on serial MRI in dementia with Lewy bodies, AD, and vascular dementia, *Neurology* **56**(10) (2001), 1386–1388.

[49] R.L. Hamilton, Lewy bodies in Alzheimer's disease: a neuropathological review of 145 cases using alpha-synuclein immunohistochemistry, *Brain Pathology* **10** (2000), 378–384.

[50] C.F. Lippa and I. McKeith, Dementia with Lewy bodies Improving diagnostic criteria, *Neurology* **60** (2003), 1571–1572.

[51] D. Galasko, D.P. Salmon, T. Lineweaver, L. Hansen and L.J. Thal.

[52] K. Gwinn-Hardy and A.A. Singleton, Familial Lewy body diseases, *Journal of Geriatric Psychiatry and Neurology* **15**(4) (2002), 217–223.

[53] Y. Trembath, C. Rosenberg, J.F. Ervin et al., Lewy body pathology is a frequent co-pathology in familial Alzheimer's disease, *Acta Neuropathologica* **105**(5) (2003), 484–488.

[54] A. Singleton and K. Gwinn-Hardy, Parkinson's disease and dementia with Lewy bodies: a difference in dose? *Lancet* **364**(9440) (2004), 1105–1107.

[55] J. Johnson, S.M. Hague, M. Hanson et al., SNCA multiplication is not a common cause of Parkinson disease or dementia with Lewy bodies, *Neurology* **63**(3) (2004), 554–556.

[56] M. Emre, D. Aarsland, A. Albanese et al., Rivastigmine for dementia associated with Parkinson's disease, *New England Journal of Medicine* **351**(24) (2004), 2509–2518.

[57] I. McKeith, T. Del-Ser, P.F. Spano et al., Efficacy of rivastigmine in dementia with Lewy bodies: a randomised, double-blind, placebo-controlled international study, *Lancet* **356** (2000), 2031–2036.

[58] I.G. McKeith, K.A. Wesnes, E. Perry and R. Ferrara, Hallucinations Predict Attentional Improvements with Rivastigmine in Dementia with Lewy Bodies, *Dement Geriatr Cogn Disord* **18** (2004), 94–100.

[59] A.J. Thomas, D.J. Burn, E.N. Rowan et al., Efficacy of donepezil in Parkinson's disease with dementia and dementia with Lewy bodies, *Int J Geriatr Psychiatry* **20** (2005), 938–944.

[60] I.G. McKeith, E.K. Perry and R.H. Perry, Report of the second dementia with Lewy body international workshop, *Neurology* **53**(5) (1999), 902–905.

[61] I. McKeith, D. Dickson, M. Emre et al., Dementia with Lewy Bodies: Diagnosis and Management: Third Report of the DLB Consortium, *Neurology* **65**(12) (2005), 1863–1872.

Immunotherapy for Alzheimer's disease

Dave Morgan*

Alzheimer Research Laboratory, Department of Pharmacology and Molecular Therapeutics, University of South Florida, Tampa, FL, USA

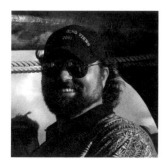

Abstract. A primary goal of research on Alzheimer's disease is to develop disease modifying therapeutics. The amyloid cascade hypothesis has focused the initial efforts on methods to reduce amyloid. One surprising approach that has shown considerable success in mouse models and has hinted at benefits in human trials is anti-Aβ immunotherapy. Schenk first showed the amyloid reducing potential of active immunization in 1999. This prompted our group and that of St. George-Hyslop to investigate whether active immunization would similarly retard the memory deficits that develop in amyloid depositing transgenic mice. Contrary to our initial predictions of premature memory dysfunction due to inflammation, vaccination protected amyloid depositing mice from developing memory deficits. Subsequent studies found that passive immunization could reverse memory deficits, even when administered for short periods. These encouraging findings led to a trial of an Aβ vaccination in Alzheimer patients. The trial was cut short due to meningoencephalitic symptoms in 6% of patients, yet, in a subset of patients, those developing brain reactive antibodies benefited from slower rates of cognitive decline. These observations have accelerated the development of passive immunization protocols and safer vaccines. At this time, anti-amyloid immunotherapy stands poised to be the first test of the amyloid hypothesis in the treatment of Alzheimer disease.

Keywords: Alzheimer disease, amyloid-β, therapeutics, transgenic, vaccine

1. Introduction

Alzheimer's disease (AD) is a significant health problem afflicting over 1% of the population in the USA and costing $100 billion, roughly 7% of the US health care costs. The expansion of human longevity and increasingly aged population predicts large increases in patients with this late life disease. This will be exaggerated when the demographic bulge known as the baby boom skews population age distributions over the next few decades. While palliative therapies may slightly delay institutionalization, disease modifying approaches to the treatment of AD are desperately needed.

As discussed elsewhere in this volume by Hardy (2005), one potential target for disease modifying therapies is the reduction of amyloid, material consisting largely of the Aβ peptide that accumulates in the brains of Alzheimer patients. A variety of avenues to reduce Aβ deposition have been described, including reduction of Aβ production, increasing the degradation of the Aβ peptide, dissolving the amyloid fibrils formed from Aβ, or enhancing the rate of Aβ clearance from the brain.

Immunotherapeutic approaches to disease modification have led to a number of successes. The only disease that has been eliminated by modern medicine, smallpox, was cured by a vaccine (200 years post-

*Corresponding author: Dave Morgan, Alzheimer Research Laboratory, MDC Box 9, University of South Florida, 12901 Bruce Downs Blvd., Tampa FL, 33612 USA. Tel.: +1 813 974 3949; Fax: +1 813 974 2565; E-mail: dmorgan@hsc.usf.edu.

Jenner). Vaccination is also closing in on a permanent cure for polio. Other forms of immunotherapy are emerging. Monoclonal antibody therapy is maturing with 16 FDA approved products such as Herceptin® and Remicade®. Immunoconjugates and chimeric proteins such as Ontak® and Etanercept® are similarly expanding the range of possibilities. Thus, experience with active immunization with vaccines and passive immunization with monoclonal antibodies is increasingly accepted as common medical practice. The question is whether degenerative diseases of the CNS would be tractable to the immmunotherapeutic approach.

2. Anti-amyloid Immunotherapy and Aβ peptides

The first demonstration that antibodies against the Aβ peptide might have some utility in modifying amyloid deposition came from *in vitro* studies by Beka Solomon and her group [38,39] as discussed elsewhere in this volume. These investigators found that anti-Aβ antibodies at low stoichiometries could prevent Aβ from forming fibrils *in vitro*. Even more important, these antibodies could disaggregate preformed fibrils, and protect neurons in culture from Aβ-induced toxicity. Subsequent work by this group has identified the EFRH epitope at positions 3–6 of Aβ as a critical target for these catalytic functions of the antibodies [15].

These early *in vitro* observations were followed by the seminal work of Schenk and colleagues, demonstrating that monthly inoculation with an Aβ vaccine preparation could lead to high anti-Aβ antibody titers, and dramatic reductions in amyloid deposition in PDAPP transgenic mice [34]. Even when initiated after amyloid deposition had occurred, the vaccine was able to slow or even reverse amyloid deposit formation. Neuritic plaques and astrocytic reactions normally observed in these mice were also quelled by the vaccine administration.

These observations were followed shortly by work demonstrating that many of the effects of the vaccine could be mimicked by passive administration of murine anti-Aβ monoclonal antibodies [5]. Moreover, these studies demonstrated that antibodies appeared to facilitate the clearance of amyloid by microglia/macrophages using an *ex vivo* tissue explant assay. Another important observation was that direct topical administration of anti-Aβ antibodies to the surface of the brain could be monitored over days and was capable of removing pre-existing amyloid deposits, not simply block their formation [2]. Thus, these early studies strongly indicated that humoral immunity was probably sufficient to slow or reverse the accumulation of amyloid, a process thought by many to be an essential feature predisposing to Alzheimer's dementia.

3. Effects of immunotherapy on learning and memory

At the time Schenk et al. published their results on amyloid deposition, the learning and memory phenotype of amyloid depositing mice was in early stages of investigation. No studies had yet correlated Aβ load with memory performance in individual transgenic mice (although multiple groups now report such observations, reviewed in [26]). We had just completed studies identifying such a relationship in our AβPP + PS1 mouse model of amyloid deposition (later published in [16]), and felt this would be an opportune model in which to investigate the effects of immunotherapy on memory performance. Based upon the inflammation hypothesis of Alzheimer's pathogenesis, we were concerned that anti-Aβ antibody opsonization of the plaques might provoke an excessive microglia/macrophage reaction which would so disrupt neural function as to prematurely cause memory loss. Thus, we started inoculating AβPP + PS1 mice at 7 months, an age when they already have amyloid deposits, and tested them for learning and memory performance at 11 months, an age before they typically develop spatial navigation deficits in a working memory version of the radial arm watermaze task.

When we tested the mice at 11 months for learning and memory, we found that all of the mice acquired the task well, learning the platform location within the maze on the first or second trial of the day, and retaining that through the 30 minute retention period. Our initial concerns that inflammation associated with the immunotherapy would disrupt memory proved unfounded. We continued treatment through 15 months of age, and tested the same mice on the same task. At this age, we found transgenic mice given the control vaccine now exhibited memory disruption, and could not learn the new platform location each day. However, the transgenic mice given the vaccine against Aβ could ultimately perform as well as the nontransgenic mice [27]. These data were published coordinately in Nature with a parallel study by Janus et al. [19], showing a similar protection from spatial navigation deficits in the TgCRND8 model of amyloid deposition with vaccination against Aβ. A third paper in that issue, Chen et al. [6] demonstrated an amyloid associated learning and memory deficit in PDAPP mice using a working memory version of the open pool water maze. As the mice aged, the deterioration of performance correlated with the amyloid loads in the individual mice, linking these two aspects of the amyloid β protein precursor (AβPP) mouse phenotype.

The active immunization against Aβ used multiple inoculations over months to demonstrate effects in transgenic mice. Part of the reason was the slow development of titers against Aβ, requiring 2–3 boosts to reach high levels using the Schenk et al. vaccination regimen [8,11,25]. The question of whether passive immunization could also benefit the cognitive deficits in the transgenic mice was addressed in two papers in 2002. Both Dodart et al. [12] and Kotilinek et al. [20] found that relatively short periods of anti-Aβ antibody injections could improve the learning and memory performance of AβPP transgenic mice. Importantly, these improvements were found in the absence of detectable changes in amyloid deposition. These data argued that there was likely some pool of Aβ, not readily detectable, that was most intimately linked to memory disturbances and was reduced by the anti-Aβ antibodies. Thus far the critical Aβ pool has not been identified. Nonetheless, these data emphasize the potency of the immunotherapeutic approach in reversing the AβPP mouse behavioral phenotype.

4. Mechanisms of amyloid lowering by immunotherapy

Certainly a straightforward hypothesis for the amyloid reducing properties of anti-Aβ antibodies is opsonization of the deposits and phagocytosis by microglia after Fc receptor activation. This was first proposed by Schenk et al. [34] and strongly supported by Bard et al. [4,5]. However, an alternative hypothesis was presented by DeMattos et al. [9]. They argued that the entry of antibody through the blood brain barrier was limited. They found that immunization with an antibody directed against the mid-domain of Aβ resulted in a massive elevation of Aβ in blood. They suggested that the amyloid lowering effects were due to trapping of the Aβ peptide in the bloodstream, increasing the net efflux of Aβ from the brain and lowering amyloid loads. Considerable evidence has accumulated supporting this "peripheral sink" hypothesis [10,21]. A third possibility for the action of anti-Aβ antibodies was actually the first to be described; the catalytic transformation of the Aβ peptide into a secondary structure less compatible with amyloid fibril formation [37].

The consensus emerging is that all three mechanisms are likely to contribute to the actions of anti-Aβ antibodies. It is important to note that the extent to which Aβ production exceeds Aβ clearance is not known in Aβ depositing mice. It is plausible that even slight changes in the production/clearance ratio may have considerable impact on the rate of amyloid deposition. The first evidence that the opsonization argument could not fully explain amyloid clearance was reported by Bacskai et al. [3]. These authors found that topical application of F(ab)$_2$ fragments against the Aβ peptide could readily clear amyloid deposits in a matter of days. Given the absence of the Fc component of the IgG, Fc receptor mediated microglial phagocytosis seemed unlikely.

Our own work has focused on the mechanisms of Aβ clearance using direct intracranial injections of monoclonal antibodies into the hippocampus and cortex of mice containing amyloid deposits. We observed a rapid clearance of diffuse and compacted deposits that is largely resolved within a week. The diffuse deposits were cleared within 24 hours [41]. This clearance was just as rapid when the antibodies are cleaved into F(ab)$_2$ fragments, or when the microglial activation was inhibited with anti-inflammatory agents (such as dexamethasone [42]). This is consistent with the catalytic dissolution hypothesis of Solomon. However, the compacted deposits required longer to be cleared (2–3 days) and their clearance was greatly reduced when F(ab)$_2$ fragments were used or microglial activation was inhibited pharmacologically. Thus, it appears that for the compacted deposits the microglial response to opsonized antigen, at least, facilitates the clearance of the fibrillar material.

When these monoclonal antibodies are applied systemically, we find murine IgG decorating the congophilic deposits in mice administered antibodies against Aβ [43]. We also detect increased activation of microglia early in the treatment regimen (detected with antibody to Fc receptors and CD45), supporting the argument that microglia/macrophages are actively clearing the Aβ deposits. Simultaneously, we find massive elevation in circulating Aβ, consistent with the amyloid sink hypothesis. These mechanisms are by no means mutually exclusive. It is likely that they additively or even synergistically contribute to the remarkably potent amyloid lowering capacity of immunotherapy. Recently, we have found that even mice started at 22 mo of age on passive immunotherapy can have

Table 1
Major events in the development of anti-Aβ immunotherapy

Year	Event	Reference
1996	Anti-Aβ antibodies catalytically disaggregate amyloid fibrils	Solomon et al. [39]
1999	Aβ vaccine reduces amyloid deposition	Schenk et al. [34]
2000	Passive immunization with anti Aβ antibodies reduces amyloid deposition; promotes phagocytosis	Bard et al. [5]
2000	Aβ vaccines protect amyloid depositing mice from memory deficits	Janus et al. [19] Morgan et al. [27]
2001	Topical anti-Aβ antibodies remove pre-existing amyloid plaques	Bacskai et al. [2]
2001	Anti-Aβ antibodies dramatically increase circulating Aβ; peripheral sink hypothesis	DeMattos et al. [9]
2002	Systemic anti-Aβ antibodies reverse memory deficits in amyloid depositing mice	Dodart et al. [12] Kotilinek et al. [20]
2003	Aβ vaccines cause meningoencephalitis in some patients participating in a clinical trial	Orgogozo et al. [31]
2003	AD clinical trial patients with high titers of brain reactive anti-Aβ antibodies benefit on measures of cognition compared to participants with low titers	Hock et al. [17]
2003-05	Autopsies from AD patients vaccinated against Aβ reveal areas of lower than expected amyloid load	Nicoll et al. [30] Ferrer et al. [14] Masliah et al. [23]

90% reductions in congophilic parenchymal amyloid plaque deposits (diffuse deposits are reduced by 50%), and reversal of memory deficits in the radial arm water maze [44]. Thus, multiple mechanisms likely mediate the potential benefits of anti-Aβ immunotherapy.

5. A clinical trial of amyloid vaccination

Based on the accumulating evidence of benefit without apparent adverse consequences in transgenic mouse models of amyloid deposition, Elan partnered with Wyeth to test an amyloid vaccine in humans in 2001. The phase 1 studies used single and multiple doses of the vaccine, demonstrating good immunological responses and tolerability of the vaccine. A phase 2a study was initiated with 375 patients at several sites. Shortly after the study was started, several patients developed symptoms of aseptic meningoencephalitis. The symptoms did not correlate with antibody titer. Ultimately, 6% of the patients in the trial developed these symptoms to varying degrees; many patients were treated with steroidal therapy and recovered [31]. Because of these adverse events, the trial was halted prematurely in early 2002, limiting its potential to demonstrate effects of immunization on Alzheimer's disease (most patients had received only 1 or 2 inoculations before truncation of the study). At present, the explanation offered for the problems encountered is that some patients developed an autoimmune cellular response to the vaccine. This led to T cell infiltration of the brain and CNS inflammation. Such a condition was observed in the cases with severe meningoencephalitis that went to autopsy [14,30].

A complete analysis of the cognitive data from the trial has not yet been reported. However, the results from the cohort of patients in Zurich have suggested that some patients benefited from the therapy. Hock et al. [17] reported that a subset of patients remained cognitively stable for 1 year after starting the trial. Because the investigators remained blind to the treatment condition, they used the anti-Aβ antibody titers in the patients of the trial to assign patients to groups. They used both a standard ELISA measurement, and a TAPIR assay, in which antisera were tested for immunoreactivity against sections from AD brain tissue. Hock et al. found that those patients with the high brain-reactive anti-Aβ titers had significantly less deterioration of cognitive performance than patients with little or no brain reactive antibody titers. Within the brain reactive antibody group, those patients with the highest levels were unchanged over 1 year of cognitive testing. At recent meetings, data were presented that this stability of cognitive performance was maintained even 2 years after the trial was truncated. Importantly, one of the patient's in the high antibody group apparently benefiting from the therapy had previously been treated for meningoencephalitis and recovered. Although only presented at scientific meetings, the full analysis of the trial has suggested some modest cognitive benefit in those patients with the highest ELISA anti-Aβ titers. However, a full TAPIR analysis of anti-Aβ antibodies from the trial participants has not been performed at this time.

6. Passive immunization of old AβPP transgenic mice

Enthusiasm for the immunotherapeutic approach has followed an oscillatory pattern with a roughly 2 year periodicity. Following the initial report by Schenk in 1999 enthusiasm peaked at the beginning of 2001 with the reports of the behavioral benefits of active immunization [19,27]. However, 1 year later enthusiasm plummeted with the premature termination of the phase 2a trial. Multiple commentaries appeared shortly thereafter, arguing that such an outcome might have been predicted, and that the trial was initiated hastily. Some even suggested, in an almost reflexive manner, that the termination of the vaccine trial somehow disproved the amyloid hypothesis of AD. The report by Hock et al. raised the level of enthusiasm. Further tests of immunotherapy that would have less propensity for developing the adverse events found in the phase 2 a trial were once again feasible. This led several groups to develop vaccines that would be less likely to provoke a cellular immune response against Aβ, often by using a non-Aβ T cell epitope [1,22] or attempting to bias the immune response to a Th2 reaction [7,35]. Others have suggested using variants of Aβ that are less likely to be toxic [36].

However, an alternative to testing different active immunization protocols is to investigate adoptive transfer of immunity using humanized monoclonal anti-Aβ antibodies. There are several advantages of such an approach; at least as a proof of principle that immunotherapy may benefit AD patients. First, the dose can be controlled. Active immunization results in highly variable responses, especially in older populations. This makes data analysis based on intention to treat problematic. It also makes dose response studies almost impossible. Periodic injections of known amounts of antibody overcome these problems. A second advantage is the treatment can be discontinued. If an adverse reaction develops, it should diminish as the injected antibodies are cleared. With active immunization, once the plunger goes down, there is no turning back. Only severe immunosuppressive therapy can be used to dampen a runaway immune response (and not always successfully). A serious disadvantage of passive immunization is the cost of monoclonal antibodies. However, this is still cost-effective when compared to the costs of institutionalization. An alternative is to consider injections of human gamma globulin. Many humans spontaneously develop low titers of anti-Aβ antibodies [18,28,29,40]. This has led to the proposal that intravenous immunoglobulin might be an effective therapy in AD [13].

A number of issues have arisen regarding the type(s) of antibody to use for passive immunization studies. Bard et al. [4] have argued that N-terminal domain antibodies (the ones most prominently formed with active immunization protocols [11,24] are the most effective *in vivo* and *ex vivo* in clearing amyloid. They also suggest that the antibody isotypes most likely to bind to Fc receptors are also the most effective antibody isotypes. Alternatively, DeMattos, Holtzman and the Lilly group argue that a mid-domain antibody with little reactivity to brain amyloid may be safe and effective [33]. Our own work has found potent effects with a C-terminal specific antibody [44].

However, even the passive immunization approach will require caution in the conduct of human trials. Pfeifer et al. [32] were the first to examine long term adoptive transfer of antibody in old AβPP transgenic mice. They reported reduced amyloid loads, but a doubling of the number of microhemorrhages in 27 mo old AβPP23 mice treated for 5 months with an N-terminal specific anti-Aβ monoclonal antibody. Our own work with a C-terminal specific antibody found a similar increase in microhemorrhage with prolonged (3–5 mo) treatment of old Tg2576 derived AβPP transgenic mice [44]. These mice had up to 90% reductions of parenchymal Congo red deposits (compacted plaques), but 3–5 fold elevation in vascular congophilic deposits (cerebral amyloid angiopathy). All microhemorrhages were in association with congophilic angiopathy. Remarkably, however, these aged mice with reduced amyloid but increased vascular leakage had learning and memory capacities equal to those of non-transgenic littermates, and far superior to the deficits found in transgenic mice given control antibody injections. Racke et al. [33] confirmed the observations of Pfeifer et al. using a different N-terminal specific antibody against Aβ, with a doubling of the extravenous hemoglobin using a severity index scoring method. However, a mid-domain antibody did not cause increased vascular leakage. Racke et al. further indicate that the mid-domain antibody does not react with brain or vascular amyloid, suggesting that the antibody binding to vascular amyloid may predilect towards microhemorrhage. However, if the TAPIR analysis, indicating that only brain reactive antibodies benefit patients cognitively, is correct, it becomes difficult to decide what type of antibody to consider for passive immunization trials.

One issue is whether vascular amyloid increases and microhemorrhage might also be the case with active immunization. Thus far, active immunization has not been investigated in old transgenic AβPP mice, in part, due to impaired immune responses to vaccines. However, the 3 autopsy reports in the Aβ vaccine trial all point to this possibility [14,23,30]. When compared to index cases that were not part of the trial, these cases from patients participating in the vaccine trial exhibited less parenchymal Aβ staining, but no reductions in vascular Aβ immunostaining. On some of the sections from the patients in the trial, the only profiles which are stained are vascular. Ferrer et al. [14] remark that the case they studied had considerable cerebral amyloid angiopathy and associated hemorrhage.

7. Conclusions

The attitudes towards immunotherapy for the treatment of AD have followed an emotional roller coaster. The initial enthusiasm was deflated by the unexpected adverse events in the clinical trial. However, the cognitive function data tantalize with suggestions that some individuals have benefited from the treatment, in spite of its abbreviated administration. Many approaches are being investigated which might avoid the adverse events associated with the active immunization trial. Passive immunization approaches are attractive because of the greater control over the anti-Aβ titers and potential to terminate the therapy. However, mouse data suggest that high anti-Aβ titers might lead to increased congophilic angiopathy and vascular leakage. Further trials of immunotherapy are already underway. One involves passive immunization with an N-terminal antibody. A second involves use of a truncated Aβ peptide vaccine to minimize T cell responses. Obviously, experience with the prior trial will dictate a cautious approach to these further studies of immunotherapeutic intervention in AD. However, assuming these trials continue to completion, they are likely to be the first therapeutic evaluations of the amyloid hypothesis in AD patients.

Acknowledgements

DM receives salary support from the NIH (AG 15490, AG 18478, NS 48335) which contributed to the preparation of this review.

References

[1] M.G. Agadjanyan, A. Ghochikyan, I. Petrushina, V. Vasilevko, N. Movsesyan, M. Mkrtichyan, T. Saing and D.H. Cribbs, Prototype Alzheimer's disease vaccine using the immunodominant B cell epitope from beta-amyloid and promiscuous T cell epitope pan HLA DR-binding peptide, *J.Immunol.* **174** (2005), 1580–1586.

[2] B.J. Bacskai, S.T. Kajdasz, R.H. Christie, C. Carter, D. Games, P. Seubert, D. Schenk and B. Hyman, Imaging of amyloid-β deposits in living mice permits direct observation of clearance of plaques with immunotherapy, *Nat. Med.* **7** (2001), 369–372.

[3] B.J. Bacskai, S.T. Kajdasz, M.E. McLellan, D. Games, P. Seubert, D. Schenk and B.T. Hyman, Non-Fc-mediated mechanisms are involved in clearance of amyloid-beta *in vivo* by immunotherapy, *Journal of Neuroscience* **22** (2002), 7873–7878.

[4] F. Bard, R. Barbour, C. Cannon, R. Carretto, M. Fox, D. Games, T. Guido, K. Hoenow, K. Hu, K. Johnson-Wood, K. Khan, D. Kholodenko, C. Lee, M. Lee, R. Motter, M. Nguyen, A. Reed, D. Schenk, P. Tang, N. Vasquez, P. Seubert and T. Yednock, Epitope and isotype specificities of antibodies to beta-amyloid peptide for protection against Alzheimer's disease-like neuropathology, *Proceedings of the National Academy of Sciences, USA* **100** (2003), 2023–2028.

[5] F. Bard, C. Cannon, R. Barbour, R.L. Burke, D. Games, H. Grajeda, T. Guido, K. Hu, J. Huang, K. Johnson-Wood, K. Khan, D. Kholodenko, M. Lee, I. Lieberburg, R. Motter, M. Nguyen, F. Soriano, N. Vasquez, K. Weiss, B. Welch, P. Seubert, D. Schenk and T. Yednock, Peripherally administered antibodies against amyloid beta-peptide enter the central nervous system and reduce pathology in a mouse model of Alzheimer disease, *Nat. Med.* **6** (2000), 916–919.

[6] G. Chen, K.S. Chen, J. Knox, J. Inglis, A. Bernard, S.J. Martin, A. Justice, L. McConlogue, D. Games, S.B. Freedman and R.G. Morris, A learning deficit related to age and beta-amyloid plaques in a mouse model of Alzheimer's disease, *Nature* **408** (2000), 975–979.

[7] D.H. Cribbs, A. Ghochikyan, V. Vasilevko, M. Tran, I. Petrushina, N. Sadzikava, D. Babikyan, P. Kesslak, T. Kieber-Emmons, C.W. Cotman and M.G. Agadjanyan, Adjuvant-dependent modulation of Th1 and Th2 responses to immunization with beta-amyloid, *Int. Immunol.* **15** (2003), 505–514.

[8] P. Das, M.P. Murphy, L.H. Younkin, S.G. Younkin and T.E. Golde, Reduced effectiveness of Abeta1-42 immunization in APP transgenic mice with significant amyloid deposition, *Neurobiol. Aging* **22** (2001), 721–727.

[9] R.B. DeMattos, K.R. Bales, D.J. Cummins, J.C. Dodart, S.M. Paul and D.M. Holtzman, Peripheral anti-A beta antibody alters CNS and plasma A beta clearance and decreases brain A beta burden in a mouse model of Alzheimer's disease, *Proceedings of the National Academy of Sciences, USA* **98** (2001), 8850–8855.

[10] R.B. DeMattos, K.R. Bales, D.J. Cummins, S.M. Paul and D.M. Holtzman, Brain to plasma amyloid-beta efflux: a measure of brain amyloid burden in a mouse model of Alzheimer's disease, *Science* **295** (2002), 2264–2267.

[11] C.A. Dickey, D.G. Morgan, S. Kudchodkar, D.B. Weiner, Y. Bai, C. Cao, M.N. Gordon and K.E. Ugen, Duration and specificity of humoral immune responses in mice vaccinated with the Alzheimer's disease-associated beta-amyloid 1-42 peptide, *DNA Cell Biol* **20** (2001), 723–729.

[12] J.C. Dodart, K.R. Bales, K.S. Gannon, S.J. Greene, R.B. DeMattos, C. Mathis, C.A. DeLong, S. Wu, X. Wu, D.M. Holtzman and S.M. Paul, Immunization reverses memory deficits without reducing brain Abeta burden in Alzheimer's disease model, *Nat. Neurosci.* **5** (2002), 452–457.

[13] R. Dodel, H. Hampel, C. Depboylu, S. Lin, F. Gao, S. Schock, S. Jackel, X. Wei, K. Buerger, C. Hoft, B. Hemmer, H.J. Moller, M. Farlow, W.H. Oertel, N. Sommer and Y. Du, Human antibodies against amyloid beta peptide: a potential treatment for Alzheimer's disease, *Ann. Neurol.* **52** (2002), 253–256.

[14] I. Ferrer, R.M. Boada, M.L. Sanchez Guerra, M.J. Rey and F. Costa-Jussa, Neuropathology and pathogenesis of encephalitis following amyloid-beta immunization in Alzheimer's disease, *Brain Pathol* **14** (2004), 11–20.

[15] D. Frenkel, M. Balass, E. Katchalski-Katzir and B. Solomon, High affinity binding of monoclonal antibodies to the sequential epitope EFRH of beta-amyloid peptide is essential for modulation of fibrillar aggregation, *J Neuroimmunol* **95** (1999), 136–142.

[16] M.N. Gordon, D.L. King, D.M. Diamond, P.T. Jantzen, K.L. Boyett, C.E. Hope, J.M. Hatcher, G. DiCarlo, P. Gottschal, D. Morgan and G.W. Arendash, Correlation between cognitive deficits and $A\beta$ deposits in transgenic APP + PS1 mice, *Neurobiology of Aging* **22** (2001), 377–385.

[17] C. Hock, U. Konietzko, J.R. Streffer, J. Tracy, A. Signorell, B. Muller-Tillmanns, U. Lemke, K. Henke, E. Moritz, E. Garcia, M.A. Wollmer, D. Umbricht, D.J. de Quervain, M. Hofmann, A. Maddalena, A. Papassotiropoulos and R.M. Nitsch, Antibodies against beta-amyloid slow cognitive decline in Alzheimer's disease, *Neuron* **38** (2003), 547–554.

[18] B.T. Hyman, C. Smith, I. Buldyrev, C. Whelan, H. Brown, M.X. Tang and R. Mayeux, Autoantibodies to amyloid-beta and Alzheimer's disease, *Ann. Neurol.* **49** (2001), 808–810.

[19] C. Janus, J. Pearson, J. McLaurin, P.M. Mathews, Y. Jiang, S.D. Schmidt, M.A. Chishti, P. Horne, D. Heslin, J. French, H.T. Mount, R.A. Nixon, M. Mercken, C. Bergeron, P.E. Fraser, P. George-Hyslop and D. Westaway, A beta peptide immunization reduces behavioural impairment and plaques in a model of Alzheimer's disease, *Nature* **408** (2000), 979–982.

[20] L.A. Kotilinek, B. Bacskai, M. Westerman, T. Kawarabayashi, L. Younkin, B.T. Hyman, S. Younkin and K.H. Ashe, Reversible memory loss in a mouse transgenic model of Alzheimer's disease, *Journal of Neuroscience* **22** (2002), 6331–6335.

[21] C.A. Lemere, E.T. Spooner, J. LaFrancois, B. Malester, C. Mori, J.F. Leverone, Y. Matsuoka, J.W. Taylor, R.B. DeMattos, D.M. Holtzman, J.D. Clements, D.J. Selkoe and K.E. Duff, Evidence for peripheral clearance of cerebral Abeta protein following chronic, active Abeta immunization in PSAPP mice, *Neurobiol. Dis.* **14** (2003), 10–18.

[22] J.F. Leverone, E.T. Spooner, H.K. Lehman, J.D. Clements and C.A. Lemere, Abeta1-15 is less immunogenic than Abeta1-40/42 for intranasal immunization of wild-type mice but may be effective for "boosting", *Vaccine* **21** (2003), 2197–2206.

[23] E. Masliah, L. Hansen, A. Adame, L. Crews, F. Bard, C. Lee, P. Seubert, D. Games, L. Kirby and D. Schenk, Abeta vaccination effects on plaque pathology in the absence of encephalitis in Alzheimer disease, *Neurology* **64** (2005), 129–131.

[24] J. McLaurin, R. Cecal, M.E. Kierstead, X. Tian, A.L. Phinney, M. Manea, J.E. French, M.H. Lambermon, A.A. Darabie, M.E. Brown, C. Janus, M.A. Chishti, P. Horne, D. Westaway, P.E. Fraser, H.T. Mount, M. Przybylski and P. George-Hyslop, Therapeutically effective antibodies against amyloid-beta peptide target amyloid-beta residues 4-10 and inhibit cytotoxicity and fibrillogenesis, *Nat. Med.* **8** (2002), 1263–1269.

[25] A. Monsonego, R. Maron, V. Zota, D.J. Selkoe and H.L. Weiner, Immune hyporesponsiveness to amyloid beta-peptide in amyloid precursor protein transgenic mice: implications for the pathogenesis and treatment of Alzheimer's disease, *Proceedings of the National Academy of Sciences, USA* **98** (2001), 10273–10278.

[26] D. Morgan, Learning and memory deficits in APP transgenic mouse models of amyloid deposition, *Neurochem. Res.* **28** (2003), 1029–1034.

[27] D. Morgan, D.M. Diamond, P.E. Gottschall, K.E. Ugen, C. Dickey, J. Hardy, K. Duff, P. Jantzen, G. DiCarlo, D. Wilcock, K. Connor, J. Hatcher, C. Hope, M. Gordon and G.W. Arendash, A beta peptide vaccination prevents memory loss in an animal model of Alzheimer's disease, *Nature* **408** (2000), 982–985.

[28] S. Mruthinti, J.J. Buccafusco, W.D. Hill, J.L. Waller, T.W. Jackson, E.Y. Zamrini and R.F. Schade, Autoimmunity in Alzheimer's disease: increased levels of circulating IgGs binding Abeta and RAGE peptides, *Neurobiol. Aging* **25** (2004), 1023–1032.

[29] A. Nath, E. Hall, M. Tuzova, M. Dobbs, M. Jons, C. Anderson, J. Woodward, Z. Guo, W. Fu, R. Kryscio, D. Wekstein, C. Smith, W.R. Markesbery and M.P. Mattson, Autoantibodies to amyloid beta-peptide (Abeta) are increased in Alzheimer's disease patients and Abeta antibodies can enhance Abeta neurotoxicity: implications for disease pathogenesis and vaccine development, *Neuromolecular. Med.* **3** (2003), 29–39.

[30] J.A. Nicoll, D. Wilkinson, C. Holmes, P. Steart, H. Markham and R.O. Weller, Neuropathology of human Alzheimer disease after immunization with amyloid-beta peptide: a case report, *Nat. Med.* **9** (2003), 448–452.

[31] J.M. Orgogozo, S. Gilman, J.F. Dartigues, B. Laurent, M. Puel, L.C. Kirby, P. Jouanny, B. Dubois, L. Eisner, S. Flitman, B.F. Michel, M. Boada, A. Frank and C. Hock, Subacute meningoencephalitis in a subset of patients with AD after Abeta42 immunization, *Neurology* **61** (2003), 46–54.

[32] M. Pfeifer, S. Boncristiano, L. Bondolfi, A. Stalder, T. Deller, M. Staufenbiel, P.M. Mathews and M. Jucker, Cerebral hemorrhage after passive anti-Abeta immunotherapy, *Science* **298** (2002), 1379.

[33] M.M. Racke, L.I. Boone, D.L. Hepburn, M. Parsadainian, M.T. Bryan, D.K. Ness, K.S. Piroozi, W.H. Jordan, D.D. Brown, W.P. Hoffman, D.M. Holtzman, K.R. Bales, B.D. Gitter, P.C. May, S.M. Paul and R.B. DeMattos, Exacerbation of cerebral amyloid angiopathy-associated microhemorrhage in amyloid precursor protein transgenic mice by immunotherapy is dependent on antibody recognition of deposited forms of amyloid beta, *Journal of Neuroscience* %**19;25** (2005), 629–636.

[34] D. Schenk, R. Barbour, W. Dunn, G. Gordon, H. Grajeda, T. Guido, K. Hu, J. Huang, K. Johnson-Wood, K. Khan, D. Kholodenko, M. Lee, Z. Liao, I. Lieberburg, R. Motter, L. Mutter, F. Soriano, G. Shopp, N. Vasquez, C. Vandevert, S. Walker, M. Wogulis, T. Yednock, D. Games and P. Seubert, Immunization with amyloid-beta attenuates Alzheimer-disease-like pathology in the PDAPP mouse, *Nature* **400** (1999), 173–177.

[35] T.J. Seabrook, M. Iglesias, J.K. Bloom, E.T. Spooner and C.A. Lemere, Differences in the immune response to long term Abeta vaccination in C57BL/6 and B6D2F1 mice, *Vaccine* **22** (2004), 4075–4083.

[36] E.M. Sigurdsson, E. Knudsen, A. Asuni, C. Fitzer-Attas, D. Sage, D. Quartermain, F. Goni, B. Frangione and T. Wisniewski, An attenuated immune response is sufficient to enhance cognition in an Alzheimer's disease mouse model immunized with amyloid-beta derivatives, *Journal of Neuroscience* **24** (2004), 6277–6282.

[37] B. Solomon, Immunotherapeutic strategies for prevention and treatment of Alzheimer's disease, *DNA Cell Biol* **20** (2001), 697–703.

[38] B. Solomon, R. Koppel, D. Frankel and E. Hanan-Aharon, Disaggregation of Alzheimer beta-amyloid by site-directed

mAb, *Proceedings of the National Academy of Sciences, USA* **94** (1997), 4109–4112.

[39] B. Solomon, R. Koppel, E. Hanan and T. Katzav, Monoclonal antibodies inhibit *in vitro* fibrillar aggregation of the Alzheimer beta-amyloid peptide, *Proceedings of the National Academy of Sciences, USA* **93** (1996), 452–455.

[40] M.E. Weksler, N. Relkin, R. Turkenich, S. LaRusse, L. Zhou and P. Szabo, Patients with Alzheimer disease have lower levels of serum anti-amyloid peptide antibodies than healthy elderly individuals, *Exp. Gerontol.* **37** (2002), 943–948.

[41] D.M. Wilcock, G. DiCarlo, D. Henderson, J. Jackson, K. Clarke, K.E. Ugen, M.N. Gordon and D. Morgan, Intracranially administered anti-Abeta antibodies reduce beta-amyloid deposition by mechanisms both independent of and associated with microglial activation, *Journal of Neuroscience* **23** (2003), 3745–3751.

[42] D.M. Wilcock, S.K. Munireddy, A. Rosenthal, K.E. Ugen, M.N. Gordon and D. Morgan, Microglial activation facilitates Abeta plaque removal following intracranial anti-Abeta antibody administration, *Neurobiol. Dis.* **15** (2004), 11–20.

[43] D.M. Wilcock, A. Rojiani, A. Rosenthal, G. Levkowitz, S. Subbarao, J. Alamed, D. Wilson, N. Wilson, M.J. Freeman, M.N. Gordon and D. Morgan, Passive amyloid immunotherapy clears amyloid and transiently activates microglia in a transgenic mouse model of amyloid deposition, *Journal of Neuroscience* **24** (2004), 6144–6151.

[44] D.M. Wilcock, A. Rojiani, A. Rosenthal, S. Subbarao, M.J. Freeman, M.N. Gordon and D. Morgan, Passive immunotherapy against Abeta in aged APP-transgenic mice reverses cognitive deficits and depletes parenchymal amyloid deposits in spite of increased vascular amyloid and microhemorrhage, *J. Neuroinflammation.* **1** (2004), 24.

Alzheimer's disease immunotherapy: From *in vitro* amyloid immunomodulation to *in vivo* vaccination

Beka Solomon
Department of Molecular Microbiology and Biotechnology, George S. Wise Faculty of Life Sciences, Tel-Aviv University, Ramat Aviv, Tel-Aviv 69978, Israel
Tel.: 972 3 6409711; Fax: 972 3 6405871; E-mail: beka@post.tau.ac.il

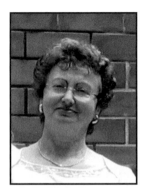

Abstract. Site-directed antibodies which modulate conformation of amyloid-β peptide (Aβ) became the theoretical basis of the immunological approach for treatment of Alzheimer's disease (AD). Indeed, antibodies towards the EFRH sequence, located between amino acids 3–6 of the N-terminal region of Aβ, found to be a key position in modulation of Aβ conformation, prevent formation of fibrillar Aβ and dissolve already formed amyloid plaques.

The performance of anti-Aβ antibodies in transgenic mice models of AD showed they are delivered to the central nervous system (CNS), preventing and/or dissolving Aβ. Moreover, these antibodies protected the mice from learning and age-related memory deficits. Development of such antibodies via active and/or passive immunization against Aβ peptide fragments has been proposed for AD immunotherapeutic strategies. Experimental active immunization with fibrillar Aβ 1-42 in hu-mans was stopped in phase II clinical trials due to unexpected neuroinflammatory manifestations. In spite of the fact that it will take considerable effort to establish a suitable immunization procedure, these results clearly strengthen the hypothesis that Aβ plays a central role in AD, stimulating a new area for development of Alzheimer's immunotherapeutics.

Keywords: Amyloid-β, site-directed antibodies, therapeutic chaperones, single-chain antibodies, EFRH sequence, immunomodulation

1. Introduction

Alzheimer's disease (AD) is characterized by progressive loss of memory and cognitive function. AD is beginning to approach epidemic proportions in the industrialized world. It is estimated by the year 2025 there will be approximately 22 million cases of AD worldwide, with at least 10 million being in the US alone [1].

The pathology of AD is characterized primarily by extracellular plaques and intracellular neurofibrillary tangles. Plaques are composed mainly of the Aβ peptide, whereas tangles are composed of the cytoskeletal protein tau [2]. He relationship between these lesions and the disease process has long been debated [3,4].

The most studied hypothesis of what leads to development of the disease is that of the amyloid cascade [5,6]; it states that overproduction of Aβ, or failure to clear this peptide, leads to AD primarily through amyloid deposition which is presumed to be involved in neurofibrillary tangles formation; these lesions are then associated with cell death, which is reflected in memory impairment, the hallmarks of this dementia. During the past ten years, the amyloid cascade hypothesis has gained strength and remains the most attractive explanation as the underlying cause of AD based on the general occurrence of amyloid pathology in the brains of all AD patients. In strong support are the mutations in familial cases of early onset AD in the genes coding for amyloid β protein precursor (AβPP) [7,8].

The hypothesis of a "cascade" has exerted considerable attraction since that process would allow for intervention at multiple and different points to slow or halt the disease process [9].

2. *In vitro* modulation of amyloid formation

Amyloid filaments, similar to those found in amyloid plaques and cerebrovascular amyloid, can be assembled from chemically synthesized Aβ under well-defined experimental conditions *in vitro*, and the effect on neural cells may be neurotoxic or neurotrophic, depending on the Aβ fibrillar state [10]. *In vitro* amyloid formation is a complex kinetic and thermodynamic process and the reversibility of amyloid plaque growth *in vitro* suggests a steady-state equilibrium between Aβ in plaques and in solution [11]. The dependence of Aβ polymerization on peptide-peptide interactions to form a β-pleated sheet fibril and the stimulatory influence of other proteins on the reaction suggest that amyloid formation may be subject to modulation.

If so-called pathological chaperones like ApoE, heparan sulfate, increase the extent of Aβ fibrils [12], we proposed site-directed monoclonal antibodies against Aβ, which decrease Aβ fibrils, as therapeutic chaperones [13–15].

Antibody-antigen interactions involve conformational changes in both antibody and antigen that can range from insignificant to considerable. Binding of high affinity monoclonal antibodies (mAbs) to regions of high flexibility and antigenicity may alter the molecular dynamics of the whole antigen [16,17]. Appropriate mAbs interact at strategic sites where protein aggregation is initiated, stabilizing the protein and preventing further denaturation [18,19]. Experimental data show that mAbs are able to stabilize the antigen by preventing aggregation and resolubilizing already formed protein aggregates [18–20]. Such antibodies were found to stabilize the conformation of an antigen against incorrect folding and recognize an incompletely folded epitope, inducing native conformation in a partially unfolded protein [20].

We demonstrated for the first time that antibodies raised against the N-terminal region of Aβ bind to preformed Aβ fibrils, leading to their disaggregation and inhibition of their neurotoxic activity [14]. Using a phage display peptide library composed of filamentous phage displaying random combinatorial peptides, we identified the 3–6 amino acid sequence of N-terminal of Aβ (Glu-Phe-Arg-His or EFRH) as the epitope of these anti-aggregating antibodies [21,22]. Blocking of this epitope by highly specific antibodies prevents Aβ self-aggregation and enables resolubilization of already-formed aggregates (Fig. 1).

3. Immunological strategies for prevention and/or reduction of amyloid plaques in AD transgenic mice

The abundant evidence that Aβ aggregation is an essential early event in AD pathogenesis has prompted an intensive search for therapeutics that target Aβ [6,23]. Several laboratories have bred AD diseased models of transgenic mice that produce human Aβ which develop plaques and neuron damage in their brains, as recently reviewed [24]. Even though they do not develop the widespread neuron death and severe dementia seen in the human disease they are used as models for the study of AD.

Recently, the immunological concept in the treatment of conformational diseases has gained more attention, and immunization approaches are being pursued in order to stimulate clearance of brain Aβ plaques [25–28]. They include both active and passive immunization techniques. Active immunization approaches employ various routes of administration, types of adjuvants, the use of modified Aβ epitopes and/or immunogenic Aβ conjugates. Passive immunization approaches include monoclonal antibodies or specific antibody fragments directed against specific Aβ epitopes. These approaches, originated from various institutions and companies, are systematically reviewed by B. Imbimbo [26].

4. Active immunization

We developed an immunization procedure for the production of effective anti-aggregating Aβ antibodies based on filamentous phages displaying on their surface the EFRH peptide as antigen. The EFRH sequence, encompassing amino acids 3–6 of the 42 residues of Aβ, was previously found to be the main regulatory site for amyloid modulation and the epitope of anti-aggregating

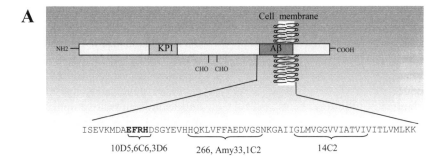

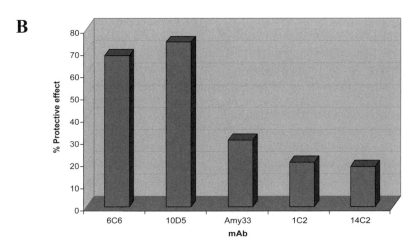

Fig. 1. A: The full-length amyloid β protein precursor (AβPP). The regions encompassing Aβ as well as the sequence of EFRH are shown below. The corresponding epitopes of the anti-Aβ antibodies are underlined. B: Protective effect of monoclonal antibodies against Aβ aggregation induced by incubation of the peptide for 3 h at 37°C. Each percentage is related to maximal binding of each monoclonal antibody to Aβ coated onto ELISA plates in the absence of soluble Aβ (100%) and calculated by comparison with the binding of the same mAbs to the residual soluble Aβ remaining after incubation at 37°C in the absence of the respective antibody [15].

antibodies [21,22]. Effective anti-aggregating antibodies were obtained by EFRH phage immunization, without adjuvant, in guinea pigs which exhibit the Aβ sequence identical to that of humans [29,30]. Filamentous bacteriophages are a group of structurally related viruses which contain a circular single-stranded DNA genome. The phages that infect *Escherichia* do not kill their host during productive infection and do not infect mammalian cells. Sera of EFRH-phage immunized animals exhibited a protective effect in preventing Aβ-mediated neurotoxicity toward PC12 cell culture and stained human amyloid plaques. Experiments in transgenic animals support the immunogenetic studies. In two different sets of experiments, we immunized the AβPP[V717I] transgenic mice (16 months old) with the EFRH-phage and analyzed them at age 21 months [31]. Amyloid burden in the brain was significantly reduced in the immunized AβPP[V717I] transgenic mice that developed anti-Aβ titers of at least 1:100, indicating that a relatively low antibody-titer may be enough to reduce reduce brain amyloid load.

Recently, double mutated hAβPP tg mice (9–10 months old), raised in the animal facility of JSW Research, Austria, were immunized with the EFRH antigens containing a different number of copies of the respective antigen. Six intraperitoneal (i.p.) injections of 10^{11} phages/mouse took place every three weeks for a total period of twelve weeks [32]. We found that phages displaying high EFRH copy numbers are more effective in eliciting humoral response against the EFRH sequence which, in turn, relieved the amyloid burden in the brains of AβPP transgenic mice and improved their ability to perform cognitive tasks.

The efficacy of phage-EFRH antigen in raising anti-aggregating Aβ antibodies versus whole Aβ shows that (a) the high immunogenicity of the phage enables production of a reasonable titer of IgG antibodies in a short period of weeks without need of adjuvant administration; (b) the key role of the EFRH epitope in Aβ formation and its high immunogenicity led to anti-aggregating antibodies which recognize whole Aβ peptide, substituting the use of Aβ fibrils.

5. Passive immunization

Another set of experiments showed that peripheral administration of antibodies against Aβ was sufficient to reduce amyloid burden in the affected mice brains [33]. The investigation confirmed that circulating antibodies were able to cross the blood brain barrier and bind to brain Aβ deposits. Despite their relatively modest serum levels, the passively administered antibodies were able to enter the central nervous system, decorate plaques and induce clearance of preexisting amyloid.

Of the antibodies tested, only mAbs 10D5, 3D6 and Pab Aβ (1-42) directed to the N-terminal regions of Aβ demonstrated efficacy *in vivo*. In contrast, mAbs 16C11, 21F12 and the control antibody TM2a, directed to other regions of Aβ, were inactive. This result is consistent with the inability of these two antibodies to decorate plaques after *in vivo* administration and explains their inability to trigger plaque clearance. These *in vivo* data confirm previous *in vitro* data [14] that only antibodies directed to the strategic epitopes involved in the aggregation process, such as EFRH, exhibit so-called 'chaperone-like' properties in dissolving amyloid plaques.

Intravenous injection of mAb266 raised against middle region of Aβ to the AD transgenic mice led to a 1,000-fold increase in the concentration of Aβ in plasma. The researchers suggest that anti-amyloid antibody decreases Aβ deposition, at least in part, by decreasing the transfer of Aβ from plasma to the CNS and increasing its transfer from the CNS to plasma without dissolving existing amyloid plaques [34].

In order to overcome low permeability of the blood brain barrier, we applied antibody engineering methods to minimize the size of the monoclonal antibodies while maintaining their biological activity. The resulting scFvs can be displayed on the surface of a phage for further manipulation or can be used as soluble ScFvs (∼ 25 kd) molecules.

We have previously shown that ScFvs raised against Aβ, which contained only variable regions of light and heavy chains of the antibodies lacking the constant region Fc, exhibit anti-aggregating properties similar to whole site-directed antibodies [35,36].

Filamentous phages displaying ScFv delivered to the CNS by repeated intranasal administrations reduced the Aβ plaque load in different regions of the brain of hAβPP transgenic mice and considerably improved the cognitive functions of treated mice. Treated mice also exhibited significantly low microglia activation [37], suggesting that passive immunization with antibodies devoid of Fc may prevent over-activation of microglia and, thus, attenuation of autoantibody triggered neuroinflammation.

6. Concluding remarks

The immunological concept described in this study was converted to a therapeutic strategy aimed at treatment of AD, as well as of other diseases caused by overproduction or wrong folding of a physiological, normal peptide.

For any immunization strategy to be effective, it needs not only to identify the specific nature of the antigen or of the epitope, but also to address the formulation and method of delivery of the antigen or antibodies as a major and critical parameter.

Active immunization with synthetic Aβ (1-42) peptide reduces Aβ plaques in AβPP transgenic mice without detectable toxicity [38], but the extension of this approach to AD patients induced a neuroinflammatory reaction in some of the study subjects, precluding further testing with the preparation [39]. Vaccination with non-toxic, small epitopes of Aβ, such as EFRH, may partially avoid the undesirable effects of neuroinflammation, e.g., by preventing T-cell activation.

On the other hand, humans may develop self-antibodies when immunized with whole or fragments of Aβ. These antibodies are capable of binding to a variety of Aβ species in the brain, thus, immunization could have contradictory effects: the desired inhibition of amyloid fibril formation versus Fc microglial over-activation leading to neuroinflammation [40].

Several strategies for prevention of neuroinflammation are under investigation. One of these is the administration of intravenous immunoglobulin (IVIG), which has well-recognized anti-inflammatory activities independent of the antigen-specific effect. A variety of explanations have been put forward to account for these activities, including Fc receptor blockade, attenuation of complement-mediated tissue damage, down-regulation of B cell responses, etc. [41].

Another approach could be passive immunization with antibodies devoid of Fc, which might prevent over-activation of microglia and, thus, attenuation of autoantibody-triggered brain inflammation [35–37,42,43].

Antibodies generated with the first-generation vaccine might not have the desired therapeutic properties to target the 'correct' mechanism, however, new clinical approaches are now under consideration.

References

[1] L.E. Hebert, L.A. Beckett, P.A. Scherr and D.A. Evans, Annual incidence of Alzheimer disease in the United States projected to the years 2000 through 2050, *Alzheimer Dis. Assoc. Disord.* **15** (2001), 169–173.

[2] D.J. Selkoe, The molecular pathology of Alzheimer's disease, *Neuron* **6** (1991), 487–498.

[3] J. Busciglio, A. Lorenzo, J. Yeh and B.A. Yankner, β-amyloid fibrils induce tau phosphorylation and loss of microtubule binding, *Neuron* **14** (1995), 879–888.

[4] J. Hardy, K. Duff, K.G. Hardy, J. Perez-Tur and M. Hutton, Genetic dissection of Alzheimer's disease and related dementias: Amyloid and its relationship to tau, *Nat. Neurosci.* **1** (1998), 355–358.

[5] D.J. Selkoe, Amyloid β protein and the genetics of Alzheimer's disease, *J. Biol. Chem.* **271** (1996), 18295–18298.

[6] J. Hardy and D. Selkoe, The amyloid hypothesis of Alzheimer's disease: progress and problems on the road to therapeutics, *Science* **297** (2002), 353–356.

[7] M.C. Chartier-Harlin, F. Crawford, H. Houlden, A. Warren, D. Hughes, L. Fidani, A. Goate, M. Rossor, P. Roques, J. Hardy and M. Mullan, Early-onset Alzheimer's disease caused by mutations at codon 717 of the beta-amyloid precursor protein gene, *Nature* **353** (1991), 844–846.

[8] E. Levy-Lahad, W. Wasco, P. Poorkaj, D.M. Romano, J. Oshima, W.H. Pettingell, C.E. Yu, P.D. Jondro, S.D. Schmidt, K. Wang et al., Candidate gene for the chromosome 1 familial Alzheimer's disease locus, *Science* **269** (1995), 973–977.

[9] M.N. Sabbagh, D. Galasko and L.J. Thal, β-Amyloid and treatment opportunities for Alzheimer's disease, *Alzheimer's Disease Review* **3** (1998), 1–19.

[10] A. Lorenzo and B.A. Yankner, Beta-amyloid neurotoxicity requires fibril formation and is inhibited by Congo red, *Proc Natl Acad Sci USA* **1** (1994), 12243–12247.

[11] J.E. Maggio and P.W. Mantyh, Brain amyloid – A physico-chemical perspective, *Brain Pathol* **6** (1996), 147–162.

[12] T. Wisniewski, E.M. Castano, A. Golabek, T. Vogel and B. Frangione, Acceleration of Alzheimer's fibril formation by apolipoprotein E *in vitro*, *Am J Pathol* **145**(5) (1994), 1030–1035.

[13] B. Solomon, R. Koppel, E. Hanan and T. Katzav, Monoclonal antibodies inhibit *in vitro* fibrillar aggregation of the Alzheimer's β-amyloid peptide, *Proc. Natl. Acad. Sci. USA* **93**(1) (1996), 452–455.

[14] B. Solomon, R. Koppel, D. Frankel and E. Hanan-Aharon, Disaggregation of Alzheimer β-amyloid by site-directed mAb, *Proc. Natl. Acad. Sci. USA* **94** (1997), 4109–4112.

[15] E. Hanan and B. Solomon, Protective effect of monoclonal antibodies against Alzheimer's β-amyloid aggregation, *Amyloid: Int. J. Exp. Clin. Invest.* **3** (1996), 130–133.

[16] S. Blond and M. Goldberg, Partly native epitopes are already present on early intermediates in the folding of tryptophan synthase, *Proc Natl Acad Sci USA* **84** (1987), 1147–1151.

[17] J.D. Carlson and M.L. Yarmush, Antibody assisted protein refolding, *Bio/Technology* **10** (1992), 86–91.

[18] B. Solomon and N. Balas, Thermostabilization of Carboxypeptidase A by interaction with its monoclonal antibodies, *Biotechnol Appl Biochem* **14** (1991), 202–211.

[19] T. Katzav, E. Hanan and B. Solomon, Effect of monoclonal antibodies in preventing Carboxypeptidase A aggregation, *Appl Biochem Biotechnol* **2** (1996), 227–230.

[20] B. Solomon and F. Schwartz, Chaperone-like effect of monoclonal antibodies on refolding of heat-denatured Carboxypeptidase A, *J Mol Recogn* **8** (1995), 72–76.

[21] D. Frenkel, M. Balass and B. Solomon, N-terminal EFRH sequence of Alzheimer's β-amyloid peptide represents the epitope of its anti-aggregating antibodies, *J. Neuroimmunol.* **88** (1998), 85–90.

[22] D. Frenkel, M. Balass, E. Kachalsky-Katzir and B. Solomon, High affinity binding of monoclonal antibodies to the sequential epitope EFRH of β-amyloid peptide is essential for modulation of fibrillar aggregation, *J. Neuroimmunol* **95** (1999), 136–142.

[23] B. Solomon and D. Frenkel, Vaccination towards prevention and treatment of Alzheimer's disease, *Drugs of Today* **36**(9) (2000), 655–663.

[24] F. Van Leuven, Single and multiple transgenic mice as models for Alzheimer's disease, *Prog Neurobiol* **61**(3) (2000), 305–312.

[25] B. Solomon, Immunological approaches as therapy for Alzheimer's disease, *Exp Opin Biol Ther* **2**(8) (2002), 907–917.

[26] B.P. Imbimbo, β-Amyloid immunization approaches for Alzheimer's disease, *Drug Dev Res* **56** (2002), 150–162.

[27] R.C. Dodel, H. Hampel and Y. Du, Immunotherapy for Alzheimer's disease, *Lancet Neurol* **2** (2003), 215–220.

[28] A. Monsonego and H.L. Weiner, Immunotherapeutic approaches to Alzheimer's disease, *Science* **302** (2003), 834–838.

[29] D. Frenkel, O. Katz and B. Solomon, Immunization against Alzheimer's β-amyloid plaques via EFRH phage administration, *Proc. Natl. Acad. Sci. USA* **97** (2000), 11455–11459.

[30] D. Frenkel, N. Kariv and B. Solomon, Generation of autoantibodies towards Alzheimer's disease vaccination, *Vaccine* **19** (2001), 2615–2619.

[31] D. Frenkel, I. Dewachter, F. Van Leuven and B. Solomon, Reduction of beta-amyloid plaques in brain of transgenic mouse model of Alzheimer's disease by EFRH-phage immunization, *Vaccine* **21** (2003), 1060–1065.

[32] V. Lavie, M. Becker, R. Cohen-Kupiec, I. Yacoby, R. Koppel, M. Wedenig, B. Hutter-Paier and B. Solomon, EFRH-Phage immunization of Alzheimer's disease animal model improves behavioral performance in Morris Water Maze trials, *J. Molec. Neurosc.* **24** (2004), 105–113.

[33] F. Bard, C. Cannon, R. Barbour, R.-L. Burke, D. Games, H. Grajeda, T. Guido, K. Hu, J. Huang, K. Johnson-Wood, K. Khan, D. Kholodenko, M. Lee, I. Lieberburg, R. Motter, M. Nguyen, F. Soriano, N. Vasquez, K. Weiss, B. Welch, P. Seubert, D. Schenk and T. Yednock, Peripherally administered antibodies against amyloid beta-peptide enter the central nervous system and reduce pathology in a mouse model of Alzheimer disease, *Nat Med* **6** (2000), 916–920.

[34] R.B. Dematos, K.R. Bales, D.I. Cummins, J.C. Dodart, S.M. Paul and D.M. Holtzman, Peripheral anti-Aβ antibody alters

CNS and plasma Aβ clearance and decreases brain Aβ burden in a mouse model of Alzheimer's disease, *Proc Natl Acad Sci USA* **17** (2001), 8850–8855.

[35] D. Frenkel, B. Solomon and I. Benhar, Modulation of Alzheimer's β-amyloid neurotoxicity by site-directed single-chain antibody, *J. Neuroimmunol.* **106** (2000), 23–31.

[36] D. Frenkel and B. Solomon, Filamentous phage as vector-mediated antibody delivery to the brain, *Proc. Natl. Acad. Sci. USA* **99** (2002), 5675–5679.

[37] B. Solomon, *In vivo targeting of amyloid plaques via intranasal administration of phage anti-Aβ antibodies*, Abstract 7TH AD/PD Conference, Sorrento, Italy, 2005.

[38] D. Schenk, R. Barbour, W. Dunn, G. Gordon, H. Grajeda, T. Guido, K. Hu, J. Huang, K. Johnson-Wood, K. Khan, D. Kholodenko, M. Lee, Z.i Liao, I. Lieberburg, R. Motter, L. Mutter, F. Soriano, G. Shopp, N. Vasquez, C. Vandevert, S. Walker, M. Wogulis, T. Yednock, D. Games and P. Seubert, Immunization with amyloid-β attenuates Alzheimer'disease-like pathology in the PDAPP mousc, *Nature* **400** (1999), 173–177.

[39] www.elan.com/News/03012002.asp?Com,ponent ID=2404&SourcePageID=149.

[40] P.L. McGeer and E. McGeer, Is there a future for vaccination as a treatment for Alzheimer's disease? Neurobiol, *Of Aging* **24** (2003), 391–395.

[41] M.C. Dalakas, Mechanisms of action of IVIg and therapeutic considerations in the treatment of acute and chronic demyelinating neuropathies, *Neurology* **59** (2002), S13–S19.

[42] B.J. Bacskai, S.T. Kajdasz, M.E. McLellan, D. Games, P. Seubert, D. Schenk and B.T. Hyman, Non-fc-mediated mechanisms are involved in clearance of amyloid-β *in vivo* by immunotherapy, *J Neurosci* **15** (2002), 7873–7878.

[43] P. Das, V. Howard, N. Loosbrock, D. Dickson, M.P. Murphy and T.E. Golde, Amyloid-β immunization effectively reduces amyloid deposition in FcR$\gamma^{-/-}$ knock-out mice, *J Neurosci* **23** (2003), 8532–8538.

Tacrine, and Alzheimer's treatments*

William K. Summers
ALZcorp, 6000 Uptown Blvd Suite 308, Albuquerque NM 87110, USA
E-mail: acasec@swcp.com

Accepted 18 March 2005

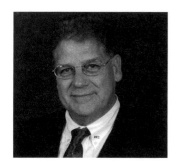

Abstract. The story of the development of tacrine began from its synthesis as an intravenous antiseptic in 1940 by Adrian Albert in Australia. In the 1970's William Summers began using tacrine in treating drug overdose coma and delirium. He felt it might have application in Alzheimer's based on work done in England by Peter Davies. In 1981, Summers et al. gave intravenous tacrine to Alzheimer's patients showed measurable improvement. Between 1981 and 1986, Summers worked with Art Kling and his group at UCLA to demonstrate usefulness of oral tacrine in treatment of Alzheimer's patients. The average length of tacrine use in 14 completing patients was 12.6 months and improvement was robust. This sparked controversy in the field. In 1993, after larger studies replicated the positive effect of tacrine, it was approved by the US Food and Drug Administration for treatment of Alzheimer's disease.

1. Introduction

In 1975, as a psychiatric resident at Washington University (St. Louis), my interest was anticholinergic delirium [33,34,39,40]. Dr. Robert N. Butler from the National Institute of Aging, at a grand rounds that year, raised the possibility that senile dementia could be the same disease as pre-senile Alzheimer's dementia [4]. This hypothesis was based on work by Dr. Robert D. Terry [45].

My work centered around a theory that cholinergic system dysfunction was the final common pathway to delirium (acute brain syndrome). This was fueled by Granacher and Baldessarini's discovery that tricyclic antidepressant overdose coma could be reversed by the acetylcholinesterase inhibitor, physostigmine [12].

My belief was that there was a threshold within the cholinergic system. Delirium resulted when this threshold was crossed [28]. Often this threshold was triggered in vulnerable, frail elderly by prescribed medications. It seemed logical that the Senile Dementia of the Alzheimer's Type (SDAT) might also represent a cholinergic system deficit.

Treating acute cholinergic deliriums proved difficult with physostigmine [12]. My personal experience with physostigmine was problematic. The beneficial effects were ephemeral. The side effects of cardiac arrhythmias and gastrointestinal side effects were common [39]. An exhaustive search in the library pointed to tacrine. On paper, it appeared to be a more suitable anti-cholinesterase.

Tacrine (tetrahydroaminoacridine, THA) has been studied for about sixty five years. In Australia during World War II, Adrian Albert Ph.D. attempted to find a safe intravenous antiseptic to treat wounded troops. His efforts were interrupted by the British production of

---
*The text was carefully edited by Ray Faber, M.D., Department of Psychiatry, University of Texas San Antonio. This work was supported by Solo Non-Profit Research Ltd.

Penicillin. Of the ninety plus derivatives of monoamine acridine synthesized, Dr. Albert was most intrigued by tacrine [1]. Tacrine is a planar three-ring acridine with minimal substitution of an amino group in the five position (Fig. 1). Chemically tacrine had flat configuration, like a frisbee, and a high pKa of 10. Thus, tacrine had the capacity to pass through cell membranes as easily as ethyl alcohol [7]. Tacrine was unique. It had a broad spectrum of arousal of the central nervous system which was credited to its reversible acetylcholinesterase inhibition [26]. Another unique feature of tacrine was that the entire structure was essential for inhibition of acetylcholinesterase [15].

In 1976, experience in humans with tacrine was limited. Samuel Gershon, M.D. working at Missouri Institute of Psychiatry had used tacrine in experimental psychosis [11]. Tacrine was able to reverse the psychosis, but physostigmine did not. Dr. Gershon had brought tacrine with him when he immigrated to the United States from Australia. Dr. Gershon enthusiastically sponsored my IND(investigational number for a drug) application with the FDA.

Shortly thereafter, I joined the faculty at the University of Pittsburgh. In 1977, I received approval to treat overdose patients with tacrine. I obtained the tacrine directly from a chemical house (Aldrich). I recall working one Saturday morning with John Fischer Ph.D., at the pharmacy school laboratory to make up the vials of tacrine used for the study. In today's world, I believe such casual innovation is not possible.

Tacrine was, as Dr. Gershon had promised, an impressive intravenous anticholinesterase. One patient had taken 10,000 mg of thioridazine (Mellaril), and he was comatose on a respirator – ten minutes of intravenous tacrine, he awoke and was able to be extubated. The patient drifted into lethargy about 12 hours later, suggesting the clinical effect of tacrine was 12 hours. The tacrine experience in reversing overdose coma in five patients was published in Clinical Toxicology [36]. If tacrine worked principally as an anticholinesterase, mixed overdose coma is a cholinergic phenomenon.

In 1976, Davies and Maloney made the discovery of a central cholinergic deficit in Alzheimer's disease [5]. This was soon confirmed by another British group [21].

In 1978, I moved to the University of Southern California in Los Angeles. Based on the new findings, I expanded the study of tacrine into Senile Dementia.

The protocol was written and approved by spring 1979. The pilot study intent was to pharmacologically confirm that memory deficits of SDAT were driven by the cholinergic system. The first patient enrolled within three months.

In designing the pilot study of tacrine and SDAT, it was found there were no appropriate psychometric instruments available. There were several instruments to measure memory deficits and make the diagnosis. However, there were no instruments to measure improvement in dementia.

In designing our own instruments we started with known validated instruments and modified them to reflect repetitive use. A global score was developed using a Swedish scale as a base [27]. This six stage scale recognized that dementia ranged from barely detectable memory deficits to bedridden and uncooperative. The late stage subjects had to be judged by the global scale alone. Earlier stage subjects could be assessed and reassessed with tests that were biased toward short term memory tasks. The simple "orientation test" was used in the middle stages of SDAT. This was a twelve item test with only one item that was repetitive. The test-retest method of presentation was important to the validity of this test. The twelve common items were presented (e.g. day, date, floor, city, etc.). The subject was asked to repeat the item immediately. This eliminated the problem of poor hearing. At the conclusion of the list of twelve items, the list was asked back. Thus memory retention of under 3 minutes was being tested. For those subjects in early states of SDAT, a complex 12 item paired-association test was developed. This "Names-Learning-Test" was modified from validated British cognitive tests of the 1970's [14]. Four separate versions of the 12 item list were made to prevent learning from repetition. It was interesting to find that a number of patients would retain items from the first list for weeks later, but could not learn items from the second list. The inter-rater reliability and comparison to commonly used instruments was later published [35].

In 1981, the results of the twelve patient pilot study was published in Biological Psychiatry [43]. This pilot was unique in dementia research. There were no restrictions on the severity SDAT or presence of concomitant illnesses. Only medications with potent anticholinergic effect were restricted.

The tacrine was given intravenously in varying doses (0.25 mg/kg to 1.5 mg/kg), because there was limited data as to what might constitute an effective dose. It was noticed that side effects were limited to nausea and diaphoresis (4 subjects) and emesis (2 subjects). These side effects seemed to be related to individual tolerance, rather that a group tolerance. For example, optimal dose was not related to the subject's age or duration of illness. The data was illogical, until the twelve subjects were separated by severity of illness with the modified

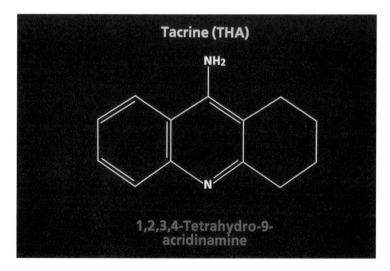

Fig. 1.

Sjögren Stage Scale. When the orientation test was separated out by stage, the beneficial effects of tacrine could be clearly seen. The peak benefit occurred from one to six hours after infusion. Nine of the twelve subjects (75%) were measurably better.

Despite positive pilot data, funding attempts languished. An NIH grant application was rejected as was an application to the State of California. My chairman refused to submit a NIH career research develop award application. In April 1981, a three-day Geriatric symposium in Los Angeles became my swan song for academic medicine [42]. The symposium, especially my research, became a focus of a press story.

Five months later, Mr. George Rehnquist contacted me. He had read about the Los Angeles symposium. He was in Knoxville, Tennessee – 2,100 miles from my office. His wife, Lucille Rehnquist, had just been diagnosed as having probable Alzheimer's. He was hopeful that I would accept his wife into my intravenous tacrine protocol.

Mr. Rehnquist was told several times that I had moved into private medical practice. He persisted. Mr. Rehnquist was told that my work was not a treatment of Alzheimer's disease. Rather it merely demonstrated that a cholinergic mechanism was involved in Alzheimer's disease. He persisted. He did not mind bringing her across the country. He did not blink at staying in Los Angeles for the month the protocol would require.

My arguments were exhausted.

In the spring of 1982, Mrs. Lucille Rehnquist received intravenous tacrine. She did remarkably well. Her data were never reported. She was the last SDAT patient given intravenous tacrine. A makeshift concoction was devised. This was phosphatidyl choline in large quantity with ophthalmic pilocarpine taken by mouth. My belief was and continues to be that Alzheimer's disease is complex. It requires a combination chemotherapy approach, much as tuberculosis or cancer does.

Also in spring of 1982, I was approached by Art Cherkin, Ph.D. He was a neurophysiologist at UCLA who championed the concept pharmaceutical synergy in cholinergic systems. He encouraged me to resume my research with tacrine. He did not view my position as a private practice physician as a problem. Dr. Cherkin introduced me to the Art Kling, M.D., who was the chairman of psychiatry at the Sepulveda VA Hospital, a division of UCLA. Dr. Kling offered me a position on the clinical faculty at UCLA. First thoughts of oral tacrine treatment of Alzheimer's disease (AD) began.

George Rehnquist would report in monthly about his wife. He always asked if tacrine could be given by mouth. Mr. Rehnquist began calling the FDA and would ask them how his wife could receive oral tacrine.

Maurice Albin, M.D., an anesthesiologist of my acquaintance at the University of Pittsburgh had told me once that tacrine could be absorbed orally [2]. Several faculty members at the Sepulveda VA, helped me prove this point.

Dr. Kling arranged for animal absorption and safety data to be developed in two species (mice and primates) [16,23]. This and other data were submitted to the FDA to amend my IND for tacrine. Bulk tacrine was manufactured by Aldrich Chemical Company in

Milwaukee for the study. It was put up in double blind fashion by a Southern California health supplement company. They also made the placebo pills. Psychometric testing was refined with the help of Larry Majovski, Ph.D. The oral tacrine protocol was approved by four Southern California private hospital IRBs. One of the hospital IRB, insisted on a change in protocol. The tacrine dose would be titrated up at the same time that a diagnostic evaluation was in progress. This change was initially aggravating. Later this was appreciated. Nonresponse to tacrine usually meant the patient would prove to not have SDAT. Because a cranial MRI was available at only one of the four hospitals, it was the only hospital used throughout the study. Curiously, this was not the hospital where the IRB insisted on modifying the protocol. All of this took 16 months. For eight months we waited for FDA approval to proceed with the oral study.

Mr. Rehnquist continued to call me frequently. He reported that my makeshift mixture was failing. Mr. Rehnquist would ask if he might urge the FDA on with a call.

A few days later I was urgently paged by my exchange. I pulled off the freeway to take a call from the FDA's, Robert Temple, M.D.

Dr. Temple verbally approved proceeding with oral tacrine. He seemed a bit perturbed with Mr. Rehnquist, and added that Mrs. Rehnquist was on a special compassionate-use IND. The thought has occurred to me more than once that Dr. Temple, who is still with the FDA, later regretted this decision . When controversy later arose around tacrine, Dr. Temple was in the center of the storm. If he had not called that day, perhaps the work on tacrine with Lucille Rehnquist would never have occurred. In that case, the whole field of cholinergic enhancement treatment of Alzheimer's disease would have been delayed if not abandoned. None of the cholinergic enhancing agents available in 1984, but tacrine, have stood the test of time.

On June 16, 1984 Lucille Rehnquist became the first human to received the oral dose of Tacrine. She did remarkably well. Lucille again did house work, cooked, and drove short distances with George in attendance. George began attending AD support groups in Knoxville with Lucille to tell his story. Soon requests to join the study began coming in from Eastern Tennessee. Because of safety concerns, the second patient was not started until eight months later. No promotion for the study was ever done. Of the 23 patients considered for the study, only two were from Southern California.

The study was economically supported by income from my private practice. This was my expensive hobby. The funds required to develop oral tacrine between 1982 and 1985 cost me about $90,000. This compares favorably with the pharmaceutical reported costs up to $897 million per product [8]. By December 1985, the study had grown beyond my means. Three approaches to fund the research developed.

First, it was discovered that our work could be patented after a visit to a St. Louis based pharmaceutical company, failed to get support. They suggested tacrine for AD could be protected under a 'use patent'. A do-it-yourself book on patents was obtained, and the arduous task of writing a patent was begun [22]. This was important, because an economically unviable treatment will have trouble making it to market. This was the sad fate of lithium carbonate which did not have an exclusive claim to the market [31].

Second, was the concept of charging the subject for research. This idea came from the New England Journal of Medicine (NEJM) [18,31]. Here the actual research drug could not be paid for by the patient, but the other costs of research could be paid for by the subjects.

Third, was to seek traditional grants and support by publishing our results to date. In May 1986, Dr. Kling suggested that a paper with our data be submitted to the NEJM. He reasoned that if accepted, this could result in funding support.

The paper was written and submitted in June, 1986 to the NEJM. In late July the manuscript was returned. It would be publishable with certain modifications. The data was updated, and "Oral tetrahydroaminoacridine in long-term treatment of senile dementia, Alzheimer type" was re-submitted in early September, 1986 [37]. Dr's Majovski, Marsh, Tachiki, and Kling were listed as co-authors because each had contributed to this paper in specific ways. To the surprise of my colleagues and I, the paper was accepted. It was given a rapid publish date of November 13th.

The editors of the NEJM called to instruct us that we were not to talk to the press about the article until after an embargo date of November 12, 1986. By Wednesday, November 5, 1986 a number of calls were received by my office. None of the calls were returned. A last minute decision to attend the Neuroscience meetings in Washington, DC was made, and the callers were told that a press conference would be held after the publication date. The press calls continued to come in.

I called the NEJM editors to report that someone had leaked the article. I wanted to make it clear that it was not me. I was surprised to find out that the leak was from the NEJM itself. Now, I was instructed to talk to the press as any callers would have a pre-print copy of the Journal, under an embargo understanding they had with major press outlets.

The press coverage was very substantial. By serendipity, three of the authors were at the Neuroscience meetings in Washington DC. As one of the media capitals of the world, this only multiplied the coverage. None of us spent much time at the meeting that year.

The paper actually reported three protocols in one study. The paper was tightly compacted into four and a third pages and written for a broad reading audience. The 1981 intravenous study had taught me that there is a personal 'best dose' for each patient. Phase I was an open label dose finding study, asking does this subject respond to tacrine. If so what is this subject's personal best dose of tacrine. To this day, important aspects of phase I are not well appreciated. First, the dose of tacrine was increased rapidly. The personal ceiling dose was determined by cholinergic toxicity. This typically was emesis with diaphoresis. The proper personal dose was the one just before toxicity. Later serum levels confirmed that this was a correct strategy with an anticholinesterase [20]. Optimal dose ranged from 25 mg tid (one subject) to 50 mg qid (two subjects). The majority of subjects were on 50 mg tid. Second, we understood that cholinergic excess was toxicity, not a side effect. When the dose was properly set, tacrine rarely gave any side-effects. Third, non-response to tacrine signaled that the dementia was due to a cause other than Alzheimer's disease [49]. This seemly bold claim bore up each time the patient was worked up in detail. Twenty-three patients were screened in Phase I. Six did not improve at any dose. Exhaustive evaluation revealed these six did not have Alzheimer's disease.

In Phase II, the design took advantage of the fact that Alzheimer's disease was unremitting and progressive. Each patient could reliably serve as their own control. This design eliminated the impact of non-study medications taken by subjects. As long as other medications were stable in both the active agent and placebo arms of the study, the effects canceled. One important exception was medications which had potent anticholinergic effect [28]. The length of Phase II was 3 weeks in each arm, which washed out short term effects that bias toward placebo. Of fifteen patients who completed the double blind crossover Phase II, fourteen demonstrated measurable positive tacrine effect.

Phase III was the third mini-study within the same paper. This was the long-term open label study. The average length of tacrine use in the fourteen completing patients was 12.6 months. This was quite a robust duration of study for the initial report of a treatment. It was felt appropriate, because tacrine had potential for long term hepatic, hematologic and neurologic toxicity. Lengthy observation on the drug was desirable. Permitting any other drug necessary to optimize health actually allowed observation of drug-drug interactions on a small population of patients. This minimized Vioxx-like surprises [49]. With this method, it was hoped that even a small study, would discovered the major adverse effects of tacrine. Indeed tacrine has now been used on a daily basis in over 300,000 patients with less than 5 deaths [32,41]. The design of inclusion of other drugs then allowing the patient to be their own control seemed effective in ferreting out adverse effects.

Reaction of researchers in the field was often negative. For example:

> "There is a scientific rationale behind THA," says Dr. Leon Thal, a researcher at San Diego Veterans Administration Hospital. "But the results are overwhelming, and when you get results like that out of the blue, the first reaction is to be skeptical." [46].

And skeptical they were.

Subsequent to the November 1986 article, the NEJM permitted publication of five of the six letters received from its vast readership [38]. All were from prominent researchers in the field. All were critical. The subsequent multicenter study, excluded my group. Instead investigation in detail of our research by the FDA and by UCLA was precipitated by researchers in the field. These investigations and restrictions by FDA minimized expansion of our work. Ultimately the integrity of the research was confirmed [9,25]. On March 28, 1989 the US patent on tacrine was issued. Tacrine now had a 17 year market value [29]. Eighteen months later the pharmaceutical company that sponsored the multicenter studies of tacrine, took a license on the patent by means of a hostile litigation against me. Four pivotal studies showed tacrine to be safe and effective [6,10,17,48].

On September 10, 1993, tacrine became the first FDA approved treatment for Alzheimer's disease [47]. The post-market experience with tacrine has been that it is much more benign that the FDA publicly proclaimed it to be [31].

Today there are five FDA approved treatments for Alzheimer's disease. Four are anticholinesterases – tacrine (Cognex®), donepezil (Aricept®), rivastigmine (Exelon®) and galantamine (Reminyl®); and the first NMDA receptor antagonist – memantine (Namenda®).

Since the discovery of tacrine, the field of Alzheimer's disease has focused much attention on the cause of the illness. Focus has been on amyloid beta-peptide as causal [13]. The competing theory has been Tau protein [44]. Much has been learned about the brain in the amyloid beta and tau protein research. To me neither of these theories seemed logical. Senile plaques and neurofibrillary tangles always struck me as tombstones derived from cellular debris. It is refreshing then to seen a shift toward new theories of etiology of Alzheimer's [19,24].

Looking to the future, I believe the oxidative injury theory will be able to explain both amyloid-beta and tau protein theories. The oxidative injury theory points to available treatments and the possibility to prevent Alzheimer's altogether [30].

I must give much credit for my story to many of the above referenced people. I most especially wish to credit Art Kling, Art Cherkin, and Ken Tachiki for inspirations, support and assistance [3].

Much credit for the tacrine's survival of the gauntlet must be given to The Wall Street Journal. The late Robert Bartley and his colleague Daniel Henninger, saw the importance in protecting tacrine, and penned a compelling set of editorials. These editorials which defended tacrine, were a risk. The risk paid off. Work on tacrine continued. The Bartley-Henninger risk has lead to the wide acceptance that neurodegenerative illness can be treated. Today there are five FDA approved treatment of Alzheimers disease and the future looks very hopeful.

References

[1] A. Albert, *The acridines; their preparation, physical, chemical, and biological properties and uses,* Edward Arnold & Co., London, 1951.

[2] M.S. Albin, L. Bunegin, Massopust and P.J. Jannetta, Ketamine-induced postanesthetic delirium attenuated by tetrahydroaminoacridine, *Exp Neurol* **44**(1) (1974), 126–129. and personal communications.

[3] Art Cherkin died in 1990 before his work really became well known. Art Kling died in 1998 in time to see much of his years of effort come to fruition. Ken Tachiki, my friend the dreamer, died in December, 2004. Robert Bartley, distinguished editor of The Wall Street Journal died in 2004. All are much missed.

[4] R.N. Butler, Mission of the National Institute on Aging, *J Am Geriatr Soc* **25**(3) (1977), 97–103.

[5] P. Davies and A.J. Maloney, Selective loss of central cholinergic neurons in Alzheimer's disease, *Lancet* **2** (1976), 1403.

[6] K.L. Davis, L.J. Thal, E.R. Gamzu, C.S. Davis, R.F. Woolson, S.I. Gracon, D.A. Drachman, L.W.S. Schneider, P.J. Whitehouse, T.M. Hoover, J.C. Morris, C.H. Kawas, D.S. Knopman, N.L. Earl, V. Kumar and R.S. Doody, A double-blind placebo controlled multicenter study of tacrine for Alzheimer's disease. The tacrine collaborative study group, *N Engl J Med* **327** (1992), 1253–1259.

[7] I.S. De La Lande and G.A. Bentley, The action of morphine and antagonists of the narcotic action of morphine on acetylcholine synthesis in brain, *Aust J Exp Biol Med Sci* **33** (1955), 55–559.

[8] J.A. DiMasi, R.W. Hansen and H.G. Grabowski, Assessing claims about the cost of new drug development: a critique of the Public Citizen and Tuberculosis Alliance reports. Tufts Center for the Study of Drug Development, Tufts University, November 1, 2004.

[9] Editorial. Dr. Summer's Victory. WSJ 25 May 1989; A16.

[10] M. Farlow, S.I. Gracon, L.A. Hershey, K.W. Lewis, C.H. Sandowsky and J. Dolan-Ureno, A controlled trial of tacrine in Alzheimer's disease: the tacrine study group, *JAMA* **268** (1992), 2523–2529.

[11] S. Gershon, Behavioral effects of anticholinergic psychotomimetics and their antagonists in man and animals, *Rec Adv Biol Psychiat* **13** (1966), 151.

[12] R.P. Granacher and R. Baldessarini, Physostigmine – its use in acute anticholinergic syndrome with antidepressant and antiparkinson drugs, *Arch Gen Psychiat* **32** (1975), 375–380.

[13] C. Haass and D. Selkoe, Alzheimer's disease. A technical KO of amyloid-beta peptide, *Nature* **391** (22 Jan 1998), 339–340.

[14] G. Irving, R.A. Robinson and W. McAdam, The validity of some cognitive tests in the diagnosis of dementia, *Brit J Psychiatry* **117** (1970), 149–156.

[15] P.N. Kaul, Enzyme inhibiting action of tetrahydroaminoacridine and its structural fragments, *J Pharm Pharmacol* **14** (1962), 243–245.

[16] A. Kling, L.J. Fitten, K. Perryman and K. Tachiki, Oral Tacrine Administration in Middle Aged Monkeys: Effect on Discrimination Learning, *Soc for Neurosci Annual Meeting* (20 October 1985), abstract No. 114.7.

[17] M.J. Knapp, D.S. Knopman, P.R. Solomon, W.W. Pendlebury, C.S. Davis and S.I. Gracon, A thirty week randomized controlled trial of high-dose tacrine in patients with Alzheimer's disease: the tacrine study group, *JAMA* **271** (1994), 985–991.

[18] S.E. Lind, Fee-for-service research, *N Engl J Med* **314** (1986), 312–315.

[19] M.E. Obrenovich, J.A. Joseph, C.S. Atwood, G. Perry and M.A. Smith, Amyloid-beta: a (life) preserver for the brain, *Neurobiology of Aging* **23** (2002), 1096–1099.

[20] T.H. Park, K.H. Tachiki, W.K. Summers, D. Kling, J. Fitten, K. Perryman, K. Spidel and A.S. Kling, Isolation and the fluorometric high-performance liquid chromatographic determination of tacrine, *Anal Biochem* **159** (1986), 358–362.

[21] E.K. Perry, B.E. Tomlinson, G. Blessed, K. Bergmann, P.H. Gibson and H.R. Perry, Correlation of cholinergic abnormalities with senile plaques and mental test scores in senile dementia, *Brit Med J* **ii** (1978), 1457–1459.

[22] D. Pressman, *Patent It Yourself,* (1st ed.), Nolo Press: Berkeley, CA, 1985.

[23] A. Rashti, S. Childers, K. Tachiki, C. Melchior, A. Steinberg and R.F. Ritzmann, Alterations in response to ethanol by tacrine and physostigmine, *Soc Neurosci* (1988), Abstract 14.

[24] C.A. Rottkamp, A.K. Raina, X. Zhu, E. Gaieve, A. Bush, C.S. Atwood, M. Chevion, G. Perry and M.A. Smith, Redox active iron mediated amyloid beta toxicity, *Free Radical Biology and Medicine* **30** (2001), 447–450.

[25] J. Scott, Alzheimer prober partly vindicated by UCLA panel, *Los Angeles Times* (9 Aug 1988), A3.

[26] F.H. Shaw and G.A. Bentley, Pharmacology of some anticholinesterases, *Aust J Exp Biol Med Sci* **31** (1953), 573–576.
[27] T. Sjögren, H. Sjögren and A.G.H. Lindgrend, Morbus Alzheimer and morbus pick, *Acta Psychiat Neurol Scand* **82**(Suppl) (1953), 1–152.
[28] W.K. Summers, A clinical method of estimating risk of drug induced delirium, *Life Sciences* **22** (1978), 1511–1516.
[29] W.K. Summers, Administration of monoamine acridines in cholinergic neuronal deficit states. United States Patent No. 4,816,456.
[30] W.K. Summers, Alzheimer's disease, oxidative injury, and cytokines, *J Alz Dis* **6** (2004), 651–657.
[31] W.K. Summers, Fee-for-service research on THA: an explanation, *N Engl J Med* **316** (1987), 1605–1606.
[32] W.K. Summers, Tacrine (THA, Cognex®), *J Alzheimer's Dis* **2** (2000), 85–93.
[33] W.K. Summers, Psychiatric sequellae to cardiotomy, *J Cardiovascular Surg* **20** (1979), 471–476.
[34] W.K. Summers, R.E. Allen and F.N. Pitts, Does physostigmine reverse quinidine delirium? *West J Med* **135** (1981), 411–414.
[35] W.K. Summers, V.L. DeBoynton, G.M. Marsh and L.J. Majovski, Comparison of seven psychometric instruments used for evaluation of treatment effect in Alzheimer's disease, *Neuroepidemiology* **9** (1990), 193–207.
[36] W.K. Summers, K.R. Kaufman, F. Altman and J.M. Fischer, THA-A review of the literature and its use in treatment of five overdose patients, *Clin Toxicol* **16** (1980), 269–281.
[37] W.K. Summers, L.V. Majovski, G.M. Marsh, K. Tachiki and A. Kling, Oral Tetrahydroaminoacridine in Long-term Treatment of Senile Dementia, Alzheimer Type, *N Engl J Med* **315** (1986), 1241–1245.
[38] W.K. Summers, L.V. Majovski, G.M. Marsh, K.H. Tachiki and A. Kling, Oral tetrahydroamino acridine in the treatment of senile dementia Alzheimer's type: Response to six letters to the Editor, *N Engl J Med* **316** (1987), 1603–1605.
[39] W.K. Summers and T.C. Reich, Delirium after cataract surgery: review and two cases, *Am J Psychiat* **136** (1979), 386–391.
[40] W.K. Summers, E. Robins and T.C. Reich, The natural history of acute organic mental syndrome after bilateral electroconvulsive therapy, *Biological Psychiatry* **14** (1979), 905–912.
[41] W.K. Summers, K.H. Tachiki and A. Kling, Tacrine in the treatment of Alzheimer's disease, *Euro Neurol* **29**(suppl 3) (1989), 28–32.
[42] W.K. Summers, J.O. Viesselman and L. Bivens, *Gerontology Symposium: Practical Issues for Family Practice, Neurology, and Psychiatry,* Bonaventure Hotel, Los Angeles, CA, April 8–10, 1981.
[43] W.K. Summers, J.O. Viesselman, G.M. Marsh and K. Candelora, Use of THA in treatment of Alzheimer-like dementia: pilot study in twelve patients, *Biol Psychiat* **16** (1981), 145–153.
[44] Y. Tatebayashi, T. Miyasaka, D.H. Chui, T. Akagi, K. Mishima, K. Iwasaki, M. Fujiwara, K. Tanemura, M. Murayama, K. Ishiguro, E. Planel, S. Sato, T. Hashikawa and A. Takashimaya, Tau filament formation and associative memory deficit in aged mice expressing mutant (R406W) human tau, *Proc Natl Acad Sci USA* **99**(21) (15 Oct 2002), 13896–13901.
[45] R.D. Terry, Dementia. A brief and selective review, *Arch Neurol* **33**(1) (1976), 1–4.
[46] M. Waldholz, A psychiatrist's work leads to a US study of Alzheimer's drug, *WSJ* (4 Aug 1987), pA1.
[47] M. Waldholz, FDA approves sale of Cognex for Alzheimer's, *WSJ* (10 Sep 1993), B5.
[48] G.K. Wilcock, D.J. Surmon, M. Scott. M. Boyle, K. Mulligan and K.A. Heubauer, An evaluation of efficacy and safety of tetrahydroaminoacridine (THA) without lecithin in the treatment of Alzheimer's disease, *Age Ageing* **22** (1993), 316–324.
[49] R. Winslow, Weighing the risks and benefits in the drug-safety debate, *WSJ* (16 Feb 2005), B1–B2.

Quality of life: The bridge from the cholinergic basal forebrain to cognitive science and bioethics

Peter J. Whitehouse*
Case Western Reserve University, OH, USA

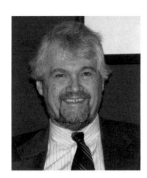

Abstract. Our paper on loss of neurons in the Nucleus Basalis of Meynert (now considered part of the cholinergic basal forebrain) in Alzheimer disease (AD) stimulated scientific interest in this little studied brain region. Our subsequent studies associated pathology in the basal forebrain with other dementias, such as Parkinson's disease, and with neurotransmitter receptor changes, such as in nicotinic receptors. We and many others worked to develop medications to treat AD through cholinergic mechanisms and eventually four cholinesterase inhibitors were approved. However the effect sizes of currently available drugs are modest and ethical issues in conducting research in dementia are challenging. In Cleveland we came to focus on the goals of improving quality of life and the importance on non-pharmacological approaches to treatment. International efforts were organized to improve the efficiency of drug development and to focus on important cultural and pharmacoeconomic issues. Eventually I became concerned about the very way we conceive AD and related concepts like MCI (mild cognitive impairment). As the hundredth anniversary of the first case approaches I am helping to organize meetings to reflect deeply on what we have learned and how to imagine creating a more positive future for persons affected by what I used to call AD.

Keywords: Cholinergic basal forebrain, Alzheimer disease, neuropathology, drug development, quality of life, bioethics, cognitive science

1. Introduction

The quality of our lives depends more on serendipity than most of us care to admit. Such is also true of the quality of one's academic career. In the 1980s, I was fortunate enough to be in the right place, with the right people, at the right time, using the right methods to ask a question about the biological substrate of the cognitive impairment of Alzheimer's disease (AD).

Our work at Johns Hopkins on the neuropathology and neurochemistry of AD and related disorders was based on concepts and approaches from the then-emerging field of systems neuroscience. A series of papers outlining the pathology in the cholinergic basal forebrain (also known as the nucleus basalis of Meynert (NBM) or the substantia innominata built on the pioneering work of Michael Johnson, Joseph Coyle, Mahlon DeLong and others at Hopkins and elsewhere. I was given the opportunity to pursue the studies by Donald Price while I rotated through neuropathology as a resident in training.

Our first challenge was to find this poorly appreciated, mysterious, and unnamed area in the human brain

---

*Corresponding author: Peter J. Whitehouse, MD, PhD, Professor, Neurology, Case Western Reserve University, 12200 Fairhill Road, Suite C357, Cleveland, OH 44120-1013, USA. Tel.: +1 216 844 6448; Fax: +1 216 844 6466; E-mail: peter.whitehouse@case.edu.

ISSN 1387-2877/06/$17.00 © 2006 – IOS Press and the authors. All rights reserved

by obtaining specimens serially sectioned through the basal forebrain area. The cholinergic basal forebrain is not a discreet nucleus, but a sheet of cells extending from the septal area dorsally to a location underneath the globus pallidus more ventrally. It was known to project widely throughout telecephalon. Components of the cholinergic basal forebrain encompass septal and diagonal band structures as well as the main portion, the NBM itself [1]. I remember well the excitement when Arthur Clark and I realized that our problem finding the NBM in our first cases of AD was not due to our anatomical ignorance but rather to the fact that most of the cells have disappeared.

Our first case published in the Annals of Neurology [2] led not only to the launch of my career but also to some limited fame in the academic and public realm. The highlight of the opportunities to inform a civic audience of our work occurred on the Oprah Winfrey show. One of my guests on the show was Dorothy French, a prima donna, married to a neurosurgery professor with AD, and had interesting ideas to share about the role of antibiotics to treat AD. The other guests included an African-American woman with AD and her family, who informed me, as we were waiting to go on stage that they never used the word AD around their mother. I interviewed this woman with dementia, and discovered that she had been lost in New York City and cared for by homeless friends. Throughout the show, Oprah persisted in asking what the difference was between senility and AD. Each time, I gave her the common expert's scientific answer, "we do not use the word senility clinically because it is an imprecise term and is ambiguous as to whether it means disease or a stage of normal aging." However Oprah was voicing the view – often found more strongly amongst African-Americans – that AD, however undesirable, was a common and hence not unexpected aspect of aging itself. As my studies of the NBM and other brain changes in AD continued, I became suspicious of the claim that AD is not a part of some people's "normal" aging. In retrospect, Oprah's perhaps wise, but at the time repetitive and vexing, question continued to haunt me as I looked for ways to improve the quality of life of older persons through clinical care and research. I also saw early in my career the need for communicating about science with the public.

Once we described the pathology in AD we examined the NBM in other diseases such as Parkinson's Disease (PD), Progressive Supranuclear Palsy, Pick's and Huntington's Disease [3–6]. My studies of the personal history of Theodore Meynert, and the nucleus he identified in his research demonstrated an interesting conceptual parallel between the brain psychiatry of his time and the biological psychiatry of ours [7]. For example, the relationships between cortical and subcortical structures were viewed as important to understanding the pathophysiology of cognitive symptoms in disease in both eras. We re-discovered that the Lewy Body had been first described in substantia innominata not the substantia nigra. Our studies of autopsy specimens from PD determined that neuronal loss occurred in the basal forebrain and hinted at a relationship between cell loss and degree of cognitive dysfunction.

The research group in Newcastle upon Tyne had already suggested that greater loss of cholinergic markers in AD related to more severe dementia. Since I had been raised in Newcastle, this friendly competition was more interesting and led to an alliance of sorts in later years. Elaine and Robert Perry, a husband and wife neurochemistry and neuropathology team from Newcastle, raised the issue of whether neurons died or merely shrank. These claims led us into computerized assessment of microscopic images to help determine the degree of pathology in various brain structures. We came to believe that shrinkage of neurons did accompany eventual death. Earlier studies in PD suggested that cell loss in the NBM might relate to bradyphrenia – slowness of thought that accompanied the bradykinesia, slowness of movement, in PD. This idea foreshadowed ideas proposed by Martin Rossor that the NBM is part of the reticular activating system involved in arousal and attention. All this early work helped accelerate research of medications to treat AD based on the cholinergic deficiency model. Could they improve memory and/or attention in patients with AD and related dementias? Thus the so-called cholinergic hypothesis was born. The strong form of the hypothesis – that loss of cells in the cholinergic basal forebrain explained most of the cognitive impairment – was often set up as a straw man to be torn down. The weak form suggested with some greater validity that the loss of cells in the NBM played some role in producing the cognitive impairment. A true and perhaps most valid test of this the hypothesis is whether drugs to benefit human beings could be developed based on this model.

I surmised early in my career that being associated with one disease, even a disease as important as AD, and one neurotransmitter, acetylcholine, arguably one of the most clinically relevant would be limiting to one's career. Hence, I started studying biominergic systems like the locus ceruleus and ventral tegmental area, as well as serotonergic raphe nuclei [8]. Here, the idea was to determine whether pathology in these structures might relate to the non-cognitive symptoms in dementia such as depression and psychosis. I also realized the need to learn more basic biological techniques than just quantitative pathology. I linked up with Mike Kuhar in Sol Snyder's Department of Neuroscience (Johns Hopkins) to learn in vitro receptor autoradiography, which allowed microscopic imaging of the binding of radioactively labeled drugs and neurotransmitters in tissue sections. We applied this approach to human autopsy tissue and characterized a variety of receptor changes in AD, PD, Huntington's disease and amyotrophic lateral sclerosis [9–12]. Perhaps our most important neurochemical finding was the loss of nicotinic binding sites in AD and PD, related to the dysfunction of neurons in the NBM [13,14]. During the Fellowship in Neuroscience, I also worked in psychiatry to enhance my clinical and research skills and began my interest in the development of drugs for AD.

These early successes led to an offer to join both the faculty at Case Western Reserve University (Case) and the staff of University Hospitals of Cleveland where I would be responsible for founding an Alzheimer Center. During my transition from Hopkins to Case, a paper appeared in the New England Journal of Medicine, claiming the dramatic benefits of tacrine (now branded as Cognex), a cholinesterase inhibitor, in patients with dementia [15]. As director of a new program in Cleveland, I became engaged in a multimember follow-up study sponsored by the National Institutes of Aging, Alzheimer's Association and Warner-Lambert Parke-Davis. Scientific and ethical concerns about the original study led to an abiding concern about conflict of interest between physicians and pharmaceutical companies, and other ethical issues centered on research in persons with dementia [16]. I was asked to serve on the FDA Central and Peripheral Nervous System Panel and was involved in the eventual decision to approve tacrine as the first drug for AD in modern times. In one sense it was wonderful to see basic research studies yield a product that could help people. However, the full unfolding of the story has, in my opinion, been less positive. Arguably, tacrine met the criteria outlined in the antidementia drug guidelines developed by Paul Leber at the FDA, but its therapeutic effects were modest at best. I somewhat reluctantly voted in favor of the approval, as I realized that this decision might lead to many "me-too" drugs. But I was also aware that if we did not approve tacrine, the industry might lose interest in developing therapies for AD.

In the ensuing years, three other drugs have been approved in the same category of cholinesterase inhibitors (donepezil or Aricept®, rivastigmine or Exelon® and galantamine or Reminyl®) and one (memantine or Nameda®) in a new category of glutamate receptor antagonists. Tacrine was an easy target to improve upon because of its liver toxicity and four times a day administration. Donepezil, developed in Japan by Eisai, ultimately became the safer once-a-day pill. It was somewhat ironic that this compound had emerged from a country that had been slowly recognizing that AD was a problem for their citizens. Vascular dementia had been thought to be more common than AD. Moreover, the Japanese pharmaceutical industry is composed of many small, usually not-research intensive companies that have a hard time competing with big multinational companies. Yet Eisai, one of the more innovative Japanese companies, was able to develop the second cholinesterase medication approved around the world and now the best selling drug to treat AD.

The need to improve the efficiency of drug development became apparent during these early days and I served as a consultant to many pharmaceutical companies and biotechnology firms. Over the ensuing years, I personally received millions of dollars in grants to support various research and educational endeavors led by the industry. One of the first grants at Case was from Warner-Lambert Parke-Davis, the marketers of tacrine. Rather than use this unrestricted grant to fund laboratory research I chose to study conflict of interest in the early tacrine trials [17].

In 1994, I formed, with over 50 colleagues from around the world, the International Working Group for the Harmonization of Dementia Drug Guidelines (IWHG) to foster global collaborations on dementia drug development and to "standardize" the regulatory approval guidelines being developed in the United States, Europe, Japan and Canada [18]. This process established a rich international network of friends and collaborators, and led to sabbaticals in Tokyo and London. It was organized around various predictable topics including domains of assessment and trial design, as well as even more challenging areas for international collaboration, cultural and ethical issues. We organized meetings in partnership with other groups such as Alzheimer Disease International, the World Federation of Neurology and the International Psychogeriatrics Association. We were the first to develop conferences on the treatment of vascular dementia and pharmacoeconomics [19].

However, as the new drugs emerged on the market, my concerns increased about the dominance of scientifically and technologically-oriented approaches to fixing AD. Find a cure became the goal, if not the obsession, of the field. Attention to the softer, human aspects of providing care was relatively neglected. I became increasingly concerned about the very way we conceptualize diseases like AD. Medicine- both in general and in the Alzheimer's field – intensified its attraction to for-profit models of research and the process of commercialization intensified. Between the time of our original work on the NBM and the approval of the last drug for AD working with industry moved from being viewed as a necessary evil beneath the dignity of many academics to a competitive arena to see who could make the most money by starting their own company or consulting with big pharmaceutical companies. Moreover, federal legislation (like Baye-Dole) began a process of undermining the very integrity of universities as relatively more independent bastions of social criticism and pursuit of knowledge. As marketing monies entered the scene, physicians found increasing conflict of interests between their professional responsibilities for putting patient concerns first and enhancing personal and organizational financial well-being.

In the basic science arena, systems neuroscience, once the dominant methodology aligned with interest in clinical/pathological studies and interests in brain/behavior correlations, was replaced by molecular biology and genetic approaches. Attention in the trial arena shifted from developing drugs to improve symptoms, to drugs to prevent and even cure the disease. Gene therapies, neural transplants and stem cells became the hypes, if not the hopes, for the future. I felt that current drugs and future research promised too much benefit to individuals and society. Direct-to-consumer advertising created not only a demand from patients for more expensive, less studied and hence less safe drugs, but also contributed to creating the very diseases from which the consumer/patient allegedly suffered in the first place. The current outpouring of concern about the power of the pharmaceutical industry, particularly in its role as a global multinational agent, is long overdue.

In the mid 1990's I left the laboratory for good, stepped down as director of Case's Alzheimer Center and steered increasingly to organizational and ethical concerns. I began to focus my NIH funded research, working with such groups as the IWGH and the National Institute on Aging Alzheimer's Disease Cooperative Study, on the concept and measurement of quality of life and ethical issues, such as informed consent in research and genetic testing [20–22]. After all, developing trustworthy information about how to improve quality of life appears to be the goal that everybody seeks, from affected persons and their families to molecular biologists and policy-makers. We tried to raise the stakes for anti-dementia drugs by asking for evidence not just for efficacy in trials but for effectiveness in practice. Moreover, I came to realize that non-biological interventions might have more profound effects on quality of life than drugs. As a result I became involved in national and local initiatives involving daycare, special care units, hospice and educational approaches. Eventually, I focused more on narrative approaches to address the cognitive challenges of aging. How could the power of stories be used to heal and relieve the suffering of those with cognitive impairment? How could multimedia approaches aid memory through reminiscence and hence improve quality of life in families affected by AD? Could advance directives, important to guiding end-of-life care, be supplemented by diary, scrap book approaches? How could computers assist caregivers? Eventually I developed with my wife and others, my most interesting organizational response to the cognitive challenges of aging. We founded The Intergenerational School, the first ever public community school based on multi-age real-life learning in community, to foster positive responses to the impairment of memory and other cognitive abilities that affect us all to one degree or another as we age. Persons with memory impairment read and garden with children from urban Cleveland attending our public school.

The excessive claims of molecular biology-driven, Nobel prize seeking, profit-driven scientists further turned me away from what I was coming to see as problematic lines of research and an uninhibited faith in the power of basic biological research. I returned in my memory to our earlier studies of the NBM and nicotinic receptors and recounted that some cell and receptor losses occurred in intellectually intact (or relatively so) normal, older individuals. I also reflected upon Oprah's penetrating question about the alleged differences between senility and AD.

Where *does* one draw the line between aging and disease I wondered? I worked on developing criteria for Aging-Associated Memory Impairment [23] and Aging Related Cognitive Decline [24]. I was linked to, but not directly involved in the American Association of Neurology's effort to develop guidelines for early recognition of AD. Ron Petersen (Mayo Clinic) led the effort to consider early diagnosis in AD in such a way that it would intensify the reification of his concept of mild cognitive impairment (MCI). Such a label threatened to create an enormous number of impaired elders who would otherwise be poised on the threshold of the AD. The label was created to tackle the laudable but challenging goal of diagnosing people earlier so as to develop treatments to prevent the emergence of AD. Seduced by the power of molecular biology, we attempted to develop (largely unsuccessfully) clinical trials that would eventually allow regulatory claims that a drug actually modified the biological progression of AD. When clinical measurement appeared to falter as an outcome measure, we turned to neuroimaging and other biological markers. Millions of dollars are now being spent trying to find a diagnostic test for AD, but all will be limited by the need to establish an arbitrary threshold on the continuum of biological changes that occur with normal aging.

Although well-motivated, these efforts – driven by the commercial engine of progress and the pathologization of aging – led to greater concern on my part, and I became increasingly critical of the concept of MCI [25–29]. I recognized that challenging this concept would also challenge the social value of the concept of another discrete category on the continuum of cognitive aging – namely AD.

We are at present thinking about our successes (and failures) over the first one hundred years of work on AD since the description of the original case by Alois Alzheimer in 1906. I and others have realized the heterogeneity of AD at all levels: genetic, biological, clinical and cultural. I have come to believe that the statement that AD is not normal aging is more political than scientific. I returned to my roots as a cognitive neuroscientist and psycholinguist to argue that AD is first and foremost *not* a brain disease, but rather a two word phrase attempting to capture a fuzzy concept – a socially constructed eponym. We can choose to use terms like MCI and AD, or challenge those labels just as we did with terms like drapeomania (a pre-civil war disease that caused slaves to run away) and homosexuality (which was abandoned by the American Psychiatric Association as a disease category in 1973).

We can hope that biological approaches can slow brain aging processes and hence treat the pathology of AD. We should not expect to find these neurological "fountains of youth" too quickly, though. Having reached the one hundredth anniversary of the disease, we need to reflect deeply on what we have learned and not merely to extrapolate our increasingly-suspect present scientific and social models of age-related cognitive dysfunction onto our already challenged future. The human race faces enormous social and health problems today and increasingly so in the near future. Ironically, my training in bioethics opened my eyes to the enormity of the moral issues facing our species, and also to the limits of a narrowly construed, academically-oriented biomedical ethics. Bioethics as envisioned by the man who coined the term, Van Rensselaer Potter, had a more global, spiritual and activist, dare I say deeper, agenda [30]. Based on the land ethic of Aldo Leopold, Potter advocated for bioethics as a bridge between science and the humanities and medicine and public health. Deterioration of our environment and challenges to our species to preserve the diversity of life cannot be corrected through mere genetic manipulations or pharmaceutical developments. Will our legacy be the decimation of our planet and the blood of countless other life forms on our hands?

How do we prioritize the challenges of what we now call AD in this more global picture in which the health and wellbeing of children and future generations around the world are increasingly threatened every day? Can we reframe AD so as to go beyond just being critical of the molecular hype that produces false hope through the promise of a pharmaceutical panacea? Can we offer a positive vision of an achievable future that we can create together? I think we can and I am trying in my own life, in my practice as a healer, and in my academic scholarship to address ways of reframing the challenges of cognitive aging. My approaches involve constructing different narratives for our individual and collective lives than currently exist. Such stories can celebrate learning about the brain and our genetic make-up. However, such future stories must also address priorities such as the fate of younger generations, especially their ability to gain an education and be productive citizens. Any minor or even major step towards a "cure" for the "diseases" of brain aging should not devalue caring as we do today in the AD field. We are all human beings living on the same planet who age and die. We must develop a global bioethic, not a narrow superficial bioethics like the one that currently dominates medicine. This global bioethic must include a concern for social justice and sustainability of diversity of life [30].

Reframing our conceptions of AD will be an essential part of this effort to create a sustainable society for the future. We are all on a trajectory towards some degree of memory loss as we age. Some will live long enough to outlive their brain's capacity to operate in the world. Some (even some with memory problems) will live long enough to contribute to intergenerational learning and share stories that celebrate life and learning even unto death. We should recognize that we all gain some wisdom as we age and that creating collective wisdom, even in the face of disease and death, is the opportunity and responsibility we all share. Better we come to die celebrating the qualities of our own lives as individuals, than we die as a species. In other words, our personal mortality is the gift to future generations for biological and cultural adaptation. Such collective wisdom will hopefully emerge in our communities of healing and of learning. My wife and I, along with others, developed the world's first intergenerational school to promote such multi-age learning [31]. Perhaps the next generation of cholinergic drugs will dramatically improve our mindfulness and attention and enhance our executive functions and wisdom. I would not bank on it, but not to worry: we have the wisdom in ourselves already, if we can only find it.

Special acknowledgement for support of this manuscript goes to the following research grants from the Shiego and Megumi Takayama Foundation and the National Institutes of Health National Institute on Aging Medical Goals in Dementia: Ethics and Quality of Life (AG/HS17511).

References

[1] J.C. Hedreen, R.G. Struble, P.J. Whitehouse and D.L. Price, Topography of the magnocellular basal forebrain system in human brain, *J. Neuropathol Exp Neurol* **43** (1984), 1–21.

[2] P.J. Whitehouse, D.L. Price, A.W. Clark, J.T. Coyle and M.R. DeLong, Alzheimer disease: evidence for selective loss of cholinergic neurons in the nucleus basalis, *Ann Neurol* **10** (1981), 122–126.

[3] D.L. Price, P.J. Whitehouse, R.G. Struble, A.W. Clark, J.T. Coyle, M.R. DeLong and J.C. Hedreen, Basal forebrain cholinergic systems in Alzheimer's Disease and related dementias, *Neurosci. Comment* **1** (1982), 84–92.

[4] P.J. Whitehouse, J.C. Hedreen, C.L. White, III. and D.L. Price, Basal forebrain neurons in the dementia of Parkinson disease, *Ann Neurol* **13** (1983), 243–248.

[5] A.W. Clark, I.M. Parhad, S.E. Folstein, P.J. Whitehouse, J.C. Hedreen, D.L. Price and G.A. Chase, The nucleus basalis in Huntington's disease, *Neurology* **33** (1983), 1262–1267.

[6] G.R. Uhl, D.C. Hilt, J.C. Hedreen, P.J. Whitehouse and D.L. Price, Pick's disease (lobar sclerosis): depletion of neurons in the nucleus basalis of Meynert, *Neurology* **33** (1983), 1470–1473.

[7] P.J. Whitehouse, Theodor Meynert: foreshadowing modern concepts of neuropsychiatric pathophysiology, *Neurology* **35** (1985), 389–391.

[8] R.J. D'Amato, R.M. Zweig, P.J. Whitehouse, G.L. Wenk, H.S. Singer, R. Mayeux, D.L. Price and S.H. Snyder, Aminergic systems in Alzheimer's and Parkinson's disease, *Ann Neurol* **22** (1987), 229–236.

[9] P.J. Whitehouse, Receptor autoradiography: applications in neuropathology, *Trends Neurosci* **8** (1985), 434–437.

[10] P.J. Whitehouse, O. Muramoto, J.C. Troncoso and I. Kanazawa, Neurotransmitter receptors in olivopontocerebellar atrophy: an autoradiographic study, *Neurology* **36** (1986), 193–197.

[11] P.J. Whitehouse, Neurotransmitter receptor alterations in Alzheimer disease: A review, *Alzheimer Dis Assoc Disord* **1** (1987), 9–18.

[12] P.J. Whitehouse, Neurotransmitter receptor alterations in Alzheimer disease: A review, *Alzheimer Dis Assoc Disord* **1** (1987), 9–18, P.J. Whitehouse, A.M. Martino, M.V. Wagster, D.L. Price, R. Mayeux, J.R. Atack and K.J. Kellar, Reductions in (^{3}H) nicotinic acetylcholine binding in Alzheimer's disease and Parkinson's disease: an autoradiographic study, *Neurology* **38** (1988), 720–723.

[13] P.J. Whitehouse, A.M. Martino, P.G. Antuono, P.R. Lowenstein, J.T. Coyle, D.L. Price and K.J. Kellar, Nicotinic acetylcholine binding sites in Alzheimer's disease, *Brain Res* **371** (1986), 146–151.

[14] K.J. Kellar, P.J. Whitehouse, A.M. Martino-Barrows, K. Marcus and D.L. Price, Muscarinic and nicotinic cholinergic binding sites in Alzheimer's disease cerebral cortex, *Brain Res* **436** (1987), 62–68.

[15] K.L. Davis, L.J. Thal, E.R. Gamzu, C.S. Davis, R.F. Woolson, S.I. Gracon, D.A. Drachman, L.S. Schneider, P.J. Whitehouse, T.M. Hoover et al., A double-blind, placebo-controlled multicenter study tacrine in Alzheimer's disease, The Tacrine Collaborative Study Group, *N Engl J Med* **327**(18) (1992), 1253–1259.

[16] P.J. Whitehouse, Interesting Conflicts and conflicting interests, *J. Amer Geria Soc* **47** (1999), 1–3.

[17] E. Kodish, T. Murray and P.J. Whitehouse, Conflict of interest in university-industry research relationships: realities, politics, and values, *Academ Med* **71**(12) (1996), 1287–1290.

[18] P.J. Whitehouse, The international working group for harmonization of dementia drug guidelines: past, present, and future, *Alz Disea Assoc Disord* **11**(Suppl 3) (1997), 2–5.

[19] P.J. Whitehouse, B. Winblad, D. Shostak, A. Bhattacharjya, M. Brod, H. Brodaty, A. Dor, H. Feldman, F. Forette, S. Gauthier, J. Hay, C. Henke, S. Hill, V. Mastey, P. Neumann, B. O'Brien, K. Pugner, M. Sano, T. Sawada, R. Stone and A. Wimo, First international pharmacoeconomic conference on Alzheimer's disease: Report and Summary, *Alzheim Disea and Associa Disord* **12**(4) (1998), 266–280.

[20] S. Post, P. Whitehouse, R. Binstock, T. Bird, S. Eckert, L. Farrer, L. Fleck, A. Gaines, E. Juengst, H. Karlinsky, S. Miles, T. Murray, K. Quaid, N. Relkin, A. Roses, P. St. George-Hyslop, G. Sachs, B. Steinbock, E. Truschke and A. Zinn, The clinical introduction of genetic testing for Alzheimer's disease, *J. Amer MedAssoc* **277**(10) (1997), 832–836.

[21] S.G. Post and P.J. Whitehouse, Fairhill guidelines on ethics of the care of people with Alzheimer's disease: A clinical Summary, *J. Amer Ger Soc* **43** (1995), 1423–1429.

[22] P.J. Whitehouse and P.V. Rabins, Quality of life and dementia, *Alzheimer Dis Assoc Disord* **6**(3) (1992), 135–138.

[23] T. Crook, R.T. Bartus, S.H. Ferris, P. Whitehouse, G.D. Cohen and S. Gershon, Age-associated memory impairment: Proposed diagnostic criteria and measures of clinical change-Report of a National Institute of Mental Health Work Group, *Dev Neuropsychology* **2** (1986), 261–276.

[24] R. Levy and P.J. Whitehouse, Report of working party of international psychogeriatric association: aging-associated cognitive decline, *Internat Psychogeiatrics* **6** (1994), 63–68.

[25] P.J. Whitehouse, MCI and AD: Different conditions or diagnostic confusion? *Geriatric Times* **4**(6) (2003), 14–16.

[26] P.J. Whitehouse, *The future of Mild Cognitive Impairment*, Fifth Issue: MCI Forum, HELP Medical Publications, France, August 2004.
[27] P.J. Whitehouse, A. Gaines, H. Lindstrom and J. Graham, Dementia in the anthropological gaze: Contributions to the understanding of dementia, *The Lancet Neurology* **4** (2005), 320–326.
[28] P.J. Whitehouse and H.R. Moody, Mild cognitive impairment: A hardening of the categories, *Dementia J.* (2005), in press.
[29] P.J. Whitehouse and E.T. Juengst, Anti-aging medicine and mild cognitive impairment: practice and policy issues for geriatrics, *J. Amer Ger Soc* **53** (2005), 1417–1422.
[30] V.R. Potter and P.J. Whitehouse, Deep and global bioethics for a livable third millennium, *The Scientist* **12**(1) (1998), 9.
[31] P.J. Whitehouse, E. Bendezu, S. FallCreek and C. Whitehouse, Intergenerational community schools: a new practice for a new time, *Educ Gerontol* **26** (2000), 761–770.

Keyword Index

$A\beta$	309
$A\beta$ oligomers	123
$A\beta PP$	91, 133, 381
$A\beta PP$ mutations	389
abnormally hyperphosphorylated tau	219
AD	309
Alzheimer disease	61, 71, 171, 195, 367, 425, 447
Alzheimer's disease	29, 53, 79, 91, 133, 163, 177, 277, 329, 381, 389, 409
Alzheimer's neurofibrillary changes	53
amyloid	91
Amyloid β	329, 341
Amyloid β-protein	163
Amyloid β-protein precursor	329, 341
Amyloid-β	133, 277, 425, 433
APOE	381
apoptosis	277
APP	163, 367
autophagy	277
bioethics	447
biomarkers	409
cathepsin	277
cerebral amyloid angiopathy (CAA)	329, 389
cerebral hemorrhages	389
cholinergic basal forebrain	447
clinico-pathological correlations	61
cognition	101
cognitive science	447
complement	271
conformational diseases	319
cortical minicolumns	79
cyclin-dependent protein kinase-5	219
dementia	389, 409
dementia disorders	61
dementia with Lewy bodies	417
diagnosis	409, 417
diagnostic accuracy rates	61
diagnostic criteria	409
diagnostic instruments	409
drug development	447
drug discovery	163
Dutch type (HCHWA-D)	329
EFRH sequence	433
endocytosis	277
endosome	277
familial Alzheimer's disease	341
Flemish APP692 disease	389
gene	341, 381
genetics	367
glycogen synthase kinase-3β	219
GSK-3β	309
HCHWAD	389
hereditary cerebral hemorrhage with amyloidosis	329
Herpes simplex virus	29
hippocampus	29
immunization	133
immunohistochemistry	271
immunomodulation	433
indomethacin	271
limbic	101
MAP1	219
MAP2	219
MCI	409
membrane attack complex	271
memory	123
mice	123
microtubule assembly	219
microtubules	177, 257
mild cognitive impairments	409
molecular misreading	319
morphometry	29
Morris water maze	123

mutation	341, 367, 373
National Institute on Aging	409
necrosis	277
neocortex	79
neural plasticity	79
neurofibrillary tangles	29, 177, 195, 219, 257
neuroimaging	409
neuropathology	447
neuropil threads	71
NFT	309
NIA	409
NIH	409
NSAID	271
olfactory system	79
operant behavioral task	123
paired helical filament	71, 171, 195, 219
parkinsonism-dementia complex on Guam	53
pathogenesis	341
pathology	133
phosphorylation	171, 177
plaques	133
plasticity	101
polyglutamine diseases	319
presenilin	381
protease	277
protein kinase A	219
protein phosphatase-1	219
protein phosphatase-2A	219
quality of life	447
rats	123
reactive microglia	271
secretases	163
self-assembly of tau	219
single-chain antibodies	433
site-directed antibodies	433
synapse	101
synapse loss	91
synaptic plasticity	91
synucleinopathies	319
tau	71, 171, 195, 219, 257, 367, 373
tau proteins	177
tauopathy	309, 319, 373
taxol	257
therapeutic	133, 425
therapeutic chaperones	433
topographic study	53
transgenic	123, 425
transgenic mice	133
ultrastructure	101
vaccine	425
vasopressin	319